REACHING TEENS

Strength-Based Communication Strategies to Build Resilience and Support Healthy Adolescent Development

Editors

Kenneth R. Ginsburg, MD, MS Ed, FAAP, FSAHM
Professor of Pediatrics
Perelman School of Medicine at the University of Pennsylvania
Craig-Dalsimer Division of Adolescent Medicine
The Children's Hospital of Philadelphia
Director of Health Services, Covenant House of Pennsylvania
Philadelphia, PA

Sara B. Kinsman, MD, PhD
Associate Professor of Pediatrics
Perelman School of Medicine at the University of Pennsylvania
Craig-Dalsimer Division of Adolescent Medicine
The Children's Hospital of Philadelphia
Philadelphia, PA

American Academy of Pediatrics
141 Northwest Point Blvd
Elk Grove Village, IL 60007-1019

American Academy of Pediatrics Department of Marketing and Publications

Maureen DeRosa, MPA, Director, Department of Marketing and Publications

Mark Grimes, Director, Division of Product Development

Eileen Glasstetter, MS, Manager, Product Development

Mark Ruthman, Manager, Electronic Product Development

Carolyn Kolbaba, Manager, Consumer Publishing

Peter Lynch, Digital Solutions Editor

Amanda Krupa, MSc, CPMW, Editor, Healthy Children.org

Regina Moi, Manager, Patient Education

Mary Claire Walsh, Managing Editor, AAP Web Sites

Sandi King, MS, Director, Division of Publishing and Production Services

Shannan Martin, Publishing and Production Services Specialist

Peg Mulcahy, Manager, Graphic Design and Production

Kate Larson, Manager, Editorial Services

Julia Lee, Director, Division of Marketing and Sales

Linda Smessaert, MSIMC, Brand Manager, Clinical and Professional Publications

Kathleen Juhl, MBA, Manager, Consumer Marketing and Sales

Mary Jo Reynolds, Manager, Consumer Product Marketing

Elyce Goldstein, Manager, Digital Content and Licensing

Sashaya Davis, Institutional Sales Manager

Video Production Team

Mark Ruthman, Producer, American Academy of Pediatrics

Robin Miller, Director and Editor, Robin Miller Videography

Kenneth R. Ginsburg, MD, MS Ed, FAAP, FSAHM, Coproducer, Content Director and Editor

Sara B. Kinsman, MD, PhD, Associate Content Director (Philadelphia)

Colette Auerswald, MD, MS, FSAHM, Associate Content Director (San Francisco)

Arvil Prewitt, Lead Camera Person

Ilana R. Ginsburg, Teen Casting Director

Talia M. Ginsburg, Teen Content Editor

Library of Congress Control Number: 2012938967

ISBN: 978-1-58110-748-7

eISBN: 978-1-58110-834-7

MA0647

The recommendations in this publication do not indicate an exclusive course of treatment or serve as a standard of medical care. Variations, taking into account individual circumstances, may be appropriate.

The American Academy of Pediatrics is not responsible for the content of the resources mentioned in this publication. Web site addresses are as current as possible but may change at any time.

Statements and opinions expressed are those of the authors and not necessarily those of the American Academy of Pediatrics.

Printed in the United States of America.

9-340/0613

1 2 3 4 5 6 7 8 9 10

Contributors

Marcos O. Almonte, MDiv
Resilience Specialist
El Centro de Estudiantes
Big Picture Philadelphia
Philadelphia, PA

Renata Arrington-Sanders, MD, MPH, ScM, FAAP
Assistant Professor
Division of General Pediatrics and Adolescent
    Medicine
Johns Hopkins School of Medicine
Baltimore, MD

Colette (Coco) Auerswald, MD, MS, FSAHM
Associate Professor
University of California, Berkeley-University of
    California at San Francisco Joint Medical
    Program
Department of Community Health and Human
    Development
UC, Berkeley School of Public Health
Berkeley, CA

Andrea R. Bailer, MSN, CRNP
Adolescent Nurse Practitioner
Advanced Practice Nurse Manager
Nicholas and Athena Karabots Pediatric Care Center
The Children's Hospital of Philadelphia
Philadelphia, PA

David L. Bell, MD, MPH
Assistant Professor of Pediatrics and Population
    and Family Health
Department of Pediatrics/Heilbrunn Department of
    Population and Family Health
Columbia University Medical Center
Medical Director, The Young Men's Clinic
New York, NY

Sandra L. Bloom, MD
Codirector, Center for Nonviolence & Social Justice
Associate Professor of Health, Management and
    Policy
School of Public Health, Drexel University
Philadelphia, PA

Larry K. Brendtro, PhD, LP
Dean, Starr Global Training Network
Albion, MI
Professor Emeritus, Augustana College
Cofounder, Reclaiming Youth International
Sioux Falls, SD

Kenisha Campbell, MD, MPH
Assistant Professor of Pediatrics
Perelman School of Medicine at the University
    of Pennsylvania
Medical Director, Adolescent Primary Care &
    Family Planning
Nicholas and Athena Karabots Pediatric Care Center
Craig-Dalsimer Division of Adolescent Medicine
The Children's Hospital of Philadelphia
Philadelphia, PA

Marina Catallozzi, MD, MSCE
Assistant Professor of Clinical Pediatrics
Columbia University College of Physicians and
    Surgeons
Morgan Stanley Children's Hospital of New York
Assistant Professor of Clinical Population and
    Family Health
Columbia University Mailman School of
    Public Health
New York, NY

Tonya A. Chaffee, MD, MPH, FAAP
Associate Clinical Professor of Pediatrics
University of California, San Francisco
Director, Teen and Young Adult Health Center
Medical Director, Child and Adolescent Support
    Advocacy and Resource Center
San Francisco General Hospital
San Francisco, CA

Liana R. Clark, MD, MSCE, FAAP
Adolescent Medicine Specialist
Philadelphia, PA
Medical Director, Global Vaccines and Policy
Merck & Co, Inc.
West Point, PA

Stephanie Contreras
Resilience Specialist
El Centro de Estudiantes
Big Picture Philadelphia
Philadelphia, PA

Alison Culyba, MD, MPH
Fellow, Adolescent Medicine
Craig-Dalsimer Division of Adolescent Medicine
The Children's Hospital of Philadelphia
Philadelphia, PA

Angela Diaz, MD, MPH
Jean C. and James W. Crystal Professor
Departments of Pediatrics and Preventive Medicine
Icahn School of Medicine at Mount Sinai
Director, Mount Sinai Adolescent Health Center
Mount Sinai Hospital
New York, NY

Nadia L. Dowshen, MD, FAAP, AAHIVS
Assistant Professor of Pediatrics
Perelman School of Medicine at the University
    of Pennsylvania
Director of Adolescent HIV Services
Craig-Dalsimer Division of Adolescent Medicine
The Children's Hospital of Philadelphia
Philadelphia, PA

Paula M. Duncan, MD, FAAP
Professor of Pediatrics
University of Vermont College of Medicine
Burlington, VT

Karyn E. Feit, LCSW
Adolescent Social Worker
Nicholas and Athena Karabots Pediatric Care Center
Family Services, Children's Seashore House
The Children's Hospital of Philadelphia
Philadelphia, PA

Carol A. Ford, MD, FSAHM
Professor of Pediatrics
Perelman School of Medicine at the University
    of Pennsylvania
Chief, Craig-Dalsimer Division of Adolescent
    Medicine
Orton Jackson Endowed Chair in Adolescent
    Medicine
The Children's Hospital of Philadelphia
Philadelphia, PA

Barbara L. Frankowski, MD, MPH, FAAP
Professor, University of Vermont College of Medicine
Pediatrician, Vermont Children's Hospital
Burlington, VT

Robert Garofalo, MD, MPH
Associate Professor of Pediatrics and Preventive
    Medicine
Northwestern University Feinberg School of
    Medicine
Medical Director, Adolescent HIV Services
Director, Center for Gender, Sexuality and HIV
    Prevention
Ann & Robert H. Lurie Children's Hospital of
    Chicago
Chicago, IL

Kenneth R. Ginsburg, MD, MS Ed, FAAP, FSAHM
Professor of Pediatrics
Perelman School of Medicine at the University
    of Pennsylvania
Craig-Dalsimer Division of Adolescent Medicine
The Children's Hospital of Philadelphia
Director of Health Services, Covenant House of
    Pennsylvania
Philadelphia, PA

Linda A. Hawkins, PhD, LPC
Adolescent Psychotherapist
Adolescent Initiative
Craig-Dalsimer Division of Adolescent Medicine
The Children's Hospital of Philadelphia
Philadelphia, PA

Cordella Hill, MSW
Executive Director
Covenant House Pennsylvania
Philadelphia, PA

Renée R. Jenkins, MD, FAAP
Professor of Pediatrics
Director, Office of Faculty Development
Howard University College of Medicine
Department of Pediatrics and Child Health
Howard University Hospital
Washington, DC

Sara B. Kinsman, MD, PhD
Associate Professor of Clinical Pediatrics
Perelman School of Medicine at the University
    of Pennsylvania
Craig-Dalsimer Division of Adolescent Medicine
The Children's Hospital of Philadelphia
Philadelphia, PA

Richard E. Kreipe, MD, FAAP, FSAHM, FAED
Dr. Elizabeth R. McAnarney Distinguished Professor
    of Pediatrics
Division of Adolescent Medicine, Golisano
    Children's Hospital
University of Rochester
Medical Director, Western New York Comprehensive
    Care Center for Eating Disorders
    Rochester Director, New York State ACT for
    Youth Center of Excellence
Rochester, NY

LTC Keith M. Lemmon, MD, FAAP
Chief, Division of Adolescent Medicine
Department of Pediatrics
Madigan Army Medical Center
Joint Base Lewis-McChord, WA
Assistant Professor of Pediatrics
Uniformed Services University of the Health
    Sciences
Bethesda, MD
Clinical Associate Professor of Pediatrics
University of Washington School of Medicine
Seattle, WA

Amanda Lerman, MD
Fellow, Adolescent Medicine
Craig-Dalsimer Division of Adolescent Medicine
The Children's Hospital of Philadelphia
Philadelphia, PA

Valerie J. Lewis, MD, MPH, FAAP, FSAHM
Adolescent Medicine Specialist, Department of
    Pediatrics
Clinical Scientist, Division of Community Health
    and Health Studies
Lehigh Valley Health Network
Allentown, PA
Assistant Professor of Pediatrics
University of South Florida Morsani College of
    Medicine
Tampa, FL

Joseph Lively
Resilience Specialist
El Centro de Estudiantes
Big Picture Philadelphia
Philadelphia, PA

Laura Collins Lyster-Mensh, MS
Policy Director, F.E.A.S.T.
Warrenton, VA

Zachary McClain, MD
Fellow, Adolescent Medicine
Craig-Dalsimer Division of Adolescent Medicine
The Children's Hospital of Philadelphia
Philadelphia, PA

Hugh Organ, MS
Associate Executive Director
Covenant House Pennsylvania
Chair, Philadelphia Anti-Trafficking Coalition
Philadelphia, PA

Jarret R. Patton, MD, FAAP
Medical Staff President-Elect
Medical Director, Outpatient Pediatrics
Lehigh Valley Health Network
Allentown, PA
Assistant Professor of Pediatrics
University of South Florida Morsani College of
    Medicine
Tampa, FL

Rebecka Peebles, MD, FAAP
Assistant Professor
Perelman School of Medicine at the University
    of Pennsylvania
Medical Director and Director of Research and
    Quality, Eating Disorder Services
Craig-Dalsimer Division of Adolescent Medicine
The Children's Hospital of Philadelphia
Philadelphia, PA

Nadja G. Peter, MD
Assistant Professor of Clinical Pediatrics
Perelman School of Medicine at the University
    of Pennsylvania
Craig-Dalsimer Division of Adolescent Medicine
The Children's Hospital of Philadelphia
Philadelphia, PA

Jonathan R. Pletcher, MD, FAAP
Assistant Professor, Pediatrics
University of Pittsburgh School of Medicine
Clinical Director, Division of Adolescent Medicine
Children's Hospital of Pittsburgh of UPMC
Pittsburgh, PA

Daniel H. Reirden, MD, FAAP, AAHIVMS
Assistant Professor of Pediatrics
Sections of Adolescent Medicine and Infectious
    Disease
University of Colorado School of Medicine
Medical Director of Youth HIV Services
Children's Hospital Colorado
Aurora, CO

Michael O. Rich, MD, MPH, FAAP, FSAHM
Associate Professor of Pediatrics
Harvard Medical School
Associate Professor of Social and Behavioral
    Sciences
Harvard School of Public Health
Director, Center on Media and Child Health
Division of Adolescent Medicine
Boston Children's Hospital
Boston, MA

Charles G. Rogers, MD
Fellow, Adolescent Medicine
Craig-Dalsimer Division of Adolescent Medicine
The Children's Hospital of Philadelphia
Philadelphia, PA

Nimi Singh, MD, MPH, MA
Assistant Professor, Department of Pediatrics
Division Head, Adolescent Health and Medicine
University of Minnesota Amplatz Children's Hospital
Minneapolis, MN

Gail B. Slap, MD, MSc, FSAHM
Professor of Pediatrics and Medicine
Perelman School of Medicine at the University
    of Pennsylvania
Associate Chair for Education, Department of
    Pediatrics
The Children's Hospital of Philadelphia
Philadelphia, PA

Jo Ann Sonis, LCSW, DCSW
Licensed Clinical Social Worker
Craig-Dalsimer Division of Adolescent Medicine
Division of Gastroenterology, Hepatology
    and Nutrition
The Children's Hospital of Philadelphia
Philadelphia, PA

Victor C. Strasburger, MD, FAAP, FSAHM
Distinguished Professor of Pediatrics
Founding Chief, Division of Adolescent Medicine
University of New Mexico School of Medicine
Albuquerque, NM

Susan T. Sugerman, MD, MPH, FAAP
Adolescent Medicine Physician
President and Cofounder
Girls to Women Health and Wellness
Dallas, TX

Oana Tomescu, MD, PhD
Assistant Professor of Medicine and Pediatrics
Perelman School of Medicine at the University
    of Pennsylvania
Craig-Dalsimer Division of Adolescent Medicine
The Children's Hospital of Philadelphia
Associate Program Director, Internal Medicine and
    Pediatrics Residency Program
Division of General Internal Medicine
Hospital of the University of Pennsylvania
Philadelphia, PA

Maria Trent, MD, MPH, FAAP, FSAHM
Associate Professor of Pediatrics
Division of General Pediatrics and Adolescent
    Medicine
Johns Hopkins University School of Medicine
Training Director, JHU Health Disparities
    Leadership in Education in Adolescent Health
    Program & DC-Baltimore Research Center on
    Child Health Disparities
Baltimore, MD

Lisa K. Tuchman, MD, MPH
Assistant Professor of Pediatrics
Division of Adolescent and Young Adult Medicine
Center for Translational Science, Children's
    Research Institute
Children's National Medical Center
The George Washington University School of
    Medicine and Health Sciences
Washington, DC

Stephen Van Bockern, EdD, MA
Professor of Education
Augustana College
Dean, Reclaiming Youth International
Sioux Falls, SD

Dzung X. Vo, MD, FAAP
Assistant Clinical Professor
Division of Adolescent Health and Medicine
Department of Pediatrics
British Columbia Children's Hospital
University of British Columbia
Vancouver, British Columbia
Canada

Zeelyna Wise
Director of Support Services
El Centro de Estudiantes
Big Picture Philadelphia
Philadelphia, PA

Michele Zucker, MD, MPH
Assistant Professor of Clinical Pediatrics
Perelman School of Medicine at the University of
    Pennsylvania
Craig-Dalsimer Division of Adolescent Medicine
The Children's Hospital of Philadelphia
Philadelphia, PA

Additional Contributors

Several organizations arranged for their young people to participate in this project.

Covenant House Pennsylvania, Philadelphia, PA
El Centro de Estudiantes, Philadelphia, PA
Larkin Street Youth Services, San Francisco, CA
YouthBuild Philadelphia Charter School,
Philadelphia, PA

Professionals from several organizations in the Philadelphia region shared their wisdom in the videos.

Adolescent Advocates, Rosemont, PA
Ahmed Ghuman, MA
Sherica Mays-Bankhead, MS, LPC
Patti Anne McAndrews, MHS, LPC, CAC
Sean Smith, MEd, AAC I
Amanda Strittmatter, MSS, LSW, AAC II

Covenant House Pennsylvania, Philadelphia, PA
Iva Bonaparte
LuCrecha Coats, MA
Bianca Cruz
Carl Hill
Denise Johnson
Ciera King
Pastor David Maddox
Robert Zindell, MS

El Centro de Estudiantes, Philadelphia, PA
David Bromley, MS Ed
Andrew Christman, MA
Matthew Prochnow, MS Ed
Helen Rowe, MS Ed
Tiffaney Whipple, MS Ed

YouthBuild Philadelphia Charter School,
Philadelphia, PA
Ameen Akbar
Ariesha Geier, MS
Jenee Lee
Simran Sidhu, MJ

The following individuals contributed to the videos as actors or participants:
Jennie Bernstein
Mei Elansary, MD, MPhil
Stephanie Grossman
Kathryn M. Murphy, RN, PhD
Samantha Powell, MD
Christopher Renjilian, MD
Melissa Riegel
Elyse Salek, MEd
Erin Sieke

To the youth we have served who have demonstrated their resilience and helped us to understand that we do our best when we facilitate them to build on their existing strengths. To the parents who have shown us that their unconditional love and consistent high expectations are the keys to their children's well-being, even through trying times.

Sara Kinsman: To John and Izzy, who have shared my greatest joy in life—next to caring for adolescents—being Izzy's mom. You have filled my life with hope and laughter. You have shown me that adversity can build new strengths and deepen our ability to help others, and the power of compassion and love. Of course, any mention of our wonderful family would not be complete without thanking Maggie and Popeye, who embody the gift of resilience.

Ken Ginsburg: To Celia, who continues to inspire me with her unyielding belief that the world can be better and that it is our job to be part of the solution. To Ilana and Talia, who are now on the cusp of adulthood and have given me joy beyond anything I had ever imagined. I deeply admire who you have become and pray that you will live life to the fullest, experiencing its abundant joys while savoring the opportunities for self-reflection and growth that come from its challenges.

The Society for Adolescent Health and Medicine congratulates the American Academy of Pediatrics on *Reaching Teens: Strength-Based Communication Strategies to Build Resilience and Support Healthy Adolescent Development*

The Society for Adolescent Health and Medicine (SAHM) wishes to congratulate the American Academy of Pediatrics (AAP) on the project *Reaching Teens: Strength-Based Communication Strategies to Build Resilience and Support Healthy Adolescent Development*. This project is a combination of text and video founded on strength-based communication. This is an important project with tremendous potential to engage all youth-serving professionals and better prepare them to communicate with youth, foster resilience, and promote positive youth development.

Founded in 1968, SAHM is a multidisciplinary organization committed to promoting adolescent health and improving the health and well-being of teenagers and young adults. The society is committed to ensuring the highest standards of care for youth; creating greater awareness of the health issues affecting this special population among health and other professionals, policy makers, and youth-serving organizations; and helping parents understand the health care needs of their adolescent children.

The Society for Adolescent Health and Medicine recognizes that the changes young people experience in adolescence create a special need for adolescent-focused health research and practice. By increasing awareness of the unique health needs of this population, we can have a positive impact on the physical, psychosocial, and overall well-being of teens and young adults around the world. Projects like *Reaching Teens* play a key role in enhancing the skills of professionals to better prepare all youth to thrive.

Again, on behalf of the SAHM Board of Directors and membership, we congratulate this group for putting together this important project. A project like *Reaching Teens* is important in promoting optimal health and well-being for adolescents and young adults everywhere.

Debra K. Katzman, MD, FSAHM
SAHM President, 2013–2014
www.adolescenthealth.org

Table of Contents

To view the collection of videos and access educational handouts,
please visit www.aap.org/reachingteens.

Acknowledgments xiii

Why It Matters to Our Future That We Reach Teens Today............................... xv
Gail B. Slap, MD, MSc, FSAHM

Foreword xvii
Paula M. Duncan, MD, FAAP

SECTION 1   ORIENTATION TO A STRENGTH-BASED APPROACH 1

Chapter 1   Introduction..3
Kenneth R. Ginsburg, MD, MS Ed, FAAP, FSAHM
Sara B. Kinsman, MD, PhD

Chapter 2   The Journey From Risk-Focused Attention to Strength-Based Care 9
Kenneth R. Ginsburg, MD, MS Ed, FAAP, FSAHM

Chapter 3   How a Strength-Based Approach Affects Behavioral Change 19
Kenneth R. Ginsburg, MD, MS Ed, FAAP, FSAHM

Chapter 4   Who's the Expert? Terms of Engagement in Adolescent Care........................25
Richard E. Kreipe, MD, FAAP, FSAHM, FAED

Chapter 5   The 7 Cs Model of Resilience..31
Kenneth R. Ginsburg, MD, MS Ed, FAAP, FSAHM

Chapter 6   The Impact of Trauma on Development and Well-being 37
Sandra L. Bloom, MD

Chapter 7   Wisdom From Model Strength-Based Programs That Work With
Youth Who Are Traditionally Labeled "At Risk"..49
Kenneth R. Ginsburg, MD, MS Ed, FAAP, FSAHM

SECTION 2   UNDERSTANDING ADOLESCENTS AND THEIR WORLD......................53

Chapter 8   Adolescent Development—Stages, Statuses, and Stereotypes.......................55
Charles G. Rogers, MD
Sara B. Kinsman, MD, PhD

Chapter 9   The Adolescent World 63
Amanda Lerman, MD
Sara B. Kinsman, MD, PhD

Chapter 10   Sex(uality) Happens: Fostering Healthy, Positive (Female) Sexuality 69
Susan T. Sugerman, MD, MPH, FAAP
Liana R. Clark, MD, MSCE, FAAP
Tonya A. Chaffee, MD, MPH, FAAP

Chapter 11   Male Sexuality 81
David L. Bell, MD, MPH
Kenneth R. Ginsburg, MD, MS Ed, FAAP, FSAHM

SECTION 3   CONNECTING WITH ADOLESCENTS AND THEIR FAMILIES................89

Chapter 12   Creating an Adolescent-Friendly Space and Service.....................................91
Angela Diaz, MD, MPH

Chapter 13   Creating a Male Adolescent-Friendly Space 99
David L. Bell, MD, MPH

Chapter 14   Setting the Stage for a Trustworthy Relationship 103
Kenneth R. Ginsburg, MD, MS Ed, FAAP, FSAHM

Chapter 15   Body Language..111
Kenneth R. Ginsburg, MD, MS Ed, FAAP, FSAHM

SECTION 4 COMMUNICATING WITH THE ADOLESCENT 119

Chapter 16   Core Principles on Communicating With Adolescents 121
Linda A. Hawkins, PhD, LPC
Kenneth R. Ginsburg, MD, MS Ed, FAAP, FSAHM

Chapter 17   Integrating the 7 Cs of Resilience Into Your Clinical Practice 133
Susan T. Sugerman, MD, MPH, FAAP

Chapter 18   The SSHADESS Screen: A Strength-Based Psychosocial Assessment.........139
Kenneth R. Ginsburg, MD, MS Ed, FAAP, FSAHM

Chapter 19   Cultural Humility 145
Valerie J. Lewis, MD, MPH, FAAP, FSAHM
Kenisha Campbell, MD, MPH
Angela Diaz, MD, MPH
Nadia L. Dowshen, MD, FAAP, AAHIVS
Kenneth R. Ginsburg, MD, MS Ed, FAAP, FSAHM
Renée R. Jenkins, MD, FAAP
Jarret R. Patton, MD, FAAP
Maria Trent, MD, MPH, FAAP, FSAHM
Dzung X. Vo, MD, FAAP

Chapter 20   Boundaries..153
Kenneth R. Ginsburg, MD, MS Ed, FAAP, FSAHM

Chapter 21   Examining Our Unconscious Biases..165
Amanda Lerman, MD

Chapter 22   Trauma-Informed Practice: Working With Youth Who Have
Suffered Adverse Childhood (or Adolescent) Experiences 173
Sandra L. Bloom, MD
Zeelyna Wise
Joseph Lively
Marcos O. Almonte, MDiv
Stephanie Contreras
Kenneth R. Ginsburg, MD, MS Ed, FAAP, FSAHM

Chapter 23   De-escalation and Crisis Management When a Youth Is "Acting Out"........187
Cordella Hill, MSW
Hugh Organ, MS
Kenneth R. Ginsburg, MD, MS Ed, FAAP, FSAHM

Chapter 24   Delivering Bad News to Adolescents...195
Daniel H. Reirden, MD, FAAP, AAHIVMS
Kenneth R. Ginsburg, MD, MS Ed, FAAP, FSAHM

SECTION 5 EMPOWERING ADOLESCENTS TO CHANGE 201

Chapter 25   Addressing Demoralization: Eliciting and Reflecting Strengths.................203
Kenneth R. Ginsburg, MD, MS Ed, FAAP, FSAHM

Chapter 26   Motivational Interviewing 209
Nimi Singh, MD, MPH, MA

Chapter 27   Health Realization—Accessing a Higher State of Mind
No Matter What..219
Nimi Singh, MD, MPH, MA

Chapter 28   Helping Adolescents Own Their Solutions 225
Kenneth R. Ginsburg, MD, MS Ed, FAAP, FSAHM

Chapter 29   Gaining a Sense of Control—One Step at a Time.......................................231
Kenneth R. Ginsburg, MD, MS Ed, FAAP, FSAHM

Chapter 30   Strength-Based Interviewing: The Circle of Courage.................................237
Barbara L. Frankowski, MD, MPH, FAAP
Larry K. Brendtro, PhD, LP
Stephen Van Bockern, EdD, MA
Paula M. Duncan, MD, FAAP

Chapter 31   Stress Management and Coping..243
Kenneth R. Ginsburg, MD, MS Ed, FAAP, FSAHM

Chapter 32   Mindfulness Practice for Resilience and Managing Stress and Pain 253
            Dzung X. Vo, MD, FAAP

Chapter 33   Helping Youth Overcome Shame and Stigma (and Doing Our Best
            to Not Be a Part of the Problem) 261
            Kenneth R. Ginsburg, MD, MS Ed, FAAP, FSAHM

SECTION 6   SUPPORTING EFFECTIVE PARENTING **273**

Chapter 34   The Professional-Parent-Teen Partnership 275
            Carol A. Ford, MD, FSAHM

Chapter 35   Preparing Parents for Their Children's Adolescence 283
            Kenneth R. Ginsburg, MD, MS Ed, FAAP, FSAHM

Chapter 36   Promoting Balanced Parenting: Warmth, Clear Boundaries,
            and Effective Monitoring 293
            Kenneth R. Ginsburg, MD, MS Ed, FAAP, FSAHM

Chapter 37   Delivering Upsetting News to Parents: Recognizing Their
            Strengths First 303
            Kenneth R. Ginsburg, MD, MS Ed, FAAP, FSAHM

Chapter 38   When Parents' Resilience Reaches Its Limits 309
            Kenneth R. Ginsburg, MD, MS Ed, FAAP, FSAHM

Chapter 39   The Importance of Self-care for Parents 315
            Kenneth R. Ginsburg, MD, MS Ed, FAAP, FSAHM

SECTION 7   MENTAL, EMOTIONAL, AND BEHAVIORAL HEALTH **319**

Chapter 40   The Role of Lifestyle in Mental Health Promotion 321
            Nimi Singh, MD, MPH, MA

Chapter 41   Friendships and Peers 327
            Sara B. Kinsman, MD, PhD

Chapter 42   Depression 339
            Sara B. Kinsman, MD, PhD

Chapter 43   Anxiety 349
            Sara B. Kinsman, MD, PhD

Chapter 44   Somatic Symptoms 361
            Sara B. Kinsman, MD, PhD

Chapter 45   Grief 375
            Alison Culyba, MD, MPH
            Sara B. Kinsman, MD, PhD

Chapter 46   ADHD in Adolescents 387
            Susan T. Sugerman, MD, MPH, FAAP

Chapter 47   Learning Differences 399
            Marina Catallozzi, MD, MSCE
            Susan T. Sugerman, MD, MPH, FAAP

Chapter 48   Perfectionism 405
            Kenneth R. Ginsburg, MD, MS Ed, FAAP, FSAHM
            Susan T. Sugerman, MD, MPH, FAAP

Chapter 49   Eating Disorders 413
            Rebecka Peebles, MD, FAAP
            Laura Collins Lyster-Mensh, MS
            Richard E. Kreipe, MD, FAAP, FSAHM, FAED

Chapter 50   Talking to Teens Who Are Using or Abusing Substances 425
            Jonathan R. Pletcher, MD, FAAP

Chapter 51   Teen Pregnancy and Parenting 439
            Charles G. Rogers, MD
            Kenneth R. Ginsburg, MD, MS Ed, FAAP, FSAHM

Chapter 52   Teen Driving 449
            Kenneth R. Ginsburg, MD, MS Ed, FAAP, FSAHM

Chapter 53   Managing Electronic Media Use in the Lives of Adolescents......................455
              Michael O. Rich, MD, MPH, FAAP, FSAHM
              Victor C. Strasburger, MD, FAAP, FSAHM

Chapter 54   Helping Teens Cope With Divorce..463
              Jo Ann Sonis, LCSW, DCSW

Chapter 55   Bullying..471
              Zachary McClain, MD
              Kenneth R. Ginsburg, MD, MS Ed, FAAP, FSAHM

Chapter 56   Unhealthy Relationships..479
              Marina Catallozzi, MD, MSCE
              Susan T. Sugerman, MD, MPH, FAAP

Chapter 57   Emotional, Physical, and Sexual Abuse...489
              Angela Diaz, MD, MPH

Chapter 58   Youth Violence..499
              Kenneth R. Ginsburg, MD, MS Ed, FAAP, FSAHM

SECTION 8   SERVING SPECIAL POPULATIONS 509

Chapter 59   Teens With Chronic Illness and Special Health Care Needs:
              A Person-Centered Approach to Communication 511
              Jonathan R. Pletcher, MD, FAAP
              Karyn E. Feit, LCSW
              Lisa K. Tuchman, MD, MPH
              Nadja G. Peter, MD

Chapter 60   Transitioning From Pediatric to Adult Care 523
              Nadja G. Peter, MD
              Karyn E. Feit, LCSW
              Jo Ann Sonis, LCSW, DCSW
              Oana Tomescu, MD, PhD
              Jonathan R. Pletcher, MD, FAAP

Chapter 61   Sexual and Gender Minority Youth...531
              Nadia L. Dowshen, MD, FAAP, AAHIVS
              Linda A. Hawkins, PhD, LPC
              Renata Arrington-Sanders, MD, MPH, ScM, FAAP
              Daniel H. Reirden, MD, FAAP, AAHIVMS
              Robert Garofalo, MD, MPH

Chapter 62   Reaching Immigrant Youth 539
              Dzung X. Vo, MD, FAAP

Chapter 63   America's Children: The Unique Needs and Culture of Military Youth.......545
              LTC Keith M. Lemmon, MD, FAAP

Chapter 64   Foster Care Youth: Engaging Foster Care Youth Into Care.................557
              Tonya A. Chaffee, MD, MPH, FAAP

Chapter 65   Youth Infected With HIV 563
              Nadia L. Dowshen, MD, FAAP, AAHIVS
              Linda A. Hawkins, PhD, LPC
              Renata Arrington-Sanders, MD, MPH, ScM, FAAP
              Daniel H. Reirden, MD, FAAP, AAHIVMS
              Robert Garofalo, MD, MPH

Chapter 66   Serving Homeless and Unstably Housed Youth 569
              Colette (Coco) Auerswald, MD, MS, FSAHM

SECTION 9   SELF-CARE FOR PROVIDERS 579

Chapter 67   Healer, Heal Thyself: Self-care for the Caregiver 581
              Oana Tomescu, MD, PhD

Chapter 68   Getting Out of the "Fast Lane"—More "Miles to the Gallon"? 593
              Renée R. Jenkins, MD, FAAP

Chapter 69   Have I Really Made a Difference? Trusting That Our Presence Matters......597
              Kenneth R. Ginsburg, MD, MS Ed, FAAP, FSAHM

INDEX 599

Acknowledgments

It would not be possible to thank all the people who supported us in preparing this textbook. We must first thank the entire staff at the American Academy of Pediatrics (AAP), who have taken this enormous project from a kernel of an idea through fruition. Some people, however, deserve special mention. We are grateful to Mark Grimes for having the vision to imagine this idea and the commitment to the well-being of teens to make it happen. Mark Ruthman has been instrumental in turning this dream into a reality; without his creative thinking and technical skills, this project simply could not exist. Eileen Glasstetter has shepherded every detail of this work, somehow managing all of the moving pieces with patience, humor, skill, and grace. Carolyn Kolbaba's resolute commitment to supporting the mission of building the resilience of children and teens continues to nurture us. And Peg Mulcahy has worked with us to design a book that visually captures the joy of working with teenagers.

We are also grateful to the AAP Adolescent Health Partnership Project (a grantee of the Partners in Program Planning for Adolescent Health), chaired by Tonya Chaffee and managed by Charlotte Zia, for its commitment to promote positive youth development. We are honored to have been part of this mission.

Next, we must offer our appreciation and respect to the leaders of the positive youth development and resilience movements who have inspired us. In particular, Rick Little and his team at the International Youth Foundation first elucidated the primary ingredients needed for healthy youth development. We have been particularly influenced by Richard Lerner of Tufts University, who was part of that team and is one of the great developmental psychologists of our time. Dr Lerner has spent decades demonstrating that positive youth development efforts indeed work. In our own field of adolescent medicine, Robert Blum and Michael Resnick have led the way and motivated us to shift from a risk-based to a strength-based approach to youth, and Karen Hein has made us understand we need to support youth so they can reach their full potential. Paula Duncan has worked tirelessly to ensure that as we offer comprehensive care, we do so through a strength-based lens while simultaneously addressing risks.

Sara Kinsman

I would like to acknowledge my many colleagues, mentors, and friends in the Craig-Dalsimer Division of Adolescent Medicine at The Children's Hospital of Philadelphia. Gail Slap has guided me at every stage of my training and development over the past 25 years. Words are not enough. Thank you, Gail. Many friends and colleagues have shared their wisdom in this work, and I would like to acknowledge their special gifts to me. Nadja Peter taught me to be thorough, very thorough; Nadia Dowshen taught me to be truly nonjudgmental; Oana Tomescu taught me how to put love into clinical medicine; Janice Hillman taught me to know who I am as a clinician; Liana Clark taught me to be candid with my patients; Bret Rudy taught me how to care deeply even when our efforts seem hopeless; Kenisha Campbell taught me the benefits of being matter-of-fact; Jon Pletcher taught me to be an advocate; Marina Catallozzi taught me to care selflessly; Dan Reirden taught me to use my sense of humor to keep balance; Len Levine taught me the importance of being true to your clinical strengths; Lisa Tuchman taught me to live balance; Valerie Lewis taught me serenity in difficult moments; Jane Subak Kennedy taught me how to respect different perspectives; Jean Anne Cieplinski-Robertson taught me that directness can be very useful; Charles Rogers taught me that you can be incredibly book smart and nice; Amanda Lerman taught me to value others' opinions; Alison Culyba taught me that you can be thorough, efficient, and kind; Zach McClain taught me the importance of a well-timed hug; Karyn Feit taught me to problem solve and not give up; Kalita Miller taught me a smile can change the direction of a day; Shirlene Brody and Nadyne Lopez taught me to stay on track (at least they tried); Carol Ford and Eileen Drames taught me to know my strengths and gave me the opportunity to colead the 5WA Inpatient Floor Team, which in turn taught me the power and joy of a well-functioning multidisciplinary team; and finally, Don Schwarz and Ken Ginsburg taught me to allow my many interests to mix together and bring goodness in a variety of ways to adolescents and their families.

Ken Ginsburg

I thank my professional mentors, Gail Slap and Donald Schwarz, who have had the experience to guide me, the knowledge to enlighten me, and the passion and love of youth to transmit to me. Above all, they have repeatedly demonstrated they care not just about my academic career but about me. I also thank the best teacher I ever had, Judith Lowenthal, who inspired me (when I was an adolescent) to grasp the potential in every young person. My first mentors and first teachers, of course, were my parents, Arnold and Marilyn Ginsburg. I learned much of what I have come to see as good parenting in their home. I was also blessed to learn about the strength of family from my grandmother, Belle Moore, who demonstrated unconditional love better than anyone I have known, except for her daughter Marilyn.

I also thank my colleagues at the Craig-Dalsimer Division of Adolescent Medicine for teaching me so much and contributing so richly to this effort. In particular, I am grateful to Carol Ford for being so very supportive of this work and for her passionate belief that supporting children and their parents in the second decade of life will have a lifelong impact. I am indebted to Sara Kinsman for consistently modeling that no effort is too great if it is necessary to facilitate healing or lessen suffering. I also must share that it is our trainees who constantly restore my energy with their idealism. There is no greater joy than to watch them become committed healers, to follow their careers, and to see their skills surpass my own. I would name each them, but you will meet many of them as you read this work.

I also must acknowledge that what I know about resilience I have learned by working with and serving resilient people. It was the people of the Cheyenne River Lakota Reservation in South Dakota who first taught me how the power of connection to family and community, as well as the commitment to making a contribution to the world, could restore balance even through difficult times. The youth of Covenant House Pennsylvania serve as a constant reminder of the tenacity and strength of the human spirit. From my colleagues who work at Covenant House, I have learned that a loving, strength-building environment that offers structure permits young people to flourish and move beyond a troubled past. I also must thank Joanna Berwind for giving me the opportunity to work with youth-serving agencies in Philadelphia to explore the impact of connections that are rooted in unconditional love and steeped in the understanding that youth are the experts in their own lives. I have also been honored to witness the strength and resilience of our nation's military-affiliated families and grateful for the opportunity to do so afforded by my work with the Military Child Education Coalition and the Child, Adolescent, and Family Behavioral Health Office (US Army Medical Command). Now I am privileged to work with Boys & Girls Clubs of America and to learn from its outstanding youth development work. Finally, I feel blessed to be given the opportunity to repay, in the smallest way, some of what I received in my current work with the National Congress of American Indians and Boys & Girls Clubs in Indian Country.

Above all, we thank the young people and their families who have let us into their lives. We are awed by the love we see every day in the parents who bring their children to us at The Children's Hospital of Philadelphia and only hope that we have served them well. We are moved by the resilience and wisdom of the youth we have served. In sharing their wisdom, they have demonstrated they are indeed poised to lead us into the future. It is our job to make sure they are fully prepared to do so.

Why It Matters to Our Future That We Reach Teens Today

Reaching Teens is an action-oriented road map linking today's adults with tomorrow's successors. Drs Ginsburg, Kinsman, and colleagues create for us a multimedia toolbox grounded in evidence and infused with trust in our capacity as adult learners and abiding respect for the teens we serve. *Reaching Teens* challenges those of us trained in traditional risk- or problem-focused models to hear the strong, healthy heartbeats in the midst of adolescent trauma or illness and to communicate the power of that strength back to its youthful source. Empowered youth become emotionally and physically healthier adults prepared to innovate and to repair our world.

Learning to listen and respond with honest optimism is no easy task, and Drs Ginsburg and Kinsman accompany us step-by-step through the process. *Reaching Teens* recognizes the differences in our learning styles, practices, and contexts. It allows us to choose written, oral, visual, individual, and group strategies that best suit our styles. We can transition from one strategy to another seamlessly, without losing pace or progress, and we can maneuver between sections and chapters when we seek help with specific issues. *Reaching Teens* is about teens and it is for us, the professionals who work with them. It is meant to be a living document that adapts as we gain in confidence and skill.

The brilliance of *Reaching Teens* is its science and humanism. It is designed to guide us today as we keep a steady eye on the generation that will lead us tomorrow. *Reaching Teens* is the art of healing at its best, produced by the finest team of professionals imaginable. These authors have enriched my life immeasurably, and they make life happier and healthier for thousands of teens daily. Join them on this journey as you read, listen, watch, and learn. Best of all, enjoy the positive change that awaits you.

— Gail B. Slap, MD, MSc, FSAHM

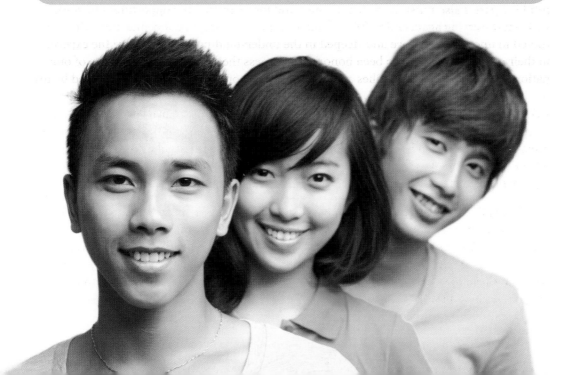

Foreword

Paula M. Duncan, MD, FAAP

In 1987, after 3 years in practice in Vermont, I informally asked my patients how I could better serve adolescents. One 16-year-old girl said, *"Well, you know you are always saying, 'Don't do this and don't do that.' I could be sitting in my room on a Friday night NOT doing drugs, NOT having sex, NOT drinking and driving…NOT doing ANYTHING and being perfectly miserable. You could try to figure out what kids need to 'say yes' to and start talking about that too."* That teen moved out of my care to a happy and successful life, but I have never forgotten her wisdom.

Another 16-year-old girl entered my world and provided me with a front-row seat for a 3-year longitudinal course in "what it takes to turn your life around." In addition to actually doing that work, she generously spent some of her time thinking about "what helped and what didn't." Her experiences and thoughts demonstrated that the strength-based approach was the key.

- *"I didn't think I had any strengths until someone pointed them out to me."*
- *"I would say it was not just one adult really caring about me that made the difference. My list would include some people who had no idea how much they helped me—just by treating me with a positive attitude and respect."*
- *"My advice to people trying to help kids like me would be to just never give up. It might be the 99th time that we are finally able to start to turn things around."*
- *"It would be a great help if adults interacted with teens in a way that supported their strengths rather than just talked about what wasn't going well for them."*

This young woman has also thrived, and she remains for me the real-life embodiment of what the literature in positive youth development and resilience demonstrates. As reflected in her words, focusing on strengths allowed her to make the changes only she could make.

We have to start the conversation by clearly stating that focusing on and reinforcing existing strengths is not just a "positive" approach that feels good, it is an important strategy to approach and mitigate risks. It is a sound strategy to turn kids' lives around.

Why We Need This Approach

- It is related to better outcomes for kids in overall health and well-being, which is summarized and explicated in the positive youth development and resilience literatures.
- Many of our best intentions may not translate into meaningful encouragement and guidance because the young people can see our mouths moving but not really hear what we're saying.
- There should be some explicit assessment of a youth's developmental trajectory, similar to what is done for younger children. Developmental milestones for teens can be identified through an evaluation of their strengths.
- All youth can benefit. For those youth coming back from one or even a couple of bad decisions, its influence can be lifesaving, but even youth who are avoiding serious risk behaviors may not be thriving and may need help staying on course. Our goal has to be that *all* youth will thrive!

We can help parents and guardians benefit from this approach as well, giving them feedback on what they're doing right whenever we see it. Such input also provides direction on what they are trying to get their teens to "say yes" to. As one parent said, *"I knew what I didn't want them to do, but I wasn't sure what I specifically was hoping they would do."* A framework like the Bright Futures developmental tasks, the 7 Cs of resilience, or Brendtro's Circle of Courage lets parents routinely and easily do a "spot-check," asking

"Does my teen have opportunities to grow in each of these areas: relationships with family, friends, and other adults; a chance to get good at things; an opportunity to do something for someone else; and a chance to make independent decisions?" There are many things for parents to learn about supporting healthy emotional development, and interactions between professionals and parents shouldn't stop because of a child's private visit in the examination room. We professionals have a role in supporting parents to be the kind of caregivers they want to be.

Why It Feels Different and Why It Works

My experience and research with my colleague Dr Barbara Frankowski have most closely exposed me to the use of the Circle of Courage covered in Chapter 30. It is one of the many strength-based approaches offered in this text. I would like to share with you, based on working with hundreds of clinicians and evaluating their experience in implementing a strength-based approach, the essence of why I think this approach not only works for youth but nourishes us.

- Because it's full of hope—honest hope linked to specific messages that the young person recognizes.

    "When youth have these things in areas of their life, things generally work out better for them, and I can't help but notice that you have strengths (or have made some progress) in every single one of these areas."

    This actually provides the young person, and sometimes family members, with a more balanced view of the young person and his or her situation. One family medicine physician told me, *"I especially use this approach when I have an adolescent patient who might need to walk out of my office with a new perspective on him- or herself."* A rural pediatrician noted how it changed the conversation in a visit when she had the young person enumerate the grandmother's strengths as a way to defuse a standoff.

- Because it changes the conversation. Some clinicians have found that using this approach adds a new dimension to their professional lives. It can help set up an alliance in which patients, parents, and clinicians can function as collaborators trying to address a concern, rather than adversaries focused on making the adolescent "change" or "behave." The most exciting aspect of this work has been the shift that clinicians notice when they begin to interact with youth and families with a new attitude.

    As Brendtro says, *"In the middle of the word encouragement is 'courage,' which is what all of us need to just keep going in tough times or to be able to make a change."* When we're talking strengths we're talking heart to heart.

Why This Book Matters

Dr Ken Ginsburg is a master of strength-based pediatrics and adolescent medicine. He approaches each youth with focused positive attention and caring and then speaks the language of hope. Dr Sara Kinsman is one of the nation's most skilled clinicians in serving youth with chronic pain and emotional trauma. In this textbook filled with video explanations and examples, they share with us their best and most effective language and strategies. Additionally, the voices of nearly 30 of some of the country's most renowned adolescent practitioners infuse this work with varied viewpoints and experience gained from working with diverse populations over decades. In keeping with one of the core principles of strength-based work—adolescents are the best experts in their own lives—teen wisdom and testimony are incorporated throughout the videos. Together, the professionals and teens address a question posed by clinicians, educators, parents, and guardians.

"How can I learn to do this? I believe that this is the best way to approach an adolescent, but I'm not sure what to say or how to think about things from this strength-based perspective."

My own focus in this work has been the use of the strength-based approach in primary care practice, especially within the preventive services visit. Because they may seem to be polar opposites, my challenge has been to consider how we complement our responsibility to assess youth risk taking with an assessment and promotion of healthy adolescent development. Just because our education as clinicians has focused appropriately on honing our ability "to describe and document the heck out of disease symptoms" to reach the correct diagnosis and institute the best treatment plan, nothing says we wouldn't benefit from acquiring a few skills in this complementary assessment of strength.

The Vermont work in the early 2000s and the national work that followed demonstrated that many of our colleagues already assessed youth for some aspects of healthy development (*"How is school going? How are you getting along at home?"*) and believed in shared decision-making when a health behavior change was needed. They found that adding in the following 2 steps provided a comprehensive and efficient approach:
1. Including a more systematic assessment of development or strengths
2. Providing the young person (and his or her parent or guardian if the youth agrees) with a very brief summary statement about the youth's progress on adolescent developmental and opportunities for growth

"I want to review with you some of the strengths you have that I've learned about as we've been talking this morning." Then after the young person knows you see him or her as a whole person, the young person may be more willing and receptive to your advice. *"I'm concerned about the fact that you're having unprotected sex, and I hope you'll be willing to discuss that with me."*

Another reason for my excitement about *Reaching Teens* is because I believe that shared decision-making is an essential part of the strength-based approach, and here you will find many examples of how to partner with young people and their parents. When young people have joined with you in arriving at a plan, they have ownership over that plan. When they have been treated as experts in their own lives and have determined their readiness to change, they are invested in the process.

Link to Bright Futures: Preventive Services Guidelines

The information contained in *Reaching Teens* is also timely for clinicians implementing *Bright Futures: Guidelines for Health Supervision of Infants, Children, and Adolescents,* 3rd Edition. Bright Futures contains the US Health Resources and Services Administration–supported pediatric well-child and preventive care guidelines specifically referenced in the Patient Protection and Affordable Care Act.

The primary reason for using these approaches is to benefit people on all sides of the "helping" conversation. The authors have given their most effective strategies, yet each reader is the expert on what will work for his or her patients, clinical situation, or family. These ideas are meant to be helpful but never prescriptive. I thank Drs Ginsburg and Kinsman as well as the American Academy of Pediatrics for unifying these writings, videos, and examples into one publication. As I see it, *Reaching Teens* offers the strategies that will allow you to implement that part of Bright Futures that focuses on developmental assessment and counseling with adolescents. I see this work as a how-to manual for communicating with teens in a way that will build on their strength while addressing their risks.

A Step Forward for Each of Us

This body of work is not just for health professionals. I genuinely believe that all of us who serve youth can grow from deeply engaging in exploring how we can better reach teens and support their families. Hopefully it will give each of us the opportunity to find the ideas, words, and approaches that match our depth of caring.

Bright Futures Guidelines: A Renewed Commitment to Strength-Based Care

Although a youth development assessment was always implicit in the preventive services visit and developmental surveillance was included at those visits on the American Academy of Pediatrics Bright Futures periodicity schedule, *Bright Futures: Guidelines for Health Supervision of Infants, Children, and Adolescents*, 3rd Edition, describes this component comprehensively and with more specificity.

Strengths and the use of strength-based approaches are highlighted in 3 parts of the Bright Futures guidelines.[1]

1. In the "Promoting Child Development" theme, Table 6 (page 71) contrasts the deficit model with the strength-based model.

2. There is explicit guidance on assessing a young person's progress on the developmental tasks of adolescence starting at age 7 years and continuing through adolescence. The "Surveillance of Development" section of each visit from ages 7 to 21 years includes guidance to determine whether the youth is making progress on some or all of the following developmental tasks measures:

   a. Engages in a positive way in the life of the community

   b. Demonstrates increasingly responsible and independent decision-making

   c. Demonstrates physical, cognitive, emotional, social, and moral competencies

   d. Forms a caring, supportive relationship with family, other adults, and peers

   e. Engages in behaviors that provide well-being and contribute to a healthy lifestyle

   f. Displays a sense of self-confidence, hopefulness, and well-being

   g. Demonstrates resiliency when confronted with life stressors

3. Each of the 11- to 21-year visits includes 5 priority areas for assessment and counseling. The strength/developmental tasks are identified for explicit attention.

   a. Social and academic competence (connectedness with family, peers, and community; interpersonal relationships; school performance)

   b. Emotional well-being (coping, mood regulation and mental health, sexuality)

These visit chapters also include examples of questions to elicit strengths, as well as phrases and anticipatory guidance concepts that may be helpful. Patient and parent questionnaires, anticipatory guidance handouts, and documentation forms are all designed to match the chapters in the guidelines, making it easy for clinicians to gather information from youth about development and strengths and to document counseling about these issues. More information about Bright Futures is available at http://brightfutures.aap.org.

Reference

1. Hagan JF, Shaw JS, Duncan PM, eds. *Bright Futures: Guidelines for Health Supervision of Infants, Children, and Adolescents*. 3rd ed. Elk Grove Village, IL: American Academy of Pediatrics; 2008

Orientation to a Strength-Based Approach

This section sets the tone for this work. First, the "Introduction" (Chapter 1) will present the core philosophical principles that guide *Reaching Teens.* It will also introduce you to how to navigate through this work, which is far more than a textbook. As a body of work that hopes to build your skill set in communicating with teenagers, we felt that the written word alone could not suffice. Therefore, you will be able to hear expert and youth testimony and witness demonstrations to reinforce material presented in text. In "The Journey From Risk-Focused Attention to Strength-Based Care" (Chapter 2), both the history and rationale of a strength-based approach to youth will be presented. Although it may seem intuitive that people will best feel empowered when we recognize their existing strengths, this premise was considered quite innovative at one time. Because we

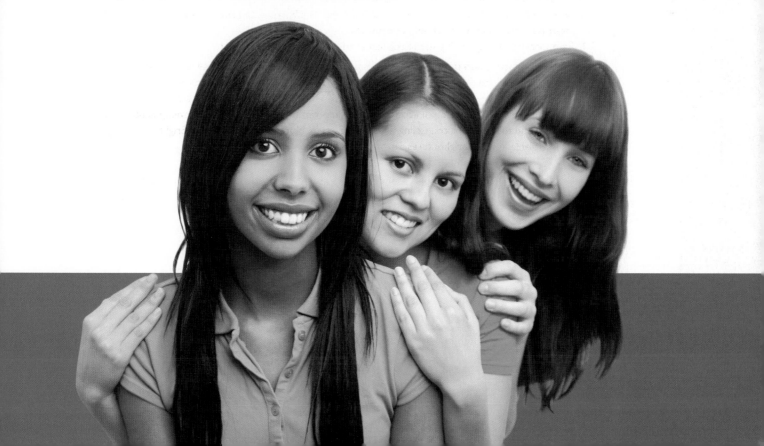

cared so deeply about the well-being of youth, we naturally focused on mitigating their risks. Now we understand that one of the most effective ways to address risk is to build on existing strengths. You will see how the positive youth development and resilience movements forms the framework for strength-based communication and interventions. Then "How a Strength-Based Approach Affects Behavioral Change" (Chapter 3) will contextualize how many of the approaches suggested in *Reaching Teens* fit into an overall strategy to apply these frameworks and promote positive behavioral change in youth. Then, in "Who's the Expert? Terms of Engagement in Adolescent Care" (Chapter 4), you will see how recognizing teens as the greatest experts on their own lives—one of the core principles of positive youth development—better positions you to engage in a shared decision-making process with them. In "The 7 Cs Model of Resilience" (Chapter 5) you will be introduced to a comprehensive model that captures the key ingredients youth need to thrive in good times and rise above adversity in challenging times. Next, in "The Impact of Trauma on Development and Well-being" (Chapter 6) you will learn how toxic stress affects behavior. Fundamental to our supporting youths' resilience is our first understanding how adversity impacts their lives. Finally, in "Wisdom From Model Strength-Based Programs That Work With Youth Who Are Traditionally Labeled 'At Risk'" (Chapter 7), you will be able to hear directly from program staff and participants about what they believe works to facilitate change in youth.

CHAPTER 1

Introduction

Kenneth R. Ginsburg, MD, MS Ed, FAAP, FSAHM
Sara B. Kinsman, MD, PhD

 Related Video Content

1.0.1 Why Do We Focus so Heavily on Communication When We Consider Impacting on the Health and Well-being of Teens?

■ Why Focus on Reaching Teens?

Adolescence is a time of great promise and potential, when each young person strives to answer the fundamental question, "Who am I?" It is the stage when youth are learning to navigate their environment, imagining what independence may look like, and considering how they might contribute to the world. It is the time when teens begin to explore intimate relationships that will hopefully prepare them to have healthy and satisfying adult lives.

> While we guide youth to avoid risk behaviors, our greater goal is to prepare them to thrive and to position them to be fully prepared to lead us into the future.

Although adolescence is a time of inspirational possibility, it is also a stage of potential peril. Teens struggle to individuate from their parents and discover how they are just like—and so very different from—them. This can lead to rebellion. Peers take on a pivotal importance as young people try on different personas and experiment with new behaviors. For these reasons, among others, the greatest threats to adolescents' lives and well-being are tightly linked to their behavior.

The teen years are the time when both healthy and dangerous lifelong habits are formed. **1.0.2**

Adolescence is often framed as a time of fierce independence, when adult guidance is rejected. In fact, adolescents are hungry for guidance. Although parents are ideally situated to offer their wisdom and experience, they are also the people from whom youth are programmed to wrest independence. This means that youth-serving professionals have a crucial role both in directly guiding teens and in supporting parents so that they can optimize their influence.

Reaching Teens: Strength-Based Communication Strategies to Build Resilience and Support Healthy Adolescent Development offers strategies and approaches that we hope will enhance your ability to effectively serve youth.

■ Our Philosophical Framework

There are several core principles drawn largely from the positive youth development and resilience frameworks that guide this work.

- While we guide youth to avoid risk behaviors, our greater goal is to prepare them to thrive and to position them to be fully prepared to lead us into the future.
- Youth have inherent strengths to be recognized and developed, and the best way to address risk may be to build on these existing strengths.

- Young people need to feel valued. They need to know that they matter. When adults genuinely listen to their views and recognize that they are the experts on their own lives, it empowers them to make healthy decisions.

- Youth thrive when they have strong, healthy connections with adults who believe in them unconditionally and hold them to high expectations. Ideally, youth have those connections with their parents. When they do, then healthy connections with other adults expand that protection. When they don't, healthy connections with other adults take on a critical importance.

 • Parenting an adolescent can be challenging, but parents remain the most important force in young people's lives. Sometimes professionals can do the greatest good by supporting effective parenting.

- It is our connection with youth that positions us to guide them. Key to that connection is that adolescents know that we genuinely like them and that they consider us worthy of their trust. 1.1

- Ideally, healthy development is supported from early in infancy. When it is not, adolescents are still capable of healing and do so best when caring adults trust in their capacity to right themselves and offer appropriate support and guidance.

- Most risky adolescent behaviors (including substance use, self-mutilation, violence, Internet addiction, and a host of other problems) serve at least partly as coping strategies that help youth manage uncomfortable stressors. If we help youth to develop a repertoire of alternative coping strategies, we will diminish their need to turn to these worrisome quick fixes. **25.9**

 • When we work with youth who have experienced trauma and are exhibiting acting-out behaviors, it is important to approach them with the unspoken mindset of "What happened to you?" rather than "What's wrong with you?" In fact, because trauma is so prevalent, and we never know someone's full past, it is wise to approach all youth with this nonjudgmental, supportive mindset.

■ Navigating Reaching Teens

The Content

The goal of *Reaching Teens* is to enhance both your comfort and skill in communicating with teenagers so that you are better positioned to guide them. Therefore, it offers basic principles of strength-based communication, approaches to connect with youth, and specific strategies and brief interventions to deal with issues likely to arise as you serve adolescents and their families. It is not intended to prepare you to become a counselor or therapist, although we hope it will enhance your journey if that is your path.

Certain strategies and approaches presented in this text, including trauma-informed care, motivational interviewing, mindfulness, stress management techniques, and others, have a full literature of their own. We hope that exposure to the repertoire of ideas here will pique your interest for deeper exploration of those strategies that you believe would work best for you.

The written word is not the most naturalistic way to convey concepts in communication. Therefore, although *Reaching Teens* anchors all of the strategies in written chapters to orient you, it then offers you video materials that allow for deeper explanations, alternate views, youth input, and demonstrations. Some video materials are oriented to parents or youth so that you can see how we might directly explain these concepts and/or so that you might repurpose these brief films for direct viewing by the parents and teens you serve.

Reaching Teens knows you are the expert on your own practice. It does not suggest replacing your style with any approach offered here; rather, it offers a repertoire of strategies you may choose from to supplement your own. In fact, you will note intentional redundancy where different experts may cover the same topic, and at times may even offer conflicting views.

Reaching Teens is divided into 9 sections, each with several chapters.

Section 1—Orientation to a Strength-Based Approach sets the philosophical tone and rationale for strength-based, trauma-informed, communication.

Section 2—Understanding Adolescents and Their World prepares you to consider the developmental milieu and environmental contexts that affect teens.

Section 3—Connecting With Adolescents and Their Families offers strategies to build trustworthy and effective relationships.

Section 4—Communicating With the Adolescent offers essential strategies and approaches to reach youth and facilitate behavioral change.

Section 5—Empowering Adolescents to Change offers specific strategies that use a shared decision-making model to empower youth to make wiser decisions and healthier choices.

Section 6—Supporting Effective Parenting considers how we as youth-serving professionals can support parents to most effectively monitor and guide their children.

Section 7—Mental, Emotional, and Behavioral Health includes strategies to help youth navigate a variety of specific psychosocial and environmental challenges.

Section 8—Serving Special Populations addresses the specific needs of unique populations.

Section 9—Self-care for Providers recognizes that this work is emotionally challenging, and sometimes exhausting and demoralizing, and that unless we care for ourselves with the same degree of commitment with which we care for others, our capacity to serve over a lifetime will be diminished.

The topics are interrelated and, therefore, are cross-referenced throughout. You may choose to start with general approaches to the adolescent (eg, building trust, or motivational interviewing) or you may first choose to dive into a topical area such as substance use. The cross-referencing allows you to begin with a general communications strategy and then link directly to a specific topic for illustration. Conversely, if you begin with a topical area, you may then wish to refer to those strategies that will help you forge a connection or effectively convey a message.

If you use the electronic text to navigate *Reaching Teens,* you will have live links that will allow you to review other chapters, link to resources, download chapters, or view videos. Some links will be imbedded within the text, and a full set will be presented as a menu at the end of each chapter. (See www.aap.org/reachingteens.)

Informed by the Best Available Evidence

Reaching Teens draws from the best of existing evidence to develop applied, theoretically based communication strategies. It is important, however, to understand that many of the techniques shared in this work have not been formally studied and therefore do not meet the highest standards of evidence. We hope that researchers dive deeply into how best to engage teens; however, the current literature is scant and much of what we believe involves difficult to study constructs. For example, a wide body of research demonstrates that a sense of connection with positive adults and peers is a core element that determines a young person's well-being. However, there isn't literature that clearly evaluates the varied ways in which to forge connections. Part of the reason this literature is sparse is because of how difficult it is to truly measure the essential ingredients of connection, such as trust, respect, and positive regard. In fact, we recognize many of these concepts are even difficult to clearly define.

In a subject area steeped in the nuances of human interactions, we choose not to be limited by the standards of being research-based, but will consistently be informed by the best of existing evidence, including expert opinion. Further, we are rooted in the theoretical constructs of the positive youth development and resilience movements.

Is This Work Just for Health Professionals?

No. *Reaching Teens* is written to benefit all professionals who serve youth. It is not designed to teach you to do therapy; rather it hopes to enhance your already existing therapeutic skills. Most of the material is written by adolescent medicine physicians and their colleagues. Consequently, many of the topics have a bias toward presentations that occur in a health care setting, but we hope that all professionals will consider how to apply the lessons learned in their practice setting. Most topics are not health specific at all, although they do impact on physical, emotional, or mental health. Even those heavily health-focused areas have applications in a counseling, youth programming, or educational setting. For example, youth with chronic disease interface in all of those settings.

Continuing Education and Building a Better Practice

This work can only begin to enhance your skills in communicating with adolescents and their families. Communication skills are built over a lifetime of service, with each interaction offering a new challenge and opportunity for growth. If you do not occasionally struggle with issues around communication, then you are not human. The key to continued growth is practice, self-reflection, and safe and ongoing feedback. We believe that some of the best feedback can come from our colleagues who are invested in our ongoing growth as well as career longevity.

Each chapter will conclude with questions that will reinforce key concepts and allow for personal reflection. These questions will also be the vehicle through which you will earn your continuing education credits if you choose to receive them (see www.aap.org/reachingteens). Each chapter will also offer discussion questions in a section called "Group Learning and Discussion" so that you can work with your colleagues to dive deeper and consider how the lessons best apply to the youth you serve. Ideally, your group can use this for quality improvement within your practice.

Trust

As you consider adding new strategies to your communications repertoire, it is important to know that you will be trying them on for size and will likely have varying levels of success. Rest assured that even the adolescent medicine "experts" who offer their wisdom here also are not uniformly successful. No strategy works for all youth, which is why it is so helpful to have a variety of approaches from which you can draw. Please do trust, however, that when you use a strength-based approach, at the very least you are empowering teens to make good decisions, even if the outcomes are not clearly evident to you at the moment.

We all end our days sometimes wondering if we have made a difference. You do not always see the results of the seeds that you plant, but trust that when your guidance is given in a deeply respectful manner, it often takes root.

■ Related Video Content

1.0.1 Why Do We Focus so Heavily on Communication When We Consider Impacting on the Health and Well-being of Teens? Ginsburg.

1.0.2 The Second Decade of Life Impacts Health and Well-being Over the Life Span. Ford, Auerswald, Diaz, Jenkins.

1.1 Why Working With Teenagers Inspires Us. Catallozzi, Bell, Arrington-Sanders, Diaz, YouthBuild.

1.2 You Only Have to Be Yourself to Work With Youth. Ginsburg.

1.3 Mental, Emotional, and Physical Health and Education Are All Interrelated as We Consider the Conditions Needed for Youth to Thrive. Diaz.

12.6 Do Not Assume Poor Youth Are Destined to Have Poor Outcomes: Access to Services Strongly Influences Outcomes. Diaz.

14.1 Checking in on Yourself: What About Your Own Adolescence Might Flavor Your Interactions With Youth? Ginsburg.

18.2 How a Comprehensive Assessment Positions Us to Develop and Prioritize Interventions. Ford.

25.9 Behaviors Must Be Seen in the Context of the Lives Youth Have Needed to Navigate. Auerswald.

CHAPTER 2

The Journey From Risk-Focused Attention to Strength-Based Care*

Kenneth R. Ginsburg, MD, MS Ed, FAAP, FSAHM

 Related Video Content

2.0 The Journey From Risk-Focused Attention to Strength-Based Care

■ Why This Matters

Psychosocial and behavioral problems are the greatest contributors to adolescent morbidity and mortality. In fact, nearly 80% of mortality in adolescents aged 14 to 24 is related to behavior, driving home the importance of risk reduction and prevention efforts.[1] Consequently, a great deal of attention has been paid to targeted risk-based approaches to prevention. However, our goal for adolescent health must not be limited to the absence of risk or the reduction of mortality, it must include the cultivation of those strengths we know position young people to take their place as contributing members of society.[2-4]

> The strength-based and risk-based approaches must not be seen as competing paradigms. We must draw from the wisdom and experience of both schools of thought to create the strategies most likely to produce youth poised to become tomorrow's productive citizens.

Healthy youth development is most likely to be achieved when both risk factors (such as poverty, dysfunctional family life, toxic stress, and violence exposure) are low and protective factors (such as meaningful connections to adults, safe and adequately resourced schools, and ample community-based programming) are stably in place. In fact, a growing body of research has demonstrated that positive youth development (PYD) and resilience-based strategies designed to develop youth capabilities are also promising means to simultaneously reduce risky behaviors.[5-10]

Our challenge, therefore, is to address risks while building on existing strengths, and, when necessary, to generate opportunities for youth to develop new competencies.

■ Risk Versus Strength

The strength-based and risk-based approaches must not be seen as competing paradigms. We must draw from the wisdom and experience of both schools of thought to create the environmental milieu and communication strategies most likely to produce youth poised to become tomorrow's productive citizens.

---

*Parts of this chapter were previously published in Ginsburg KR, Carlson EC. Resilience in action: an evidence-informed, theoretically-driven approach to building strengths in an office-based setting. *Adolesc Med State Art Rev.* 2011;458–481, xi.

A Brief History: The Journey From Risk-Focused Attention to Strength-Based Care

Because behaviors explain a disproportionate amount of youth morbidity and mortality,[1] initial research efforts focused on uncovering risk factors that led to unhealthy and unsafe behaviors. It became clear that "risk factors" existed that increased the likelihood people would engage in destructive behaviors that limited their ability to make substantial contributions to society.[2] Health policy and programs were developed to target those risk factors, and generations of youth professionals were taught to attempt to mitigate those risk factors.

Over time it became equally as clear that not everyone who had been exposed to risk factors participated in destructive behaviors or "failed." Some became contributing, successful, healthy members of society despite exposure to the very same risks. In fact, it seemed that the challenges in their lives seemed to hone their passion and develop their empathy. The question of why some people "fail" and others are able to thrive despite challenges stirred a great deal of interest.[3,4]

Resilience research explored the "protective factors" that reduced the likelihood of negative outcomes and enhanced the likelihood of desired outcomes.[5-9] An easy temperament and high intelligence were protective, but supports and circumstances around children's lives also made a large difference in who overcame adversity. A repeated finding was that having a meaningful, trusted connection with at least one caring, competent adult was the core of resilience.[10,11] Ideally, that adult was a parent, but other adults could compensate if they served as role models in settings where parents were unavailable or ineffective. Other important sources of support were found in communities and schools.[12] Research also demonstrated that resilience was uneven; a person might be highly resilient in one area and vulnerable in another.[13] Further, the myth of the invulnerable child was dispelled, as there was a limit to how much exposure to adversity any person could be expected to handle even with ample supports.[14]

The emergence of clear protective factors held potential to transform our approach to risk. If we could learn to create and promote the protective factors in young people's lives, it might magnify the potential to change their life trajectories. However, the resilience framework was limited because it specifically explored how to work with youth that were inherently "at risk" by virtue of their exposure to adverse circumstances.

The PYD framework took the concept of protective factors a step further. It was interested in ALL youth and the consideration of what homes, schools, communities, and spiritual centers could do to contribute to healthy youth development. A popular mantra of PYD became Karen Pittman's call to action: "Problem-free *isn't* fully prepared. And fully prepared *isn't* fully engaged."[15] The goal was no longer only to help youth overcome adversity or avoid risks; it was for youth to thrive. Rick Little[16] and Richard Lerner and colleagues[17] developed a model that helped people conceptualize the ingredients a young person needed to be fully prepared: confidence, competence, character, connection, and contribution. The Search Institute,[18] in parallel, developed a model that described 40 essential assets young people needed to develop to their potential, and worked with communities to ensure those assets existed in their children. The Communities That Care model empowered communities to use evidence-informed and evidence-based interventions to support the development of healthy children and adolescents.[19]

Research continued to accumulate on the positive effects of PYD-based programming. Catalano and colleagues[20] conducted a literature review of successful PYD programs. Results indicated that PYD programs led to improvements in interpersonal relationships, where youth increased skills in empathy, caring, communication, and overall quality of relationships. Positive youth development programs also impacted youth self-efficacy by increasing their self-esteem, helping them achieve confidence and self-identity, and helping

A Personal Journey

I have been working with youth labeled "at risk" since I was 19 myself. The 2 groups I worked with, Native American youth in South Dakota and homeless youth on the streets of New York City, were navigating challenges that would have killed me. I was moved by their depth and inspired by their strength.

I began training in adolescent medicine in 1990 and was taught the power preventive care had when we assessed for risk and intervened before crises took hold. Two facts informed every interaction I had. First, nearly 80% of what killed kids was behaviorally related. Second, many teens who had killed themselves had seen a medical doctor in the very few weeks or days before they acted. I presumed they often presented with a hidden agenda, and never wanted to miss a covert plea for help. Armed with this information, I approached every visit prepared to uncover risk and then guide the youth away from tragedy. I would assess my patients for risk, give them key facts on what needed to change, invite them to take action, and refer them when appropriate to services.

In my gut, I felt that it wasn't good enough to hope that the youth I cared for would be risk-free. More importantly, no matter how warm or empathetic I tried to be, there was still a degree of shame in the room. How could there not be when the focus of our interactions centered on what the teen was doing wrong? I had warm relationships with my patients, and felt honored to be in their lives, but something didn't feel right about having as a goal that they would avoid risk.

Of course I wanted them to avoid risk, but I wanted them to thrive, to be prepared to take over our world.

I was inspired by some of the leaders in adolescent medicine who were asking us to look beyond risk factors and to instead build protective factors. (Specifically, I listened with rapt attention to the words and findings of Drs Karen Hein, Robert Blum, and Michael Resnick.) I began to explore the resilience and youth development movements for these protective factors and to consider how we could apply these strategies in our offices. A consistent finding was that "connection" is key to resilience: connection to parents, schools, community programs…maybe even to us.

The answer to creating connection that spoke to me came from the training I received years earlier at Covenant House. Central to our mission is to serve each youth with "absolute respect and unconditional love."

Love?!?! Love was not on any of my board exams.

I think love is about listening. Listening in a way that really hears the story in context and that looks for a person's inherent strengths as they navigate their world. Are they resilient? Respectful, despite being looked down upon by others? Full of compassion, despite having received little themselves?

When I asked kids who turned their lives around what worked, I was repeatedly told that the pivotal moment was when a youth worker made them understand they weren't trash. Love for me became about hearing people's stories and telling them back in a way they had never heard before. It was about taking demoralized youth and giving them the gift of realizing they were worthy of admiration.

I found that once I gave myself permission to see the best in youth and to visualize their risk in the context of understanding that each person does their best to play the hand he is dealt, my relationship with my patients became deeper, and far more fulfilling. More importantly, I was better positioned to engage them in a productive behavioral change process.

Now I find myself training others. When my students present a teen to me, their opening line has to be, "This is _____, and what I love about her is _____." Nontraditional, I know. But they have to do the work of sitting with another human being and seeing the best in her. Strength in the midst of adversity; resourcefulness in the midst of scarcity. Respect. This allows my trainees a different view, and combats the "otherness" that we use to separate ourselves from those we are meant to heal. It allows us to begin one of the most important conversations we can have with our trainees: how to love while maintaining boundaries.

It allows me to go and meet a whole human being instead of a problem.

them experience independence and self-control. Positive youth development programs were also found to foster development of cognitive competencies, such as abstract and reflective thinking, creativity, and problem-solving. Participation in programs gave youth a sense of purpose and oriented them toward success so that they maintained healthy goals and expectations and had hope for the future. This change in belief patterns resulted in higher academic aspirations, motivation, commitment to schooling, and increased academic achievement. Youth involved in PYD programs not only made improvements within themselves, they also increasingly contributed to and engaged with families, communities, and society.

One study particularly worthy of attention is Lerner and colleague's[21] 4-H study of PYD. It was a longitudinal study that sought to understand the processes involved in the emergence of PYD. It focused on understanding the developmental pathways of youth and identifying how the strengths and development of youth are enhanced by their contexts (eg, out-of-school programs). This study was the first to empirically verify the existence of the PYD constructs (ie, the "Five Cs" of competence, confidence, character, connection, and contribution). They also studied the impact of out-of-school time and youth development programs (ie, programs exemplified by the 4-H club) on resilience and PYD. Central to the 4-H philosophy is that caring, competent adults facilitate programming, but youth are central to the planning and implementation of programming. Simultaneously, they also looked at the reduction of risk and problem behaviors, including smoking, drinking, bullying, and depression. The results demonstrated that youth that participated in a PYD program had better grades, greater expectations to go to college, and higher self-esteem. Participants also had higher levels of civic engagement and contributed more to their communities. Finally, they were less likely to experience depression or engage in risk behaviors such as tobacco use, alcohol use, and bullying.[21]

A Healthy Environment Creates a Healthy Person

The link between developmental assets and health has become clear. Researchers from multiple disciplines, including psychology, sociology, nursing, public health, social work, and medicine, have demonstrated that enhancing positive factors reduce the likelihood youth will engage in a number of destructive behaviors and have better health and developmental outcomes.[22–24]

Youth in PYD programs have demonstrated a lower risk of having personal, social, and behavioral problems, including decreased substance use, violence, truancy, school and peer problems, high-risk sexual behavior, and smoking.[20,21,25]

A sentinel study using data from the National Longitudinal Study of Adolescent Health examined adolescent risk and protective factors for emotional health, violence, substance use, and sexual behaviors among adolescents from 7th through 12th grades.[26] It found that parent-family and school connections were protective for each of these behaviors, and follow-up studies subsequently found that various dimensions of connectedness protected youth from both genders and varied racial and ethnic backgrounds against a wide range of risk behaviors.[26]

■ Bringing Strength-Based Practice to Our Offices

Once those factors that contributed to resilience and healthy youth development were shown to be linked to health outcomes, the movement to apply these frameworks in health care settings gained momentum. For example, *Bright Futures: Guidelines for Health Supervision of Infants, Children, and Adolescents* calls for the use of strength-based approaches in the adolescent health supervision visit.[27]

Youth professionals that choose to incorporate a strength-based approach do not necessarily need to add a new component to their visits if they already address behavioral concerns, guide youth away from risk behaviors, and promote healthy development. Rather, the incorporation of these techniques offers a way to reframe and prioritize their guidance.[28,29]

The use of strength-based communication strategies allows us to elicit the teen's strengths, which in turn positions us to

1. Teach youth to recognize and capitalize on their strengths.
2. Make suggestions to boost strength areas that are lacking or deficient.
3. Engage youth in a discussion about needed behavior change.
4. Have structured discussions about behavior change (eg, motivational interviewing).[30]

When we use a strength-based approach with teens, we communicate that we expect them to engage in positive behaviors. Youth are portrayed in society, and too often treated, as risk takers engaging in bad behavior. This often distorted perception of youth impacts the way multiple systems view, react to, and act toward all adolescents. And, in turn, the way adults treat youth (ie, having low expectations of them) impacts the way youth behave. A strength-based approach allows us to convey high expectations even while addressing risk. It engages youth in a respectful change process that recognizes they remain the greatest experts on their lives.

The benefits of our using strength-based techniques in practice is not limited to our interactions with youth. As parents/caregivers witness a model of effective communication, they are taught to think about teens differently, and what they witness may be tried at home.

There are many proponents of applying the lessons and principles of the resilience and PYD movements to our offices. Currently, there is not yet a strong evidence base of how to do this effectively while being sensitive to practical time pressures. **This volume brings together adolescent medicine, nursing, and social work expertise as well as professionals from community-based agencies to consider how to assess for and mitigate risk while simultaneously working to build and reinforce protective factors in the lives of youth.** It brings together the existing evidence base with the wisdom and expertise of seasoned practitioners. Our teens ultimately deserve the rigorous outcomes research that will make it easier to "manualize" and disseminate practical strength-based approaches.

■ Advocating for Strength-Based Practices Beyond Our Offices

Reframing Adolescence

First, we should shine a light on the toxic messages youth endure. Adolescents in our society have been (wrongly) acculturated to view their developmental stage as universally a time of storm and stress. Youth receive messages that they are troublesome, even dangerous. Minority and other marginalized youth receive even higher doses of these caustic messages.

To begin to grasp why these messages can subvert positive development, it is helpful to understand adolescence from both the developmental perspective and from a vantage point rooted in resilience theory. Key to understanding adolescent development is knowing that the fundamental questions of adolescence are "Who am I?" and its corollary "Am I normal?" When the answers to these questions are "I am another person's fear" and "Normal kids are those who adults worry about," healthy development is undermined.

Resilience theory holds that "youth live up or down to our expectations of them," giving defeating messages of low expectations a high magnitude of importance.

Undermining messages are everywhere. Books abound that portray how crazy teens are, and popular media reinforces an image of teens as self-indulgent, risky, and even dangerous. Even exciting findings about the teen brain are sometimes presented in ways that suggest teens are all impulse and no control. Public health messages that hype teen sexuality, drug use, and violence present an overriding message: "Crisis in America!!!" This hyperbole may catch people's attention, but this mentality promotes a dangerous and inaccurate view of adolescence that harms youth. The more we allow these negative images to circulate, the more youth will do what it takes to match them; the more uncomfortable they will feel with themselves when they don't; and the greater difficulty they will have navigating peer relationships when they choose to do the right thing.

With the best of intentions, we want to illuminate the problems of youth: "Did you know that X% of teens have sex before the end of Grade Q?" "An alarming Y% of adolescents use drugs." "Over Z% of teens drop out before graduating high school." "Binge drinking is a growing problem on campuses; X% of freshman say they have blacked out after a night of drinking." "Parents, you'll want to hear the startling finding of a new study on teen sexuality, right after these messages...." Then the story airs: "Crisis in our community, 38% of teens _____." When the expert then asks, "Where are the parents?" and talks about "kids nowadays," youth learn that adolescents are supposed to frighten us.

Social marketing experts understand the power of the media in shaping self-perceptions and behaviors. Dr Jeff Linkenbach of Montana State University has created a vigorous response to popular messages about adolescents. With www.mostofus.org he strives to teach communities and policy makers that drive the self-perception of youth to transform how youth are portrayed.[31] The bottom line is that we have to make doing the right thing seem normative rather than odd. What if the binge drinking story said, "Although X% of college freshmen say they are drinking to dangerous levels on the weekends, the good news is that most teens are choosing better ways of spending their weekends." What if the story on school dropouts sounded more like this: "Clearly some kids are not able to be successful, and Z% are leaving. The good news is that most teens are working hard to keep their stake in the future." Imagine how much better youth who wanted to delay sexual activity would feel if stories on teen sexuality ran like this: "Despite the fact that popular shows focus on teens having sex, in a recent study, less than half of teens were choosing to have sex by Grade Q."

■ Putting It Together: Supporting Community-Based Youth Development Strategies

What Can We Do Within Our Communities?

- Notice the acts of generosity and compassion shown by youth and spread these good news stories. Don't notice only the heroic acts, but also the everyday acts; recognize kindness and contribution as the norm.
- Advocate for the positive portrayal of youth in the community. Ask for a shift away from media coverage where only the highest achievers and delinquents get airtime.
- Advocate for public health messages that don't just tell kids what not to do but fervently tell kids what to do; recognize that most youth are already doing the right thing.
- Advocate for enrichment programs in communities and schools, especially in those areas most at risk that currently only have prevention programs. This doesn't mean you should suggest the risk-based programs should be cut.

- Give youth opportunities to contribute to our communities. When they're out there serving others, their value will be noticed and they'll receive those vital reinforcing displays of gratitude.
- Work with parents so that young people have appropriate role models, rules, and boundaries that ensure safety. If these are seen as normal in your community, adolescents will have less reason to rebel.

We also have the credibility to advocate that the lessons of PYD and resilience inform how schools, programs, and communities interact with youth. There is a growing body of solid science about what strategies produce positive developmental outcomes for youth that can guide those who design and implement youth programming. We need only advocate that the science be applied and that intervention evaluations continue.

■ Core Principles of Positive Youth Development

- Young people will come to our programs or offices for the content offered, but what will determine whether their experience will shape their lives and prepare them to make meaningful societal contributions is the human context in which that programming is delivered: It is about the people, it is about us.
- The connection to a supportive, caring, and competent adult is the key to building resilience in youth. That adult needs to believe in the youth unconditionally while holding them to high expectations because youth live up or down to the expectations caring adults set.
- Unconditional belief does not imply a valueless acceptance of every choice. It is about accepting the youth as he is, rather than remaking him into an image you'd prefer. It is about communicating that you are not going anywhere; you can be counted on. Ideally, parents are the key adults in their children's lives. When parents are effective, other caring adults add extra layers of protection. When they are not, our roles take on critical importance.
- High expectations are not about grades or performance. They certainly can be about demonstrated effort, tenacity, "stretching," and thinking outside of the box. They must be about character, integrity, and honesty.

Then, that adult must interact with the young person in a way that will help them achieve mastery. The following core principles are worth considering as we strive to impact youth well-being in our offices and community programming:

- Young people need to feel valued. They need to know that they matter. When adults genuinely listen to their views and recognize that they are the experts on their own lives, youth learn to believe their opinions matter. In a program this means that youth should help to develop, evaluate, and improve the program. In our offices it means that they drive the agenda and determine their readiness to change.
- Youth are often the best teachers and role models of other youth. The more opportunities we give older youth to support younger people, the more they will know how much they matter. It is especially vital to allow teens to serve as models. Teens who know they are role models are more likely to behave in the manner we hope for.
- Adults can be both instructive and supportive from the sidelines, but teens should choose and carry out activities as independently as possible if they are to become more competent and confident. Nothing discourages their efforts to achieve mastery more than an adult who steps in and says, "Let me do that for you," when they can do it themselves. Failure is a great teacher when it feels emotionally and physically safe. Ideally, we put into place boundaries that ensure safety and then allow freedom to navigate within those boundaries.

- Ideally, healthy development is supported from early in infancy. When it is not, adolescents are still capable of healing and do so best when caring adults trust in their capacity to right themselves and offer appropriate support and guidance.
- Most of the adolescent behaviors that we fear (including substance use, self-mutilation, eating disorders, Internet addiction, and a host of other problems) serve as coping strategies that help youth manage uncomfortable stressors. If we help youth develop a repertoire of alternative coping strategies, we will diminish their need later to turn to these worrisome quick fixes. Youth watch our own behaviors closely and how we model adaptive strategies to stress matters.

If we apply these core principles to our daily interactions with youth, they will guide young people to build the competencies and confidence they need to become successful adults that are in control of their lives and capable of making wise decisions.

•• Group Learning and Discussion ••

We all want to mitigate risk. Many of us were trained in recognizing and briefly addressing problems. As a group, have a frank discussion on the limitations of this approach. How does it flavor our interactions? Our views of youth? Their views of us? Their belief in their potential to change? Then discuss how an approach that addresses risk but that builds on strength might create a different milieu in our offices.

Continuing Education

If you are applying for continuing education credits, a test is available online. For more details, visit www.aap.org/reachingteens.

◼ References

1. Centers for Disease Control and Prevention (CDC). Youth risk behavior surveillance—United States, 2009. *MMWR Morb Mortal Wkly Rep*. 2010;59(SS-5):1–142
2. Garmezy N. Vulnerability research and the issue of primary prevention. *Am J Orthopsychiatry*. 1971;41(1):101–116
3. Rutter M. Protective factors in children's responses to stress and disadvantage. In: Kent MW, Rolf JE, eds. *Social Competence in Children. Primary Prevention of Psychopathology*. Vol 3. Hanover, NH: University Press of New England; 1979:49–74
4. Masten AS, Wright MOD. Cumulative risk and protection models of child maltreatment. In: Rossman BBR, Rosenberg MS, eds. *Multiple Victimization of Children: Conceptual, Developmental, Research and Treatment Issues*. Binghamton, NY: Haworth Press; 1998:1–7
5. Masten AS. Resilience in individual development. Successful adaptation despite risk and adversity. In: Wang MC, Gordon EW, eds. *Educational Resilience in Inner-City America: Challenges and Prospects*. Mawah, NJ: Lawrence Erlbaum Associates, Inc; 1994:3–25
6. Fergus S, Zimmerman MA. Adolescent resilience: a framework for understanding healthy development in the face of risk. *Annu Rev Public Health*. 2005;26:399–419
7. Rutter M. Resilience: some conceptual considerations. *J Adolesc Health*. 1993;14:626–631, 690–696
8. Werner EE, Bierman JM, French FE. The children of Kauai: a longitudinal study from the prenatal period to age ten. Honolulu, HI: University of Hawaii Press; 1971
9. Donovan JE, Jessor R, Costa FM. Structure of health-enhancing behavior in adolescence: a latent variable approach. *J Health Soc Behav*. 1993;34(4):346–362
10. Resnick MD, Harris LJ, Blum RW. The impact of caring and connectedness on adolescent health and well-being. *J Pediatr Child Health*. 1993;29(suppl 1):S3–S9

11. Eccles JS, Early D, Fraser K, Belansky E, McCarthy K. The relation of connection, regulation, and support for autonomy to adolescents' functioning. *J Adolesc Res*. 1997;12:263–286

12. Sanders MG. The effects of school, family, and community support on the academic achievement of African American adolescents. *Urban Educ*. 1998;33:385–409

13. Luthar SS, Zigler E. Vulnerability and competence: a review of research on resilience in childhood. *Am J Orthopsychiatry*. 1991;61(1):6–22

14. Masten AS. Ordinary magic. Resilience processes in development. *Am Psychol*. 2001;56(3):227–238

15. Pittman KJ. *The power of engagement*. In: *Youth Today*. Washington, DC: The Forum for Youth Engagement; 1999. http://www.forumfyi.org. Accessed August 28, 2012

16. Little RR. What is working for today's youth: the issues, the programs, and the learnings. Paper presented at: The Institute for Children, Youth, and Families Fellows' Colloquium, Michigan State University; 1993; East Lansing, MI

17. Lerner RM, Lerner JV, Almerigi JB, et al. Positive youth development, participation in community youth development programs, and community contributions of fifth-grade adolescents: findings from the first wave of the 4-h study of positive youth development. *J Early Adolesc*. 2005;25(1):17–71

18. Search Institute. 40 Developmental Assets for Adolescents. http://www.search-institute.org/developmental-assets/lists. Accessed July 22, 2013

19. Hawkins JD, Catalano RF, Arthur MW, et al. Testing communities that care: the rationale, design and behavioral baseline equivalence of community youth development study. *Prev Sci*. 2008;9(3):178–190

20. Catalano RF, Hawkins JD, Berglund ML, Pollard JA, Arthur MW. Prevention science and positive youth development: competitive or cooperative frameworks? *J Adolesc Health*. 2002;31(suppl 6):230–239

21. Lerner RM, Lerner JV, Phelps E, et al. The positive development of youth technical report: the 4-H study of positive youth development: report of the findings from the first four waves of data collection: 2002–2003, 2003–2004, 2004–2005, and 2005–2006. Medford, MA: Institute for Applied Research, Tufts University; 2008. http://www.4-h.org/uploadedFiles/About_4-H/Research/4-H-study-of-positive-youth-development.pdf. Accessed July 22, 2013

22. Bernat DH, Resnick MD. Healthy youth development: science and strategies. *J Public Health Manag Pract*. 2006;(suppl):S10–S16

23. Kreipe RE. Adolescent health and youth development: turning social policy into public health practice. *J Public Health Manag Pract*. 2006;(suppl):S4–S6

24. Pittman KJ. What's health got to do with it? Health and youth development: connecting the dots. In: *Forum Focus*. 2005;3(2):1–4. http://www.forumfyi.org/files/ForumFocusHealth.pdf. Accessed July 22, 2013

25. Pittman KJ, O'Brien R, Kimball M. *Youth Development and Resiliency Research: Making Connections to Substance Abuse Prevention*. Washington, DC: Center for Youth Development and Policy Research; 1993

26. Resnick MD, Bearman PS, Blum RW, et al. Protecting adolescents from harm: findings from the national longitudinal study on adolescent health. *JAMA*. 1997;278(10):823–832

27. Hagan JF, Shaw JS, Duncan P, eds. *Bright Futures Guidelines for Health Supervision of Infants, Children, and Adolescents*. 3rd ed. Elk Grove Village, IL: American Academy of Pediatrics; 2008

28. Duncan PM, Garcia AC, Frankowski BL, et al. Inspiring healthy adolescent choices: a rationale for and guide to strength promotion in primary care. J Adolesc Health. 2007;41(6):525–535

29. Ozer EM, Adams SSH, Lustig JL, et al. Can it be done? Implementing adolescent clinical preventive services. *Health Serv Res*. 2001;36(6 pt 2):150–165

30. Frankowski BL, Leader IC, Duncan PM. Strength-based interviewing. *Adolesc Med State Art Rev*. 2009;20:22–40

31. Linkenbach J. Montana model of social norms. http://www.mostofus.org. Accessed July 22, 2013

■ Related Video Content

2.0 The Journey From Risk-Focused Attention to Strength-Based Care. Ginsburg.

■ Related Web Site

MOST of Us
www.mostofus.org

CHAPTER 3

How a Strength-Based Approach Affects Behavioral Change

Kenneth R. Ginsburg, MD, MS Ed, FAAP, FSAHM

 Related Video Content

3.0 How a Strength-Based Approach Supports Behavioral Change

■ Why This Matters

Adolescent health and well-being are largely determined by behaviors. In fact, nearly 80% of mortality is behaviorally related and a substantial amount of morbidity is associated with emotional health and behavioral decisions.

The impact of encouraging positive behavioral choices during adolescence reaches far beyond the teen years. Thinking patterns formed in adolescence may persist and affect adult emotional well-being. Many behaviors that deeply affect health (eg, cigarette use and other addictions, sexual habits) may begin in adolescence, and many health habits (eg, exercise, nutrition, appropriate sleep, relaxation strategies) that will heavily influence physical and emotional health begin in adolescence.

Our role in helping young people make and sustain healthy choices affects health far into the future.

The strength-based interviewing and assessment techniques suggested throughout much of this textbook are designed to support positive behavioral change by forging connections, building confidence, and fostering motivation. Similarly, some of the skills discussed, such as developing positive coping strategies or solving problems one step at a time, reinforce positive behavioral decisions.

> **Many habits and behaviors that will heavily influence lifelong physical and emotional health begin in adolescence. Therefore, the impact of encouraging positive behavioral choices during adolescence reaches far beyond the teen years.**

■ Stages of Behavioral Change

Behavioral changes are not usually "events," rather they are active or passive decisions made over time that can be supported or undermined by life circumstances, media, peers, family, and helping professionals.

The process of behavioral change is posited in many different theoretical frameworks, but Prochaska's transtheoretical model of behavioral change (TTM) is a helpful tool to conceptualize this process in adolescents.[1] The TTM suggests that individuals proceed through a series of stages as they attempt to change aspects of their lives, and it offers important insights into the factors that inhibit or promote positive change at each stage. The TTM predicts youth progress through the following stages of change:

1. Precontemplation (youth has no intention of changing or denies need for change)
2. Contemplation (youth is considering change and weighing perceived costs and benefits)
3. Preparation (youth is actively planning to change)
4. Action (youth is making an attempt to change)
5. Maintenance (youth is solidifying change and resisting relapse)

One of the key concepts within TTM is decisional balance. This involves a weighing of costs and benefits, or pros and cons of any behavior.[2] The relative weight of the pros and cons helps determine a person's readiness to move forward in the behavioral change process. If the perceived benefits (pros) of a behavior outweigh the perceived costs (cons), it may make no sense to a person to consider thinking about change (ie, she will not move beyond precontemplation). She moves toward contemplation when the decisional balance is more even, and is ready for action when the cons of the behavior are seen as outweighing the benefits. A person will likely only maintain a new behavior when the benefits of the new healthy behavior consistently outweigh the perceived benefits of the replaced behavior. One can assess an individual's progress through these stages not only by tracking behavior, but also by evaluating changes in confidence and in relative weighting of the costs and benefits of change.

A youth may be at a different stage of change for various behaviors. Interactions can be most effective if the stage of change is identified for the targeted behavior and appropriate information and support is offered to move the young person toward the next stage.[3] At the earlier stages, awareness of the causes and consequences of a behavior, or the perception of available alternatives, can influence an individual's progress.[4] But forward movement can be paralyzed by a person's belief that he is incapable or unworthy of change. Once a person has decided to move forward, it is critical that he has the skills to do so, because a motivated person who lacks skills will find frustration. Some of those skills should involve adaptive behaviors to replace the benefit of the old behaviors. Further, if a person is to maintain a behavior, support and reinforcement from others can be important, and the skills to resist pressure to return to destructive behaviors may be critical.

■ Adjusting Interaction Approach Based on Stage of Change

An assessment that includes an area to be addressed as well as a stage of behavioral change allows us to better hone our interactions.

- During *precontemplation*, the young person may be unaware of a problem altogether, not grasp the consequences of her behavior, or be demoralized about her ability to change. At this stage, it is important to both give information and build confidence if needed. It makes sense also to get an idea of what benefits and costs the adolescent sees in her current behavior.
- During *contemplation*, the young person is beginning to consider change and determining if the change is likely to be worthwhile. We may be most effective by helping the youth understand the benefits of alternative behaviors. It is also important to help her gain the confidence to believe that if she takes positive action, she will likely succeed. This may be an opportune time to begin introducing skills.
- During *preparation*, the young person is seriously considering taking action. It is particularly important here that she is equipped with appropriate skills. No matter the level of motivation, the change process will fail without the concrete skills (eg, getting condoms, knowing how to put them on) and negotiation skills (eg, dealing with partners who say condoms are not natural) a youth needs to be able to put her plans into operation.

- When an adolescent has decided to take *action,* it is particularly important that negative learned behaviors are replaced with positive ones. Because many behaviors have effectively reduced stress, the adolescent needs positive strategies that also ameliorate stress. Otherwise, the decisional balance will weigh in favor of the former behavior.
- If the teen has already tried out new behaviors and is trying hard to *maintain* those behaviors, it is important that positive reinforcement comes from parents, peers, and you. Without this reinforcement, the adolescent may relapse in response to negative influence or long-held low expectations or critical self-appraisal. Here might be the time to reassess pressures that may be destructive and reinforce the navigational skills that will allow her to continue forward movement.

■ Reaching Teens: Infused With Strength-Based Strategies Designed to Promote Positive Behavioral Change

Many strength-based techniques included throughout this work hold the potential to promote positive change. As you consider each technique suggested throughout this text, it may be helpful to consider how it could reinforce your ability to promote positive change. A few examples are offered here.

Strategies That Position You to Be an Agent of Change

- *Setting the Stage for Trustworthy Interactions:* This strategy builds the type of relationship where an adolescent and family consider a professional trustworthy enough to be an ally in the behavioral change process (see Chapter 14).
- *Understanding Youth Are Experts in Their Own Lives:* Our goal is to influence youth behavior, not to impose our views. Adolescence is a time where the developmental imperative is answering the question, "Who am I?" Therefore, having a sense of control over their decisions and views is essential. When they feel controlled they rebel. When we value the expertise they have, they may invite us into their lives. When we acknowledge that only they have the wisdom and experience to know how to navigate their own circumstances, they will be more likely to join with us to consider how to move forward (see Chapter 4).
- *Motivational Interviewing:* This method facilitates an adolescent to consider the pros and cons of a given behavior in order to develop discrepancy between her current behaviors and goals. The entire premise is to move adolescents toward positive behavioral change (see Chapter 26).
- *Eliciting and Reflecting Strengths:* This technique focuses on building a teen's confidence in his belief that he can change. It is particularly useful for teens who may be demoralized or who see themselves as powerless or unworthy to initiate change (see Chapter 25).
- *Circle of Courage:* This approach is another technique that elicits, reflects, and builds strengths while exploring 4 key youth assets: Mastery, Belonging, Independence, and Generosity (see Chapter 30).

Strategies That Offer Strength-Building Skills

- *Social Skills to Navigate Peer Culture:* If a youth has decided to choose positive behaviors and activities, but his peer group has not, his decisional balance will likely weigh against positive movement (ie, being good vs losing friends). If he is equipped with skills that allow him both to make healthy choices *and* successfully navigate peer culture, he is more likely to initially take action and maintain the positive behaviors, even in the face of pressure to revert to old behaviors (see Chapter 41).

- *Reinforcing Parental Strategies for Effective Discipline and Monitoring:* Young people become demoralized when they see no connection between their action and consequences. Youth who feel "controlled" learn that their choices don't matter. Parents who know how to appropriately discipline teach children that their behavior leads to consequences; good behavior leads to rewards and increasing freedoms and responsibility while poor behavior requires parents to tighten the reins out of concern for safety. Youth who understand that the choices they make matter may be more likely to choose their behaviors wisely (see Chapter 36).
- *Taking Control—One Step at a Time:* A young person can want to do the right thing but become demoralized as she considers how overwhelming the process of change may be. This will cost her the needed confidence to even contemplate change. If she is facilitated to break the process of change into smaller component parts, she may achieve a better sense of control over her choices (see Chapter 29).
- *Mindfulness:* Young people can become stuck in the stories of their past or paralyzed as they contemplate their future. This can prevent them from conserving the energy needed to take action in the present (see Chapter 32).
- *Positive Coping Strategies:* Because many worrisome behaviors reduce stress, a young person needs effective positive strategies that also lower stress. Otherwise, the social risks will continue to offer very real benefits that outweigh the costs. In primary prevention, youth develop a repertoire of activities and skill sets that serve as positive stress-reduction strategies. In secondary prevention, an adolescent already engaging in a negative behavior is guided to build positive coping strategies. A person with existing positive strategies may never "learn" the benefit of negative quick fixes. A person using negative behaviors for stress reduction may shift her decisional balance if positive behaviors consistently offer relief (see Chapter 31).

●● Group Learning and Discussion ●●

This chapter serves as a "landing page" for a variety of behavioral change strategies. Your group should have a general discussion on how to adjust interaction style based on stage of behavioral change. Then you should focus on one of the specific strategies to build your skills.

■■■■■■■■ Continuing Education ■■■■■■■■■

If you are applying for continuing education credits, a test is available online. For more details, visit www.aap.org/reachingteens.

■ References

1. Prochaska JO. Decision making in the transtheoretical model of behavior change. *Med Decis Making.* 2008;28(6):845–849
2. Velicer WF, Prochaska JO, Fava JL, Norman GJ, Redding CA. Smoking cessation and stress management: applications of the transtheoretical model of behavior change. *Homeost.* 1998;38:216–233
3. Prochaska JO, Velicer WF. The transtheoretical model of health behavior change. *Am J Health Promot.* 1997;12:38–48
4. Prochaska JO, DiClemente CC, Norcross JC. In search of how people change. Applications to addictive behaviors. *Am Psychol.* 1992;47(9):1102–1114

■ Related Video Content

3.0 How a Strength-Based Approach Supports Behavioral Change. Ginsburg.

1.0.2 The Second Decade of Life Impacts Health and Well-being Over the Life Span. Ford, Auerswald, Diaz, Jenkins.

CHAPTER 4

Who's the Expert? Terms of Engagement in Adolescent Care

Richard E. Kreipe, MD, FAAP, FSAHM, FAED

 Related Video Content

4.0.1 The Keys to Working With Teens: Respect, Listening, and Recognizing Their Expertise
4.0.2 Recognizing Youth as the Experts in Their Own Lives Is More Than Humble or Respectful, It Is a Good Strategy for Engagement and Promoting Positive Behavioral Change

■ Why This Matters

In 1904 G. Stanley Hall[1] coined the phrase "storm and stress" to capture what he considered 3 key elements of adolescent development: conflict with parents, mood disruptions, and risky behavior. This viewpoint dominated the view of adolescence for many adults. In 1959, focusing on identity development, Erikson[2] framed the primary task of adolescence in terms of confusion or diffusion of identity versus achieving a stable identity; leaving adolescence without a stable identity was posited to lead to isolation, rather than interpersonal connections, in adulthood.

> **Adolescents are the experts in their own lives. But adults have a role in providing support and guidance to the emerging young adult.**

The phrase "generation gap" embodied the cultural conflict of the 1960s and 1970s between adolescents and "the establishment." Flashpoints of conflict were an emerging "sexual revolution" and the use of illegal drugs, such as marijuana and hallucinogens, reflecting an emerging emphasis on counter-cultural individual freedoms (slogans included, "do your own thing" or "don't trust anyone over 30" or "make love not war"). However, large population studies of adolescent males by Offer[3] demonstrated that for most, adolescence was NOT a time of turmoil. Nevertheless, the approach to adolescents by adults throughout most of the 20th century was influenced by a negative view of adolescence and an emphasis on authoritarian harm avoidance and risk reduction.

Over the last 3 decades, a growing body of evidence underscores the benefit of adults developing partnerships with adolescents in a positive youth development approach that emphasizes adults honoring, respecting, and valuing each adolescent's emerging identity to increasingly support autonomy. This strength-based approach is linked both to a reduction in health risk behaviors and to an increase in health-promoting behaviors. As noted by Pittman, "problem-free is not fully prepared."[4]

Thus key outcomes of healthy adolescent development include the emergence of a youth who has an affirmative sense of self (character) by acquiring competence in a variety of domains through meaningful connections with peers and adults in which the adolescent makes meaningful contributions and gains confidence. In so doing a healthy youth gains skills in coping and control (mastery). In every aspect adolescents are the experts in their own lives. But, in every aspect, adults have a role in providing support and guidance to the emerging young adult.

■ Putting Principles Into Action

Three principles can be used to engage youth as their own "expert."

1. **Self-determination theory (SDT)** focuses on individuals becoming motivated to initiate health-related behaviors and maintain them over time. In SDT, developing a sense of *autonomy* and *competence* are considered critical to self-regulate and sustain behaviors through *internalization* and *integration*. Interactions with adults that support an adolescent's emerging sense of autonomy and confidence as change agents are key. A sense of *relatedness* to the professional is also crucial to internalization. Thus connecting with adolescents and gaining their trust increases the likelihood that they will respond to suggestions to change.[5]

2. **Nurturant-authoritative approach** emphasizes the importance of combining nurturance (with attention to support of the youth's emotional experience) and an authoritative stance (with the professional serving as an authoritative not authoritarian presence—expert in matters related to health and well-being) in which youth learn about their condition, have limits set, and are able to partner with adults. This balances subjective with objective, and affective with definitive attention to an adolescent's needs.

3. **Mindfulness** involves reflection and self-awareness by practitioners to examine their belief systems and values, deal with strong feelings, make difficult decisions, and resolve interpersonal conflict.[6] It requires critical informed curiosity ("beginner's mind"); openness to new ways of perceiving common presentations with the goal of delivering compassionate, informed care; committed to making correct decisions; understanding the patient; and relieving suffering.[6] Mindful practitioners tend to form "a tacit bond with the youth that transcends professional roles"[6] (see Chapter 32).

Each of these elements can empower an adolescent to function as her or his own expert in promoting and sustaining mental and physical health. In the next section, 3 different cases, each with an eating disorder, will illustrate the application of these in practice. A consistent health concern, anorexia nervosa, is chosen to focus emphasis on the 3 principles that engage youth to become their own "expert."

■ Case 1. Self-determination Theory and Autonomy Support: "You Just Don't Understand"

Michele is a 15-year-old cross-country runner brought to Dr Brown's office by her parents because of restrictive anorexia nervosa. They express a mixture of worry, frustration, anger and fear regarding her mounting resistance to their escalating requests, bargaining, and threats to remove her from the cross-country team. They want her physician to prescribe a high-calorie diet and to restrict her from compulsive exercise so that she gains weight.

1. Rather than respond to the parents' request, Dr Brown says to Michele, *"It sounds like there's been a lot of conflict at home about your eating and exercise. I'm interested in what you have to say about that."* (Michele needs to be the focus of attention, with authentic interest in her perspective, more than facts.)

2. Michele responds, *"What's to say? I'm fat...."* (Key issue: Michele is feeling fat.)

3. Her parents immediately interrupt to emphasize that she is not fat, but Dr Brown raises his hand to stop them. (Need to break patterns of parental behavior that do not support autonomy—even "dysfunctional" autonomy. Also demonstrates to Michele that Dr Brown is prepared to break down barriers to self-expression raised by others.)

4. Leaning in toward Michele to make direct eye contact with her, Dr Brown invites her to continue, *"You were saying that you feel fat. Tell me more about that feeling."* (Nonverbal cues to encourage Michele to open up and to demonstrate that she was being listened to at an emotional level. This emphasizes that she is the "expert" on her feelings.)

5. With downcast eyes and withdrawn body image and affect, Michele describes her "disgusting" body image, links it to her low self-esteem, and expresses a desire to lose weight both to feel better about herself and to become a faster runner. (Important potential points of connection between Dr Brown and Michele and motivators in treatment and recovery are being established.)

6. Dr Brown responds by saying, *"I hear that you feel fat and the only way to feel better about yourself is to lose weight. But you also feel like no one understands because all you hear your parents say is to eat more and to exercise less. You really want to make the cross-country team and the fastest girls on the team are all thinner than you."* (Nonjudgmental acceptance of Michele's subjective experience, emphasizing the "positive" reasons driving her behaviors that are viewed by others as "dysfunctional," but are actually very functional.)

7. Michelle responds, *"Way thinner. Our best runner is super-skinny. I wish I could be like her…."* (More evidence of linking losing weight with being a faster runner.)

8. Dr Brown continues, *"So, you believe if you would be allowed to lose more weight you would feel better about yourself AND be a better runner. But, you've already done such a good job of following your plan to lose weight and get faster that your parents and coaches are worried about your health. Sounds like you're stuck. Am I on the right track?"* (Acknowledges Michele's ambivalence and synthesizes the dilemma that she is facing. Tension with parents: "being allowed to." Acknowledgment that she has followed her plan: "done a good job." Adults are concerned about her: "parents and coaches are worried." Health is the major focus of the interaction.)

9. Michelle regains her composure, looks up for the first time, and says *"Yes. I don't like all the fighting, but I'm afraid that if I start to eat that I won't be able to stop and will get huge."* (Verbalizes the dilemma and demonstrates insight.)

10. When her parents say, *"Honey, you've got a long way to go before you get huge,"* Dr Brown turns away from Michelle and toward them and says *"For you to help Michelle, it will be important to listen very carefully to what she says about her feelings. If she says that she feels fat, she feels fat. If she says she is afraid of getting huge, she is afraid of getting huge. There is nothing rational about the feelings associated with an eating disorder. Feelings just are. Trying to reassure her by telling her that she has nothing to worry about when she expresses a worry is NOT reassuring. Listening to her worries—without judging them in any way—can actually help to lessen them. One parent told me, 'I finally realized that I have two ears and one mouth, so I need to listen twice as much as I talk.' Your job actually will get easier if you focus more on listening to what's happening for Michelle. You don't have to figure everything out. Michelle is smart, she doesn't like all the conflict, and she needs to be at the center of any treatment plan that's going to be successful."* (Directing comments to Michele's parents in her presence serves 2 purposes, it educates them about how to support autonomy and it demonstrates to Michelle that Dr Brown is interested in supporting her autonomy.)

11. Dr Brown then says to Michele, *"I'd like to help you and your family with this, but first I need to examine you to check your blood pressure, pulse, and temperature, and listen to your heart and figure out where your metabolism is. You say that you want to continue to run cross-country, but it would not be fair to you or your family or your team to keep running if you are not healthy. You say that you feel fat and I accept that because only you know how you feel. You're the expert about how you feel. But I'm the expert on health, so we need to work together."* (Emphasizes an understanding of the concerns

of the patient and parents and clarifies the role of the physician and the development of a partnership.)

■ Case 2. Nurturant-Authoritative Approach: "I Want to Get Taller and Stronger"

Sean is a 13-year-old whose father was placed on a very low-fat diet, lipid-lowering drugs, and aerobic exercise regimen after a heart attack. Sean's mother expressed concern that he had become a "health freak," eliminating snacks, eating only low-fat vegan foods, and following an "extreme" exercise video routine twice a day. With a body mass index (BMI) at the 90th percentile previously, over the last year neither Sean's height nor sexual maturity increased, and his weight decreased to a BMI at the 25th percentile. Sean wants to become a Navy Seal, does not want to get fat, and asks about medications to help him get taller and stronger.

Key points to discuss with him, alone, would include

1. Positive reinforcement for Sean paying attention to his health and reducing his BMI, which can be very difficult during puberty.

2. Need for a detailed food journal to determine the nutritional adequacy of Sean's intake. This would allow the health professional to support Sean's goal of being "healthy," but also provide opportunities to give specific feedback about ways in which the diet could improve. Although his BMI has decreased dramatically, neither his height nor his sexual maturation has increased, suggesting nutritional inadequacy.

3. Emphasis that although there are medications that help kids grow taller and stronger, they would not be indicated in his case because of his inadequate nutritional intake. Moreover, his failure to grow taller or mature sexually should be noted explicitly— although he is undoubtedly already aware—and linked to his diet and exercise. If Sean were to improve his intake of calories with a balanced meal plan, he would grow and mature, precluding any need for medications.

4. Focus on getting taller rather than gaining weight. Although getting taller and gaining weight are linked, paying attention to the former brings into play all of the elements of self-determination theory noted above. It also prepares Sean to accept a "sports nutrition approach," balancing intake and output. If the professional cannot provide authoritative information about how to ensure adequate intake without excessive exercise, then referral to a dietitian who has a physical fitness focus would be appropriate. Such referral would send a strong nurturant-authoritative message.

5. Although there may be evidence of an eating disorder, labeling Sean's condition as such would be of little value. He has already begun his journey to be an expert at controlling his body, but has overcompensated and is now at an unhealthy place at the other end of the spectrum. Nurturing all that he has done to reduce his BMI, while also providing factual information from an authoritative stance increases the likelihood Sean will settle somewhere between the 2 extremes.

■ Case 3. Mindfulness: "Healer, Know Thyself"

Traci is a 17-year-old with bulimia nervosa for 3 years, following a 2-year history of anorexia nervosa, and sexual abuse at age 13. She returns for a follow-up visit. Since developing bulimia nervosa, she has maintained a stable weight, but intermittently engages in self-injurious behaviors and high-risk sexual behaviors, smokes cigarettes, sometimes gets drunk at parties on weekends, and recently stopped taking her selective-serotonin reuptake inhibitor pills because "they weren't working." She also refuses to be in therapy because "I've had four different shrinks and none of them helped." As her pediatrician since childhood, you recognize a pattern of self-destructive behaviors that you find personally frustrating, have begun to believe that she is help-rejecting, and are considering referring her to an internist since she will turn 18 in 10 months.

In adolescent health care, much attention is paid to the adolescent patient, but relatively little to the professional providing the care. Mindfulness is both a discipline and attitude of the mind[6] that facilitates professionals supporting adolescents perceiving themselves as experts in their own lives. Adolescents often present significant counter-transference challenges to professionals; patients with chronic behavioral conditions can be especially frustrating. Traci has a 5-year history of an eating disorder, transforming from anorexia to bulimia nervosa after sexual abuse. She has a pattern of self-destructive and help-rejecting behaviors. Referral from pediatric to adult care is understandable but could also be perceived as rejecting.

Key points in Traci's care

1. Traci returns for follow-up, so her health professional is doing something right. The fact that the patient is not changing does not mean that nothing is happening during visits. A mindful professional who is self-aware could say to Traci, *"It's good to see you today. When I saw your name on the schedule today, I got to thinking about your case, and my sense is that you aren't making any progress toward recovery. Maybe the problem is that what I expect and what you expect are different. Or maybe you are making progress in ways that I am not aware of, and I'm just looking at the wrong outcomes."* This would demonstrate to the patient reflection and self-awareness.

2. When Traci reports repetitive self-destructive behaviors, the professional could focus on maintaining a "beginner's mind," attempting to listen to the patient's history as if it were the first time it was heard. A beginner's mind frees a professional from the bounds of past experiences and allows new perceptions to emerge. Being approached in such a manner may alter Traci's openness to see things differently.

3. When Traci discusses self-injurious behavior, curiosity would lead a mindful professional to not ask her why she engages in such behavior, but a more in-depth exploration of the experience itself: what she feels before, what she feels during, what she feels afterward, things that trigger and things that prevent the behaviors. This could lead to insight for the patient, understanding for the professional, and more compassionate care and mutuality (see Chapter 49).

•• Group Learning and Discussion ••

Group Reflection
1. How does our practice interact with adolescents? Do we deliver information lecture-style or do we allow them to come to their own conclusions? Do we tend to take an "I'm an adult and I know best" approach, or do we listen attentively to their views, recognizing that only they know what they are feeling and experiencing?
2. What might it mean to practice with a shared decision-making model?

Group Activity
Dr Kreipe offered examples of young people with disordered eating. As a group, consider picking another challenging issue (eg, sexual promiscuity, drugs, truancy) and consider how the 3 frameworks (mindfulness, self-determination theory, nurturant-authoritative approach) could help your practice serve teens.

▪▪▪▪▪▪▪ Continuing Education ▪▪▪▪▪▪▪

If you are applying for continuing education credits, a test is available online. For more details, visit www.aap.org/reachingteens.

▪ References

1. Hall GS. *Adolescence: Its Psychology and Its Relation to Physiology, Anthropology, Sociology, Sex, Crime, Religion, and Education.* Vols I & II. Englewood Cliffs, NJ: Prentice-Hall; 1904

2. Erikson EH. *Identity and the Life Cycle. Selected Papers.* New York, NY: International Universities Press; 1959

3. Offer D. *The Psychological World of the Teenager: A Study of Normal Adolescent Boys.* New York, NY: Basic Books; 1969

4. Pittman KJ, Martin S, Yohalem N. Youth development as a "big picture" public health strategy. *J Public Health Manag Pract.* 2006;(suppl):S23–S25

5. Williams GC. Improving patients' health through supporting the autonomy of patients and providers. In: Deci EL, Ryan RM, eds. Handbook of Self-Determination Research. Rochester, NY: University of Rochester Press; 2002:233–254

6. Epstein RM. Mindful practice. *JAMA.* 1999;282(9):833–839

▪ Related Video Content

4.0.1 The Keys to Working With Teens: Respect, Listening, and Recognizing Their Expertise. Kreipe.

4.0.2 Recognizing Youth as the Experts in Their Own Lives Is More Than Humble or Respectful, It Is a Good Strategy for Engagement and Promoting Positive Behavioral Change. Bell, Catallozzi, Auerswald, Ginsburg.

4.1 Listen to Us: We Understand Our Lives Best. Youth.

4.2 When We Are Out of Balance, We Try to "Fix" Rather Than Understand Youth. Singh.

4.3 Older Children and Adolescents Are Capable of Participating in Health Decisions. Peter.

26.2 Motivational Interviewing: Making Sure to Uncover the Teen's Perspective. Singh.

28.1 Teens Told What They "Should" Do Will Lose the Ability to Learn What They Can Do. Rich.

35.8 Listening: The Key to Guiding Your Child. Ginsburg.

CHAPTER 5

The 7 Cs Model of Resilience

Kenneth R. Ginsburg, MD, MS Ed, FAAP, FSAHM

 Related Video Content

5.0 Applied Resilience: The 7 Cs Model of Resilience

■ Why This Matters

The positive youth development (PYD) model is committed to building strengths or assets so youth are prepared to thrive. Resilience advocates are committed to helping youth overcome adversity. In order to best support youth to lead us into the future, we need strategic thinkers from multiple disciplines to work together to create the developmental milieu that will allow ALL children and teens to thrive through good and challenging times.

The 7 Cs model offers a common language across disciplines that could be an important step to breaking down silos as we work together to prepare our children and teens to thrive.

Currently there are several resilience paradigms and models of youth development that have great merit. However, if we could use a common language across our disciplines, it would be an important step to breaking down our silos. The 7 Cs model is relatively simple and incorporates the key elements of youth development, resilience, and even effective parenting.

■ History of the Cs

Rick Little and colleagues[1] proposed the initial 4 Cs: competence, confidence, (positive social) connection, and character as theoretical latent constructs. Eccles and Gootman,[2] among others,[3,4] reviewed evidence from research and practice that stress using 5 Cs (also including contribution) and furthered our understanding of the development of these constructs and the goals and outcomes of community-based programs aimed at enhancing youth development. Lerner and colleagues[5] were the first to confirm the existence of the 5 Cs through the 4-H study. They found that young people who display attributes of PYD also display the original 4 Cs and made impressive contributions (the 5th C) to themselves, their families, communities, and society. Pittman and colleagues,[6] through The Forum for Youth Investment, linked and synthesized the research on development, resilience, competence, prevention, and engagement. They promote broadening the field's definition of positive youth outcomes to include the 5 Cs of confidence, character, connection, competence, and contribution. Two more Cs, coping and control, have been added here because they are particularly key for youth displaying resilience.[7,8]

The resilience movement is tightly linked to and largely overlaps with the PYD philosophically, but it focuses on the importance of recovery from and overcoming adversity.[9] Although coping is usually included as a part of competence-building in PYD programs, it is highlighted in the 7 Cs model as one of the best ways of reducing risks and of overcoming adversity. Positive coping strategies allow youth to manage stress without turning to risk behaviors, which often serve as quick and easy, but dangerous, fixes. Finally, one of the keys to a person's willingness to enter the positive behavioral change process is to have self-efficacy (the belief in one's ability and skills to tackle a problem). The final C, control, includes self-efficacy because people with control understand that the actions they take can determine, or at least alter, their destiny. Control also allows 2 other principles associated with positive outcomes to be included in the model: delayed gratification and locus of control. People with an internal locus of control believe that what happens is related to their choices and behaviors; those with an external locus of control view themselves as being controlled by outside forces.[10–13]

■ The 7 Cs

Confidence: Confidence is earned through demonstrated and reinforced competence. Every child and adolescent is *already* doing something right. It is our job to help youth recognize what they are doing right so they can begin to trust in their capabilities. This will enhance their sense of self-worth and self-efficacy.[14,15] Confidence may be an important starting point for positive behavior because a young person who lacks confidence may be demoralized and can't imagine taking the steps necessary to make wise decisions. Adults can help youth gain confidence by noticing, eliciting, and reflecting on their existing strengths. Noticing the strengths of youth is especially important because one of the central themes of the PYD framework is that children live up or down to adults' expectations.[16] In fact, parents' and teachers' expectations of youth have been shown to relate to their academic performance.[17]

Competence: Competence is about possessing the skills that will prepare someone to succeed in school, in a future vocation, and within a family. Youth also need to possess peer negotiation skills to safely navigate their world and coping skills to avoid risks and recover from stressors. It is the role of adults both to model and develop skills in youth as well as to notice, reinforce, and build on existing competencies. Conversely, adults can undermine a young person's sense of competence when they view a youth as inherently a problem, or try to "fix" a situation rather than guide a young person to find his own solutions. A sense of competence is earned through experience and helps create the important self-perception that one can set and achieve goals.

Connection: A meaningful connection with adults is one of the core protective factors and the one most tightly linked to resilience.[18] Young people will be resilient if the important adults in their lives believe in them unconditionally and hold them to high expectations. Connections with family, school, community, and culture, are key as youth need multiple layers of connection to thrive. Social reinforcement from peers, family, school, and the community impact behavior.[19] Connection is impacted by changing family dynamics, and is also affected by the increased independence and autonomy experienced during adolescence.

Character: Character is about having an understanding of behavioral norms, recognizing the perspective of others, and grasping how your behavior impacts other people, as well as having moral standards and self-awareness. Youth develop character intrinsically and through observation of others. Parents, other adults, and a young person's best friends all act as role models and impact the positive, responsible behavior of youth. In the end, it is character that ensures one's "assets" will be used for the greater good. Children who have a good sense of themselves, respect for others, and an appreciation for the bigger world around them are on their way to becoming stable, responsible adults. Character traits such as self-regulation and tenacity are also associated with success.

Contribution: Youth who possess the protective traits associated with confidence, competence, connection, and character are poised to make contributions to themselves, their families, communities, and society.[20] When we ask youth to offer their input into programs and policies that affect them, we value and reinforce their contribution. Those who experience the personal rewards of service tend to feel better about themselves and may be more comfortable asking for help in time of personal need because they will have learned that those who give do so not out of obligation or pity, but because they gain something themselves. Contribution offers the opportunity to learn valuable leadership skills and gain a sense of purpose and accomplishment. Youth who contribute will be surrounded by appreciation, rather than condemnation or low expectation, and will want to continue to earn gratitude. Youth benefit when they learn that people expect the best from them.

Coping: Children who learn to cope effectively with stress are better prepared to overcome life's challenges. The best protection against unsafe, worrisome behaviors may be to possess a wide repertoire of positive, adaptive coping strategies. In primary prevention, we create opportunities for children and families to develop positive coping strategies and teach them coping skills they can employ when most challenged. In secondary prevention, we work with people already engaged in worrisome behaviors and invite them to consider replacing those behaviors with others that will also reduce stress, but will do so safely and productively. Adults, especially parents, need to model appropriate coping strategies because children are watching them very closely.

Control: Control (or self-efficacy) is about believing in one's own ability to avoid risky behaviors in the face of temptation.[21] Having a sense of control over one's environment leads to having the capacity to act independently and is related to a sense of purpose/future. Discipline should teach that one's actions lead directly to outcomes (ie, demonstrated responsibility is rewarded with increasing trust and privileges). Parents who make all of their children's decisions deny them opportunities to learn self-discipline and self-responsibility. Parents can teach and model self-control and impart the importance of delayed gratification. Youth who live in unsafe environments or who have met with repeated failures lose a sense of control, begin to believe they do not have the ability to impact on their destiny, and may become demoralized.

The 7 Cs model offers an overview of the assets and circumstances, and supports a young person needs for optimal development and for resilience. It is a comprehensive model created by advocates and researchers from multiple disciplines. It is not designed as a model for clinicians to follow precisely in an office setting; rather, we support a teen's overall resilience and positive development through specific interactions that also support positive behaviors.

■ The 7 Cs Are Infused Throughout *Reaching Teens*

The PYD and resilience frameworks inform *Reaching Teens*. Specific examples in which the 7 Cs model is incorporated into this work are included below. The examples are meant to be illustrative rather than comprehensive.

Confidence is one of the keys to moving a young person from precontemplation to contemplation. *Reaching Teens* covers how to recognize and build on someone's existing strengths in an effort to build confidence (see Chapter 25).

Teaching young people skills supports their **competence.** Care is taken not to undermine competence by communicating with youth in ways that allow them to set the agenda and reach their own conclusions (see chapters 26 and 28).

Character is reinforced when we notice what adolescents are doing well and suggest they have contributions to make to their family, school, and community environments.

Connection is promoted when we support family bonding, school engagement, and healthy relationships with peers. By focusing on building supportive and trustworthy relationships, we thereby enhance our own connection with youth (see Section 3). Meta-analyses suggest that it is the therapist and not the treatment per se that is most responsible for therapeutic progress.[22] Although not all youth-serving professionals are therapists, we are engaging youth in behavioral change processes and our connection with them is key to their progress.

Adolescents' sense of **control** is enhanced when we help them learn to solve problems they had previously felt they could not handle (see Chapter 29). It is furthered when we support parents to implement appropriate discipline and monitoring strategies (see Chapter 36).

Coping and stress management may be the key skill set needed if one is to avoid risk behaviors and recover from adversity (see chapters 31 and 32).

We appreciate adolescents' **contribution** when we value them as experts on themselves (see Chapter 4).

●● Group Learning and Discussion ●●

Download the "Are We Building Resilience in the Youth We Serve?" handout, read the reflective questions, and create an agenda to address those areas that may require further development in your practice setting. It may be that the first step is to flag those areas that may require further development, and then set a priority list of which areas are most urgent to address.

Discuss as a group whether different disciplines in your setting use different terminology to describe goals when working with youth. Consider whether a shared language would better facilitate care in your setting. If your group response is affirmative, then consider whether the 7 Cs of resilience could meet your needs.

For a deeper dive into how the 7 Cs can fold into a practice, read and discuss Dr Susan Sugerman's chapter, "Integrating the 7 Cs of Resilience Into Your Clinical Practice" (see Chapter 17).

■■■■■■■■ Continuing Education ■■■■■■■■

If you are applying for continuing education credits, a test is available online. For more details, visit www.aap.org/reachingteens.

■ References

1. Little RR. What is working for today's youth: the issues, the programs, and the learnings. Paper presented at: The Institute for Children, Youth, and Families Fellows' Colloquium, Michigan State University; East Lansing, MI; 1993
2. Eccles JS, Gootman JA. *Community Programs to Promote Youth Development*. Washington, DC: National Academy Press; 2002
3. Roth JL, Brooks-Gunn J. Youth development programs: risk, prevention and policy. *J Adolesc Health*. 2003;32:170–182
4. Lerner RM. *Liberty: Thriving and Civic Engagement Among American Youth*. Thousand Oaks, CA: Sage Publications; 2004
5. Lerner RM, Lerner JV, Almerigi JB, et al. Positive youth development, participation in community youth development programs, and community contributions of fifth-grade adolescents: findings from the first wave of the 4-H study of positive youth development. *J Early Adolesc*. 2005;25(1):17–71

6. Pittman KJ, Irby M, Tolman J, Yohalem N, Ferber T. *Preventing Problems, Promoting Development, Encouraging Engagement: Competing Priorities or Inseparable Goals?* Washington, DC: The Forum for Youth Investment, Impact Strategies, Inc; 2003

7. Ginsburg KR, Jablow MM. *Building Resilience in Children and Teens: Giving Kids Roots and Wings*. 2nd ed. Elk Grove Village, IL: American Academy of Pediatrics; 2011

8. Lemmon K. Recognizing and responding to child and adolescent stress: the critical role of the pediatrician. *Pediatr Ann*. 2007;36(4):225–231

9. Masten AS. Resilience in individual development. Successful adaptation despite risk and adversity. In: Wang MC, Gordon EW, eds. *Educational Resilience in Inner-City America: Challenges and Prospects*. Hillsdale, NJ: Erlbaum; 1994:3–25

10. Shoda Y, Mischel W, Peake PK. Predicting adolescent cognitive and self-regulatory competencies from preschool delay of gratification: identifying diagnostic conditions. *Dev Psychol*. 1990;26(6):978–986

11. Rotter JB. *Social Learning and Clinical Psychology*. Englewood Cliffs, NJ: Prentice-Hall; 1954

12. Rotter JB. Generalized expectancies of internal versus external control of reinforcements. *Psychol Monogr*. 1966;80(1):1–28

13. Lefcourt HM. Internal versus external control of reinforcement: a review. *Psychol Bull*. 1966;65(4):206–220

14. Bandura A. *Social Foundations of Thought and Action*. Englewood Cliffs, NJ: Prentice Hall; 1986

15. Bandura A. Perceived self-efficacy in cognitive development and functioning. *Educ Psychol*. 1993;28(2):117–148

16. Pittman KG, Martin S, Yohalem N. Youth development as a 'big picture' strategy. *J Public Health Manage Pract*. 2006;(suppl):S2–S25

17. Mistry RS, White ES, Benner AD, Huynh VW. A longitudinal study of the simultaneous influence of mothers' and teachers' educational expectations on low-income youth's academic achievement. *J Youth Adol*. 2009;38:826–838

18. Resnick MD, Bearman PS, Blum RW, et al. Protecting adolescents from harm: findings from the national longitudinal study on adolescent health. *JAMA*. 1997;278:823–832

19. Akers RL, Krohn MD, Lanza-Kaduce L, Radosevich M. Social learning and deviant behavior: a specific test of a general theory. *Am Sociol Rev*. 1979;44:636–655

20. Lerner RM, Lerner JV, Phelps E, et al. The positive development of youth technical report: the 4-H study of positive youth development: report of the findings from the first four waves of data collection: 2002–2003, 2003–2004, 2004–2005, and 2005–2006. Medford, MA: Institute for Applied Research, Tufts University; 2008 http://www.4-h.org/uploadedFiles/About_4-H/Research/4-H-study-of-positive-youth-development.pdf. Accessed July 22, 2013

21. Bandura A. Self-efficacy: toward a unifying theory of behavioral change, *Psychol Rev*. 1977;84(2):191–215

22. Wampold BE. The psychotherapist. In: Norcross JC, Beutler LE, Levant RF, eds. *Evidence-Based Practices in Mental Health: Debate and Dialogue on the Fundamental Questions*. Washington, DC: American Psychological Association; 2006:200–208

■ Related Video Content

5.0 Applied Resilience: The 7 Cs Model of Resilience. Ginsburg.

5.1 Building Resilience in Your Child: The 7 Cs Model of Resilience. Ginsburg.

5.2 A Brief Presentation of the 7 Cs Model of Resilience. Ginsburg.

12.10 "Trust? What's the Point?...I Guess It's That People Kept Pushing." Adolescent-Friendly Services Never Give Up on Youth. Youth.

25.1 Covenant House Staff Share How Recognizing Strengths Positions Them to Support Progress. Covenant House PA.

25.2 YouthBuild Staff Share How Recognizing Strengths Positions Them to Support Progress. YouthBuild Philadelphia.

25.3 Young People Speak of the Power of Being Viewed Through a Strength-Based Lens and the Harm of Low Expectation. Youth.

39.2 Modeling Resilience for Your Children: Defining and Defending Your Priorities. Sugerman.

48.4 Because We Need to Learn How to Recover From Failure, Adolescence Needs to Be a Safe Time to Make Mistakes. Ginsburg.

61.20 Youth Testimony: "This Is How to Address Me" (and Much More): Guidance From a Young Transgender Person. Youth.

66.15 Testimony From a Young Woman With a History of Unstable Housing: My Path Toward Becoming a Youth Advocate. Youth.

66.16 Testimony From a Young Man With a History of Unstable Housing: "Pain Is Like a Teacher"—Recovery and Resilience. Youth.

Also see Chapter 17, "Integrating the 7 Cs of Resilience Into Your Clinical Practice," for a series of videos in which Dr Susan Sugerman discusses how resilience principles are incorporated into her adolescent practice.

■ Related Handouts/Supplementary Materials

Building the 7 Cs of Resilience in Your Child (parent handout)
Are We Building Resilience in the Youth We Serve? (handout for youth-serving agencies and practices)

CHAPTER 6

The Impact of Trauma on Development and Well-being

Sandra L. Bloom, MD

 Related Video Content

Refer to Chapter 22 for related video content.

■ Why This Matters

If we are committed to *Reaching Teens* using a strength-based approach that builds resilience, we must be equally as committed to understanding risk factors and the environmental and social forces that drive so much risk. Toxic stress and trauma are key underlying factors that explain much of the behavior we hope to address in order to prepare young people to thrive.

> **The magnitude of young people's exposure to overwhelming stress is so great and such a threat to national well-being that the issue must be addressed as a major public health threat.**

The numbers of youth exposed to overwhelming events during critical developmental periods is astonishingly high and requires us to take a public health approach that focuses on addressing the problems of the young people who have already been affected by traumatic events, building in resiliency skills for those already at risk, and educating everyone.[1]

The American Academy of Pediatrics (AAP) published a sentinel article in 2012 crafted by Jack P. Shonkoff, MD; Andrew S. Garner, MD, PhD; and the AAP Committee on Psychosocial Aspects of Child and Family Health, the AAP Committee on Early Childhood, Adoption, and Dependent Care, and the AAP Section on Developmental and Behavioral Pediatrics that elucidated "The Lifelong Effects of Early Childhood Adversity and Toxic Stress."[2,3] It called for action to prevent the experiences in children's lives that expose them to toxic levels of stress and steps to mitigate their consequences. Most importantly, it recognized that youth-serving professionals had a key role in addressing this issue.

This chapter is written as an orientation to the toll trauma takes on its victims. Chapter 22 will go one step further by discussing trauma-informed practice. It is worth noting, however, that much of *Reaching Teens* is trauma informed, as it is steeped in recognizing youth as experts in their own lives and recognizes that we are obligated to take the respectful steps needed to earn their trust and avoid instilling further shame or triggering reactions that are rooted in a trauma history.

■ A Word About Vocabulary

Currently, we have a problem with the English language in that there is no word that encompasses the topic of severe stress in childhood. The word "trauma" is being used as a shorthand term for far more complex phenomena. The best way to think about the broader concept is that there is a stress continuum, more like the continuum that we understand goes from excellent health to terminal illness, with no absolute points of demarcation and, until death, the possibility of moving back and forth on that continuum. Movement along that continuum is determined by many different factors, such as the state of preexisting health, the age of the person, the nature of the disease process, and a multitude of socio-cultural factors.

Similarly, in the last few decades we have learned a great deal about the continuum of stress moving from positive stress to tolerable stress, toxic stress, and traumatic stress. Stress and health interact in complex ways so that, taken together, exposure to stress can be seen as a vast public health problem, particularly when too much stress is experienced in childhood.

Positive stress produces short-lived physiological responses that promote growth and change and are necessary for healthy development. Going to school for the first time, taking tests, performing a new activity, preparing for a big game, applying for college, going off to college—all of these and many other stressors experienced by children and young people can be stressful but are challenges that promote the young person's abilities to deal with a changing world.

Tolerable stress occurs as the result of a more severe, longer-lasting difficulty, such as the loss of a loved one, a natural disaster, or a frightening injury. The stress is serious enough to activate the body's stress-management system, but if the activation is time-limited and sufficient social support buffers the young person's central nervous system, the brain and other organs recover without long-term negative effects.

Toxic stress, on the other hand, is associated with prolonged and intense activation of the body's stress response to such an extent that it can change the very architecture of a young person's brain with problematic long-term consequences. Many factors determine the ways in which toxic stress affects a developing child—the nature of the stressor, the age of the child, the level of preexisting health and mental health, the family situation, the number and extent of protective factors that exist within the child and the child's environment. Because human children are dependent on adult care for such an extended period, any experience of disrupted attachment can increase the likelihood that the child will experience toxic stress (Figure 6.1). Toxic stress exposure is being used as a way of

---

FIGURE 6.1
EFFECTS OF TOXIC STRESS ON BRAIN DEVELOPMENT IN EARLY CHILDHOOD

Impairs connection of brain circuits and in extreme cases, results in smaller brain development.

May cause development of low threshold for stress, resulting in overreactivity (chronic hyperarousal).

High levels of stress hormones, including cortisol, can suppress body's immune response.

Sustained high levels of cortisol can damage the hippocampus, responsible for learning and memory. Cognitive deficits can continue into adulthood.

Verbal abuse from parents and from peers has been shown to interfere with development of gray matter and white matter.

understanding the profound effects of situations, such as child physical abuse, sexual abuse, neglect, witnessing domestic violence, and being exposed to community violence, particularly when these events are repetitive, even chronic.[1,2]

Traumatic stress occurs when a person experiences or witnesses an event that is overwhelming, usually life-threatening, terrifying, or horrifying in the face of helplessness. As with toxic stress exposure, the effects of traumatic stressors will be multi-determined and therefore are highly individual. The young person's preexisting vulnerability, the nature of the stressor, the child's immediate reactions to the event or events, and what happened after the event or events may play a contributing role in determining the complex outcomes that we witness in practice (Figure 6.2). Traumatic events that may be experienced directly by young people include, but are not limited to, violent personal assault (sexual assault, physical attack, robbery, mugging), being kidnapped, being taken hostage, terrorist attacks, torture, incarceration, natural or human-made disasters, severe automobile crashes, or being diagnosed with a life-threatening illness. For children, sexually traumatic events may include developmentally inappropriate sexual experiences regardless of whether there was threatened or actual violence or injury. Witnessed events include, but are not limited to, observing the serious injury or unnatural death of another person due to violent assault, accident, war, or disaster or unexpectedly witnessing a dead body or body parts. Events experienced by others that are learned about include, but are not limited to, violent personal assault, serious accident, or serious injury experienced by a family member or a close friend; learning about the sudden, unexpected death of a family member or a close friend; or learning that an attachment figure has a life-threatening disease.

FIGURE 6.2
COMPLEX OUTCOMES OF TRAUMATIC STRESS

Hyperarousal	Second injury
Memory problems	Loss of social support
Deficits information processing	Avoidance
Survivor guilt	Shattered meaning
Intrusions	Attitude change
Emotional dysregulation	Reenactment
Developmental interference	Maladaptive coping

Allostatic load is the term being used to describe the wear-and-tear on the body and brain resulting from forces such as poverty, bigotry, chronic hunger, and lowered socioeconomic status. All can have a profound effect on development and later health outcomes secondary to the constant stress on the child and on his or her caregivers, even in the absence of perceivable traumatic events.[4,5]

In families with multiple problems, toxic stress, traumatic stress, and allostatic load may interact in a complex manner, potentially creating a wide range of problems for the young people in the family.

■ How Big a Problem Is This?

The magnitude of young people's exposure to overwhelming stress is so great and such a threat to national well-being that the issue must be addressed as a major public health threat.

Adverse Childhood Experiences: A Public Health Nightmare

Adversity can be defined as a state, condition, or instance of serious or continued difficulty. It implies that the person who experiences adversity is under conditions of chronic stress, but individuals vary greatly in their response to adversity. Children often experience adverse experiences, sometimes over many years, and this exposure can have very detrimental effects on the body, mind, and spirit. However, the capacity to bounce back from adversity, also known as resilience, often is a response to adverse childhood experiences.

Nonetheless, one sobering illustration of the enormity of the problem posed by exposure to toxic stress comes from the Adverse Childhood Experiences (ACE) Study done by Kaiser Permanente and the Centers for Disease Control and Prevention.[6] The purpose of the study was to examine the impact of exposure to toxic levels of stress across the life span. So far, this is the largest study of its kind to examine the long-term health and social effects of adverse childhood experiences. The researchers asked 18,000 willing participants—all members of the Kaiser HMO in San Diego—if they would take a survey. Most of the participants were white, 50 years of age or older, and well educated, representing a solidly white, middle-class population.

An adversity score or ACE score was calculated by simply adding up the number of categories of exposure to a variety of childhood adversities that the person had experienced before the age of 18. These categories included severe physical or emotional abuse; contact sexual abuse; severe emotional or physical neglect; living as a child with a household member who was mentally ill, imprisoned, or a substance abuser or living with a mother who was being victimized by domestic violence; or parental separation/divorce (Figure 6.3). So, for example, you could interview a young woman and find out that she was sexually abused by an uncle, her parents were divorced, her mother was hospitalized for depression, and her father drank heavily and used drugs. Her ACE score would be at least 4—score 1 point each for sexual abuse, parental divorce, mental illness in her mother, and substance abuse in her father. Or a young man tells you that his father spent time in prison when he was growing up, his mother was a drug addict and neglected him, and his stepfather beat him. His ACE score would be 5—score 1 point for living with someone as a child who was in prison, another for his mother's drug addiction, 1 each for emotional and physical neglect, and 1 for physical abuse.

FIGURE 6.3 ACES CATEGORIES	
ABUSE	**HOUSEHOLD**
• **Physical abuse**	• **Mental illness**
• **Sexual abuse**	• **Substance abuse**
• **Emotional abuse**	• **Domestic violence**
• **Physical neglect**	• **Parental separation/divorce**
• **Emotional neglect**	• **Incarceration**
I POINT/CATEGORY—ADD TO GET TOTAL ACE SCORE	

Returning to the original ACE Study of this largely white, middle-class, older population, almost two-thirds had an ACE score of 1 or more, while 1 in 5 was exposed to 3 or more categories of adverse childhood experience. Two-thirds of the women in the study reported at least one childhood experience involving abuse, violence, or family strife. The researchers compared the ACE score to each person's medical, mental health, and social health data and found startling and disturbing associations. The higher the ACE score, the more likely a person was to suffer from one of the following: smoking, chronic obstructive pulmonary disease, hepatitis, heart disease, fractures, diabetes, obesity, alcoholism, intravenous drug use, depression and attempted suicide, teen pregnancy, sexually transmitted infections, poor occupational health, and poor job performance. Worse yet, the higher the ACE score, the more likely people were to have a number of these conditions interacting with each other. In other words, the higher the ACE score, the greater the impact on a person's physical, emotional, and social health.

According to the study findings, if you are a woman and have adverse childhood experiences, your likelihood of being a victim of domestic violence and rape steadily increases as the ACE score rises; if you are a man, your risk of being a domestic violence perpetrator also rises. The study showed that adverse childhood experiences are surprisingly common, although typically concealed and unrecognized, and that adverse childhood experiences still have a profound effect 50 years later, although now transformed from psychosocial experience into organic disease, social malfunction, and mental illness.

Other Exposure to Violence Among Children

A replication of the ACE Study—one that would take into account, for example, the other kinds of exposure that inner-city children have, in addition to the existing categories of adversity—is badly needed, but has not yet been attempted. We do know, however, that many children who live in conditions of urban poverty are exposed to dreadful experiences. A 1998 study of 349 low-income black urban children (aged 9–15) revealed that those who witnessed or were victims of violence showed symptoms of post-traumatic stress disorder (PTSD) similar to those of soldiers coming back from war.[7] The Justice Department recently supported the most comprehensive nationwide survey to date of the incidence and prevalence of children's exposure to violence.[8] The findings are extremely disturbing, confirming that most of our society's children are exposed to violence in their daily lives (>60% in the past year). Nearly half of the children and adolescents had been assaulted at least once in the past year. We have not even begun to address the long-term public health effects of this kind of violence exposure, nor have we dealt with the fact that in less than 20 years, the number of children with incarcerated parents has increased by 80%.[9] We have not yet begun to reckon with the fact that, as of 2001, 1 in 6 black males had been incarcerated, and that, if current trends continue, 1 in 3 black males born today can expect to spend time in prison during his lifetime.[10]

■ Psychophysiological Pathways to Problems

Exposure to toxic and traumatic stress often has long-term consequences for young people because of the many ways in which overwhelming stress interferes with healthy function, even while the physiological responses to these very events are intended to promote human survival. We do not have space here to fully explain the nature of the stress response, so we will summarize the key concepts.

Prolonged Dependency and Attachment Needs

Immature human beings are helpless for a longer period of their lives than any other species. This dependency has necessitated an extensive attachment system between adults and offspring that results in devastating deficiencies whenever the young person fails to receive this kind of protection. This reality poses a particular problem for modern family organization simply because in the past there was a much higher caregiver-to-child ratio than exists today. Because of the nature of our society, children have far fewer opportunities to bond with reliable and available adults. This shortcoming becomes a more pervasive problem in adolescence when the desire to separate from primary caregivers is developmentally natural but the only available relational substitutes are peers.

Fight–Flight–Freeze

The basic internal physiological protective mechanism, present in all mammals, is called the fight–flight–freeze response.[11] This is not a planned, deliberately thought out reaction, but a rapid-fire, automatic, total body response. When we perceive that we are in danger, our bodies make a heroic and rapid response. Numerous neurotransmitters and hormones produce massive changes in every organ system. The brain sends instantaneous signals to the adrenal glands to secrete epinephrine or, as it is also called, adrenaline. At the same time, the brain releases a kindred substance, norepinephrine, which affects only the brain itself. Likewise, increased amounts of steroids flood into the bloodstream, as well as opioid substances that are pain relievers.

In the fight or flight part of the response, heart rate, blood pressure, and respiratory rate increase along with alertness and vigilance. Simultaneously a decrease occurs in feeding, reproductive activity, and immune response. This radical adjustment is in the service of survival, preparing us to make an immediate response to the dangerous situation. When this reaction is a response to a real danger, is time-limited, and is effective, it is lifesaving and highly adaptive. Problems arise only when this reaction is evoked in the absence of any threat, when the threat is prolonged, or when the organism can do nothing to protect itself from the threat. Then, the chemicals related to this response keep pumping out, negatively affecting our bodies and brains.

If there is no chance for survival if we try to run or fight, we may automatically freeze. The freeze response activates a very different sequence of autonomic nervous system arousal, slowing the heart rate, causing us to fall over and thus preserve blood flow, and even simulate death so that a predator loses interest.[12]

Chronic Hyperarousal

The stress response is lifesaving in a true emergency. But, under conditions of chronic stress, something goes wrong as the body attempts to cope with a chronic overload of physiological responses. The effectiveness of the response diminishes, and the body becomes desensitized to some of the effects of the neurohormones and hypersensitive to others. The entire system can become dysregulated in many different ways. This results in a set of highly dysfunctional and maladaptive brain activities. The person experiences this as a state of chronic hyperarousal. Essentially, the baseline level of arousal for the person has changed and they cannot control their own responses to stimuli.

We all have a "volume control" over our level of arousal. If we are in a lecture hall and hear a noise at the back, we cease paying attention to the speaker and swivel our heads to appraise the source of the noise. Once we are assured that the noise was just a latecomer and that there is nothing to fear, our level of arousal rapidly returns to normal and we are able once again to attend to the lecturer. Our reaction is quite different if we hear a sound, turn our heads, and see a man with a gun heading toward the front of the room. In this case we become hyperaroused. This is a clear and present danger, and the fight–flight–freeze response is triggered within each of us.

Young people who have been severely or repeatedly traumatized may lose this capacity to modulate their level of arousal. Their reaction to the benign latecomer is quite similar to their reaction to the threatening stranger. They stay hyperaroused and guarded; they are unable to calm themselves down even when they see that there is no danger. They feel embarrassed by their response, while at the same time they are irritable, angry, and frightened for no apparent reason. They are prepared to fight or flee, even though there is no danger. They may also become flooded with memories, images, and sensations that are overwhelming. As a result, they are likely to feel they are "going crazy."

This reaction can be triggered by almost anything. Once we have experienced a stimulus that evokes fear, we become "fear-conditioned," a state that is incredibly powerful and difficult for the logical centers of the brain to override.[13] Because of the vast associational network of our brains, we can pair fear with virtually anything. This happens at the time of the frightening event, beyond conscious control, and very quickly. Later the person is usually not consciously aware of the connection between the fear-provoking stimulus, and the fear response has become completely automatic.

Each episode of danger connects to every other episode of danger in our minds, so that the more danger we are exposed to, the more sensitive we become to danger. With each fight-or-flight experience, our mind forms a network of connections that is triggered by every subsequent threatening experience or stimulus. Because we are so intelligent, these connections can be very widely linked to any stimulus that is paired with the dangerous experience.

Alcohol, drugs, sexual activity, violent acting out, risk-taking behavior, eating excessively, inducing vomiting, purposely hurting the body, exercising, over-involvement in work—all of these behaviors can temporarily produce some relief from this highly unpleasant state of hyperarousal. The problem, of course, is that the relief is only temporary. After withdrawal from alcohol or other drugs, or other behaviors, the agitation rebounds with even greater ferocity. All of these behaviors can become habitual, even addictive, in such a situation.[14] In this way, coping skills that were initially highly adaptive become maladaptive habits (see Chapter 31). Pair chronic hyperarousal with the failure to integrate all information during a traumatic experience and it becomes easy to understand otherwise perplexing symptoms.

■ Failure of Integration

The hallmark characteristic of a healthy adult brain is integration of multiple complex functions. It takes at least 22 years for the human brain to achieve the wondrous network of associations that typifies healthy human maturity. Under normal conditions, the brain is constantly integrating the elements of every component of experience—behavior, emotions, sensations, and knowledge. As healthy adults, that integration occurs seamlessly and unnoticeably. In the immature human, the brain is still establishing the neural connections that will ultimately allow that seamless integration. Throughout that long developmental period, the brain is particularly vulnerable to the effects of stress because of the powerful chemical action of the stress hormones, particularly epinephrine, cortisol, and the beta-endorphins.

Under extreme stress, the brain stops properly integrating the components of experience. The psychophysiological mechanism that describes this loss of integration is called *dissociation.* Dissociation appears to be a central part of many traumatic experiences and is viewed by some as a state—a special type of consciousness that we all have access to under normal and traumatic conditions—and by others as a trait, that is, a characteristic quality or property of an individual that may be heritable. There is still debate in the field about exactly what dissociation is and how important it is in understanding PTSD. However, like the stress continuum, dissociation falls along a continuum that goes from normal dissociation (as seen in daydreaming) to acute dissociation (commonly referred to as shock) to a wide variety of problematic and more maladaptive forms of pathological dissociation.[15,16] As an acutely adaptive state, dissociation prevents a vulnerable and frightened human being from literally dying of fright. But in the longer term, the loss of integration creates significant and complicated problems.

The failure to fully integrate all the aspects of experience at the time of an overwhelming event helps to explain the multiplicity of symptoms that may occur afterward. The failure to integrate one or more sensations that were occurring at the time of the event can result in a wide variety of sensory intrusive experiences known as flashbacks. These commonly are experienced in the form of haunting images, voices, or even hallucinations involving sense of smell. Often missed are the flashbacks that are lodged in the bodily experience of the event or events, commonly known as body memories. Many persistent and repetitive physical symptoms actually represent unintegrated body experiences that occurred during the overwhelming event. Dissociated emotions are very common, resulting in impaired emotional regulation, emotional numbing, and inappropriate emotional responses, particularly when reminded of something traumatic from the past. Dissociated knowledge is evident in the many forms of amnesia that accompany trauma. Dissociated behavioral sequences are recognizable when a trauma survivor compulsively repeats behavioral sequences from the past that lead to *traumatic reenactments.*

Complicating this further are the cognitive impairments that accompany high levels of arousal, most particularly the "speechless terror" that characterizes moments of exquisite fear. During these times, the brain becomes incapable of properly encoding experience in words, leaving the victim with a void that has been called the "black hole of trauma"[17], and thus disabling the person from speaking about, or even thinking about, the worse aspects of an experience.

After a traumatic event, most people experience *acute stress,* and if they come to medical attention may be diagnosed with *acute stress disorder*, which by definition must occur within 4 weeks of the traumatic event and be resolved within that 4-week period. Calling this a disorder may be a bit of a stretch, since so many people experience this after an overwhelming event.

According to the *Diagnostic and Statistical Manual of Mental Disorders, Fifth Edition (DSM-5)*, published by the American Psychiatric Association (APA) and regarded as the standard for diagnoses, if acute stress-related symptoms persist for longer than a month, then a person is suffering from PTSD. If so, the person has experienced or witnessed a traumatic event; is suffering from intrusive re-experiences, such as nightmares and flashbacks; actively avoids encountering reminders of the traumatic event; and experiences symptoms of increased physiological arousal.[18]

Complex PTSD or *developmental trauma disorder* as of this writing are not yet officially considered diagnoses as defined by the APA. Nonetheless, people working in this field believe it is necessary to understand the very complex changes in a person's body, mind, identity, personality, relationships with others, ability to differentiate right from wrong, and meaning-making that may be the result of exposure to toxic stress and disrupted attachment beginning in childhood, or to chronic, severe interpersonal violence that occurs at any age.[19]

■ The Good News: Parents and Other Adults Can Be Protective

We may not be able to prevent every bad occurrence that happens to young people, but the good news is that a relationship with one adult in a child's life may make all the difference in whether or not he or she ends up following a positive life trajectory. The basis of this may turn out to be related to yet another biological adaptation recognized in primates and humans, particularly among females, called "tend and befriend" and sometimes called "appeasement."[20] This happens when someone addresses a threat from another person by offering them something they might want or that would therefore change the emotional dynamic away from immediate danger, while allowing the threatening other to remain in control of the situation.

Research suggests that, by virtue of differential parental investment, female stress responses have selectively evolved to maximize the survival of self and offspring. As a result, females are more likely to respond to stress by nurturing offspring, exhibiting behaviors that protect them from harm and reducing neuroendocrine responses that may compromise the health of their offspring (the tending pattern), and by befriending (affiliating) with social groups to reduce risk. Researchers of social animals and humans hypothesize that females create, maintain, and use social groups, especially relations with other females, to manage stressful conditions and that these attachment processes chemically counteract the negative impact of the stress hormones.

The well-being of our children depends on many more adults—inside and outside of the family—adopting the strategy of "tend and befriend," especially with young people facing the most adversity. Any of us can make a difference in a young person's life. Central to the notion of positive stress is the availability of a caring and responsive adult who helps the child cope with the stressor, thereby providing a protective effect that facilitates the return of the stress response systems back to baseline status. When buffered by an environment of stable and supportive relationships, positive stress responses are a growth-promoting element of normal development.

Thus the essential characteristic that makes this form of stress response tolerable is the extent to which protective adult relationships facilitate the child's adaptive coping and a sense of control, thereby reducing the physiological stress response and promoting a return to baseline status.

■ Pulling It Together: What Might Trauma Look Like in Our Young Patients or Clients?

The presentation of trauma and our response as caring adults who serve youth will be covered more thoroughly in Chapter 22 on trauma-informed practice. Here we wish to briefly establish how a state of hypervigilance or dissociation needed for survival might look in a teen we serve.

- It may be harder to forge a trusting relationship, because the young person has not experienced adults as consistently safe.
- Parents and teachers may describe the youth as easily upset, easily provoked, or highly reactive.
- The youth may display what others consider to be inappropriate emotions and behavior.
- The young person may be triggered by traumatic reminders in the environment, and the emotional responses may be occurring during an altered state during which the youth experiences flashbacks.
- The youth may be diagnosed as hyperactive or oppositional defiant.
- The teen may appear inattentive as he is focused on internal stimuli or hyperattentive to "danger signals" of which adults are not aware.

- A common post-traumatic presentation is dissociation. This may be reported as "lying," which represents a confabulated reality produced to replace actual events that are too difficult to recall, or "zoning out," which represents a behavior that has proven to be adaptive during unimaginable moments.

Recognizing these presentations allows us to better serve without judgment and to approach youth with the mindset of "what happened to you?" rather than "what is wrong with you?" It allows us to see resilience where others may view ineptitude, an oppositional personality, or brokenness.

●● Group Learning and Discussion ●●

This chapter provides the basis of understanding on how stress affects physiology and behavior. Chapter 22 on trauma-informed practice offers strategies to better assess and serve traumatized youth. Consider reading these chapters together and having your group participate in the group learning and discussion exercises suggested in Chapter 22.

▬▬▬▬▬▬ Continuing Education ▬▬▬▬▬▬

If you are applying for continuing education credits, a test is available online. For more details, visit www.aap.org/reachingteens.

■ References

1. Bloom SL, Farragher B. *Restoring Sanctuary: A New Operating System for Trauma-Informed Systems of Care*. New York, NY: Oxford University Press; 2013

2. Shonkoff JP, Garner AS; American Academy of Pediatrics Committee on Psychosocial Aspects of Child and Family Health, Committee on Early Childhood, Adoption and Dependent Care, Section on Developmental and Behavioral Pediatrics. The lifelong effects of early childhood adversity and toxic stress. *Pediatrics*. 2012;129:e232–e246. http://pediatrics.aappublications.org/content/129/1/e232.full

3. Garner AS, Shonkoff JP; American Academy of Pediatrics Committee on Psychosocial Aspects of Child and Family Health, Committee on Early Childhood, Adoption and Dependent Care, Section on Developmental and Behavioral Pediatrics, et al. Early childhood adversity, toxic stress, and the role of the pediatrician: translating developmental science into lifelong health. *Pediatrics*. 2012;129:e224–e231. http://pediatrics.aappublications.org/content/129/1/e224.full

4. McEwen BS, Gianaros PJ. Central role of the brain in stress and adaptation: links to socioeconomic status, health, and disease. *Ann N Y Acad Sci*. 2010;1186:190–222

5. Marmot M. *The Status Syndrome: How Social Standing Affects Our Health and Longevity*. New York, NY: Holt; 2004

6. Felitti VJ, Anda RF. The relationship of adverse childhood experiences to adult medical disease, psychiatric disorders, and sexual behavior: implications for healthcare. In: *The Impact of Early Life Trauma on Health and Disease: The Hidden Epidemic*. Lanius R, Vermetten E, Pain C, eds. New York, NY: Cambridge University Press; 2010:77–87

7. Li X, Howard D, Stanton B, Rachuba L, Cross S. Distress symptoms among urban African American children and adolescents: a psychometric evaluation of the Checklist of Children's Distress Symptoms. *Arch Pediatr Adolesc Med*. 1998;152:569–577

8. Finkelhor D, Turner H, Ormrod R, Hamby S, Kracke K. Children's exposure to violence: a comprehensive national survey. *Juv Justice Bull*. 2009; October. http://www.ncjrs.gov/pdffiles1/ojjdp/227744.pdf. Accessed July 22, 2013

9. Glaze LE, Maruschak LM. Parents in prison and their minor children. *Bur Justice Stat Spec Rep*. 2008;NCJ 222984. http://bjs.ojp.usdoj.gov/content/pub/pdf/pptmc.pdf. Accessed July 22, 2013

10. Mauer M, King RS. *Uneven Justice: State Rates of Incarceration By Race and Ethnicity.* Washington, DC: The Sentencing Project; 2007. http://www.sentencingproject.org/doc/publications/rd_stateratesofincbyraceandethnicity.pdf. Accessed July 22, 2013

11. Cannon WB. *The Wisdom of the Body, Second Edition.* New York, NY: W.W. Simon; 1939

12. Levine P. *Waking the Tiger: Healing Trauma: The Innate Capacity to Transform Overwhelming Experiences.* New York, NY: North Atlantic Books; 1997

13. LeDoux JE. Emotion as memory: anatomical systems underlying indelible neural traces. In: *The Handbook of Emotion and Memory: Research and Theory.* Christianson SA, ed. New York, NY: The Guilford Press; 1992:269–288

14. van der Kolk BA, Greenberg M. The psychobiology of the trauma response: hyperarousal, constriction, and addiction to traumatic reexposure. In: *Psychological Trauma.* van der Kolk, ed. Washington, DC: American Psychiatric Press; 1987:63–88

15. van der Kolk BA. The body keeps the score: approaches to the psychobiology of posttraumatic stress disorder. In: *Traumatic Stress: The Effects of Overwhelming Experience on Mind, Body and Society.* van der Kolk BA, McFarlane AC, Weisaeth L, eds. New York, NY: The Guilford Press; 1996:214–241

16. van der Kolk BA. The complexity of adaptation to trauma self-regulation, stimulus discrimination, and characterological development. In: *Traumatic Stress: The Effects of Overwhelming Experience on Mind, Body and Society.* van der Kolk BC, McFarlane AC, Weisaeth L, eds. New York, NY: The Guilford Press; 1996:182–213

17. Pitman RK, Orr SP. The black hole of trauma. *Biol Psychiatry.* 1990;27(5):469–471

18. American Psychiatric Association. *Diagnostic and Statistical Manual of Mental Disorders.* 5th ed. Arlington, VA: American Psychiatric Association; 2013

19. Ford JD, Courtois CA. *Treating Complex Traumatic Stress Disorders in Children and Adolescents: An Evidence-Based Guide.* New York, NY: The Guilford Press; 2013

20. Taylor SE, Klein LC, Lewis BP, Gruenewald TL, Gurung RAR, Updegraff JA. Biobehavioral responses to stress in females: tend-and-befriend, not fight-or-flight. *Psychol Rev.* 2000;107:441–29

■ Related Video Content

See Chapter 22.

CHAPTER 7

Wisdom From Model Strength-Based Programs That Work With Youth Who Are Traditionally Labeled "At Risk"

Kenneth R. Ginsburg, MD, MS Ed, FAAP, FSAHM

 Related Video Content

7.0 "What Works": Collective Wisdom From 3 Model Strength-Based Programs

Reaching Teens is, at its core, a work designed to prepare you to apply the principles of positive youth development (PYD) and resilience theory in your interactions with adolescents and their families. It is intended to enhance your ability to use strength-based communication strategies to engage youth and their families in a shared decision-making process that will support their positive behaviors.

These core principles and strength-based communications are also central features of many youth programs. These youth programs stand in sharp contrast to those that approach youth as problems to be solved, or as discipline cases to be controlled. Both might enroll youth labeled "at risk," but the experience of those youth may be quite different depending on program philosophy.

Youth who make it despite exposure to adversity are those who have had at least one adult who cares about (loves) them unconditionally and holds them to high expectations. That adult is ideally a parent. When it is, then extra adults, such as program staff, are additive. When a parent is unable to fill that role, then other adults, such as professionals and program staff, are critically important.

Strength-based programs understand that although youth might come for content, (eg, tutoring, basketball, education, shelter), what makes a difference in whether or not the program will help them to thrive is the style with which they interact with adults. A healing environment is created when the staff is committed to making youth feel cared about. It is largely about relationships—connections. As we consider whether a program will provide a healing and growth-oriented context, we return to those 2 most basic principles of resilience. First, youth who make it despite exposure to adversity are those who have had at least one adult who cares about (loves) them unconditionally and holds them to high expectations (see Chapter 5). That adult is ideally a parent. When it is, then extra adults, such as program staff, are additive. When a parent is unable to fill that role, then other adults, such as professionals and program staff, are critically important. Second, youth live up or down to the expectations we set for them. These expectations are about effort and character; youth note whether or not we expect them to be problems.

All programs that serve youth likely adhere to the philosophy they believe will lead to the best outcomes, although their targeted outcomes might be different. Is the goal to keep them away from trouble, or to prepare them for good citizenship? To avoid risk, or to lead us into the future? It is a reasonable goal for a program that serves youth repeatedly labeled as "at risk" to keep them away from that risk. However, there are some programs that serve very similar youth who hold different expectations.

There are many resilience-based or youth development programs that build youth for leadership, as defined as being contributing members of society. One program that has been particularly well studied is 4-H. Dr Richard Lerner and colleagues[1] empirically verified the existence of the PYD constructs (ie, the 5 Cs of competence, confidence, character, connection, and contribution) by closely following the program and outcomes at 4-H. They also demonstrated that youth that participated in 4-H had better grades, greater expectations to go to college, and higher self-esteem. Participants also had higher levels of civic engagement and contributed more to their communities. Finally, they were less likely to experience depression or engage in risk behaviors such as tobacco use, alcohol use, and bullying.

Here, we wish to introduce you to 3 model programs in Philadelphia. Covenant House Pennsylvania serves marginalized and homeless and trafficked youth. It offers a wide range of services from street outreach to shelter to medical services.[*] El Centro de Estudiantes is a school that serves youth who have failed traditional classrooms and have generally been discipline problems. Many have been told they would never succeed in school. They found El Centro through word of mouth. Youthbuild Philadelphia is a 1-year program that serves youth who did not finish high school, but who wish to return to complete their education. All youth in these 3 programs would be labeled "at risk" by any measure. All 3 programs have in common a deep commitment to relationships—connection—as being the key ingredient that will engage youth and potentially turn them around.

The interview team traveled to these 3 sites with the intent of collecting input for the general work to ensure that both professional and youth wisdom and experience were included to represent the most marginalized populations. Open-ended questions (eg, "What works or doesn't work here?") were asked as a lead-in to a series of questions designed to supplement various chapters. However, the views from the staff who serve these youth and testimony from these young people about "what works" deserve to be seen in their entirety.

■■■■■■■■ Continuing Education ■■■■■■■■■

If you are applying for continuing education credits, a test is available online. For more details, visit www.aap.org/reachingteens.

---

*Dr Ginsburg is health services director at Covenant House, Philadelphia, PA.

■ Reference

1. Lerner RM, Lerner JV, Almerigi JB, et al. Positive youth development, participation in community youth development programs, and community contributions of fifth grade adolescents: findings from the first wave of the 4-H study of positive youth development. *J Early Adolesc*. 2005;25(1):17–71

■ Related Video Content

7.0 "What Works": Collective Wisdom From 3 Model Strength-Based Programs. YouthBuild Philadelphia, Covenant House PA, El Centro de Estudiantes.

7.1 Staff From Covenant House PA. Covenant House PA.

7.2 Staff From YouthBuild Philadelphia. YouthBuild Philadelphia.

7.3 Youth Advisors (Teachers) From El Centro de Estudiantes. El Centro de Estudiantes.

7.4 Resilience Specialists From El Centro de Estudiantes. El Centro de Estudiantes.

7.5 Testimony From the Executive Director of YouthBuild Philadelphia. Sidhu.

7.6 Testimony From the Executive Director of El Centro de Estudiantes. Bromley.

12.10 "Trust? What's the Point?...I Guess It's That People Kept Pushing." Adolescent-Friendly Services Never Give Up on Youth. Youth.

12.11 "Its About the People Who Are Here"—The Central Element of an Adolescent-Friendly Space. Sidhu.

16.2 It Is Good That We All Have Different Styles, But We Have to Uniformly Communicate That We Expect the Best and Know Youth Can Succeed. Sidhu.

20.3 Professionals Offer Healing "Love," But for Youth Who Have Been Mistreated or Let Down, It Is Only Safe With Clear Boundaries. Hill, McAndrews.

22.0 Trauma-Informed Practice: Working With Youth Who Have Suffered Adverse Experiences. El Centro staff, Covenant House staff.

23.0 De-escalation and Crisis Management: Wisdom and Strategies From Professionals Who Serve Youth Who Often Act Out Their Frustrations. Youth-serving agencies.

25.1 Covenant House Staff Share How Recognizing Strengths Positions Them to Support Progress. Covenant House PA.

25.2 YouthBuild Staff Share How Recognizing Strengths Positions Them to Support Progress. YouthBuild Philadelphia.

66.4 Testimony From the Executive Director of Covenant House PA. Hill.

66.6 Passing the Test: Earning the Trust of Homeless and Marginalized Youth. Bailer, Covenant House PA staff.

66.7 Homeless and Marginalized Youth: Young People Who Have Been Tested by Life Bring so Much to the World. Covenant House PA staff.

66.8 Staff Diversity: Creating a Safe Environment Where ALL Youth Feel Safe. Covenant House PA staff.

66.9 What Does Success Look Like When We Work With Homeless and Marginalized Youth? Auerswald, Covenant House PA staff.

66.10 Facilitating Homeless and Marginalized Youth to Believe in Their Potential to Achieve Success. Covenant House PA staff.

66.11 Never Make Promises to Homeless and Marginalized Youth That You Cannot Keep. Hill.

66.12 Homeless Teens: Boundaries, Rules, and High Expectations Can Be Welcomed by Underparented Youth. Hill, Covenant House PA staff.

66.13 The Importance of Understanding Boundaries (and Your Own Buttons) When Working With Marginalized Youth. Hill.

66.14 The Truth May Unfold Slowly for Youth With a History of Adults Failing Them. Hill.

Understanding Adolescents and Their World

Adolescence is a time of tremendous growth and change. To effectively work with teens, it is important to understand both adolescent development and the environmental and emotional contexts teens navigate. "Adolescent Development—Stages, Statuses, and Stereotypes" (Chapter 8) offers a whirlwind tour of the literature on the social, cognitive, emotional, and moral development of youth, but focuses on those points that affect our ability to effectively interact with youth. "The Adolescent World" (Chapter 9) offers a glimpse into the multiple environmental contexts with which they interact and drives home the hard work involved in forging an identity. Female and male sexuality (chapters 10 and 11) offer a deeper dive into the key developmental adolescent task of developing a healthy sexuality. The sexuality chapters simultaneously address avoiding perilous risk behaviors sometimes associated with sexual awakening.

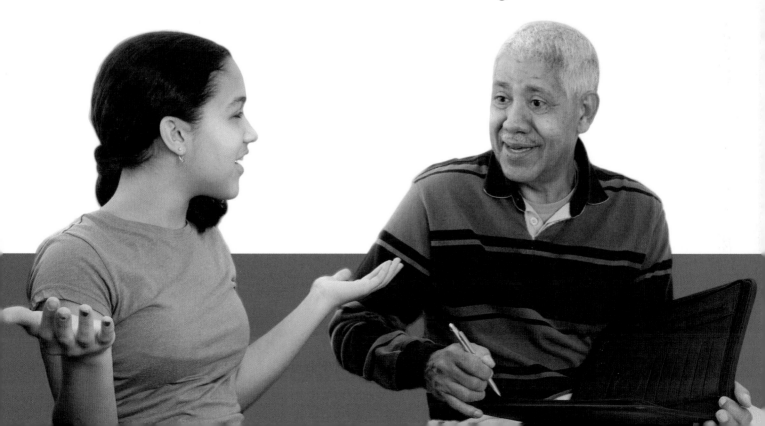

CHAPTER 8

Adolescent Development— Stages, Statuses, and Stereotypes

Charles G. Rogers, MD
Sara B. Kinsman, MD, PhD

 Related Video Content

8.0 Adolescent Development 101

■ Why This Matters

Changes occurring across adolescence have important implications for parents, practitioners, and policy makers. The biological, emotional, and social development that occurs between childhood and adulthood raises important questions: In what ways do young people change from childhood to adulthood? What are the primary developmental tasks of adolescence? Are there discreet stages or is it a continuous process? Are there different trajectories for young people in different social settings?

Professionals and parents equipped with an understanding of the complex interplay of forces that influence development will be better prepared to support young people through this critical transition.

> **Far from being a period of "storm and stress," adolescence should be a time of growth, discovery, learning, enjoyment, and preparation for the future.**

■ Physical Development

The most visible changes of adolescence are physical—early teens often look like children and develop at highly variable rates into young adults. Physical changes related to pubertal maturation have been well described by Marshall and Tanner.[1,2] These changes are closely associated with the timing of growth spurts in both height and weight. Puberty can begin as young as age 8 years in females and as late as 14 years in males. Becoming familiar with normative variations in timing is important. Early maturing and late maturing adolescents face unique individual and social challenges. For those experiencing physical maturity early, adults may assume they are older and expect more mature thinking, when in fact the teen is still chronologically, cognitively, and emotionally quite young.

The dramatic physical changes occurring during puberty contribute to construction of an adolescent's self-identity through reflected appraisals. Reflected appraisals refer to the process of a young person internalizing the impressions and stereotypes others have of them and incorporating those impressions into their identity. For example, if a young man develops the physical appearance of an athlete, those around him who expect athleticism will influence his self-perception. The links between physical, social, and identity development are of great importance.[3,4] While this chapter will be primarily focused on cognitive, emotional, and identity development, it is helpful to remember that these developmental streams are never completely separated from each other nor from the ongoing physical changes teens are experiencing.

■ Understanding Adolescence

In 1904 developmental psychologist G. Stanley Hall wrote a systematic overview of adolescence. Hall[5] defined adolescence as a period of "storm and stress." Though his theories were later expanded to reflect a more balanced view of adolescence, Hall's appreciation for adolescence as a unique time in life set the foundation for future theorists to include this period into their understanding of development.[6] Piaget, Erikson, and others started to wonder what happens during adolescence that explains the difference between a child and an adult.

Cognitive Development

In the mid-20th century, Piaget[7] proposed that children transition from concrete cognitive operations to formal cognitive operations as they mature. Concrete operational thinking allows an individual to understand and talk about tangible problems such as the number of objects they are adding, subtracting, or multiplying. Once an individual is able to think deductively from a hypothesis, she has entered what Piaget termed formal operations or abstract thinking.[7] Now she has the ability to manipulate symbols, follow theoretical assumptions, and solve, for example, algebraic equations, and physics problems and, most importantly, take prior experiences and apply them to new situations.

Why is this so important? Professionals and caretakers are most effective with young people when we take into account their cognitive development. For example, if we are talking to a teen who thinks in concrete ways, we cannot expect her to think forward and predict a hypothetical long-term consequence of her actions. However, once she is able to generate a hypothesis and link her behaviors with theoretical outcomes, her ability to identify a problem, consider solutions, and develop plans (and even contingency plans) will dramatically improve. Your discussion with her will reveal a richer understanding of the complexity of a situation and involve a back-and-forth discourse about possible outcomes and solutions.

In the decades since Piaget proposed his stage theory, several important considerations have been raised by researchers and practitioners.[8] These involve a growing understanding that different aspects of cognitive development, including acquisition of spoken and written language, executive function, working memory, and complex decision-making develop at very different rates and with varied eventual aptitudes for each individual.[8–12] Modularity and theory-theory are 2 theories of cognitive maturation that expand our understanding of cognitive development by allowing for different cognitive abilities to develop at variable rates and in relation to experience, culture, society, and environment.[8,13,14]

Modularity and Theory-Theory

Modularity theory, developed by Fodor, proposes that a person is born with innate "modules" that are discreet, self-contained systems involving particular cognitive processes.[8,13,15] For example, language and visual perception are often cited as examples of distinct cognitive modules. Information from the environment is filtered to the module, which causes a triggered cognitive process to be expressed. This trigger could be an environmental

The Teen Brain

Modern imaging techniques allow us to see the developing teen brain as never before. Here are a few key points drawn from an exciting and ever-expanding body of knowledge.

- Some of the greatest changes occur in the pre-frontal cortex, areas of the brain involved in planning complex behaviors, expressing personality, and controlling social behavior. As adolescence advances, there is an increase in white matter (the insulated, or myelinated, nerve fibers and connections throughout the brain) and a decrease in grey matter (the cell bodies of brain neurons).
- This increase in white matter appears to involve both an increase in myelination of existing connections (which speeds up nerve transmissions), and an increasing number of connections between the pre-frontal cortex and multiple other areas of the developing brain. While still exploratory, this research suggests these connections may reflect a crucial component of the neurobiological mechanisms underlying complex behaviors and decision-making.
- Early adolescence is a time of increasing sensitivity to dopamine in pathways connecting the pre-frontal cortex, the striatal system (a linking and processing hub in the brain), and the limbic system—including the amygdala (a region associated with processing emotions, regulating behaviors, supporting memory, and integrating sensory input). Dopamine is a signaling molecule that triggers specific receptors found throughout the brain, and influences many different processes, such as those listed above. Increased sensitivity to dopamine may be associated with increased sensation-seeking behaviors, reward-seeking behaviors, and goal-directed activity. Across middle and later adolescence and into adulthood, the dopamine receptors decrease in number and are redistributed away from the reward and behavior pathways.
- New studies combining insights from sociology, anthropology, and trauma studies are documenting the effects of environment and life experience on the developing brain. Research reveals that outside forces, such as trauma, nutrition, poverty, discrimination, and education, to name a few, are associated with changes in the structure and function of the brain at the level of signaling molecules, such as dopamine and serotonin, and in the ways white and grey matter are organized.

These key anatomic and molecular changes support much of what we have observed about teenagers. For example, teens are sometimes prone to emotionality and can view risk as exciting (findings thought to be linked to dopamine sensitive pathways associated with the limbic system). This increase in dopamine sensitivity may encourage early adolescents to explore, try new activities, and take calculated risks—all good things from evolutionary and developmental perspectives.

The multiplying connections leading out from the pre-frontal cortex link to multiple brain regions, including behavioral, emotional, and data processing centers. These connections may provide the neurobiological basis underlying developmental increases in inhibition, planning, delayed gratification, and social interactions that occur as adolescence proceeds.

This emerging neuroscience reinforces many longstanding behavioral strategies. For example, the adolescent brain shows increased reactivity in areas of the brain involved in risk taking and sensation seeking, such as the amygdala, peaking in early to middle adolescence. However the effectiveness of the pre-frontal cortex in regulating those areas continues to develop at least into the mid-20s. The difference in development between the 2 processes, reactivity and regulation, suggests a mechanism underlying why teens sometimes need physical space and time to calm themselves and regain control over their impulsive reactions. Many strategies suggested throughout *Reaching Teens* are designed to guide teenagers in safe spaces to reach their own conclusions at their own pace. Others are intended to protect teens from the inherent dangers associated with risky and impulsive behaviors.

Adolescent advocates must remain vigilant over how the emerging knowledge on the teen brain is used. It should elegantly present adolescence as an exciting time of growth and potential. It should be used to underscore the importance of healthy environments for brain development, including safe schools, good nutrition, adequate sleep, and the absence of toxins, including drugs. It should never be used to imply that the adolescent brain is somehow broken or "incomplete," or lead to suggestions that teens are incapable of self-regulation. It should be used to support high expectations for all youth, and for ensuring that resources are available to meet and exceed those expectations. The developing brain does not limit young people; it sets the stage for them to achieve their dreams and change our world.

influence or it could simply be expressed at a certain point in the young person's biological development.[8] A frequently used example providing support for this theory involved the observation that a person can see 2 lines of equal length next to each other, but can't perceive that they are the same length. This observation suggests that the portions of the mind involved in knowing the lines are the same length and perceiving their length are separate and discrete. The concept that various domains of cognition are discrete and don't share information, and may develop at different rates or times, can suggest partly why a young person may have difficulty perceiving social cues despite being top in her class, prioritizing tasks despite navigating complex social systems, or recognizing risky situations despite being able to explain in detail the possible risks.

The theory-theory proposes that cognitive development proceeds in the same way that scientific theory development proceeds.[8,14] This means that a young person proposes a basic theory of how the world around them works, subsequently tests that theory with real-world information, and incorporates new data into the original theory and develops a new theory or understanding. For example, an adolescent could believe that if she wants a new video game, and she has the money, then she should simply buy it. However, her belief or theory might change if, after spending money for a new game, she learns that she can't pay for gas to go visit and hang out with her friends. By understanding that a young person's decision-making or impulse control could develop inconsistently, we should not be surprised if a young person can put together a well-reasoned argument in one cognitive arena, but still be at risk for poor reasoning and decision-making in another arena. Providers can become skilled at supporting areas of cognitive development to compensate for unevenness and even find ways to trigger the development of other domains. For example, a youth counselor may notice that a teen she is working with has a well-developed ability to make good interpersonal decisions but is struggling with academics. The counselor could leverage the teen's strength to help her get tutoring while choosing friends that will support her academically.

Identity Development

It is often said the fundamental questions of adolescence are Who am I? and Am I normal? These 2 questions get to the heart of identity development. Erik Erikson[16,17] was an early theorist who proposed an 8-stage model of identity development that characterized each stage as a primary crisis or conflict that, if resolved appropriately, allowed progression to the next stage. The "identity achievement" versus "identity diffusion" stage has the strongest implications for teens. Erikson proposed that by successfully navigating this stage in life, an adolescent could develop secure and well thought out beliefs about himself and the world around him.[16,17]

James Marcia[18] further expanded the concept of identify development by proposing 4 categories of adolescent identity, which he called statuses, and applied them to Erikson's model: identity achievement, identity moratorium, identity foreclosure, and identity diffusion. Unlike stages, Marcia proposed that there was no definite progression from one to the next, and a young person could move back and forth between statuses depending on his situation and life circumstances.[19] Identity moratorium is the time when a teen can avoid choosing a firm identity, so the young person can experiment with various potential identities. This time allows an adolescent to "try on" new and creative identities, and find elements he can incorporate into his consolidated, achieved identity.[18,19] For adolescents, shifting peer groups, challenging their parents, changing hair colors and fashion styles, growing or declining interest in spirituality, and sexual experimentation are all ways that young people wrestle with developing a secure identity. It is important for adults to take the time to try to understand what young people are striving to explore and provide acceptance for this developmental process. By bridging to their world, we provide support to an adolescent's individual developmental quest. In fact, Marcia was concerned about youth who did not take time to explore their identity and prematurely adopted a set identity. He believed that these adolescents were at risk for difficulty coping when later circumstances challenged their one worldview.[18,19]

Identity statuses revolutionized traditional psychosocial development theory and started a movement toward more contextually sensitive models, which took into account how development is affected by race, minority status, acculturation, religiosity and spirituality, sexual orientation, and gender identification.[19-23] These theories allowed different aspects of a young person's identity to develop at differing rates, which affirmed that identity development is variable. It helps explain why young people can seem so mature in one area of their lives but feel unsure and incompetent in another area. Furthermore, it helps us understand why young people can appear to have settled on a fixed identity at one point in adolescence (eg, "I love sports!") yet can change dramatically several months later (eg, "I hate sports!"). Beyond just understanding that these changes occur, the concept of identity statuses helps us recognize that none of these changes are necessarily failures of development or even developmental abnormalities. They are all part of the ongoing quest for identity.

Moral Development

Kohlberg[24] expanded our understanding of moral development during adolescence. He proposed that adolescence is generally associated with the conventional stage of moral development as teens try to uphold social norms and maintain order in their adolescent social groups. The post-conventional stage reflects a young adult's ability to see beyond social norms and adhere to universal ethical principles.[24] Gilligan[25] challenged Kolberg and other's work by incorporating women's voices and perspectives in her research. Gilligan, and others after her, thought Kohlberg's model focused on competition, rights, and logic. While women also shared these interests, Gilligan found that women also valued the importance and inviolability of relationships.[25] These perspectives of moral development provided a deep appreciation for how context shapes all aspects of adolescent development.

■ Multicultural and Global Perspectives: Toward a Contextual Adolescence

The importance of culture on adolescent development has been demonstrated by cultural anthropologists who showed that almost all cultures have a socially constructed period of adolescence between the onset of reproductive ability and socially sanctioned childbearing, which was highly variable and based on cultural norms.[26,27] These cross-cultural perspectives of adolescence laid the foundation for Uri Bronfenbrenner's development of ecological systems theory, which attempted to explain how various contexts are layered from more proximal microsystems (such as family, school, peers) to more distal macrosystems (such as community, society, and culture).[28,29] Beyond simply describing these contextual layers, Bronfenbrenner showed how the respective layers could influence each other in a reciprocal fashion. For example, a young person's family would transmit their values to her, which could influence her choice of career; subsequently what profession she enters and how she carries out that profession will influence her community and culture. This becomes particularly significant when we recognize that many young people are working to forge a secure identity while facing multiple expectations and imposed stereotypes about youth. Although these stereotypes may unduly affect youths' initial self-perceptions, they are not fixed permanently. Young people have the ability to shift and change those stereotypes. They may initially take an action in defiance or reaction to the stereotypes (eg, working harder to defy an image of an unconcerned adolescent), but their actions and behaviors then alter community perceptions of youth through their interactions with their social environment.

One of the most important outcomes of Bronfenbrenner's perspective is Margaret Beale Spencer's phenomenological variant of ecological systems theory.[28] Her model recognized and defined how developmental processes, contextualized experiences, and even the unique meanings individuals develop from their unique social context are all interrelated.[20,28,30] Minority or marginalized youth are shaped by their interactions with 2 cultures: the dominant societal culture and their own culture. The interplay between the 2 cultures uniquely influences all aspects of development.[20,28,30] In addition, these complex interactions shape how providers, educators, policy makers, and researchers nurture positive youth development through a nuanced and contextually grounded understanding of resilience promoting factors.[28] Read Chapter 62, "Reaching Immigrant Youth," for a richer discussion on acculturation.

■ Conclusions

Adolescence is an exciting time in life, both for teenagers going through this transition and for those of us who have the joy of interacting with them on a daily basis. Far from being a period of "storm and stress," adolescence should be a time of growth, discovery, learning, enjoyment, and preparation for the future. As we understand adolescent cognitive, identity, and moral development in their cultural and environmental contexts, we are able to listen and appreciate what our young people are saying—both through their words and their behavior. As we gain this fuller, richer, and deeper understanding of them and their lives, we adjust our interactions and interventions to meet them at their developmental levels. By doing this, we can better provide support to young people as they navigate the steps and stages ahead, appreciating them for who they are right now and who they are becoming.

●● Group Learning and Discussion ●●

This chapter offers the base needed to interact with youth. We cannot hope to optimize our interactions with adolescents if we do not understand the complex developmental changes of this period. There are no specific "practice" exercises in this section. Rather, the knowledge gained here should universally inform how we approach youth and how we choose to incorporate each of the strategies proposed in the rest of this work.

■■■■■■■■ Continuing Education ■■■■■■■■

If you are applying for continuing education credits, a test is available online. For more details, visit www.aap.org/reachingteens.

■ References

1. Marshall WA, Tanner JM. Variations in pattern of pubertal changes in girls. *Arch Dis Child.* 1969;44(235):291–303

2. Marshall WA, Tanner JM. Variations in the pattern of pubertal changes in boys. *Arch Dis Child.* 1970;45(239):13–23

3. Smolak L, Stein JA. A longitudinal investigation of gender role and muscle building in adolescent boys. *Sex Roles.* 2010;63(9/10):738–746

4. Milkie MA. Social comparisons, reflected appraisals, and mass media: the impact of pervasive beauty images on black and white girls' self-concepts. *Soc Psychol Q.* 1999;62(2):190–210

5. Hall GS. *Adolescence: Its Psychology and Its Relations to Physiology, Anthropology, Sociology, Sex, Crime, Religion and Education.* London, England: Appleton & Co.; 1908

6. Lerner RM, Steinberg L. The scientific study of adolescent development. In: Lerner RM, Steinberg L. eds. *Handbook of Adolescent Psychology: Individual Bases of Adolescent Development.* 3rd ed. Hoboken, NJ: John Wiley & Sons; 2009

7. Piaget J. Development and learning. In: Gauvain M, Cole M, eds. *Readings on the Development of Children.* 5th ed. New York, NY: Worth Publishers; 2008

8. Gopnik A. The post-Piaget era. *Psychol Sci.* 1996;7(4):221–225

9. Huizinga M, Dolan CV, van der Molen MW. Age-related change in executive function: developmental trends and a latent variable analysis. *Neuropsychologia.* 2006;44(11):2017–2036

10. Leslie AM. Pretense and representation: the origins of "theory of mind." *Psychol Rev.* 1987;94(4):412–426

11. Perner J. *Understanding the Representational Mind.* Cambridge, MA: The MIT Press; 1991

12. Albert D, Steinberg L. Judgment and decision making in adolescence. *J Res Adolesc.* 2011;21(1):211–224

13. Leslie A. Some implications of pretense for mechanisms underlying the child's theory of mind. In: Astington JW, Harris PL, Olson DR, eds. *Developing Theories of Mind.* Cambridge, United Kingdom: Cambridge University Press; 1990:19–46

14. Gopnik A, Wellman HM. The theory theory. In: *Mapping the Mind: Domain Specificity in Cognition and Culture.* Cambridge, United Kingdom: Cambridge University Press; 1994:257–293

15. Fodor JA. *The Modularity of Mind.* Cambridge, MA: The MIT Press; 1983

16. Erikson EH. *Identity and the Life Cycle.* New York, NY: W. W. Norton & Company, Inc.; 1980

17. Erikson EH. *Identity, Youth, and Crisis.* New York, NY: W. W. Norton & Company; 1968

18. Marcia JE. Development and validation of ego-identity status. *J Pers Soc Psychol.* 1966;3(5):551–558

19. Schwartz SJ. The evolution of Eriksonian and, neo-Eriksonian identity theory and research: a review and integration. *Identity.* 2001;1:7–58

20. Spencer MB, Markstrom-Adams C. Identity processes among racial and ethnic minority children in America. *Child Dev.* 1990;61(2):290–310

21. Perry DG, Pauletti RE. Gender and adolescent development. *Res Adolesc.* 2011;21(1):61–74

22. Halverson ER. The dramaturgical process as a mechanism for identity development of LGBTQ youth and its relationship to detypification. *J Adolesc Res.* 2010;25(5):635–668

23. Lopez AB, Huynh VW, Fuligni AJ. A longitudinal study of religious identity and participation during adolescence. *Child Dev.* 2011;82(4):1297–1309

24. Kohlberg L. *The Psychology of Moral Development: The Nature and Validity of Moral Stages.* San Francisco, CA: Harper & Row; 1984

25. Gilligan C. *In a Different Voice: Psychological Theory and Women's Development.* Cambridge, MA: Harvard University Press; 1982

26. Schlegel A. A cross-cultural approach to adolescence. *Ethos.* 1995;23(1 Adolescence):15–32

27. Schlegel A, Hewlett BL. Contributions of anthropology to the study of adolescence. *J Res Adolesc.* 2011;21(1):281–289

28. Swanson DP, Spencer MB, Dell'Angelo T, Harpalani V, Spencer TR. Identity processes and the positive youth development of African Americans: an explanatory framework. *New Dir Youth Dev.* 2002;(95):73–99

29. Bronfenbrenner U. Toward an experimental ecology of human development. *Am Psychol.* 1977;32(7):513–531

30. Spencer MB. Development of minority children: an introduction. *Child Dev.* 1990;61(2):267–269

■ Related Video Content

8.0 Adolescent Development 101. Clark.

8.1 Puberty 101. Sugerman.

8.2 Development Is Uneven. Sugerman.

8.3 Adjusting Health Messages for Different Developmental Stages: Using Smoking as an Example. Diaz.

28.0 Facilitating Adolescents to Own Their Solution: Replacing the Lecture With Youth-Driven Strategies. Ginsburg.

35.2 Even During Your Toughest Parent-Teen Moments, Remember That Your Teen Loves You so Much, It Hurts. Sugerman.

35.4 The Teen Brain: A Balancing Act Between Thoughts and Emotions. Catallozzi.

CHAPTER 9

The Adolescent World

Amanda Lerman, MD
Sara B. Kinsman, MD, PhD

■ Why This Matters

Some adults regard young people as living in an easygoing world free of serious responsibility. Their basic needs are often still provided by adults, and they seem to spend their time in unproductive ways: hanging out, watching TV, playing games, and messaging each other minute-to-minute. Parents, teachers, and other adults marvel at how much time teenagers expend in seemingly inconsequential activity. They may continually ask, "What did you do with the whole day?" More than likely, adolescents will not be able to explain fully what they "accomplished," and their uninformative responses may further the adult's view that teens "waste time" in trivial activities. Similarly, adults often struggle to understand how adolescents can get so concerned, excited, or upset over seemingly small matters. Bewildered, they may blame hormones.

> **Adults have all been through childhood and adolescence, and their own memories may be helpful in relating to young people. Personal experience, though, can grant a false sense of complete understanding. The adolescent world has challenges that adults have forgotten about, play down, or even repress.**

It can be hard as an adult to see young people's world through their lens. In her 1988 novel, *Cat's Eye,* which explored relationships between female childhood friends, Margret Atwood illustrates this phenomenon, writing:

> "Little girls are cute and small only to adults. To one another they are not cute. They are life-sized."[1]

Adults have all been through childhood and adolescence, and their own memories may be helpful in relating to young people. Personal experience, though, can grant a false sense of complete understanding. The adolescent world has challenges that adults have forgotten about, play down, or even repress. Still few adults would voluntarily step back in life to relive the joy of middle school. Remembering the very real challenges that come with transitioning from childhood to adulthood can help us better understand and empathize with the ways adolescents negotiate their world.

■ Activities, Interests, and Identity Formation

Just as little children need time to play and learn about their world,[2] the unstructured time spent by adolescents is critically important for their social development. Adolescents need to explore their world and their place in it. When they spend hours "hanging out" with people their own age, they are learning how to communicate with peers and develop social skills. This is a time of trial and error. Adolescents learn that they cannot control their friends' comments or behaviors and that unlike most family members, classmates are not always interested in being fair, kind, or supportive. Meanwhile, most adolescents start to identify attributes in peers who are "good matches"; recognizing these qualities can guide them toward the people their age who can become enduring and reliable friends and extend their social world beyond the family.

Other activities also irk parents. They worry about excessive time and energy spent changing clothes, perfecting hairstyles, and scrutinizing their bodies. When young people obsess over their physical appearances, though, they are not being shallow—they are beginning to think about how they present themselves to the world. They are trying on different identities to see what is comfortable and what feels "like me." When teenagers develop keen interest in idols—celebrities, actors, musicians, sports stars—they are not just mimicking pop culture, they are aligning themselves with different role models to see how they fit. When youth jump from one activity to another, they are not necessarily "quitters"; they may be exploring their various abilities. When adolescents join subcultures—musical subcultures like goth, punk, or hip hop; lifestyle subcultures like vegan or gamer, or, in past years, hippie; or fraternities, sororities, clubs, or other groups—they are not just blindly following or seeking acceptance, they are also trying on identities as they search for their true selves. All of these endeavors may seem frivolous to adults, but they present adolescents with opportunities to create, problem solve, and develop in multiple ways. What seems a waste of time to some adults may actually be critical to youth development, since even more daunting than figuring out the external world is discovering one's own identity.

The focus on the external—appearance, image, and association—can make these pursuits appear useless, misguided, or even harmful, but the surface is simply the easiest place to start. Initial attempts toward defining and redesigning their public face may represent the first move teens make from a passive sense of self based on predetermined characteristics (such as biological sex or skin color) toward active identity formation. Deeper introspection, self-adjustment, and growth can follow.

Similarly, young people do not just investigate and assimilate existing culture—they play an active role in reinventing it. Children and adolescents have long been regarded as being "socialized" by the world in which they are raised, but there is now evidence that this process is not unidirectional. Sociologists have observed that growing minds do not just absorb and mirror the culture they experience—they appropriate and reshape it.[3] Adolescents are molded by their world, and they in turn rearrange the cultures they encounter. We all see examples of this every day. Young minds create most new language—slang, which ultimately becomes canonized in the *Oxford English Dictionary*. Young hearts have fueled societal change throughout history: consider their role in the French Revolution or the American civil rights movement. Young people challenge adults not because they are hormone-crazed, irrational, or delinquent, but because they see novel solutions, embrace change, and fight for progress even when it requires upheaval of the current order.

■ More Difficult Than You May Remember

The lives of adolescents may not involve many bills to pay, but they contain an enormous amount of uncertainty and can include overwhelming stress. Some youth endure significant hardships such as bullying, abuse, abandonment, poverty, homelessness, and other life-threatening adversities. Others struggle with mental or physical illness. We can readily feel for teens who are visibly suffering, but it is not always clear when young people are in distress. The warning signs that an adolescent is hurting can be subtle or simply different from what we might expect. Adolescents struggling with major depression, for example, may display the profound sadness seen in depressed adults. Unlike adults, however, they are just as likely to exhibit irritability, or even rage, as the main symptom of depression. This can evoke our anger rather than our support.

Teens may be embarrassed or ashamed to reveal their pain, may struggle to put their feelings into words, or may have no idea what they are experiencing. If young people do not respond when asked "What's wrong?" it may be because they have no answer to the question.

The most disadvantaged youth, who may have the greatest need, may also be the most easily misunderstood. Some grow up lacking basic necessities and may see no reason to hope for a better life. As compassionate citizens, we lament the substandard education provided by their underfunded schools, the tragic shortcomings of the foster care system, or their inconsistent access to quality health care, but our concern may not be apparent to them. They may notice instead the uneasiness they inspire in other people in stores, on the street, or on public transit. The greatest obstacle to meeting their potential may be when they internalize these low expectations.

The challenges of adolescence are not limited to the sickest, most troubled, or most disadvantaged teens. The stress of this transitional period can be oppressive to youth in any setting. Even if an adolescent does not directly experience hardship, they know of others who have and have become aware of the unfairness of suffering. These realizations are unsettling as an individual transforms from viewing the world as a child to holding the more complex worldview of adults.

Struggling to make sense of the world's harsh realities can be terrifying, especially since modest life experience makes it hard to recognize all its possibilities. The classic 1986 film *Stand By Me* sensitively captures the unmitigated feelings of youthful inexperience. It tells the tale of a formative weekend expedition embarked upon by 4 young friends in late summer before starting junior high school. The main character narrates the tale from adulthood. As the picture opens, he explains:

> "I was living in a small town in Oregon called Castle Rock. There were only twelve hundred and eighty-one people. But to me, it was the whole world."[4]

Seen through the frame of a man in middle age reflecting and redefining his experiences as a 12-year-old boy, the emotional moments in the picture are far more poignant. As he recounts the plot, the narrator implicitly tells the story of youthful innocence, reminding audiences what it actually felt like to be young, inexperienced, and unaware of the size of the world beyond a small town. Decades later it can be near impossible to conjure up that feeling, to un-know what one now knows and remember how real teenage anxieties and heartaches felt. With a limited view of the world at large, every problem can loom large—each family quarrel can seem insurmountable, each test can threaten to determine lifetime potential for success or failure, and each interpersonal conflict can forebode a lifetime of social rejection.

Columnist Dan Savage's "It Gets Better" Web video campaign, created in 2010 to "show young LGBT people the levels of happiness, potential, and positivity their lives will reach—if they can just get through their teen years,"[5] highlights the truncated perspective that all teenagers experience. The movement features videos created by lesbian, gay, bisexual, and transgendered (LGBT) adults reflecting on the difficulties of their teen years and telling the hopeful tales of how much better their lives became after adolescence—after graduating from the high schools that circumscribed their social experiences, after gaining independence from judgmental family units, after moving on from intolerant home communities. The lesson on perspective, created specifically to address the particularly intense isolation frequently experienced by LGBT youth, can be extended to all young people. The worlds of adolescents are limited. Without broader outlook, the bullying, judgment, or condemnation of a few individuals can seem like rejection by the whole world, and, without greater context, everyday pressures can be crushing.

Clearly not every young person struggles with sexual orientation, or with bullying, but they all have different and unique challenges. Adolescent worlds exist in infinite varieties representing the brilliant diversity of young people, but they are all constrained by a short lifetime of previous experiences. As they emerge from childhood into an awareness of the complexity of the world, young people know that they have only a few years before they have to navigate it independently. In the best situations, teenagers have adults around them that empower them to find their own dreams and encourage them to excel, but the broad array of possibilities can be dizzying. If adults are not careful with their messages, it can seem to young people that any misstep could be catastrophic.

■ Here's What to Do

As new members of society, adolescents are charged with the task of making sense of the world around them and, even more daunting, with figuring out how they fit into it. Rather than fearing their potential for innovation, we can foster it. Young people are not yet vastly experienced in the world, but they have a tremendous amount to contribute. When we make assumptions about adolescents' thoughts, feelings, and experiences, we risk misunderstanding and hindering their potential to develop positive connections with adults and the broader community. To engage adolescents, and to bridge the generational gap, we can start by accepting that they have a unique perspective. If we challenge our assumptions about adolescents and break out of our own memories and biased perspectives, we can forge more meaningful connections with the teens in our lives. When we are open to adolescents and their individual outlook instead of lecturing or insisting they conform, we will empower them to use their energy and innovation to repair our world.

●● Group Learning and Discussion ●●

This chapter reminds us of the complexity of the lives of youth. We cannot hope to influence their behavior if we do not understand the world they must navigate. There are no specific "practice" exercises in this section. Rather, the insights gained here should universally inform how we approach youth and how we propose they initiate positive behavioral changes in their lives.

There is a likelihood, however, that this chapter reminded you of the complexity of your own "adolescent world." This gives you an opportunity for self-reflection. When you understand your own adolescence, you are one step closer to understanding the adult you have become. You also may more readily note where you are "stuck"—to better comprehend why certain situations or people make you reactive or apprehensive. In particular, you may better grasp why certain adolescents you care for might trigger buttons within you that were installed long ago. When you are equipped with these insights, you are better prepared to serve youth.

■■■■■■■■ Continuing Education ■■■■■■■■■

If you are applying for continuing education credits, a test is available online. For more details, visit www.aap.org/reachingteens.

References

1. Atwood M. *Cat's Eye*. New York, NY: Doubleday; 1988
2. Ginsburg KR; American Academy of Pediatrics Committee on Communications, Committee on Psychosocial Aspects of Child and Family Health. The importance of play in promoting healthy child development and maintaining strong parent-child bonds. *Pediatrics*. 2007;119(1):182–191
3. Corsaro WA. *The Sociology of Childhood*. Thousand Oaks, CA: Sage Publications; 1997
4. Reiner R. *Stand By Me* [videorecording]. Burbank, CA: RCA/Columbia Pictures Home Video
5. Savage D. It Gets Better Project. What is the It Gets Better Project? http://www.itgetsbetter.org/pages/about-it-gets-better-project. Accessed June 25, 2013

Related Video Content

9.0 The Adolescent World: Who Said Anything About the Teen Years Being Care Free? Youth.

9.1 The Adolescent World: Navigating School Pressures. Youth.

9.2 The Adolescent World: Navigating Relationships at Home. Youth.

9.3 The Adolescent World: Navigating a Stressful Environment. Youth.

9.4 The Adolescent World: Being Held to Low Expectations. Youth.

9.5 The Adolescent World: Building a Family When the One at Home May Have Let You Down. Youth.

9.6 The Adolescent World: Comfort With Diversity. Youth.

9.7 The Adolescent World: A Time of Fun and Discovery. Youth.

25.9 Behaviors Must Be Seen in the Context of the Lives Youth Have Needed to Navigate. Auerswald.

35.9 Thoughts on Parenting: The Voice of Adolescents. Youth.

41.5 Peers and Friendships: The Voice of Youth. Youth.

48.5 Teen-Produced Song: Paper Tigers. Youth, Toro.

CHAPTER 10

Sex(uality) Happens: Fostering Healthy, Positive (Female) Sexuality

Susan T. Sugerman, MD, MPH, FAAP
Liana R. Clark, MD, MSCE, FAAP
Tonya A. Chaffee, MD, MPH, FAAP

 Related Video Content

10.0 Sexuality: A Normal Aspect of Adolescent Development

■ Why This Matters

Sexuality is a normal human condition.
Development of sexual characteristics, feelings, urges, and eventually behavior is as normal as the acquisition of other assets such as physical strength or abstract thought. Because of its relatively "late" introduction along the developmental spectrum (as well as the associated implications), sexuality can feel like a newer, "bigger," and sometimes overwhelming concept to adolescents and their parents. Adopting an approach that acknowledges human sexuality as healthy, normal, and necessary allows a young person to incorporate sexual capacities into their lives in appropriate, adaptive ways.

> **We have the unique privilege of being able to positively influence how teens approach sexuality. While we must always teach them to protect their physical and emotional safety, we are equally responsible to help them learn to accept and honor their sexual thoughts, feelings, and interests without shame. By providing accurate information and support for healthy decision-making, we can promote teens' readiness for positive, mature, and developmentally appropriate sexual experiences.**

Teens deserve to respect and honor their sexuality. Adolescents' curiosity and excitement about their changing bodies and emerging sexual feelings are normal. Armed with accurate information delivered in an appropriate developmental context, young people can become not just respectful and appreciative, but also proud and protective of this gift we call sexuality.

■ Why You? The Role of the Adult Professional

We have the unique privilege of being able to talk frankly and honestly about both sexuality and sex with teenagers, parents, and communities. We understand that sexuality encompasses much more than sexual intercourse. Emotions, attractions, and relationship development are coupled with physical connections in a somewhat complicated muddle that we can help our teens work through. We have the opportunity to recognize the risk for confusion, shame, and insecurity commonly associated with teen sex and instead help them understand their experiences, learn to make healthy decisions, feel proud of who they are, and protect themselves from the potential dangers that can occur with sexual experimentation and experience.

Put It in Context: Who, What, When, Where, Why and (Most Importantly) How to Talk About Sex

Who: Consider all aspects of the teen when approaching conversations about sexuality. Take into consideration a teen's developmental attributes, incorporating your assessment of any significant disparities between her physical appearance and emotional maturity (eg, a well-developed 13-year-old girl may appear fully mature physically but not be emotionally). A young person's family situation (including current living environment, parent dynamics, as well as family background) colors her readiness to hear and use information and advice about sexual behaviors. Assess the role of peer and media influence on that particular teen's perceptions and experiences, taking into account the cultural context in which she encounters issues around sexuality.

What: Prioritize providing accurate, factual information in developmentally appropriate ways. Use correct terms for body parts and sexual functions, acknowledging euphemisms, slang, or "pet" names only to clarify and educate about proper terminology in context. Provide as much information as a particular teen is "ready" to hear and understand, but also leave the door "open" for further questions. Find ways to introduce decision-making skills (eg, role plays, choreographed conversations, "what if's").

When: Give the right information at the "right time" and "right place." There will be times to offer education and times to respond to requests for information, advice, and reality checks. Your approach will vary according to whether the context involves a "push" (didactic curriculum setting, anticipatory guidance, etc) or a "pull" (direct query from a teen, current or anticipated need, response to a crisis, etc).

Where: Location matters when considering how to provide sexuality education and support for teens. A classroom environment dictates a different approach than a one-on-one clinical encounter, a school counselor's office, or a youth group retreat.

Why: If responsible adults, and most importantly parents, do not discuss healthy sexuality with teens, who will? We leave them to learn from the media, Internet, and peers.

How: Talking about sex can be difficult for many people, including parents and teenagers, let alone clinicians! *How* you communicate sexuality information to young people matters as much as *what* you say. Remain open-minded and nonjudgmental of the teen's perspective, even if you have concerns about her behaviors. Also, it is important to avoid putting your agenda ahead of the teen's. The goal for the communication needs to be to help guide the teen toward *her* making healthy choices for herself. Sometimes we can be more directive than facilitative. In discussing sexuality, we must recognize that we are facilitating the teen along her sexual path with the aim of helping her stay healthy and safe along the way.

When appropriate, offer parents the opportunity to discuss their views on adolescent sexuality *in front of the teen and before discussing sex with the teen privately.* Ask parents to share their wishes and expectations for their teen's sexual development over time. Consider asking how they would respond if their teen's experiences differ from what they hope for them. Most adults parenting teens today are not as naïve as adolescents presume; many were teens during very sexually "rebellious" times themselves. They may or may not have had sex during adolescence. But they most likely know someone who did. Many parents embrace this opportunity to "publicly" offer reasoned advice to their child without being accused of lecturing.

Offering parents the chance to discuss sexuality honestly in front of their child is instructive from multiple standpoints. You gain the opportunity to observe parent-child interactions as well as their level of communication about sex. It lets parents know you are all on the same team, with the common goal of helping the teen become a sexually healthy adult. Often teens are surprised to find that parents may be more accepting and understanding than previously expected. Further, speaking clearly and honestly in this way reassures parents about your approach to sexuality education, earning their trust for when you later meet confidentially with their child. Above all, it allows you to model for parents and their children how to have appropriate and productive conversations around a very sensitive topic. When you are speaking together with both parent and adolescent, you should foster open communication about general sexuality topics, but be careful not to confront the teen about any of her specific past behaviors in front of her parents at this time.

Some examples are included below.
- Set the stage for open communication about sexuality.
  — Normalcy. *"During the teen years it's very common to have sexual feelings about people you like or find attractive. The good thing to know is that there are many ways that teens choose to act on these normal feelings. Some choose touching and closeness without going any further and some move to having sex. The important thing is for you to figure out what feels right for you and make decisions that support your choices. I'll also be here to help you with your choices and questions along the way."*
- Present information in a manner that is matter-of-fact and without value-laden connotations.
  — Shaving. *"Your pubic hair is there for a reason. In addition to protecting you from friction (rubbing from clothing or other people), it can increase sensation (think about whiskers on a cat). When you shave, you increase your risk of ingrown hairs and even severe skin infections; I encourage you to consider NOT shaving, at least inside the bikini line."*
- Find opportunities to bring up common concerns that may be hard for teens to ask on their own.
  — Masturbation. *"Some people (males and females) like what happens when they touch themselves in their private areas. Some don't like it or worry it is not an appropriate thing to do. It's a very personal and private decision. Either way, it's important to know that you won't hurt yourself or cause any damage if you do it."*
- Speak as if you presume she has normal curiosity and motivation to protect herself.
  — Sexting. *"Wanting someone to think you're sexy or desirable is normal. But sending pictures of yourself can cause you a lot of bad consequences. Can you think of reasons I would say that? (Example: What do you think could happen if someone even accidentally forwards a naked photo of you to other people?")*
- Keep the conversation light-hearted (and possibly humorous) but always respectful.
  — Respectful limit-setting. *"Sometimes a guy might want to 'take things to another level' with you because sex has been built up as the most amazing thing ever. But take it from me, amazing sex comes from waiting until you're ready. If he is and you're not,*

well it might be amazing for him, but you'll only have an 'eh' experience and that is so not cool. You can honor his sexuality by letting him know you're flattered, but that you don't want to have sex."

- Look for opportunities to "ask" not "tell" teens about sexuality.
  — Asking open-ended questions such as *"What do you consider to be a healthy relationship?"* and *"When do you think you will be ready for sex?"* reveals where teens are in their sexual development. For example, a response like *"when I'm 18-years-old"* is very concrete (and may or may not be very realistic). By comparison, *"when I meet the right person"* or *"when I fall in love"* demonstrates a more mature understanding of intimacy and love (but may still benefit from guidance in thinking through the details of "readiness" and "love").

■ Guiding Teens to Empowered, Healthy ▶ 10.6 Sexuality

Priority one. Teach them to love themselves and put their needs first and foremost. *The most important relationship they have is the one they have with themselves.* When people understand, accept, and value (eg, *love*) themselves, they are in a position to develop the knowledge, skills, and motivation to take good care of themselves.

Leave *nice* at the door. Girls are often socialized to be nice at all costs when they like someone. As such, they can quickly learn to ignore their needs, wants, and desires in favor of a partner's. It is important to teach them to leave being *nice* at the door and be authentic in sharing their likes and desires with a partner. Even if the partner gets upset or disagrees with where they are or what they feel, it is important for them to remain true to what is right for them and not capitulate to make someone else happy.

Self-validation promotes prevention of pain and shame. When they prioritize their needs and their safety, they are better able to prevent, avoid, and resolve painful, difficult, or shameful situations in life generally and with regard to their sexuality specifically. Helping teens work toward an understanding of who they are and what they need to do to remain in control of their sexuality and sexual experiences goes a long way toward preparing them to have healthy intimate relationships with others.

Assume the best. Assume teens care about themselves as much as their parents do. They just may not have developed a mature understanding about what they need and how to protect themselves. Just as with other developmental skills, it becomes the job of the adults in their lives to help support them through this time of learning and skill-building until they are able to better care for their own needs.

Young people need to know they're normal. Ultimately, our youth need *reassurance that they are normal* and that having sexual feelings, and eventually experiences, is expected. They need *information* about the physical as well as emotional changes they will experience through puberty and beyond. Our children need a *place to go* for accurate, developmentally appropriate information they can understand and use in real time. They may go back to the same question at a later time, but from a different perspective.

Set positive expectations and provide guidance on how to achieve them. Help young people understand that they deserve to have great sex, then explain what this means and why this is so hard to do as a teen or even a young adult. Review the benefits of healthy, loving, sexual intimacy (physical pleasure, emotional connection, stress relief, etc). Also include the potential negatives (not just disease or unplanned pregnancy, but also threats to relationship stability, heartbreak, damage to reputation, loss of trust of parents, pain during sex, and possibly increased stress). Motivational interviewing techniques can help young people understand the advantages of delaying sexual activity until they are more mature and prepared (remind them how much more mature they feel today than they did 2 to 3 years ago, and how much more mature and capable they will feel in the near future) (see Chapter 26).

Avoid dated "dating" language. If we presume the words "dating" or even "talking" mean what they did when we were teens, we miss the opportunity to have conversations with teenagers about the reality of sex and love in their lives. Gone are the days when "hooking up" after a movie meant meeting friends for ice cream. Be aware that the landscape of their language and phrases changes on every second Tuesday at secret teen meetings intentionally designed to keep adults confused and out of the loop. Spend time with teenagers who are willing to educate you about the terms they use to describe their relationships, the typical progression of relationships, and the standards or expectations regarding how teens interact sexually in their communities.

Keep conversations gender neutral. Allow for the possibility that a young person may be attracted to men, women, or both. Most often, it is not necessary to identify whether a teen's partner is male or female. Use gender-neutral language when counseling about diseases or offering support around sexual concerns: *"Anyone who is intimate with another person can get these diseases,"* or, *"Do you have any questions or worries about your sexual feelings or experiences that you want to discuss today?"* Stay focused on promoting healthy, supportive, safe relationships regardless of a teen's choice of partners.

Teach relationship literacy. Unlike the generations that preceded them, today's teens live in a world where, more and more often, there is opportunity (or pressure) for physical intimacy prior to or even independent of emotional intimacy. Emphasize communication and problem-solving within relationships as critical tools for maintaining healthy adult connections throughout life, not just with partners, but even with friends, bosses, coworkers, and their communities. Emphasize the importance of building healthy relationship skills as a priority over sexual skills, especially for young people who may not be equipped to handle the consequences of sex.

Prepare teens to prevent, recognize, and respond to unhealthy relationships. Teens need concrete explanations and examples of the differences between healthy, controlling, and abusive relationships. Whether with friends or intimate partners, adolescence is a time when young people learn to differentiate between relationships that *feel good to them* and those that *are good for them*. Often they do not recognize when their relationships become unhealthy or dangerous until it is too late. Educate yourself on the typical patterns and warning signs of concerning relationships. Be willing to explore with teenagers why they think their relationships may or may not be good for them, and have resources to provide support if they find themselves (or a friend) needing help to get out of an unhealthy relationship situation (see Related Resources and Chapter 56).

Life isn't like the movies. Teens need to hear from credible professionals that, unlike Hollywood, where it takes 1 to 2 minutes of screen time between the first kiss and waking up naked in bed together, most sexual relationships evolve over time. Help teens understand the value of a slow, patient progression through the stages of emotional and physical intimacy. Remind them it doesn't have to be all or nothing.

Don't limit sexuality conversations. Often when providers discuss sex ▶ 10.3 with adolescents, the conversation starts with asking whether or not they have had sexual intercourse, and then moves to a lecture on birth control methods and condom use. But more important, in many cases, this simple protocol is to instead help them learn to make healthy sexual decisions. Asking a teen who has not had sex. *"How do you think you will know that you're ready to have sex?"* can initiate a great conversation about sexual readiness and concrete factors that the teen may want to establish in her relationship before moving to intercourse. With sexually active teens, queries about the whys of their sexual relationship and what positives they get from them can also help them explore the health of their sexual relationships.

Abstinence from what? Adolescents deserve honest conversations with supportive adults about exactly *what* they should be abstaining from and concrete advice about *how* to make that happen. Ask, *"Are there ways to be sexual without having sex?"* From there, a discussion of outercourse, a lost concept for many adolescents, can be helpful. Outercourse encompasses everything that can be done sexually without penetrative intercourse. Help them understand that sexuality includes everything from making eye contact across a crowded room (or cyberspace) to sexual intercourse. Explain how discussing limits and boundaries in detail with a partner in advance of any sexual contact promotes communication and strengthens the ability to self-regulate the progression of sexual expression within a relationship.

Safety is nonnegotiable. Use techniques such as motivational interviewing or staged conversations to help teens understand the potential dangers of being too trusting, allowing themselves to be left alone with someone, sending inappropriate photos or texts, having contact without condoms, etc. Provide education for preventing, recognizing, and responding to potential or real dangers. Work with teens to develop safety plans, including code words to use with parents, friends, or roommates, when they find it necessary to get out of an uncomfortable situation without losing face. For more information about code words, see Chapter 41, page 335.

Nobody's perfect. Negative sexual experiences are best avoided, but when they happen, help young people use them as learning opportunities. Especially in the context of sexual trauma, let them know their future does not have to be defined by bad things that happened in the past. Direct them toward support resources, therapists, and other programs that help them cope and recover from difficult experiences.

What their parents really need to know... Most parents of today's teenagers are not as naïve as adolescents presume. They experienced their own adolescence during a time of significant changes in social and cultural expectations about sex. Even if they prefer their children not become sexually active, they want the best for their children and don't want to see them come in harm's way. They may not need the details of how much "tongue" was involved in each kiss (they certainly won't want to share the details of their own sex lives). But, they do need reassurance their teens won't get a disease, become pregnant, or be abused.

Teach teens to use their parents wisely. Explain to teenagers that their parents are on their team. Remind them that their parents have wisdom to offer based on their own experiences (*"What year was it when your parents were your age? What was happening in the world at that time?"*). Offer to broker difficult conversations and resolve unnecessary secrets that may be causing friction or distance between a teen and his or her parents. When appropriate, strategize with teens how they use their time with you as an excuse to bring up difficult subjects with their parents even later that same day.

Build your own toolkit. Find resources in your community, such as clinics, hotlines, therapeutic specialists, and support groups, to make available to the young people you work with. Create a list of favorite Web resources to share with them. Consider having books available for them to read or even purchase for more information and support on difficult topics.

■ Pointers for Parents: Raising Sexually Healthy Children 56.7

Parents matter. It is the privilege, right, and responsibility of parents to facilitate the development of healthy sexuality in their children. Most parents have the same goal for their children that they have for themselves—to grow up to be good people who can take good care of themselves. It is the job of parents to be a source of information and wisdom about sexual issues, to support developmentally healthy sexuality, to recognize and respond to unhealthy or unsafe sexual experiences, and, most importantly, to monitor and defend the safety of their children when possible and appropriate.

Don't blame teens for being normal. Our children live in a highly sexualized society where they are exposed to sexual language, images, and behaviors before they are developmentally prepared to handle them. Kids didn't "ask" for hormones at age 12, but they are stuck learning how to handle their changing bodies and urges in a society that shows them "yes" but tells them "not now."

Don't discredit love. Understand the importance of romantic attachments in a teenager's life and the intensely strong feelings that they generate, even if your definition and perspective of love differ from your child's.

Don't abstain from educating your own children. If you don't educate them, someone else will. They learn from behaviors and attitudes modeled by other adults, from the media and popular culture, and certainly from peers. Stand up and let your own views be counted as part of their sex education.

Talk about sex early and often. They don't always hear you. They may not always believe you. They often don't remember, especially if they weren't ready to hear you. (But they are often listening when they are pretending not to be.)

Avoid sexuality conversations that are all *"don'ts."* Parents often recount that they speak to their teens often about sex. Yet generally those conversations are all about the *"don'ts."*

- *Don't* have sex.
- *Don't* get pregnant.
- *Don't* get a disease.

It's *don't, don't, don't.* But what gets left out are the *"do's."* What can they *do* to be sexually healthy with a partner that they care about? How can they decide whether a partner is interested in them as a person or just as a potential sex partner? What ways can they address peer or partner pressure to be sexual when they don't feel they are ready? These topics need to be part and parcel of any discussion of healthy sexuality. Give them some things they can do!

▶ **10.5**

Right time, right place. Provide accurate information in developmental context. Meet them where they are. A young child asking, *"What does sex mean?"* may wonder what the teacher meant when she said, *"line up by sex"* for recess. Find out exactly what the question is, then try to give an honest answer that meets that need.

Be real. Dispel myths and rumors. Provide accurate information. Use simple language, but respect their intelligence and curiosity. Above all, avoid talking down to children and teens about sex.

Empower your children. Let them know they deserve to feel honored in their relationships, to have their own space, to keep their friends, to include their family, and to feel good about who they are. Teach them to expect a give-and-take, but that, in the end, a good relationship helps you to be more of who you already are and feel even better about it.

Set positive expectations. Let your children know they deserve to have great sex. Discussing what's good about sex will help them to have positive standards by which to judge sexual experiences. Help your kids know *why* sex is worth waiting for and give them some realistic guidance about how they will know when it might be worth moving forward.

Use the media (the good, bad, and the ugly). Use topics presented in daily media sources and popular teen culture as springboards for theoretical conversations about sex and relationships. Avoid proclamations and judgments, even about fictional characters; your children will anticipate your reacting to them in the same way should they ever be in that situation. Consider role-playing through a situation presented on TV as collaborative, nonjudgmental thought processing; it will provide insight into your child's view of the world and give you the opportunity to offer your ideas for them to reflect on.

Live by example. If you have a good relationship, let your children know it. Let them witness you and your partner having a disagreement and working it out; let them see you kiss and make up.

Teaching kids about sex doesn't mean parenting without values. Acknowledging sexuality is not the same as condoning or giving permission to have sex. Helping their children understand that sexual thoughts and feelings are normal gives parents the opportunity to follow up with conversations about *how* (and from *what*) to be abstinent as well as how to regulate their impulses and urges. It opens the door to continued conversation about how to be safe and responsible when their adolescents begin to engage in intimate physical or sexual activities.

You have 2 ears and 1 mouth. Listen more than you talk. Be the sounding board that helps developing teens come to their own good decision about their sexual behaviors. Engaging kids in conversation about sexuality goes much further toward developing independent decision-making than lecturing about what they "should" and "shouldn't" do.

Ask, don't tell. Find out what your child is thinking when talking about their relationships or sexual experiences. What does it mean to have a boyfriend or girlfriend at what age? Listen to what it means to the teen at that time. The teen's level of understanding and participation may actually be appropriate for her developmental level. Understand, don't judge. It is also helpful to talk about her friends and her relationships. Teens can be more chatty about their friends than about themselves, but listening to what their friends are doing will offer insight into how your teen herself feels.

Don't ask too many questions, or you won't get any information at all. Provide a respectful place for sharing what she is willing to share (excitement of first love, feeling valued, wanted, desired by someone else in a very different, intensely intimate way).

Keep it generic. Being willing to speak in generalities allows conversations about difficult subjects like sex to move forward without getting anyone too uncomfortable. Let your children know that you know of people that had certain experiences when they were younger, that you have been in difficult situations or know others who have been, and that you're not afraid to discuss those things on some level. Avoid interrogating your teen about what exactly they did or didn't do sexually; you don't want them to demand details about your love life, either. Keeping things on a surface level gives permission to continue the discussion over a greater breadth (and possibly depth) of topics and allow you to communicate more honestly about sex in ways that may very well be helpful one day.

Adolescence is for practice. The teenage years are great for learning about relationships. What is the difference between a crush and real love? Between a "boyfriend" or "girlfriend" and a friend who is a boy or a girl? What belongs on Facebook and what doesn't? How does he treat you when you're alone compared to when your friends or parents are around? Does she keep a confidence or tell all her friends about it the next day? Without a few battle scars, how will we know a good relationship when we see it? On the other hand, major mistakes that change our lives (like disease or unintended pregnancy) are best avoided.

Things that are hard are not without value. Help your teen learn from his or her mistakes. The goal is to learn to develop and maintain healthy relationship skills. Protecting your children from every trauma may not bring the message home, as well as the lessons learned from experiencing a broken heart themselves.

Beware of the "D" word. Children fear *disappointing* their parents more than just about anything else in the world. While you should let children know when their behavior is dangerous or wrong, be very clear that there is nothing they could ever do that would make you stop loving them. Reassure them that after your blood pressure comes down, you still want what's best for them and you will see they find help when they need it. Avoid getting into situations where their fear of your disappointment or anger keeps them from coming to you when they need you the most.

Be clear that safety is nonnegotiable. Think about your bottom-line priorities for your children. Chances are nothing matters more to you than their safety. Be very clear, and repeat often, that nothing matters more than knowing they are going to be okay. Establish a code word they can use to get your attention and help when they need to get out of a potentially dangerous or uncomfortable situation. Set a standard for protecting themselves from disease and unwanted pregnancy regardless of whether you agree with their decision-making about sex. Make sure that they know they can come to you for help if something goes wrong.

Find a surrogate. Talking about sex is difficult. When necessary, identify and encourage them to ask for help from other trusted adults; it doesn't always have to be you.

Build your own toolkit. Create a list of Web resources about sexuality that you believe offer sound information and advice. Consider keeping books at home that support your values about sexuality while providing accurate information. Find resources in your community, such as clinics, hotlines, therapeutic specialists, and support groups, in case you or your children need more help.

●● Group Learning and Discussion ●●

Mikayla is a 16-year-old female who's coming to see you for routine acne follow-up. Her mother asks to speak with you privately prior to the appointment. She explains that she is aware of her daughter's interest in using birth control pills to help with her acne and is willing to consider this, but she is worried her daughter will see it as permission to have sex. Her mother believes Mikayla's assertion that she and her boyfriend are not having sex, but is worried about how being on the pill may change this.

1. Whom do you put in the examination room first? Mikayla alone? Mikayla and her mother together? Discuss the potential benefits and difficulties of each approach.
2. How would you explain the role of hormonal therapy in this situation?
3. How much time would you allow for discussion of sexuality in a routine acne follow-up visit?
4. Collaborate with colleagues about ways to approach the subject of sexuality in front of teens and parents (individually and together) to earn trust from each.
   a. Do you speak differently to teens when the parent leaves the room?
   b. How can you avoid the "we have a secret" mentality when reuniting a parent and teen to wrap up your assessment and recommendations at the end of an adolescent visit?
5. Role-play for your colleagues how you anticipate the conversation going between you and the mother, you and the teen, and between all 3 of you in the same room.

Kayla, age 13, has been brought in by her parents after they found out she sent a picture of her breasts to a boy from school over the weekend. They have lectured her about sexting and why it is dangerous. They want you to reinforce this message and find out what else she may have been doing. They would like her tested for sexually transmitted infections while she is here. In the meantime, they have taken away her cell phone, her computer, and her privileges to be out with friends for the next month.

1. Consider the developmental attributes of early to middle adolescence.
   a. How would you assess whether Kayla's thoughts about sexuality are consistent with her developmental staging?
   b. How would you assess whether the sexting was an impulsive teenage mistake or a sign of underlying behavioral or emotional concerns?
2. Role-play with colleagues on how you would counsel Kayla and her parents and how your approach would differ depending on your answers to the question above.

●● Group Learning and Discussion, continued ●●

Miranda, age 17, is upset that her younger sister Shannon, age 15, is having sex. Miranda feels obligated to tell her parents what is going on and asks your advice.

1. Consider the following as you formulate your response:
   a. How do Miranda's own feelings about sexuality play into this situation?
   b. What do you think is her responsibility given the circumstances?
   c. How can you help Miranda to be a supportive big sister?
2. Role-play the conversation from different perspectives (whether Miranda may be simply jealous, bossy, appropriately concerned about safety, etc).

■■■■■■■■ Continuing Education ■■■■■■■■

If you are applying for continuing education credits, a test is available online. For more details, visit www.aap.org/reachingteens.

■ Related Video Content

10.0 Sexuality: A Normal Aspect of Adolescent Development. Clark.

10.1 All Adolescents Are Sexual Beings Deserving of Guidance. Clark.

10.2 We Must Teach Teens That Sexuality Is so Much More Than Sex. Clark.

10.3 "How Do You Know if You're Ready?" Talking to Teens About Delaying Intercourse. Clark, Jenkins, Chaffee.

10.4 Parents as (Positive or Negative) Role Models: Helping Youth Discuss What They Have Learned About Relationships at Home. Chaffee.

10.5 "Don't, Don't, Don't!" Does Not Adequately Educate Youth About Healthy and Safe Sexuality. Jenkins.

10.6 Case: A Comprehensive Office-Based Conversation on Healthy Sexuality With a Teen and her Mother. Sugerman.

8.1 Puberty 101. Sugerman.

11.1 Your Gender Does Not Limit Your Ability to Address Healthy Sexuality With Any Teen. Catallozzi, Bell.

11.2 Why Addressing Sexual Behavior During Adolescence Affects Health and Well-being Over the Life Span. Ford.

11.7 Who Should Get Tested for HIV and Other STIs? Reirden, Garofalo.

18.11 SSHADESS Screen: Pearls on Asking About Sexuality. Dowshen, Diaz, Pletcher, Reirden.

18.17 Case: SSHADESS Screen Reveals Teen Feeling Uncomfortable With Sexual Experience. Lerman.

56.5 Healthy Relationships Include Communication About Your Sexual Needs. Clark.

56.6 Assessing the Health of Sexual Relationships. Chaffee.

56.7 Case Example: Talking About Relationships as Part of a Sexual Health Visit. Sugerman.

■ Related Handouts/Supplementary Materials

Pointers for Parents: Raising Sexually Healthy Children

Relationship Requirements (from the heart and the head)

Your most important goal: Love and Protect Yourself

Visit www.ahwg.net for more patient and parent handouts (see below).

■ Related Web Sites

Advocates for Youth

www.advocatesforyouth.org

Great information for parents, teens, educators, physicians, and advocates. Encourages responsible decisions about reproductive and sexual health.

The Adolescent Health Working Group

www.ahwg.net

Various resources and toolkits offered by the Adolescent Health Working Group for providers, youth, parents/caregivers, and educators on many teen issues, including adolescent sexual health from the Adolescent Health Working Group.

Amy Schalet, PhD

www.amyschalet.com

Lead author of the "ABCD paradigm" (**A**utonomy, **B**uilding healthy relationships, **C**onnectedness, and **D**iversity) promoting conversations between teens and adults (parents/guardians) about appropriate readiness for sexuality.

Bedsider

www.bedsider.org

Simple, straightforward guide to birth control options and how to use them effectively.

StayTeen.org

www.stayteen.org

An initiative for teens sponsored by The National Campaign to Prevent Teen and Unplanned Pregnancy.

Iwannaknow.org

www.iwannaknow.org

Sexual health information for teens and young adults for facts, support, and resources to answer questions, find referrals, and get in-depth information about sexual health, sexually transmitted infections, healthy relationships, etc. A site of the American School Health Association.

Love Is Not Abuse

www.loveisnotabuse.com

Loveisrespect.org

www.loveisrespect.org

Parenting Teens

www.parentingteensonline.com

Articles for parents on adolescent health, teen sexuality, risk behaviors, mental health, and media safety.

Physicians for Reproductive Choice and Health

www.prch.org/arshepdownloads

Offers modules for providers on suggested practices for adolescent reproductive and sexual health care.

Center for Young Women's Health, Boston Children's Hospital

www.youngwomenshealth.org

Comprehensive information about everything from puberty to periods, birth control pills, polycystic ovary syndrome, pregnancy prevention, and more.

■ Related Resources

Berman L. *Talking to Your Kids About Sex: Turning "The Talk" Into a Conversation for Life.* New York, NY: DK Publishing; 2009

Ginsburg K. *Building Resilience in Children and Teens: Giving Kids Roots and Wings.* 2nd ed. Elk Grove Village, IL: American Academy of Pediatrics; 2011

Ginsburg K, Fitzgerald S. *Letting Go with Love and Confidence: Raising Responsible, Resilient, Self-Sufficient Teens in the 21st Century.* New York, NY: Penguin Group; 2011

Harris RH, Emberly M. *It's Perfectly Normal: A Book about Changing Bodies, Growing Up, Sex, and Sexual Health.*, Somerville, MA: Candlewick Press; 2009

Richardson J, Schuster MA. *Everything You Never Wanted Your Kids to Know About Sex (But Were Afraid They'd Ask): The Secrets to Surviving Your Child's Sexual Development from Birth to the Teens.* New York, NY: Three Rivers Press; 2004

Schalet AT. *Not Under My Roof: Parents, Teens, and the Culture of Sex.* Chicago, IL: University of Chicago Press; 2011

CHAPTER 11

Male Sexuality

David L. Bell, MD, MPH

Kenneth R. Ginsburg, MD, MS Ed, FAAP, FSAHM

■ Why This Matters

Healthy sexuality is central to healthy development. Healthy sexuality is tightly linked to both an individual's sense of self and ability to enter into an intimate partnership. Consequently, a great deal of attention is focused on helping adolescents develop healthy sexuality while avoiding the risks that are often associated with sexual awakening.

An objective observer of our approach to sexuality would likely note a marked disparity between the attention given to males and females. Males are looked at rather monolithically, almost as predators, and little regard is noted of the complexity of their thoughts and fears, and less is made of them as individuals capable of having intimate relationships. We can and must do better.

> **We need to address the constraining myth: "Males only want sex, not intimacy." Many sociology studies disprove this concept. Both emotional and physical intimacy are core human needs that, when fulfilled, enhance our physical and mental health.**

■ Disparities

Why is there such a difference in the attention given to male versus female sexuality? It may be that female development comes with an "event"—menstruation—for which young women need to be prepared. It may be that girls tend to ask more questions, while boys may tend to grow more silent with the advent of adolescence. The fear of pregnancy may come into play, with girls needing to be "protected." It may be that girls are being prepared to be mothers and that communication and intimacy are considered essential ingredients of motherhood (and not fatherhood?). Perhaps it is that we view boys so narrowly when it comes to their sexuality that we don't think there is much to talk about. We do not feign to be able to understand the complex interplay of factors that makes us treat boys and girls differently here, we only call for male sexuality to be given the attention it deserves.

■ Animal Urges 11.14

As long as we treat young males as animals we will keep them in "cages" that prevent them from reaching their potential in intimate relationships.

Consider the prevailing boxes in which we place the genders. Young women are seen as prey and men as predators. Think for a moment about how often you have heard a phrase that conveys these essential notions.

"Boys have only one thing on their minds."

"Boys think between their legs."

"Look at that boy, he's on the prowl."

Remember that adolescence is a time when youth are figuring out the answer to the fundamental question, "Who am I?" and its corollary question, "Am I normal?" Further recall that one of the key principles of resilience theory is that youth live up or down to the expectations we set for them. When we understand these contexts, it becomes even clearer that there is great potential harm in simplifying male sexuality into animalistic urges. Civility seems out of the range of something to be discussed, intimacy is not even worthy of consideration. Confusion and complexity of feelings make no sense. Youth who feel as if they want to delay their entrée into the sexual world feel abnormal.

■ Intimacy Is Masculine: Involved Fatherhood Is an Expression of Masculinity

We cannot both lament the absence of fathers in the lives of their children and perpetuate the myth of males as operating primarily to fill their animal urges. Sexuality is tied to intimacy. Intimacy is critical to relationships. Relationships are essential to building and maintaining healthy families. Fathers should be expected to be full and equal partners in families.

A first step in transforming the conversations and low expectations of boys is to commit to not raising boys to think that intimacy is feminine. They need to know that strong men address feelings, masculine men attend to the feelings and needs of their partners, and there is no more masculine role than to be an involved, engaged parent. Next, we need to address the constraining myth: "Males only want sex, not intimacy." Many sociology studies disprove this concept. Males want intimate relationships as well. Both emotional and physical intimacy are core human needs that, when fulfilled, enhance our physical and mental health.

■ First Things First: Understanding the Mechanics

Boys may be less likely to ask the questions, but they still need the answers. For this reason, we should address the following topics routinely, much as females are taught about breast development and menstruation.
- Pubertal development
- Masturbation
- Frequent erections
- Nocturnal emissions
- Ejaculation

■ Parents' Role in Sexuality Education

Many parents are squeamish about discussions about sexuality. Some fear that discussions give implicit permission to start having sex. Professionals can help parents understand their vital role in discussions around respect and intimacy. We can guide them that when they do not choose to have these discussions they relinquish this part of their son's education to their peers, the media, or even pornography.

■ Sex Is Not a Singular Act

Sexual awakening is an expected, healthy phase of development. As long as sex is equated only to intercourse, we will have a lot of youth rushing toward it. This may be particularly true for boys, who receive so many messages that they should be "doing it." If "it" is intercourse, the message is clear. When we have honest, open discussions about the wide range of sexual behaviors, "it" has many meanings. When sexual awakening is considered a journey that may begin with hand-holding and that progresses through kissing, more intimate touching, and finally with intercourse, we give young people permission to move slowly along a path that is satisfying and physically and emotionally safe. When our conversations are limited to intercourse, we should not be surprised when our youth move quickly toward intercourse in response to their natural sexual maturation.

How to Make Love to a Woman 11.5

The truth is that male and female sexuality are different. Although we cannot sort out what part of that is biologically ingrained versus a response to socialization, a difference remains. Male pleasure tends to be more focused on the genitals, whereas female pleasure involves more erogenous zones and focuses more on the relationship.

Boys need to better understand female sexuality in order to give them permission to both develop their own sense of intimacy and to slow down. A good conversation starter (or shocker!) is to ask a young man if he wants to talk about how to be a great lover. At first, he may be embarrassed at even broaching the topic, but will usually agree to the conversation with both anticipation and hesitation. He likely will come to the conversation with the expectation that female sexuality clearly parallels male sexuality.

Once granted permission to have the conversation, a good opening line is *"What part of a guy do you think a woman thinks is sexiest?"* You'll enjoy the answers. Depending on age, the answers tend to range from genitals to certain muscle groups (buttocks, shoulders, chest, arms.) Tell them that the answer women usually give is "eyes." After a moment of disgust, most boys will say *"What? Uh…Why?"* This is your opportunity to begin the conversation about intimacy and respect. *"When they look into your eyes they see if you are listening to them, respecting them, and valuing their opinion. Most of making love to women is about your relationship."* Then you can proceed to have conversations about sensuality and female erogenous zones. This will reinforce the fact that the best lovers do not focus on intercourse but on sensuality, intimacy, and communication. It also may decrease their self-imposed and externally reinforced pressure to rush toward intercourse as they realize that moving slowly makes them better lovers.

Men Have Feelings Too

It is important to ask about and discuss the relationships young men have. Rarely do many young men have a safe and trusted space to speak honestly and truthfully about how they feel about their relationships. They honor and appreciate the opportunity to be heard. It is also important to foster conversations about the overall health of their sexual relationships.

Males Have a Variety of Attractions 11.12

The lack of acceptance of men who have sex with men and men who have sex with both men and women comes at a high cost. More men are gay than self-identify as gay, and more men have sex with men than report it. The fact that there is not the same acceptance of the fluidity in sexuality as there is with females may contribute to men keeping their behavior secret.

It is important for professionals to discuss relationships without regard to the gender of the partner. One approach to discussions assessing sexual behavior and relationships starts with a general rule to keep the gender of the partner neutral. For example, how many partners have you had sex with in the past 2 months? Were they female, male, or both? Inquiries about sexual orientation and sexual attractions can happen organically based on their answers or reactions to the initial questions. Even asking the open-ended question about different sexual behaviors and sexual partners, when done with an accepting tone, signals that the professional is open to the discussion.

As stated previously, our cultural beliefs and biases about men's sexuality create unhealthy emotional and behavioral "cages" for adolescent males and men throughout life. Here are a few beliefs and biases that have significant broad mental health and psychosocial consequences that affect males regardless of their sexual identities or orientation, in many cases even if one is heterosexual or "straight." (1) You must continually prove your heterosexuality or your "manhood" or always face doubts by others if you act in any way outside of the box of being a heterosexual male. (2) "Men are always ready for sex." If a young man does not have sex, is not ready for sex, or does not want to have sex with a particular woman, he and others might question his sexual orientation. This can continue throughout the life span. Males are many times under pressure to perform in sexual relationships to prove themselves, sometimes with a mild to high degree of coerciveness. Their reputation in their peer group is tied to their sexual activity. (3) Most men have concurrent multiple partners. If you don't, your core masculinity is in question. This myth persists despite evidence that most men and women report similar numbers of partners in the past 12 months. Anecdotally, many young men that have reported having many partners and always being ready for sex report that sex loses its enticement after a while. They want more from the relationships than just sex.

Cultural fears of being seen as or called non-heterosexual even impact on men's friendships. In many male relationships, homophobia plays some role in the degree of nonsexual intimacy or in limiting the demonstration of culturally allowed or sanctioned affection. Strong or close friendships, if a male has them, can offer safe havens to jokingly mock these cultural sanctions (see Chapter 61).

Males Have Worries Too 11.11

A good strategy in addressing males' sexual concerns is to normalize their questions and concerns. Use phrases such as, *"Many guys have asked that same question...; Many guys have told me that...."* This strategy helps to keep the dialogue open and lets the individual avoid isolation or embarrassment.

Penis Size

Our culture gives mixed messages about penis size, making this a disclosed or undisclosed concern for many men. A common retort is *"It's the not the size, but the motion of the ocean that counts."* Many times this response is given without exploring the context of the concerns. Ask why they are concerned. Ask if anyone they have been sexually intimate with has remarked about their size. Ask if they are comparing their size to anyone else's size—in their personal life, in magazines, or on videos. An honest discussion about penis size can help ease many worries. It may also be helpful to put their concern to rest with knowledge that flaccid penis lengths rarely predict erect penis lengths. In addition, knowing that the average flaccid penis length is 1 to 4 inches and average erect length is 5 to 7 inches may put their concerns into perspective.

A common issue raised by health educators is that one size condom fits all. Even though demonstrations confirm that a condom can fit over one's skull or arm or the melon of choice, the unspoken story is that skulls, arms, or melons of any type do not have the same nerve innervations or infrastructure as the penis. The best message for males is to find the brand and type of condom that fits and feels the best and then to use them consistently.

Pleasure

On average, males are more apt to experience the immediate physical pleasure of orgasms. However, young men may disclose an inability to experience orgasms. Often a solution is to discuss the consistent use of condoms. Motivational interviewing strategies (see Chapter 26) can reveal anxiety about pregnancy or infections after an unprotected sexual episode. We can facilitate young men to understand that condoms diminish anxiety and increase pleasure overall and in the long term.

Sexual Functioning

Many adolescent and young males can experience episodes of sexual dysfunction. It is important to normalize the occasional episode to diminish the possibility of a self-perpetuating cycle of dysfunction. However, young men with repeated experiences with dysfunction deserve a full history and examination. A good clue that a young man's erectile dysfunction is likely to be related to anxiety or stress is when they continue to awaken with erections.

Young men with chronic disease or mental health issues, particularly those on certain medications, may be at risk for erectile dysfunction. Their experiences with sexual dysfunction may be a factor in poor adherence to their medication regimens, so it may be worth exploring this issue whenever a young man is not being adherent.

Young men also worry about premature ejaculation. Although this is a common phenomenon for all men, it is particularly prevalent for adolescents. They may be particularly worried if they are exposed to locker room banter that exaggerates sexual performance or pornography that portrays unrealistic sexual acts. Although older adolescents will sometimes raise these issues, most young men keep their fears and anxieties about this silent. Therefore, it can be a point to raise routinely, *"Most young men ejaculate before they wish they would. Control comes with age."* It also might be worth reinforcing that because condom use minimally decreases sensation, it may delay ejaculation. There are Web sites available that teach men how to slow down ejaculation (www.nlm.nih.gov/medlineplus/ency/article/001524.htm and www.wikihow.com/Stop-Premature-Ejaculation). It is beyond the scope of this chapter to teach these strategies here, but health professionals should achieve a comfort level with this subject manner. History and conversations should include

- Asking about the quality of his relationship and the history of sexual relationships
- Asking if there are any observed patterns; for example, if there are any specific relationships where premature ejaculation occurred more often
- Normalizing the occurrence of premature ejaculation at some point for most males
- Discussing the importance of becoming aware of his levels of sexual arousal
  — Explain that males can manage their levels of sexual arousal with practice by
    ♦ Deep breathing
    ♦ Becoming aware and changing muscle tensions
    ♦ Changing focus of body sexual sensations from the penis to other areas of the body
    ♦ Changing positions and thrusts
    ♦ Changing masturbation practices—primarily to learn to slow the process

■ Birth Control Is a Shared Responsibility

We need to have conversations about birth control and self-protection with males just as we address these topics with women. They need to understand that parenthood is something so important that it needs to be delayed until they can offer a baby the sense of security and stability it deserves (see Chapter 51). They cannot assume that the young woman is handling birth control. Ideally, they will share this responsibility. At the least, they have to take personal responsibility over their procreation and safety.

This means that we should hold conversations with young men about effective condom use and about the ineffective practice of withdrawal. Conversations about condoms need to include

- Where to find them
- Checking the expiration date
- Which ones to use (latex)
- Size options (to their comfort)
- How to open the packages (no teeth)
- How to put them on (closing the tip and slowly rolling them down to be sure you know which way they roll)
- How and where to take them off (away from their partner)
- How to discard them

We also need to ask youth how often they use them. *"Did you use a condom the last time you had sex." "How many times did you use a condom out of the last 10 times you had sex?"* Then assess their desire to use condoms more regularly and ask them what makes a difference in whether or not they use a condom. Expect the following answers:

> *"Are you kidding? Always!"*
>
> *"Not if I'm with my girlfriend, but if I'm with someone else."*
>
> *"If I have them."*
>
> *"They don't feel right."*
>
> *"It's not natural."*
>
> *"They break anyway."*
>
> *"If a girl makes me wear them, I know not to trust her,"* or *"I don't want her to think I don't trust her."*
>
> *"It ruins the mood."*

Depending on the answer, you can assess their motivation to use condoms more consistently using motivational interview techniques: *"What is good about using condoms?"*; *"What is bad about using condoms?"* Using the "importance" ruler *"on a scale of 1 to 10, 10 being 'absolutely yes' and 1 being 'not at all,' how motivated are you to always use condoms?"*

"Why did you pick that number instead of a (2 numbers below their choice)? What would it take to move you to a (1–2 numbers above their choice)?" (See Chapter 26 for more information on motivational interviewing.)

Then directly and honestly address some of the barriers they may have previously stated:

"If I have them." If possible, dispense condoms. If this is not possible in your setting, refer to a center where condoms are accessible. Suggest that the young man keeps condoms with him routinely.

"It ruins the mood." This can be somewhat true. Discuss, however, how the consequence of not protecting oneself ruins many moods. If the young man is in a relationship, ideally condom use can become part of the sexual ritual.

"If I trust her." One of the biggest barriers to condom use is that they are sometimes viewed as a sign of mistrust. Instead we have to help youth understand that condom use is a sign of mutual respect. Further, when the elimination of condom use is viewed favorably, as a sign of growing trust, it makes it very hard to reinstitute their use if suspicion begins to enter the relationship. A policy of "condoms always" prevents these uncomfortable interactions.

"It's not natural." "You are absolutely right, we are not designed with latex on us. However, it also doesn't feel good or natural to have an STI."

"It doesn't feel right." In this case, a professional can have a frank conversation about finding a brand that fits right, and more effectively transmits heat. Further, it is an opportunity to talk about the fact that the decreased sensation delays ejaculation. Don't ask directly about their experience. Just state, in a matter-of-fact manner, *"You are right that it doesn't feel as good. But the truth is that it feels just as good when you cum, and you'll last longer. Most guys your age cum faster than they'd like and often before their partner has reached orgasm. Guys who wear condoms have decreased sensation—like you said—last longer because of it, and may be better lovers."*

"They break anyway." This is an opportunity to discuss proper size and placement of condoms. It is also an opportunity to have a conversation about lubrication and/or female sexuality. Talk about the importance of foreplay in producing female lubrication and how a male can assess a female's readiness for intercourse by assessing the presence of lubrication with his fingers.

In the case of men who have sex with men, many of the above conversations also apply. But here, the importance of lubrication is even more critical.

●● Group Learning and Discussion ●●

Sexuality is an uncomfortable subject for many of us to discuss generally. It may be even more uncomfortable to discuss with adolescents. However, when we do not, then we leave adolescents' sexuality unduly influenced by peers and media. In the case of young men, this might mean that relationships and intimacy will never be discussed. In the case of young men with same-sex attractions, this might mean an ongoing and unnecessary isolation. In the case of adolescents with sexual anxieties, this will mean their fears and sense of inadequacy will build.

Break into pairs and practice discussing healthy male sexuality with the following young men.

Scenario 1
A 16-year-old male who presents for his yearly sports examination. He denies ever having sexual intercourse.

Scenario 2
A 19-year-old male who presents with anxiety. After confidentiality is assured, he blurts out that he is having tremendous discomfort because of his attractions to his college roommate.

Scenario 3
A 17-year-old male who presents with premature ejaculation.

■■■■■■■■ Continuing Education ■■■■■■■■

If you are applying for continuing education credits, a test is available online. For more details, visit www.aap.org/reachingteens.

■ Suggested Reading

Chandra A, Mosher WD, Copen C, Sionean C. Sexual behavior, sexual attraction, and sexual identity in the United States: data from the 2006–2008 National Survey of Family Growth. *Nat Health Stat Report.* 2011;3(36):1–36

Herbenick D, Reece M, Schick V, Sanders SA, Dodge B, Fortenberry JD. Sexual behavior in the United States: results from a national probability sample of men and women ages 14–94. *J Sex Med.* 2010;7:255–265

Levant RF. Toward the reconstruction of masculinity. In: Levant RF, Pollack WS, eds. *A New Psychology of Men.* New York, NY: Basic Books; 1996:230–51

Martinez G, Copen CE, Abma JC. Teenagers in the United States: sexual activity, contraceptive use, and childbearing, 2006–2010 National Survey of Family Growth. *Vital Health Stat 23.* 2011;1–35

Ott MA. Examining the development and sexual behavior of adolescent males. *J Adolesc Health.* 2010;46:S3–S11

Pathela P, Hajat A, Schillinger J, Blank S, Sell R, Mostashari F. Discordance between sexual behavior and self-reported sexual identity: a population-based survey of New York City men. *Ann Intern Med.* 2006;145:416–25

■ Related Video Content

11.1 Your Gender Does Not Limit Your Ability to Address Healthy Sexuality With Any Teen. Catallozzi, Bell.

11.2 Why Addressing Sexual Behavior During Adolescence Affects Health and Well-being Over the Life Span. Ford.

11.3 Promoting Condom Use in Young Men. Bell.

11.4 Masturbation: If Parents Ignore It and Professionals Ignore It, Who Will Discuss It? Campbell.

11.5 Young Men Need to Learn That Respecting Women and Understanding Female Sexuality Enhances Their Ability to Be Good Lovers. Ginsburg.

11.6 Sensitively Performing a Male Genital Examination. Ginsburg.

11.7 Who Should Get Tested for HIV and Other STIs? Reirden, Garofalo.

11.8 Beyond Risk Management: Discussing Intimacy and Healthy Sexuality. Chaffee.

11.9 Model Discussion With Young Man on Healthy Male Sexuality. Bell.

11.10 A Comprehensive Approach to Discussing Healthy Male Sexuality. Bell.

11.11 Male Concerns About Sexual Dysfunction and Infertility. Bell.

11.12 Avoiding Labels: Exploring Attractions, Behaviors, and Orientation. Hawkins, Arrington-Sanders.

11.13 Teaching Young Men About Sexually Transmitted Infections. Bell.

11.14 Refuting the Damaging Myths About Male Sexuality. Bell.

11.15 If We Are to Build Strong Men Destined to Be Good Husbands and Fathers, We Need to Raise Our Sons With Love and Affection. Bell.

Connecting With Adolescents and Their Families

If we are to enter adolescents' lives, they need to understand that we genuinely care for them and are worthy of their trust. Although trust is something that is built over time, an initial impression can make a difference, especially for a marginalized teen. Sadly, many adolescents become used to being judged and held to low expectations, making it necessary for us to demonstrate that we expect the best of them. "Creating an Adolescent-Friendly Space and Service" (Chapter 12) describes how we can create an environment welcoming to teens. "Creating a Male Adolescent-Friendly Space" (Chapter 13) discusses some specific strategies to welcome young men to our services and then engage them in our care. "Setting the Stage for a Trustworthy Relationship" (Chapter 14) offers a strategy to initially address some

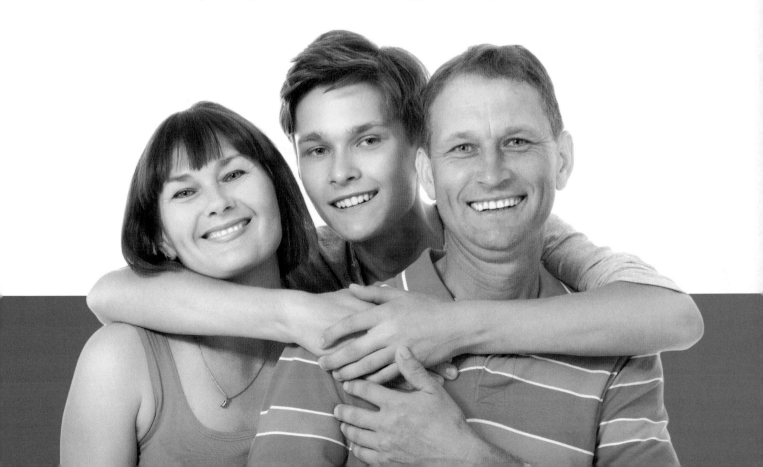

of the major issues teens and families consider as they extend their trust to you. The words that a professional might use to engage a teen are only a portion of what is communicated. "Body Language" (Chapter 15) describes how we can reinforce or undermine our connection with youth through nonverbal communication.

CHAPTER 12

Creating an Adolescent-Friendly Space and Service

Angela Diaz, MD, MPH

 Related Video Content

12.0 Creating an Adolescent-Friendly Space

■ Why This Matters

Adolescents are full of promise and yet remain at risk and, as a group, face significant health disparities. Many people believe adolescents are naturally robust and need minimal, if any, health care. In reality, large numbers of teens have serious health problems—even more have significant health needs, including need for mental health services.[1-3] Thus in 1997 the American Medical Association classified adolescents as a population developmentally at the "crossroads" of good and poor health, and this remains true today.[4]

Here are a few examples of unmet needs.

> **Adolescent health concerns are as much emotional and behavioral as they are physical. Having comprehensive, integrated services under one roof is the ideal solution. Even if you don't have all the services under one roof, you can still create an adolescent zone of safety where you can ask about each teen's life, including about their health and behaviors, their emotional and family life, and their environment. Never forget that the most important thing under the roof is the people who are committed to serving adolescents with unconditional love, nurturance, and absolute respect.**

- 1 in 5 adolescents has a significant health problem, and many more have significant needs, yet very large numbers forgo care.[5]
- At least 20% of teens have significant mental health problems; yet only 1 in 5 of these will get the services they need.[6]
- 9% of all 10- to 17-year-olds and 12% of poor 10- to 17-year-olds have limitation of activity due to a chronic health condition.[7]
- Despite the need for health care, adolescents and young adults make fewer physician visits compared to other age groups. The percent of total physician visits by teens is 9.1% compared to teens representing 15.5% of the population.[8]
- Black and Latino adolescents and young adults face even higher disparities, despite their greater need and lower health status.[9,10]
- Despite the opportunity adolescents present us for health promotion, they lack the preventive education and interventions they need.[11]

We should strive toward ensuring greater health equity. This requires the careful consideration of adolescent-specific needs in terms of service design and approach.

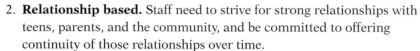

■ A Framework for Creating an Adolescent-Friendly Environment

To be adolescent friendly, services should strive to be

1. **Staffed by teen-friendly people.** Teens know when they are valued versus held to low expectations. Staff need to like teens and have both the skills to communicate with them and to hold a sense of purpose to deliver high-quality services to them.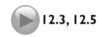

2. **Relationship based.** Staff need to strive for strong relationships with teens, parents, and the community, and be committed to offering continuity of those relationships over time.

3. **Accessible.** Sites need to be geographically and financially accessible, easily identifiable, and easy to access for services both by appointment and walk-in.

4. **Safe.** A "safe space" is welcoming and warm, with art and furniture that communicate teens are welcome.

5. **Non-stigmatizing.**

6. **Confidential.**

7. **Adolescent specific.** This is ideal, but may not always be possible. When it is not possible, consider creating an adolescent space or time.

8. **Holistic, comprehensive, coordinated, and interdisciplinary.** Either directly or through a network of connected organizations, the services should focus on wellness, health education, prevention, and primary care, while also offering acute and tertiary care.

9. **Based on a bio-psycho-socio-cultural-spiritual approach.**

Services should be accessible (geographically and financially), easily identifiable, and easy for a teen to get into.

Adolescence is a time of increasing independence, yet adolescents are still learning how to navigate the world on their own. In the past, they may have been taken to a professional by a parent and may be unused to acting on their own behalf. They may be unsure of exactly where to go for care or how to access it.

A Safe Place With No Attached Stigma

Adolescents require a "safe space" that is welcoming, with art and furniture for teens, and with no stigma attached to help seeking.

Seeking care for the first time under their own steam may be scary, intimidating, and strange for any teen. Even those who are not visiting for the first time, or who are accompanied by a parent, still have a lot to learn about what is expected and how to talk about concerns and problems. The physical environment is very important. It helps if it is attractive and colorful, but even very humble surroundings are okay as long as the place has positive messages for youth. The kind of messages that are on the walls as posters, or as artwork, or are found in brochures can signal to teens that the place is a safe place where they can talk about any issue. A safe space is a place that encourages kids to talk about any issue they have on their mind. Posters—not just about sex, drugs, and rock and roll, but also about safety, abuse, and trauma; about lesbian, gay, transgender, and questioning youth; about cultural identity, race, and racism; about education, careers, and work; about aspirations and dreams—tell the young person that this is a place where everyone is welcomed and anything can be discussed.

Non-stigmatizing means that not only should a teen not feel labeled for walking in the door but also that it should not be apparent to others who are in the waiting area for which particular services the adolescent has come. For example, having specific days or clinic areas designated for teen pregnancy or for eating disorders, will create a potentially stigmatizing and embarrassing situation for teens seeking those services.

Confidentiality Is a Cornerstone of Adolescent Health Care

Because adolescent health involves highly personal and sensitive subjects, such as sexuality and sex, many adolescents need assurance that they can talk confidentially with their provider. As a result, privacy is recognized as one of the cornerstones of adolescent health care. Some teens can talk to their parents and some cannot. Confidentiality laws level the field so all teens can get the services they need. Otherwise, many teens would elect not to get necessary care out of fear of disappointing adults in their lives or even receiving recrimination.

Confidentiality protection helps ensure that teens get the services they need. It is essential that professionals familiarize themselves with their state confidentiality laws. We can advocate for strengthening confidentiality laws when this will improve teens' access to services.

Providers need to discuss confidentiality with the adolescent and their parents from the beginning of their relationship, and they should also discuss the fact that confidentiality is conditional and describe when the provider is required by law to inform a parent or the authorities (see Chapter 14). For example, confidentiality will not be maintained when the patient's safety or that of others is threatened, such as in abuse situations, or when a patient is suicidal or homicidal.

Confidentiality protection does not leave families out of the equation. While the primary relationship is between the professional and the youth, parents are also important clients in adolescent care. Providers should also talk to teens about including their parents in their health care decisions and facilitate it when necessary. Confidentiality laws help some teens come for help, and eventually the provider can help the teen to better communicate with his or her parents. Handled correctly, confidentiality does not interfere with the parent-teen relationship but instead, over time, has the potential to strengthen that relationship. The key is to provide confidential care to teens while at the same time helping parents feel involved and included.

How I Ensure That I Can Have a Private Conversation With Each and Every Adolescent

First discuss confidentiality with the teen—and with the parent if he or she is present. When a parent is present with the teen, I ask the teen and the parent how I can be of help and then proceed to take the nonconfidential history from the teen and involve parents in medical history, family history, or any place where I think they may be helpful.

Then I ask the parents or other adult to go to the waiting room explaining, *"So that I can continue to talk with your child and do a physical exam, and when I am finished I will invite you back to join us."*

When alone with the teen I proceed with the sensitive issues. I say that I will be asking the teen questions that I ask every teen. Then I ask about family relationships (including abuse and neglect), stresses and pressures the teen may feel, peer relationships, romantic relationships, and others. Sensitive issues, such as relationships, emotional well-being, and sexuality, are so personal that it is always better to communicate directly with the teen without a third person in the room. And because of this, when addressing a teen who does not speak your own language, it is better to use a professional translator who is familiar with the work if you can, and, if not, colleagues or other staff who are sensitive to the issues raised in working with teens. I try not to use the teen's family or friends.

Adolescent-Specific Services

Services should be adolescent specific, if possible, and should be easy to navigate.

Staff who offer adolescent-friendly services will be able to engage with young people in a developmentally appropriate manner that understands the changing lives of young people from early to late adolescence. Providers need to understand the strengths, language, behaviors, worries, and concerns of teens. In many ways, adolescents can be viewed as a culture group with subcultures within it, or as a cluster of culture groups. In my experience, some key characteristics of adolescents as a group are that they

- Like to be respected
- Like to be liked
- Like to be talked with not talked to
- Don't like other people knowing their business unless they tell
- Don't like to be shamed and are proud
- Are not likely to volunteer information unless asked
- Are generally modest
- See beyond the surface
- Feel vulnerable, not invincible

Teens will respond if asked directly about their lives in a nonjudgmental manner. They need to be given permission to talk. If we don't ask, generally they won't tell. In one large national representative study of teens,[12] most reported that their providers frequently failed to ask them about issues such as sexual risk, violence, abuse, and other risk factors. Among those considered at highest risk, one-third had not discussed what they wanted to with their provider and only 12% had discussed everything they wanted to. Yet these issues often have a tremendous impact on health.[13] So the provider should learn to be comfortable asking direct questions about all aspects of the teen's life.

Holistic, Comprehensive Care

Services should be holistic, comprehensive, coordinated, and interdisciplinary, and should be rooted in a bio-psycho-socio-cultural-spiritual approach.

Adolescence is a time of experimentation, and the health of adolescents is shaped largely by interrelated behavioral and social factors. Teen health is determined by a complex interaction of physical, behavioral, emotional, familial, and social-environmental variables and, in many ways, the health problems of teens are social morbidities.

For example, the following risk factors are reported among high school students[14]:

- 7.5% had had intercourse before age 13, and 17.5% reported their last intercourse was unprotected.
- 28.7% had persistent sadness and 17.6% reported they had had suicidal thoughts/plans.
- 16% reported abnormal weight loss behavior.
- 8.2% were currently frequent smokers, 28.7% reported problem behavior with alcohol, and more than 20% had used marijuana in the past month.
- 21.8% engaged in 2 or more fights in the past year and 18.5% had carried a weapon in the past month.

Furthermore, these risks are highly interrelated. For example,

- 43.6% of those who had intercourse before age 13 had problem alcohol behavior.
- Of those who reported that their last intercourse was unprotected: 43.5% reported frequent sadness, 25.8% reported abnormal weight loss behaviors, and almost 46% had problem drinking.

Adolescents often have multiple needs and concerns. However, they do not have the experience to sort out these various needs. They have not learned to think of their health needs in terms of the silos by which many health services are organized and their health concerns are as much emotional and behavioral and value driven as they are physical. For many who are seeking care independently for the first time, they may have a worry or crisis that is driving them to seek care.

Having comprehensive, integrated services under one roof is the ideal solution. But, if you don't have all the services under one roof, you still must ask comprehensively about each teen's life, strengths, assets, and interests, including not just health and behaviors, but emotional and family life, and environment. That's the heart of serving adolescents. ▶ 12.9

Regardless of where you serve teens, a model of care rooted in a bio-psycho-socio-cultural-spiritual approach provides the framework to engage each aspect of an adolescent's life.

•• Group Learning and Discussion ••

This group learning and discussion experience is going to begin with a field trip. If your group is large, you may need to break into groups of 3 to 5. Go outside of your setting and reenter it wearing the lens of a teen coming in for the first time.

1. Is the front desk staff prepared to receive the youth in a universally respectful, nonjudgmental manner? Will the teen feel as if staff likes young people?

2. Will the teen feel stigmatized on entry? Will it be clear that coming to this site or attending this particular session means that he or she carries a specific diagnosis, or has a particular problem?

3. As the teen sits in the waiting room, what messages will be received by looking at the décor, the colors, and the posters? Will people who look like him or her be present or absent in the messaging on the posters? Will adolescents be depicted in a positive or negative light? Will the message be "Danger: Teens at Risk!!!"? Can there be a message, "Teens are wonderful, they just may need a little help."?

4. As teens wait for your services, will they have something to do or will there only be magazines available targeted for children or preteen girls?

5. Would a young man feel as welcomed as a young woman?

6. As the teen sits in your waiting area, will he or she be alone or are enough adolescents present that a tipping point has occurred where they feel welcomed? If you serve few adolescents, have you considered creative scheduling to cohort them so they feel less isolated?

Process your findings together and develop a strategy to address any shortcomings. Above all, ask your group to consider whether you are currently using a problem-focused approach or a strength-based bio-psycho-socio-cultural-spiritual approach.

■■■■■■■■ Continuing Education ■■■■■■■■

If you are applying for continuing education credits, a test is available online. For more details, visit www.aap.org/reachingteens.

■ References

1. Diaz A, Peake K, Surko M, Bhandarkar K. Including "at-risk" adolescents in their own health and mental health care: a youth development perspective. *Soc Work Ment Health*. 2004;3(1–2):3–22

2. McManus MA, Shejavali KI, Fox HB. *Is the Health Care System Working for Adolescents? Perspectives from Providers in Boston, Denver, Houston, and San Francisco*. Washington, DC: Maternal and Child Health Policy Research Center; 2003

3. Fairbrother G, Scheinmann R, Newell K, Klein J, Osthimer B, Dutton M. *In Their Own Voices: A Report on Health Care from Low-Income Adolescents in New York City*. New York, NY: New York Academy of Medicine, University of Rochester, and Children's Defense Fund; 2004

4. American Medical Association. *American Medical Association: Guidelines for Adolescent Preventive Services*. Chicago, IL: American Medical Association; 1997

5. Ames N. Medically underserved children's access to health care: a review of the literature. *J Hum Behav Soc Environ*. 2008;18(1):64–77

6. Kataoka SH, Zhang L, Wells KB. Unmet need for mental health among U.S. children: variation by ethnicity and insurance status. *Am J Psychiatry*. 2002;159(9):1548–1555

7. McManus MA, Fox HB. *Making the Case for Addressing Adolescent Health Care Fact Sheet No 3*. Washington, DC: National Alliance to Advance Adolescent Health; 2007

8. Ziv A, Boulet JR, Slap GB. Utilization of physician offices by adolescents in the United States. *Pediatrics*. 1999;104(1);35–42

9. Elster A, Jarosik, J, VanGeest, J, Fleming M. Racial and ethnic disparities in health care for adolescents: a systematic review of the literature. *Arch Pediatr Adolesc Med*. 2003;157:867–874

10. Vo DX, Park MJ. Racial/ethnic disparities and culturally competent health care among youth and young men. *Am J Mens Health*. 2008;2:192–205

11. McManus MA, Fox HB, Maloney SK, Diaz A, Morris A. *Strengthening Preventive Care to Better Address Multiple Health Risks Among Adolescents*. Washington, DC: The National Alliance to Advance Adolescent Health; 2010

12. Schoen C, Davis K, Scott Collins K, Greenberg L, Des Roches C, Abrams M. *The Commonwealth Fund Survey of the Health of Adolescent Girls*. New York, NY: The Commonwealth Fund; 1997. http://www.commonwealthfund.org/Publications/Fund-Reports/1997/Nov/The-Commonwealth-Fund-Survey-of-the-Health-of-Adolescent-Girls.aspx. Accessed June 26, 2013

13. Klein JD, Wilson KM. Delivering quality care: adolescents' discussion of health risks with their providers. *J Adolesc Health*. 2002;30:190–195

14. Fox HB, McManus MA, Arnold KA. Significant Multiple Risk Behaviors Among U.S. High School Students. Washington, DC: The National Alliance to Advance Adolescent Health; 2010

■ Related Video Content

12.0 Creating an Adolescent-Friendly Space. Diaz.

12.1 Creating an LGBTQ-Friendly Space. Dowshen, Arrington-Sanders, Hawkins.

12.2 Creating an Immigrant Youth-Friendly Space. Vo.

12.3 Ensuring a Space Without Judgment or Low Expectation so Risks and Hopes and Dreams Will Be Shared. Campbell.

12.4 Texting: Availability, Education, and Reminders Beyond Our Walls. Diaz.

12.5 Love and Respect Are Key Ingredients to Creating an Adolescent-Friendly Space. Diaz.

12.6 Do Not Assume Poor Youth Are Destined to Have Poor Outcomes: Access to Services Strongly Influences Outcomes. Diaz.

12.7 A Teen-Friendly Private Practice: Resources, Referrals, and Physical Setting. Sugerman.

12.8 A Diverse Environment Is a Safe Environment. Ginsburg.

12.9 Youth With a History of Homelessness or Unstable Housing Share What They Need From Youth-Serving Agencies. Youth.

12.10 "Trust? What's the Point?…I Guess It's That People Kept Pushing." Adolescent-Friendly Services Never Give Up on Youth. Youth.

12.11 "It's About the People Who Are Here"—The Central Element of an Adolescent-Friendly Space. Sidhu.

13.0 Creating a Welcoming Space for Young Men. Bell.

34.1 Professionals Support Parents by Creating a Space Where Teens Can Receive Caring, Objective Guidance Without Fear of Judgment or Punishment. Diaz.

CHAPTER 13

Creating a Male Adolescent-Friendly Space*

David L. Bell, MD, MPH

 Related Video Content

13.0 Creating a Welcoming Space for Young Men

■ Why This Matters

When we make a space adolescent friendly, we signal our desire and commitment to meet teen's needs and expectations. However, many of our environments are designed with greater attention to female adolescents. Although many of the concepts and strategies to creating teen-friendly spaces apply to all adolescents, males are worthy of particular attention both because they rarely get it and because it may take a greater effort to engage them in preventive services.

> **Young men want someone who speaks *with* them, not *at* them, who pauses to listen *to* them, not to think of the next topic to spew at them through an unrequested lecture.**

■ The People Matter Most

We are the most critical element. To make a teen male-friendly space, the people matter the most—from the front desk staff, to mid-level assistants, to the professionals. Males are keenly vigilant about how we treat them and how we communicate with them. They quickly sense whether they are deemed worthy of respect—or disdain. They take note of whether their needs seem to have been considered.

Their first impressions of the service's friendliness are likely made based on the choice of words and tones of voices of our telephone staff and our front desk staff. First impressions are also made as they observe how we treat and talk to each other and to other teens present in the office. Our interactions generate important initial and ongoing impressions that determine the perceived safety and friendliness of our spaces.

Most importantly, males want respectful, knowledgeable, and genuinely caring professionals. They want, as we all do, to be asked questions in a respectful manner. As importantly, they want someone that listens to them in an open, nonthreatening, personable, nonjudgmental manner. They want someone who speaks *with* them, not *at* them, who pauses to listen *to* them, not to think of the next topic to spew at them through an unrequested lecture. In addition, making the interview feel like an easy conversation creates

---

*Chapter 12, "Creating an Adolescent-Friendly Space and Service," addresses the general needs of adolescents, including males. This chapter focuses specifically on meeting the needs and expectations of males.

a safe place to ask questions about a range of topics, including those related to health, relationships, and stress.

For most males, the professional's gender does not matter as long as the above characteristics and traits are present. A minority of males cares about the gender of the provider, and their comfort level varies idiosyncratically with the types of conversations they want to have or, in the case of a health setting, their comfort level with the genital examination.

The Place Matters Too

Clean settings are generally important and contribute to a sense of order and well-being. In a medical setting, it is important to use universal precautions. Patients want to see that the office is clean, that the staff is using clean equipment, and that the clinician washes his or her hands and uses gloves appropriately. Youth have stated that they feel safer when they see staff opening clean needles and syringes from their packaging.

Empowering messages for both males and females can create and connect youth to a welcoming environment. Pictures, posters, bulletin boards, and magazines that are interesting to males are the "last" touches to make the ultimate male-friendly space. These pictures and posters should include males, whom the youth population can relate to according to age, race, and ethnicity.

Sometimes messages framed only to females support and reinforce our culture's negative biases toward males. Males receive so many messages that they care little about relationships, education, or childrearing. Strive to find posters and materials that promote positive messages and display affirming images of men. An example of a campaign that framed messages that speak to both males and females in all types of relationships in the important area of relationship violence is, "It is my strength not to hurt," a campaign by the organization Men Can Stop Rape.

Magazines are good ways to occupy time while waiting. Choose a few popular magazines that interest males, like sports, technology, car and motor, and male fashion magazines. If possible, choose a variety of magazines, so the young men do not believe you have simplistic or stereotyped views of who they might be or where their interests lie.

Recruitment

All of the above elements are important to any efforts to increase male use of services, but isolated males will not feel comfortable and may not return. "Recruiting" new males to your program can be easier than one initially imagines. Assuming young women primarily use your program or site, consider word-of-mouth marketing from females. Ask the females to recruit new males by spreading the news about the male services provided. Similarly, count on word of mouth from the males. Males that have good experiences will suggest your site to their friends, cousins, and sports mates.

The Health Setting

The Male Genital Examination

As adolescent providers, it is important to talk initially with the patient clothed. Sometimes the examination may be performed clothed while only exposing the body areas being focused on at the time. In other settings, according to the resources, and youth and clinician preferences, patients can be examined in gowns. Males, in general, if getting undressed will likely feel more comfortable keeping their underwear on until the time when their genitals are examined. This can alleviate the unwanted, anxiety-provoking erection, which can be uncomfortable for both the patient and clinician. If a young man gets an erection during the examination, it is important to complete the examination in a respectful and composed manner. It is inappropriate and unnecessary to walk out because of the erection or to get a chaperone immediately, assuming you do not perceive sexual intentions.

Sexual arousal research demonstrates that males can get sexually aroused for a variety of reasons. Genital arousal can occur apart from sexual desire. It can be due to environment cues—that they are naked in front of another person or that there are tactile sensations caused by a gown moving in the breeze or from the examination itself. Adolescents get erections particularly easily, and sometimes just worrying about the possibility will cause an erection.

After he has gotten dressed, acknowledge that many males get erections during the genital examination. Ideally, do this in a casual, matter-of-fact way, ▶ 11.6 while also reviewing the rest of the visit. *"I enjoyed meeting you today because of X. You were concerned about Y, which I hope we addressed to your satisfaction. Your exam was normal today (or today we found). You are growing normally in terms of your height and weight. Your sexual development is right on track as you grow into a man. You got an erection during the exam, as many young men do. That is further evidence that your sexual development is normal. One other thing you asked me to take note of is Z, which we can discuss."*

Use of Chaperones

Both patients and clinicians have the right to request chaperones, if there are perceived concerns about comfort, safety, or legal allegations. Like the presence of chaperones during a pelvic examination for a female patient, the chaperone does not have to directly observe the examination or the patient's genitalia. Their presence is for understanding and hearing the nature of the communications and interactions during the examination, preferably while sustaining a significant degree of privacy for the patient.

■ Concluding Thoughts

Creating a safe and friendly space for male adolescents is a core element of communicating that we are respectful of their needs and committed to meeting their expectations. First and foremost, it creates a welcoming and positive space. Perhaps above all, it creates an environment in which males can share their feelings honestly and explore issues that many in our culture do not believe they are capable of or interested in addressing. Given the right environment, males are not the monosyllabic beings they are perceived to be. They have a range of feelings that need to be processed and stresses they need to learn to manage. They will show us this side of themselves when they know that we genuinely consider it a pleasure and honor to serve them.

●● Group Learning and Discussion ●●

This group learning and discussion experience is going to begin with a field trip. If your group is large, you may need to break into groups of 3 to 5. Go outside of your setting and reenter it wearing the lens of a 15-year-old boy coming on his own for the first time.

1. Is the front desk staff prepared to receive him in a universally respectful, nonjudgmental manner?

2. As he sits in the waiting room, what messages will he receive by looking at the décor, the colors, and the posters? Will people who look like him be present or absent in the public health messaging on the posters? Will people who look like him be depicted in a positive or negative light?

3. As he waits, will he have something to do or will he only have magazines available targeted for children or preteen girls?

4. As he sits in your waiting area, will he be alone or have you recruited enough males that a tipping point has occurred where males feel welcomed? If you serve few males, have you considered creative scheduling to cohort them so they feel less isolated?

Process your findings together and develop a strategy to address any shortcomings.

■■■■■■■ Continuing Education ■■■■■■■■

If you are applying for continuing education credits, a test is available online. For more details, visit www.aap.org/reachingteens.

■ Suggested Reading

Armstrong B. Health promotion with adolescent and young adult males: an empowerment approach. *Adolesc Med State Art Rev.* 2011;22:544–580, xii

Ginsburg KR, Slap GB, Cnaan A, Forke CM, Balsley CM, Rouselle DM. Adolescents' perceptions of factors affecting their decisions to seek health care. *JAMA.* 1995;273:1913–1918

Kapphahn CJ, Wilson KM, Klein JD. Adolescent girls' and boys' preferences for provider gender and confidentiality in their health care. *Adolesc Health.* 1999;25:131–42

Men Can Stop Rape Strength Campaign. http://www.mencanstoprape.org/A-Comprehensive-Approach-The-Strength-Campaign. Accessed June 25, 2013

■ Related Video Content

13.0 Creating a Welcoming Space for Young Men. Bell.

11.6 Sensitively Performing a Male Genital Examination. Ginsburg.

11.15 If We Are to Build Strong Men Destined to Be Good Husbands and Fathers, We Need to Raise Our Sons With Love and Affection. Bell.

CHAPTER 14

Setting the Stage for a Trustworthy Relationship

Kenneth R. Ginsburg, MD, MS Ed, FAAP, FSAHM

> ▶ **Related Video Content**
>
> 14.0 Setting the Stage for a Trustworthy Relationship With Teens and Their Parents

■ Why This Matters

Both the greatest joy and challenge of caring for adolescents is forming a meaningful connection that will foster an honest, communicative relationship. Adults who care for adolescents serve as a critical layer of protection when we assess them for emotional well-being and risk behaviors. In order for us to fill this pivotal role, adolescents need to consider us trustworthy enough to share their personal information, and their parents need to be supportive of our role.

> **During the first moments of a new visit, adolescents are deciphering whether or not you are going to pass their critical "trustworthy test."**

Although trust is something that builds over time, the first few moments of an encounter can be used to help teens and families understand our role and consider why we may be deserving of their trust. ▶ **14.10**

■ Setting the Stage With Adolescents

There is an unfair and inaccurate perception that adolescents lie to adults. The truth is that they can be very honest when they judge adults to be trustworthy. In particular, adolescents in or near crisis often search for a responsible adult with whom they can disclose their concerns. For adolescents not in crisis, selectively withholding information may be adaptive. Regardless, the take-home message adolescents should have is that your office can be a safe place where they can seek help and guidance if and when they need it.

During the first moments of a new visit, adolescents are deciphering whether or not you are going to pass their critical "trustworthy test." Some may even ▶ **14.9** have life experience that has taught them to build protective barriers surrounding them. These few moments can be used to begin to build trust if you openly discuss the parameters of the relationship and your approach to serving teens. This investment may help form a therapeutic alliance, enhance your ability to gather a more accurate history, and even increase your efficiency over the long term.

The biggest barrier to investing the time in "setting the stage" is time itself. This strategy does take several minutes before you address the presenting concerns. However, there is an efficiency that comes from averting crises and addressing problems early on. It is important to realize that this conversation only needs to happen once in the initial visit and then be followed by brief booster reminders in future visits.

Another real concern to consider is that every time a question is asked in a safe, therapeutic setting, the potential exists that a crisis or problem will be uncovered. For this reason, it is imperative to have referral strategies in place both to deal with the reality of time limitations and to magnify your effectiveness.

12.7

Key Elements Adolescents Need to Hear to Extend Their Trust to You

The ideas presented here are based on clinical experience and research that elicited adolescents' desires regarding health care. Many of the suggestions are really about style of interaction. You have a relationship with the teens you serve and know what works within your community. Approach each of the key elements presented by considering how they should be adapted to fit your style and practice.

Much of what follows suggests how to begin a relationship with youth you meet as adolescents. Your initial approach to teens you have known during childhood may be quite different. It may even feel unnecessary to spend any time building trust, because the relationship is well seasoned. On the other hand, their desire to please you may influence them to withhold information, much like they would from their parents. Further, getting honest answers to private questions may prove to be difficult precisely because of how much they care about your opinion of them or because they have grown accustomed to you always including their parents in summary discussions. Therefore, consider marking a transition in your relationship where you acknowledge their growth and changing needs, and then reinforce some of the following points much as you would with a new client or patient.

For purposes of illustration, a medical visit will be described. But the key elements are important in many other settings.

What Can You Do for Me?

The first point adolescents need to understand is your role within the context of their lives. By explaining that you are part of a team of responsible adults who care about them and want them to thrive, your adolescents will understand who you are and that you can offer much more than keeping them physically healthy. In fact, if they expect that you are only interested in their physical health, they will have no reason to trust your guidance when it comes to their emotional and behavioral health. It may be helpful to start the visit by explaining how you think of health differently, and, with their permission, would like to address their health in a broader way.

What Will This Visit Be Like?

Adolescents should understand your goal is to help them transition into being their own spokesperson and advocate. They should understand this transition takes place gradually and with the support of their parents. Some settings begin this transition by separating adolescents from their parents throughout the visit in an effort to promote adolescent independence. I would suggest parents are present from the onset so that they understand both the social contract you will be creating with their adolescent and their important role in their adolescent's care. Adolescents are more likely to trust the process, the social contract, and your relationship with them if their parents hear your commitment to privacy and a teen-centered practice and agree to it in their presence. Otherwise, the adolescent may be faced with a parent who will greet them after the visit with, *"What did you talk about in there?"* followed by, *"Why don't you want to tell me?"*

Next, the standard structure of each visit can be explained. For example, you might begin by stating, *"I would like to talk about the way our visits will work. I will always start by asking you questions including any concerns you might have today. I am also going to ask you the questions directly, because I want you to learn how to tell your story to a professional. However, I am glad your parents are in the room because they are our teachers. I don't expect you to know all the answers to the questions I'll be asking. For those questions that you are unsure of, we can turn to your mother/father and ask them to teach us both. Your job is to listen to what your parents say so you can learn and answer these questions next time. Sound like a good plan?"* This conversation will also put parents at ease because their role as teachers and experts is clarified.

Why Do You Need to Ask Personal Questions?

Young people need to understand why they are being asked questions different from those they expected or were prepared to answer. Most adolescents made their appointments because of forms they needed completed. In a medical setting, their greatest focus may be their anxiety about having their bodies examined. Many will have no expectation of a psychosocial assessment of their overall well-being.

Start by explaining that you will be asking them private questions because you want them to be prepared to thrive. Helpful segue may include asking adolescents, *"If you were able to spend private time with young people, what kind of questions would you ask?"* Their answer may be highly informative; the first thing that comes to their mind may reveal their greatest concern.

Honesty

It is important for all adolescents to understand that your setting is a place where honesty is necessary and appreciated. Most adolescents are accustomed to having relationships where adults do not offer full disclosure or honesty. In fact, many might be all too familiar with the use of fear tactics to scare them into behaving "appropriately." As a result, many teenagers learn not to trust what adults say and may automatically categorize you as "just like the rest of them."

A starting point is for adolescents to know they can get honest information in your office. Information abounds on the Internet, but teens are not sure which information is valid. You should be seen as a trusted judge. Further, it may be helpful to indicate that you will share what you know and be honest about what you don't know regarding any questions they may ask. Then pledge to find the answers to things you don't know, and assure them you will not withhold information about their health from them at any time.

Service With Respect and Without Judgment 12.3, 14.5, 14.10

Adolescents need to be reminded that our aim is to serve them in a nonjudgmental way. They need to believe that not only are you worthy of their trust but that you respect their choice to not respond to certain questions. Their expectations and experiences with adults may include judgments and punishment. This is particularly true of adolescents who come from marginalized groups. They expect to be judged, as do adolescents with a history of engaging in worrisome behaviors. On the other end of the spectrum, and sometimes the hardest youth to engage, are well-resourced young people who have learned to project themselves as well put together or problem-free.

It is helpful for adolescents to realize that you understand disclosures are solely by choice and signify the adolescent's wish to move forward. Thus, express your appreciation and respect of any disclosure they may choose to make. This appreciation stands in sharp contrast to the condemnation youth often feel when they share information.

Adolescents need to understand that your nonjudgmental stance does not mean you condone every behavior. Instead it demonstrates that while behaviors can be judged healthy or unhealthy, the adolescents who choose to engage in them are not judged. Through this dialogue, teens may come to understand that your job is to help them be prepared to make the best choices. Words are only one source of information teens use to determine if they are being judged. Teens' vigilance can be triggered or mitigated by body language (see Chapter 15).

■ Privacy and Limits of Confidentiality 14.3

Confidentiality is the cornerstone of adolescent care because it allows for open communication between the young person and the professional. Specific laws vary by state and should be reviewed. Many clinicians are taught to explain privacy as follows: *"The relationship in this room will be kept confidential. That is, unless I thought you were going to hurt yourself or hurt someone else, or if an adult is or was going to hurt you."* There are numerous ways in which this script could be misunderstood.

First, many teens misinterpret the word "confidential" as denoting "confidence." To prevent misinterpretation, you might state, *"The word you might hear that describes our relationship is "confidential," that really just means "private."* In other words, *"I'm not interested in spreading your story or your business around. In fact, I can't because it's illegal for me to do so."* Because the word "secret" denotes shame or stigma, do not use it to explain privacy.

Next, the limits of privacy also require clear explanations. Your first step is to understand your state laws around privacy so you can communicate them clearly. In general, most states agree that it is the clinician's obligation to seek intervention immediately if there is imminent potential of serious harm to any teen (eg, they are thinking of killing themselves or hurting someone else badly or killing them, or are or were abused in any way). If, however, we stick to the standard script, adolescents may interpret "unless you are going to harm yourself" very differently from what we believe we are communicating. A 14-year-old likely knows you think cigarettes and drugs are "harmful." Similarly, a 16-year-old probably believes you think having sex or being truant from school is harmful. For these reasons, being very explicit about the limits of privacy from the onset and all of those areas (sex, drugs, etc) that are protected under confidentiality will help establish the climate of your relationship and define what is considered "safe" to disclose.

To further lessen adolescents' anxieties about privacy, it is critical that we understand that adolescents worry about disclosures to a variety of people. It is helpful to emphasize that this is not just about having the choice about privacy with their parents or caregivers, it is also about a commitment that you will not share their information with their friends, teachers, community members, other office staff, or law enforcement officers.

Explain to adolescents that, although you guarantee them privacy, your goal is to promote open communication within their family, especially in times of crises. This is also a key element of engaging the family. Tell the adolescent that if there were a problem, you may ask for their permission to involve their parents. However, reassure them that, unless one of the issues you included as a limitation to privacy existed, they will continue to remain in charge of their information and it is their choice whom to engage.

You might consider saying to the adolescent while their parents are still in the room, *"Suppose you had a problem and you and I had to work together to address this problem. Who else would we want on this team? Who would be the most important person or people to guide you?"* This is an opportunity to gain insight into the social context of the family. The adolescent will paint for you a snapshot of who they consider their most vital support. Although this will not always include the parents, it likely will, especially if they are present. When the adolescent does acknowledge the parent as a vital support, you can agree that their parent is the key person in their lives.

At this point you can turn to the parent and say, *"For this strategy to work* [emphasize the word *strategy*], *it is important for your son to know that we would work together as a team to keep him safe or help get him out of trouble. It may be useful for us to work together to create rules or boundaries to help your son thrive. However, if we could agree together that there will be no punishment for anything that comes up in my office, I believe your son will learn that this office is a place to get out of trouble without fear of getting into trouble."* Obtaining everyone's verbal agreement in each other's presence further confirms the social contract and builds mutual trust.

■ Setting the Stage With Parents 14.5, 14.8

(Note that efforts to engage parents were interspersed throughout setting the stage with the teen as noted above.)

Parents go through a tough transition in professionals' offices during adolescence. Previously, their role was to speak for their children and receive professional advice on behalf of their children. Suddenly they are asked to leave the room and are only told private information with their teen's assent. If parents are simply asked to step out of the room or if their child's visit is started without them present, they may feel that you are overstepping your role into "parenting." Further, they may feel that "secrets" are being kept from them.

For these reasons, the parents or caregivers of your adolescents need to understand their role within the context of your relationship with their child. They need to understand that you recognize that they are the most important people in their adolescents' lives and deserve to know about their children's health. The key to establishing a trusting relationship with them is their understanding that you are employing a strategy, including confidentiality, that will enable their adolescents to receive responsible guidance from another adult. This strategy relies heavily on mutual trust between you, the parent, and their child.

To minimize the possibility that parents will reject the notion of confidentiality, it is helpful to explain that children often worry about disappointing parents, and, therefore, sometimes withhold important information. Further, adolescents may believe that their parents will suspect they are already engaging in or are about to engage in a behavior by merely asking to be informed about it. Having another adult in their life with whom they can discuss sensitive issues does not mean they no longer love, trust, or need their parents.

If parents can agree ahead of time in front of their adolescents that your role is to be a guide and teacher, then your office setting will more likely become a place where adolescents will safely share information. Essentially, these adolescents will learn that they can disclose information that will help them avoid further trouble without fear of punishment. Once the purpose of the adolescent's visit is clear, confidentiality has been discussed, and you have ascertained the parents' concerns, you can then ask them to kindly step out of the room.

•• Group Learning and Discussion ••

 14.2

Reflect as a group on the following points:
- Do all teens who seek services in our office understand their privacy rights? Would they be clear that this is a place to get honest, accurate information? Would they fear being judged?
- Do parents of adolescents have a clear sense of their important role, or might they feel alienated or marginalized?
- Do all of our office staff understand privacy rights?
- Most people are trained to say, *"All information will be kept confidential unless you are going to hurt yourself or hurt someone else, or someone else is hurting you."* Discuss how a young person can misunderstand this phrase and why we need to be more explicit about privacy rights if we are to optimize adolescent disclosure.

Practice

Setting the stage for a first visit with a teen, being sure to cover the following points:
- Your philosophy about health
- Parents' important role as teachers
- Honesty
- Judgment
- Privacy rights
- The important role of parents in the event a problem is revealed

Setting the stage with an adolescent when you have an existing relationship

Overcome the barriers to investing the time to "set the stage":
- Discuss how an initial time investment in setting the stage might actually save practice time.
- Prepare a referral list for a variety of crises. This will lessen the almost universal unconscious bias that makes us avoid questions to save time and/or avoid the feeling of inadequacy that comes from knowing about a problem but feeling powerless to do anything about it.

▉▉▉▉▉▉▉ Continuing Education ▉▉▉▉▉▉▉

If you are applying for continuing education credits, a test is available online. For more details, visit www.aap.org/reachingteens.

▉ Suggested Reading

Berlan ED, Bravender T. Confidentiality, consent, and caring for the adolescent patient. *Curr Opin Pediatr.* 2009;21:450–456

Ford C, English A, Sigman G. Confidential health care for adolescents: position paper of the society for adolescent medicine. *J Adolesc Health.* 2004;35(2):160–167

Ford C, Thomsen SL, Compton B. Adolescents' interpretations of conditional confidentiality assurances. *J Adolesc Health.* 2001;29:156–159

Ford C, Millstein SG, Halpern-Felsher BL, Irwin CE. Influence of physician confidentiality assurances on adolescents' willingness to disclose information and seek future health care: a randomized controlled trial. *JAMA.* 1997;278(12):1029–1034

Ginsburg KR, Menapace AS, Slap G. Factors affecting the decision to seek primary care: the voice of adolescents. *Pediatrics.* 1997;100(6):922–930

Ginsburg KR, Slap GB, Cnaan A, et al. Adolescents' perceptions of factors affecting their decisions to seek health care. *JAMA.* 1995;273(24):1913–1918

■ Related Video Content

14.0 Setting the Stage for a Trustworthy Relationship With Teens and Their Parents. Ginsburg.

14.1 Checking in on Yourself: What About Your Own Adolescence Might Flavor Your Interactions With Youth? Ginsburg.

14.2 Case: Setting the Stage. Catallozzi.

14.3 Confidentiality for Adolescents in Health Care Settings. Ford.

14.4 Setting the Stage for a Long-term Partnership: Focus on Youth With Chronic Disease. Pletcher.

14.5 Setting the Stage for a Health Professional-Parent-Teen Partnership. Sugerman.

14.6 Central Elements of Setting the Stage: Honesty, Withholding Judgment, and Respect. Dowshen, Strasburger, Vo, Bell.

14.7 Case: Social Worker Setting the Stage. Feit.

14.8 Confidentiality Positions Professionals to Support Parents. Jenkins, Diaz.

14.9 Making Inroads With Youth Who Put Up Barriers. Arrington-Sanders.

14.10 What Makes Adults Worthy of Our Trust: The Youth View. Youth.

12.3 Ensuring a Space Without Judgment or Low Expectation so Risks and Hopes and Dreams Will Be Shared. Campbell.

12.7 A Teen-Friendly Private Practice: Resources, Referrals, and Physical Setting. Sugerman.

12.10 "Trust? What's the Point?…I Guess It's That People Kept Pushing." Adolescent-Friendly Services Never Give Up on Youth. Youth.

18.2 How a Comprehensive Assessment Positions Us to Develop and Prioritize Interventions. Ford.

18.3 A Strategy for Incorporating a Comprehensive Psychosocial Screen Into the Office Visit. Pletcher.

18.15 Case: SSHADESS Screen Reveals Bullying. Lewis.

37.0 Delivering Upsetting News to Parents: Recognizing Their Strengths First. Ginsburg.

CHAPTER 15

Body Language

Kenneth R. Ginsburg, MD, MS Ed, FAAP, FSAHM

 Related Video Content

15.0 Body Language Conveys Respect or Judgment, Openness or Mistrust, and High or Low Expectations

■ Why This Matters

We need to build relationships based on trust if we are to guide teens to make wise and healthy choices. Without trust, adolescents will withhold personal information and maintain barriers that limit genuine engagement.

> **Precisely because low expectation—in the guise of fear, derision, or judgment—is transmitted through body language, it may be the most critical tool in leveling the power dynamic, conveying genuine comfort, and communicating positive regard.**

The words we use to earn trust (see Chapter 14) can be reinforced or undermined by our body language. In fact, more communication is conveyed through body language than the spoken word.[1] Whereas spoken words contain critical content, their meaning can be shaped by delivery style, including the way speakers stand, gesture, and look at the person. Although the face and body both contribute to conveying an emotional state, when the face and body communicate conflicting emotional information, people are biased toward the emotion expressed by the body.[2]

It may be particularly important to consider the messages our bodies communicate when we serve marginalized youth because they have learned to be hypervigilant to others' judgments and intentions.

■ How Marginalization Increases One's Sensitivity to Body Signals

All adolescents are held to low expectations, often seen as a potential source of trouble or danger, especially when they are together in groups. However, marginalized adolescents, in particular, are often judged quickly for their appearance or group membership. In this context, the term "marginalized" refers to being out of the mainstream for one reason or another. Marginalized groups include all racial minorities, gender atypical sexual minority youth, adolescents in poverty and those experiencing unstable housing, obese youth, and teens with disabilities, among others. All of these groups have in common the experience of others signaling lower expectations to them. Some groups may become used to engendering fear as they note people checking their wallets or crossing the street, while other groups may notice scoffing, staring, or giggling when they walk past. It is critical to understand here that many of these judgments are delivered through body language.

The Toxic Effects of Being a Recipient of Judgment

To begin to understand how deeply judgment can affect the well-being and self-perception of marginalized youth, we need to consider its impact both from a developmental and resilience perspective. Adolescent psychosocial development is most easily summarized by recalling that the fundamental task of adolescence is answering the question, "Who am I?" Imagine the impact if part of that answer becomes, "I am someone who is feared" or "I am someone worthy of ridicule." Next, recall that one of the core principles of resilience theory is that young people live up or down to the expectations set for them. What does it mean for the predicted behavior of a young person when he is made to absorb the expectation that he will cause trouble?

Powerlessness as a Consequence of Marginalization

A sense of powerlessness is an eventual consequence of receiving judgment and derision. Further, one may begin to attribute power to those who actively or passively, consciously or unconsciously, send belittling messages.

Consider now how a marginalized youth feels about those in power as he becomes increasingly powerless in response to prolonged exposure to low expectations. Hurt? Resentful? Angry? The youth could reasonably be expected to desire power himself. Next, consider his personal experience with power, especially relative to people whom he perceives hold the power. He has learned that others fear him. At first that was likely painful, but later he may have learned to take advantage of that fear to gain a measure of personal power. He learned he could be intimidating.

Some marginalized adolescents have an "attitude"—a personality style that can be aggressive, dismissive, or sarcastic. It is a style that implies they are impervious to pain, that others' opinions really do not affect them. Adult caregivers serving adolescents with an aggressive or overly nonchalant attitude may become aggressive or frustrated. One could imagine them saying, *"Don't have that attitude with me!"* or *"Don't you see I'm trying to help you?"* However, those types of responses will backfire because they reinforce the sense of shame that is likely driving the behavior. Further, when youth have had a history of trauma, they can be highly reactive and can be triggered by demeaning words.

A first step in more effectively addressing the attitude is to come to awareness that it is an attempt to gain a sense of power in a world that feels resistant to sharing power. It is a defensive posture that says, "I have been hurt by people like you and I will not allow myself to be vulnerable now." A second step is to approach all youth from a strength-based perspective because many have little experience with someone expecting the best in them (see Chapter 25). Genuine positive regard and affirmation go a long way in eliminating the need for a defensive posture. Next, be clear that you know you have to earn their trust. Strategies for doing so verbally are offered elsewhere (see Chapter 14).

Precisely because low expectation—in the guise of fear or judgment—is transmitted through body language, it may be the most critical tool in leveling the power dynamic, conveying genuine comfort, and communicating positive regard.

Are These Issues Really Present in the Office Setting?

The teens who present in your office are not likely to arrive with conscious assumptions that you will be racist, homophobic, or judgmental of their life circumstances, disability, or body habitus. More likely, they are coming to complete a task (such as getting forms completed), discuss specific problems, or be cleared for sports participation. They are likely not coming anticipating an opportunity to delve deeply into their psychosocial and environmental contexts or to join with you in a positive behavioral change process.

In order to make our visits more effective, teens need to understand the potential opportunity your setting offers. The first step toward this is in setting the stage for a trustworthy interaction. The second step may be having them come to an unconscious realization that you are somehow different than the adults they normally encounter. This is where body language enters the equation. If they are used to adults fearing them or being closed to considering what they have to say, body language that conveys something very different than these norms can be transformative.

How Can I Relate to Youth From Other Cultures or Life Circumstances?

Many of the issues that we need to consider as caregivers serving youth from different cultures are covered in Chapter 19. However, no matter how personally aware we may be of cultural issues, we still will likely have to navigate through assumptions youth make about us because of our gender, race, or sexuality. Even if, for example, we are acutely sensitive to power differentials or racism, a teen may assume that we hold certain views if we are from a majority culture. It is the reality of what we bring into the room. It is vital to remember here that we are all "other" to someone. Regardless of your background, there will be adolescents who make assumptions of how you feel about them based on your external characteristics.

We must not become demoralized or disempowered by the fact that we are also victims of these assumptions. Nor should we believe that the means to mitigate these potential barriers is to match ourselves to adolescents from similar backgrounds or sexualities. There is a tremendous opportunity to have an added impact by overcoming those assumptions. If a person has received toxic or belittling assumptions from people who share certain characteristics with you, your interaction might be healing when you display the highest regard. In fact, when teens were asked what would make them feel safe from racism and prejudice, they did not suggest that they be assigned to caregivers that matched their demographic. Rather, they agreed that they preferred to receive care from centers with racially diverse staff. They stated that they looked for diversity when determining if they would be treated fairly. They wanted to note diversity in the center both "up front," referring to support staff, and "in the back," referring to professional staff, and they wanted to see that they were all talking and getting along. In other words, they called for a diverse staff with shared power, rather than one in which races were segregated by positions of varied status.[3] Further, what really made teenagers feel they would be treated fairly within the centers was to observe positive interactions among diverse staff. According to the youth, therefore, none of us as individuals have to be different than who we are; it is in our totality that we need to represent diversity.

■ Body Language 101

It is beyond the scope of this text to teach the specifics of body language. Rather, the goal here is to bring you to awareness that unintentional signals you may be sending through your gaze, movements, and posture can affect your interactions, particularly with marginalized youth. Resources are offered for you to consider a deeper dive into the subject.[4–10]

Many aspects of body language vary by culture. For example, some cultures value eye contact and see an inability to maintain a gaze as a sign of discomfort or shiftiness. Other cultures consider prolonged eye contact deeply disrespectful. Different cultures and ethnicities maintain a different zone of body space within which a person is seen as intrusive or inappropriate and beyond which a person might be viewed as distant or cold. It takes a great deal of sensitivity and cultural humility to adapt to the various cultures you are likely to encounter.

Because body language varies so much by culture, this is an area that may best be learned among your colleagues. Not only will they have a grasp of the population you serve, they may be able to offer insight into how your body reflects your emotional state. Although you cannot realistically be expected to change your emotional and instinctual reactions, some of which may be authentically protective, you can learn to control them to make it more likely that your gaze, posture, and movements will engender trust and safety by reflecting the genuine concern and openness you have for each of your teens.

There are some relatively universal signals people subconsciously send that convey judgment, fear, and domination. It is important to note here that many body language movements may be overinterpreted or misinterpreted. For example, crossed arms and legs really may signify defensiveness or fear, but they also might just be a comfortable position one takes when relaxed. The point of this discussion is not to make you self-conscious or label your emotions; rather, it is for you to consider how a youth could perceive your body signals.

▶ 15.1

Following are some brief thoughts to consider for further reflection and exploration.

Power

One of the core principles of this text is that young people are the experts in their own lives. If we are to adhere to this principle, then our challenge is to facilitate their own wisdom and to engage them in a shared decision-making process. A first step is to think about how our offices are designed and how our body language supports or undermines this principle. Examine your office space and consider whether it is set up in a manner that communicates that you are the authority or that there are 2 experts in the room—one with the wisdom that comes from life experience and professional training and one with the wisdom that comes from navigating his or her own environment.

Do you sit behind a desk in a chair that speaks of authority and privilege? Is your room set up so that your back faces the teen as you record her statements. These limitations in your physical environment can be remedied by moving your chair out from behind the desk, by using similar chairs, or even occasionally by trading chairs. If possible, restructure your room so that a computer never stands in the way of your ability to listen fully. Consider a round table where you will sit at the very same level as the teen and where no position around the table denotes greater authority or power.

Hand motions can also convey dominance. For example, pointing or waving fingers can be determined as condescending or even aggressive. Hands folded with the fingers laced together can be interpreted as "crowning" a sign of regal dominance, particularly if you lean back and place your hands atop your head.

Body stance can also display a desire to take control or even to signal aggression. For example, males who stand chest to chest with hips aligned in parallel to another male signal aggressive intent. It is unlikely that you as a caregiver will assume this stance. However, because you might receive it from a hostile youth or even angry parent, you should be prepared to deescalate the tension. Merely sitting down or pivoting your body away will break that power dynamic. With the changes in position, you signal that you are okay with not being dominant and prefer to return to routine interactions.

Fear

Many marginalized youth have grown to consider it normative for others to fear them. Your perceived fear may trigger the defensive attitude or their own sense of powerlessness.

A defensive position may make a teen assume that you fear him or her. A person who is intimidated will tend to cover those parts of the body that could be damaged by an attack. The chin is lowered, protecting the neck. The groin is covered with knees together, crossed legs, or covered with hands. The arms may be crossed or held across the chest. A person may place a physical object in front of him or her to act as a barrier. This barrier could be as small as a file or as large as a table.[8]

In contrast, open body language signals that you are relaxed. Particularly for youth who engender fear as a survival tactic (eg, gang-affiliated youth), your genuine comfort as displayed through open body language can go a long way toward allowing those teens to reveal their more authentic side.

Body Space

It is particularly important to be sensitive to the cultural background of the teen, as acceptable body space varies widely by culture. Spatial violations set off our emergency system in preparation for dealing with a potential threat. Marginalized youth, adolescents who live in dangerous environments, and youth who have been traumatized may by hypervigilant to their personal body space. In fact, they may instinctively be reactive and take an offensive stance when their space is violated. Space itself can deescalate the reactivity and reduce the tension (see Chapter 22). On the other hand, too great a distance can be perceived as aloofness or even fear.

Gaze

Eye contact can trigger a range of emotions that are cultural and context specific. Some cultures consider eye contact a prerequisite to a respectful conversation and assume that someone who won't look you in the eye has something to hide or doesn't consider you worthy of their attention. Other cultures consider anything but a fleeting gaze to be deeply disrespectful.

Judgment

There may be no more universal need in working with youth than to create a genuinely nonjudgmental stance. Nonjudgmental body language techniques include having a relaxed body (eg, uncrossed arms and legs) and keeping your body oriented toward the adolescent. A further key is to listen with full attention without reacting to the content being shared, or appearing to evaluate it for its merit. Listening with full attention usually includes open body language with little movement. When the listener is still, it implies he is forgetting about everything else except the person speaking. The attentive listener might also lean forward with head tilted. He may use short phrases such as *"uh huh,"* or *"tell me more,"* but does not react with either words or facial expressions that give away his opinion. In contrast, closed body language (crossing arms and legs, assuming a defensive posture) and facial grimaces signaling disgust or eyebrow creases conveying worry will likely stifle conversation. Similarly, a young person might stop sharing when she becomes aware that she is being evaluated. A classic sign that one is evaluating another is the steepled hands clasped together, as if in prayer, with both hands pressed together, or with linked fingers and index fingers pointing upward. The upward pointing fingers may touch the lips. Another movement that signals an "evaluation" is ongoing is the stroking of the chin or other part of the face.[8]

Signaling Openness and the Desire to Serve

Because of adolescents' need to assert independence, they may reject suggestions made with an authoritarian or controlling tone and posture. It is not unusual for teens to receive advice while being told what they must do. The body language associated with the kind of advice that insists on a specific action includes finger pointing and other signals of dominance. Rather than a dominating or defensive body language, consider communicating that you are receptive to their views. Hands out with palms up signals that you are welcoming their input and that you have a desire to serve rather than dictate.

•• Group Learning and Discussion ••

Body language and the power dynamic in your practice are ideal (albeit difficult!) topics to be discussed among your colleagues. Prior to the discussion(s), consider exploring some of the resources that follow to learn more about the specifics of body language so you can expand your repertoire. The following questions may help you consider how to create both a teen-friendly space and have more effective interpersonal interactions:

- Could our front desk staff unintentionally be signaling judgment to our marginalized youth or their parents?
- We understand that youth gain a sense of personal safety and perceive they are more likely to be treated fairly when they see a diverse staff at all levels of an organization that communicate productively and congenially with each other. Do we go out of our way in our setting to both optimize diversity and demonstrate healthy relationships among ourselves? What could we do to make our positive interactions more visible to youth?
- As we examine our office spaces, do they seem like an environment where we would promote shared decision-making with teens and families? What simple modifications could be made to convey our openness to this model?
- Consider for each of the cultures you serve how body space and eye contact might differ. Are there any other issues related to body language that need to be modified based on the background of your teens and families?
- After ensuring a zone of safety within the group, first discuss how each of you use your tone and body language to welcome teens and convey your positive regard and openness toward them. Then share strategies you each use to calm a situation where hostility might be escalating. Finally, consider discussing amongst yourselves how each of you might unintentionally signal fear, disagreement, or judgment.

To optimize this experience, consider practicing with a partner.

■■■■■■■■ Continuing Education ■■■■■■■■

If you are applying for continuing education credits, a test is available online. For more details, visit www.aap.org/reachingteens.

References

1. O'Daniel M, Rosenstein AH. Professional communication and team collaboration. In: Hughes RG, ed. *Patient Safety and Quality: An Evidence-Based Handbook for Nurses.* Rockville, MD: Agency for Healthcare Research and Quality; 2008

2. Meeren HK, van Heijnsbergen CC, de Gelder B. Rapid perceptual integration of facial expression and emotional body language. *Proc Natl Acad USA.* 2005;102(45):16518–16523

3. Ginsburg KR, Menapace AS, Slap GB. Factors affecting the decision to seek health care: the voice of adolescents. *Pediatrics.* 1997;100(6):922–930

4. Sinke CB. A tease or threat? Judging social interactions from bodily expressions. *NeuroImage.* 2010;(49):1717–1727

5. Hills L. Reading and using body language in your medical practice: 25 research findings. *J Med Pract Manage.* 2011;26(6):357–362

6. Ouellette RW. Approaching an upset person: body language and verbal communications. *J Healthc Prot Manage.* 2010;26(1):100–104

7. Levin RP. Body language speaks volumes. *Am Dent Assoc.* 2008;139(9):1262–1263

8. Changingminds.org. Using Body Language. http://changingminds.org/techniques/body/body_language.htm. Accessed June 25, 2013

9. Navarro J. *What Every Body Is Saying.* New York, NY: Harper Collins Publishers; 2008

10. Ekman P. *Emotions Revealed: Recognizing Faces and Feelings to Improve Communication and Emotional Life.* New York, NY: Henry Holt and Company; 2007

Related Video Content

15.0 Body Language Conveys Respect or Judgment, Openness or Mistrust, and High or Low Expectations. Ginsburg.

15.1 Specific Messages Conveyed Through Body Language. Hill, Ginsburg, Bailer, Feit.

15.2 Commenting on the Body Language of a Young Person. Feit.

19.5 A Diverse Workforce Generates a Sense of Safety and Security in Youth. Trent, Ginsburg, Hill, Lewis.

Communicating With the Adolescent

This text hopes to build your repertoire in using resilience-focused, strength-based strategies to promote adolescent health and well-being. The previous section focused on the early connection that sets the tone for communication. Here, we go a step further to offer both general strategies and specific skills for effective communication. First, a brief overview to the basics of communication is offered in "Core Principles on Communicating With Adolescents" (Chapter 16). Next, "Integrating the 7 Cs of Resilience Into Your Clinical Practice" (Chapter 17) will offer a brief overview into how the core elements of resilience can be reinforced in our visits. "The SSHADESS Screen: A Strength-Based Psychosocial Assessment" (Chapter 18) is a verbal behavioral screen that starts by contextualizing risk within a broad initial understanding of the young person's strengths. "Cultural Humility" (Chapter 19) understands that we are all "other" to somebody and that the only way that we can be uniformly respectful to

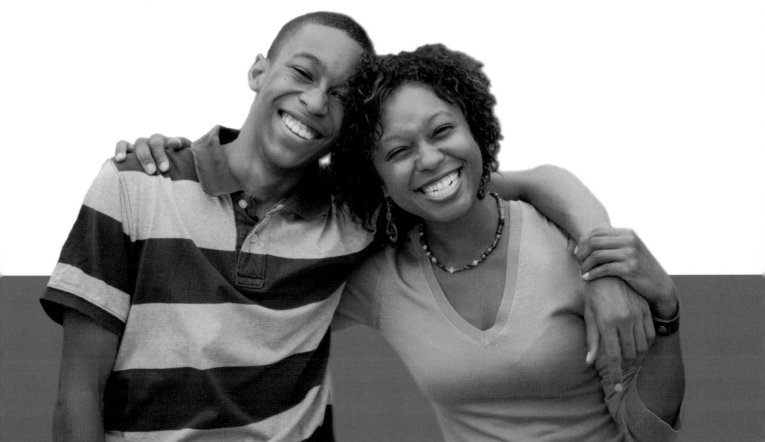

people is to consistently be prepared for them to teach us about their culture and environment. A critical first step in being culturally humble is having an awareness of your own unconscious biases. Even as we make decisions about diagnoses or treatment plans, these biases can play a part. "Examining Our Unconscious Biases" (Chapter 21) looks at thinking patterns and assumptions we may have that can interfere with our ability to objectively evaluate evidence and draw the most appropriate conclusions. "Trauma-Informed Practice: Working With Youth Who Have Suffered Adverse Childhood (or Adolescent) Experiences" (Chapter 22) speaks to the special needs of youth exposed to toxic stress and trauma. It covers how your interaction style can prevent defensive reactive responses and help guide youth towards healing. "Boundaries" (Chapter 20) is a critically important chapter in a body of work that states "unconditional love and absolute respect" are key to reaching youth. We must not be afraid of the word "love," but we must be very clear about what it means and must practice love with boundaries both to be protective of our own emotions and to prevent youth from becoming reliant on us in a way that could interfere with their own autonomy. Next, "De-escalation and Crisis Management When a Youth Is 'Acting Out'" (Chapter 23) offers strategies to restore calm to a youth whose anxiety, anger, or frustration may be building. Finally, "Delivering Bad News to Adolescents" (Chapter 24) acknowledges our own internal struggles with being the bearer of difficult news and offers approaches to conveying information in a supportive manner.

CHAPTER 16

Core Principles on Communicating With Adolescents

Linda A. Hawkins, PhD, LPC
Kenneth R. Ginsburg, MD, MS Ed, FAAP, FSAHM

 Related Video Content

16.0 Communicating With Teens 101

■ Why This Matters

How many times have you heard, *"You can't trust what a teen says."*? Why do so many adults think teens are difficult to talk to and impossible to get to open up? Professionals who work closely with teens do not usually hold these negative views. We have found teens to be very forthcoming. Too honest at times! Further, we have grown to understand that it is healthy for teens to be somewhat reserved in their disclosures until they have built a solid and trustworthy relationship. In fact, isn't it appropriate for all of us to keep our most intimate information private, making rare exceptions for those people who have earned our trust?

> **It is healthy for teens to be reserved in their disclosures until they have built solid trustworthy relationships.**

Professionals who follow some core principles of communication will find it easier to witness the very best of youth. They will also be better positioned to meet the needs and expectations of adolescents as they join with them in a shared decision-making process to guide them toward healthier behaviors and wiser choices.

■ Communication 101

Reaching Teens is, at its core, a text on strength-based communication; therefore, many communication principles are covered in great depth elsewhere. This chapter can be thought of as a landing page from which you can explore each of these topics. In some cases where the topics do not have their own designated chapter, a brief discussion is offered here.

■ Setting the Tone

Are We Trustworthy?

It is not reasonable to expect a teen to tell us the most personal details of their lives just because we are professionals. We have to earn that trust; it doesn't just come because we have a specific title. While that takes time, we can "set the stage" initially by addressing some major concerns. This forms the template for a trustworthy relationship with both teens and their families. This is covered in full in Chapter 14.

Are We Respectful?

No one wants to be a problem to be solved. Instead, every youth needs to be seen in the context of their strengths. There is no stronger way to convey respect than to listen. Just to listen. Respectful listening recognizes that the speaker is the expert in his or her own life and views the speaker through a positive lens that notices foremost their strengths. Respectful listening can also hear what is *not* being shared by a youth, to hear where clarification and questions can be added. The key here is to gain permission to explore further. An example of this would be, *"I noticed that you haven't mentioned much about how school is going for you right now. Is it okay for me to ask how that part of your life feels?"*

33.3

Body Language

The words that we say convey only a small portion of what we communicate. In fact, our body language can reinforce or undermine our intended messages. All youth are hypersensitive to adult hypocrisy and pick up on body language signals. However, marginalized and/or traumatized youth who have consistently absorbed judgmental glances, altered body language, and even fear triggered by their presence, are hypervigilant to body language. All too often our busy schedule has us entering a room with a million things on our mind. Our youth deserve our full attention, including looking them in the eye and offering a handshake as a sign that we are happy to see them. This is covered in greater depth in Chapter 15.

■ Learning About Behavior

Address Risks, but Always While Recognizing Strengths

Choosing to use a strength-based approach with youth does not make you blind to risks. To the contrary, one of the best ways of addressing risk is to build on existing strengths. Our goal is to fully understand and appreciate the skills a young person possesses, and then use those strengths to mitigate risk and to build skill sets where they need further development. Therefore, as we interview youth to screen them for risks, it is important to contextualize their risks within their environments, while clearly also eliciting their strengths, hopes, and aspirations. The SSHADESS Screen is offered in *Reaching Teens* as a brief interview that explores risks within a broader context (see Chapter 18).

18.1

Stories Are Like Onions

The goal of an interview or assessment is not to get to the root of every problem or to gain full disclosure on every thought, feeling, or risk exposure. It is to have a therapeutic discussion that guides you on where to focus your energies, and on where and how to facilitate progress while leaving the young person feeling safe, comfortable,

18.7

and engaged. If it leaves her feeling vulnerable or exposed, it may be your last interaction and may increase her stress, which, in turn, might drive her to familiar negative coping strategies. Your goal is to uncover a layer at a time, safely, respectfully, and therapeutically. This approach allows a young person to slowly realize the benefit of disclosure and determine how and when to continue to move forward as she continually builds her trust in you.

Being an Open Book Is Not Always a Good Sign

Because so many young people can be reserved or monosyllabic, it is easy to congratulate ourselves when a young person offers us full disclosure. Often a young person is open and forthcoming with information precisely because we have set the stage for a trustworthy relationship. However, we have to remain vigilant to the possibility that an adolescent pouring out her thoughts and feelings could be in crisis. It can be normal for a teen to be reserved; it can be normal for a teen to be open and gregarious. However, youth in acute crisis can be less likely to use an "editor" and can reveal themselves too easily. Further, a youth who lacks relationships with adults can become too easily attached before taking you through an appropriate trust-building and testing process. In situations like this, it is fair to suggest that a youth save some information for the next appointment so they don't flood the first visit with excessive information and then leave wishing they had held some back. A way to suggest this could include, *"It sounds like there have been a lot of challenging events in your life, and I'm honored that you feel that you can trust me with this information. I'd like to push the pause button on all that you are sharing so that I can continue to build the trust in our working relationship and continue to assure you that I'm worthy of your trust."*

Never Diminish a Feeling

"Don't worry about it." "Just get over it." "It's not that big a deal." This is the type of advice youth often receive from friends and families. It belittles their concerns. It is diminishing. Instead, let young people know you hear their concerns and will explore them. Reassure them that based on their existing strengths (after you have appropriately elicited them), you believe they will get through this. See if the young person has overcome a similar challenge in his life, and point out how he used his strengths at that time. In a health setting, if after careful consideration and attention you believe there is no problem, then it can be therapeutic to say, *"After a thorough evaluation, I am not concerned because _____. What concerns are you left with?"* However, the elimination of your concern may not quickly eliminate the youth's worries. You might add, *"We've talked through the possibilities, and we know there isn't a dangerous medical concern on the top of the list today. I appreciate this understanding may not take away the worried feeling right away, and that's okay. I'm still here to listen."*

Never Say, "I Understand"

You don't. A person in crisis can respond angrily and defensively—*"How could you understand, you've never been _____."* Instead, ask for help in your journey toward understanding. Reinforce that the adolescent is the expert and you are requesting the opportunity to learn. Try, *"I can't imagine what you have been through, tell me what it has been like for you."* Or, *"Teach me what I need to know to care for you."*

Helping Youth Express Their Emotional Thoughts

Some youth do not yet have language for an experience they are trying to share. Offer some options to help them teach you about themselves so you do not have to try to "guess" their feelings. For example, *"I have heard from some folks who have described similar experiences and they shared feelings like hurt, worried, confused, or scared...do any of those words fit with the feelings you had in your situation?"*

Listening for the Unspoken Signals

Why Now?

It is not unusual for a young person to present with a concern that has been ongoing. It can be useful to directly ask, *"It sounds like this has been going on for a while. Tell me why you are coming in now."* The answer might elucidate the meaning of the problem and uncover a change in the environment or mounting anxiety about the issue.

Sometimes a youth decides to share an important part of themselves with us many weeks or months into our working relationship. For marginalized and/or traumatized youth, there is a clear testing period where they are deciding if we are worthy of their most valuable information. Frequently, this information can include unsafe and unhealthy experiences they have had or are currently grappling with, including substance use and/or unsafe sexual practices or physical abuse. Do not be surprised if several months into your work with a youth, they admit that some or much of what they shared with you has not been true. Consider it an incredible day when you have passed their tests, and asking "why now" is also important, *"Thank you for sharing all of this valuable information about yourself with me today and letting me know that I passed your tests of trust. Can you let me know some of the things that I did that let you know that you can trust me so that I can be sure to continue them?"*

What Are You Worried About?

Especially in a health setting, a young person's fears may be driving their symptoms. It is not unusual for them to withhold their deepest worries, assuming you can sense them. The easiest way to allay their hidden concerns is to directly ask, *"What are you worried might be going on?"* Sometimes just addressing an unwarranted fear can change the quality, intensity, or experience of the problem. This is also a wonderful way to learn about any myths or misinformation the youth has about their body, their health, or their behaviors.

The Body and Mind Are Integrated

Stress will often manifest with physical symptoms, such as fatigue, bellyaches, headaches, chest pain, or limb and joint pain. It is critical that we address stress' role in how our bodies function and feel. However, there is a real danger of a young person hearing, *"I think you're crazy"* or *"I think you're faking"* when we discuss stress after she has told us how her body is feeling. We have to integrate the body and mind in a way that is respectful and informative. Sometimes continued attention to the experience teens are having with their body will keep them engaged with you as the story of background stressors reaches consciousness and safely unfolds over time. Strategies for serving youth with body-mind conditions are offered in Chapter 44.

How Can We Best Serve?

Information or Support?

Not every young person needs the same thing. Young people with an internal locus of control, meaning they have the sense that they can control their environment, may only need information. These youth will bring a lot of questions into your office and may not leave a lot of space for you to ask additional questions, and that's going to be okay for them. Teens with an external locus of control, who do not feel that what they do has proven to make any difference, may need a higher level of support. They may even sometimes need for an authority figure to initially take charge. These youth will hope that you will ask the important questions leading you to the good options or answers for their concerns. Our ultimate goal, however, is to facilitate them to know how to take control a step at a time (see Chapter 29).

Boundaries

People who care deeply are the best at serving others. But caring deeply also can leave professionals depleted and ultimately may lead them to experience burnout. Further, in order to keep your relationships with youth therapeutic, it is critical that they know that you care but also that they should not become reliant on you. They must remain the experts on their lives and the person most committed to their progress. Your most effective role may be coaching youth on healthy decision-making and facilitating them to find skills in themselves that they didn't yet know they possessed.

Appropriate boundaries must not be seen as something that limits inter-actions, but rather as something that preserves our therapeutic relationships and our capacity to remain compassionate over a lifetime of service (see Chapter 20).

▶ 20.0

Respecting Adolescent Wisdom and Experience

Youth Are the Experts in Their Own Lives

Only the young person sitting in front of you fully understands their environ-mental context. Only adolescents will know what will work and what might not be feasible in the world they navigate. A first step toward joining with a teen in a healing process is to recognize that expertise. Recognizing, acknowledging, and speaking about this early on can prove to enhance the boundaries and the partnership in your relationship. You may have the degree, but the youth is the expert on herself. This can sound like, *"I have spent many years studying how to serve young people. Similarly, you have spent many, many years studying your life and your experiences. Together, I think we can make a great team for your health and wellness."* Once you do, you will serve her with more humility. You will naturally draw from her expertise to guide you on how best to facilitate her progress. A richer discussion is offered in Chapter 4.

▶ 4.0.1

Shared Decision-Making

We demonstrate that we believe that they really are the experts in their own lives when we engage them in shared decision-making. This is more than a philosophical approach to youth; it is eminently practical. When we determine what is best, it sets a young person up to not follow our instructions and then be considered "non-adherent" (in a professional setting) or "defiant" (at home). When we guide youth in a shared decision-making process, we each take our reasonable roles. Adolescents are the experts on their lives; know what they can handle, and at what pace; decide what they are willing to do; and determine who is going to help them with their plan once they leave our office. We have life experience, professional expertise, and a commitment to ensuring safety and furthering wise, healthy decisions. Together, each comfortable in our roles, we can come up with plans that the young person is motivated and prepared to follow.

■ Addressing Behavior

People Are Hungry for Brief Interventions

It might be best for a young person to engage in a long-term therapeutic healing process with someone, but it is not always possible. Some young people are resistant to that level of engagement until they have a successful experience with a compassionate and competent healing provider under their belt.

Reaching Teens is not a manualized text on therapy, rather it offers approaches to engagement, assessment techniques, shared decision-making and motivational strategies, and brief intervention techniques. This creates a starting point for youth to have those first successful experiences with you that may allow other important health and wellness providers to join in the youth's care.

Bringing Attention to an Issue Is a Start

The first step of addressing a problem is acknowledging that it exists. Something as simple as saying, *"I am concerned about…"* or *"I am confused about how…"* begins the process where a teen may consider behavioral change. For example, *"You mentioned earlier that you are excited about starting a new job soon, but you are still enjoying smoking marijuana every day and sleeping in late. I'm confused about how you are going to be able to enjoy all of those things together."*

Behavior Changes a Step at a Time

Sometimes a solution seems so obvious to us. But if we want a healthy decision to be long-lasting, the young person needs to own the decision to change and determine his own readiness and pace of change. Several "stages of change" theories exist, but one that has been used extensively with teens is Prochaska and DiClemente's transtheoretical model of change. It is the backbone of motivational interviewing. Motivational interviewing is rooted in the understanding that people are the experts in their own lives and determine their own readiness to change by considering the benefits of change versus both the benefits and downsides of staying with familiar habits. Further, it states that any change has to start from where the youth currently stands and can only happen one step at a time. See Chapter 26 for an overview and strategies.

Shifting Language Subtly to Begin Consideration of Change

People sometimes use language that constrains the possibility of change; even a subtle shift of language can therefore hold profound meaning. It can also be used as a starting point to facilitate a person to challenge her own assumptions. For example, *"This always happens to me"* or *"I never"* can allow you to state, *"Really, always?"* This can begin the process of the young person shifting and considering the possibility of change. *"Well, not always. If I _____, then sometimes it doesn't happen."* Similarly, even asking a young person to add the word "yet" after a self-defeating statement can open awareness to the possibility of change. For example, *"I am just a dropout, I'm no good at school,"* could be transformed into, *"I am just a dropout, I'm no good at school—YET."*

Sometimes a young person's words don't match the facts. Some professionals may interpret this as lying, leading to the potential for an adversarial, condescending, or dismissive encounter. Instead, we can try to shift our understanding of the youth's statement as a stepping-stone in preparation for more consistent behavioral change. For example, when asking a youth if he has had unprotected sex recently, an answer of *"No, I use condoms all the time"* seems contradictory to the lab results showing a sexually transmitted infection.

Honoring that the story the youth is sharing is part of his behavioral change process can be a powerful and supportive tool if you say, *"You mentioned that you are using condoms all the time and it sounds like that is definitely your goal. Your test result showed that there was a time recently when that goal wasn't as easy to achieve. Do you remember what made that time harder than others to use a condom? Then, together, we can figure out ways to use that challenge to keep your goals on track."*

Demoralized Youth Do Not Believe in Their Potential

Some youth have repeatedly failed to improve their situations because of internal and/ or external barriers, or have absorbed undermining messages from others. These youth may be hopeless or demoralized and, therefore, may not even be receptive to considering healthier choices. A first step may be to listen to their stories with the aim of understanding the context of their lives and the strengths they have demonstrated in navigating through those challenges. After eliciting those stories, professionals can reflect them back to youth so they can better see their own strengths even amidst stressful circumstances and dangerous choices they have made to survive their realities. For many youth, you may be the first adult who is going to listen to their story, believe what they have to say, and tell them that they are a valued person. Through active respectful listening, you will find places to reflect back to wise choices they made, healthy options they considered, and strong behaviors they are activating (like coming into your office). When they are equipped with a better understanding of what they are already doing right, they might be better prepared to take further steps. At the least they will know that professionals do not see them only as risk-taking problems to be solved (see Chapter 25).

Young People Have to Own Their Choices: First, They Have to Understand Your Suggestions

Adults often tell adolescents what to do based on wisdom and experience but fail to remember that this can drive teens toward rebellion. When we lecture young people, it backfires for 3 reasons. First, if lecturing is part of their lives outside of our office, they have already tuned us out as soon as they saw the lecture coming…or before out of fear that one was on the way. Second, it can be condescending. Third, a lecture is inherently abstract in nature—linking a long-term outcome with a series of intermediate steps. Preteens and early adolescents cannot yet think abstractly, and all people in the midst of crisis cannot think abstractly. Instead, we have to deliver messages in concrete ways, facilitating youth to figure things out and, therefore, own the solutions (see Chapter 28). A first step to being able to talk to adolescents in a way they can understand is to grasp how cognitive development changes during adolescence and determine where the youth currently stands on the developmental trajectory (see Chapter 8).

▶ **28.0**

If a Young Person Is to Take on a Problem, It Must Not Feel Overwhelming

As long as a problem feels too big to handle, a person will avoid addressing it, assuming it is not manageable. Developmentally, youth may not be capable of considering and mapping out, in the right order, ways to break down a problem into smaller pieces. For these reasons, a key communication strategy is to help an individual realize that every problem has its component parts, and that only one piece of the problem needs to be tackled at a time. Similarly, in the case of long-term planning, only one step needs to be taken at a time. After one step of the journey is taken, the destiny seems more attainable. The first part of the comprehensive coping strategy offered here is to make a problem

▶ **31.2**

seem manageable. Several brief intervention strategies, based on breaking large decisions or problems into component parts, are also offered.

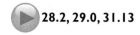 **28.2, 29.0, 31.13**

■ Humility

Cultural Humility

We do not need to be matched to the youth we serve by race, culture, ethnicity, gender, or sexual orientation. What we need to be is deeply respectful. One of the most important means to demonstrate respect is to strive to understand how someone's beliefs, attitudes, and actions are shaped by their environment and culture. It is impossible to be truly culturally "competent," if competency is defined as having a facile understanding of cultural nuances and perspectives. However, it is possible to be culturally humble. One of the greatest ways to demonstrate humility is to be a genuine learner. People appreciate informing someone who is able to say, *"Tell me about you,"* *"Tell me what I need to know to care for you,"* *"Teach me."* This discussion continues in greater depth in Chapter 19.

■ Check in on Your Assumptions

Even the best listeners make assumptions about what another person means by the words they are saying. We also might believe that we understand the underlying meaning of non-verbal communication. However, we are often wrong, and, therefore, can misread a teen's mood or arrive at a plan that doesn't meet the teen's needs. For example, an adolescent sitting with her arms crossed and looking distant might be angry toward you or dismissive of your presence. But she also might be replaying a difficult morning at home and feeling particularly vulnerable, or she may be feeling especially nervous because she wants to ask you something very important. Your assumption could make you feel angry and defensive, when what the girl really needs from you is support. It is helpful to check your assumptions. Statements such as, *"It seems to me you might be feeling _____. Am I right or totally off-base?"* or the more open ended, *"Can you tell me what you're feeling now"* can be highly productive.

■ Apologies Can Go a Long Way 16.1

Even when our intentions are pure, we all say and do the wrong thing sometimes. Even if we are convinced our actions or words are masterful, a young person can still take offense. It matters less how the message was intended and more how it was received. One of the most effective strategies to defuse tensions and restore a therapeutic interaction is to apologize. Even if you believe you did everything right, you can always apologize for the experience someone had and how your words were received. Similarly, when you receive a complaint about colleagues, you do not have to feel badly for not defending them or feel as though you have "thrown them under the bus" when you apologize for the way the young person felt. If there is a feeling in the air that you cannot explain, it can be helpful to preemptively apologize to stem rising tension: *"It seems like you are upset about something, is there anything I may have done—or not done—that I could make right?"*

You might even consider highlighting how much you care about serving adolescents well by acknowledging you might not always get it right without their guidance. This might be particularly helpful in the beginning of a relationship with a traumatized or marginalized youth who has been conditioned to quickly react to affronts or reject services. *"As I'm getting to know you better, I'm going to make some mistakes. I'll let you know in advance that I'll apologize when I know that I've made a mistake, but, if I miss a mistake that I've made, please tell me so. You can say, 'nope, you got it wrong.' And we can fix things as we go."* This is a great way of reminding the youth that they are the experts on themselves, they are partners in the working relationship with you, and their input in their care is vital to their health and wellness.

Starting Off on the Right Foot

Sometimes the best apology happens before tension has risen. If you know a young person has been kept waiting, starting out with, *"I am so sorry that you have been waiting for so long"* can diminish rising frustration. You might add, *"I try so hard to give youth what they need and that makes keeping a tight schedule really difficult sometimes. I want you to know that I'm going to stay late to make sure you get your full appointment time, is it okay for you to stay late with me or do you want me to add another appointment to my schedule next week to give you the full time you deserve?"* This last example points out that you are going to disrupt your own schedule to make up for your lateness and honors that the youth might *not* be able to stay beyond the original time they scheduled for their appointment. We can't ask youth to be productive members of our society with jobs and responsibilities and then presume that they can spend any unexpected extended time in our offices.

■ Communication During Crises

Getting Through It

The first goal of crisis intervention is to prevent a tragic consequence. It may be that after an assessment for intent to harm self or others, our major role is to assure a young person that they will get through this. That may seem implausible to him. That is why it can be so critical to help him understand your commitment to support him and to build over time his capacity to deal with the issues that created the crisis. Seeing the crisis while also exploring means he has used to navigate past difficulties can help him see competencies he has forgotten he possessed. The goal during crisis is to first ensure safety and then to make an adolescent feel both connected and competent (see chapters 5 and 17).

De-escalation

All of us who work with adolescents will experience crises in which youth will have difficulty containing their emotions. When we try to "control" the situation, it can drive youth toward a state of even more heightened emotions. On the other hand, when we listen respectfully, we can defuse both passions and tensions. It is not uncommon during these situations that a youth just needs to feel "heard," and honoring his feelings can be the most important therapy you can give. Offering a reflection of what the youth is saying demonstrates that you are listening, a precious gift when a youth is hurting. *"It sounds like this feels really overwhelming and unfair," "You are describing a really sad situation,"* or *"All of what you are describing should not have happened; I'm so sorry it did."* When listening and validating are not all that the youth needs, you need to activate your skills for crisis management and/or call in resources for additional support. A variety of strategies are offered in Chapter 23.

Seeking Help Is an Act of Strength

It can be difficult to guide a teenager to seek professional guidance. Our challenge is to transform help-seeking from being viewed as a source of shame or stigma into being a source of pride. Teens may feel ashamed that they can't handle their own problems or worry that going for help confirms they are weak. It is important for them to understand that, to the contrary, seeking help is an act of strength because strong people know they are capable of feeling better, and will take the steps to get there. Further, no one wants to be pitied, and teens may assume professionals will look down on them. They need to understand that professionals who work with youth do so because we care for and respect them. This is covered in much greater depth in Chapter 33.

It needs to be noted here that some cultures do not value the concept of counseling, therapy, or the engagement of other people outside of the family for support. These situations should be respected, and additional support should be framed in ways that are culturally respectful.

●● Group Learning and Discussion ●●

This overview summarizes points offered in greater detail elsewhere. Pick a communication strategy for which your group would benefit from further development, and then see that chapter for suggested group learning activities.

■■■■■■■ Continuing Education ■■■■■■■

If you are applying for continuing education credits, a test is available online. For more details, visit www.aap.org/reachingteens.

■ Suggested Reading

Prochaska JO, DiClemente CC. Stages of change in the modification of problem behaviors. *Prog Behav Modif.* 1992;28:183–218

Robinson PJ, Gould DA, Strosahl KD. *Real Behavior Change in Primary Care: Improving Patient Outcomes and Increasing Job Satisfaction.* Oakland, CA: New Harbinger Publications, Inc.; 2010

Stuart M, Lieberman JA. *The Fifteen Minute Hour: Practical Therapeutic Interventions in Primary Care.* New York, NY: Saunders Publications; 2002

■ Related Video Content

16.0 Communicating With Teens 101. Hawkins.

16.1 The Power of an Apology to "Reset" a Relationship. Hawkins.

16.2 It Is Good That We All Have Different Styles, But We Have to Uniformly Communicate That We Expect the Best and Know Youth Can Succeed. Sidhu.

16.3 Kids May Not Understand What They Don't Understand; Therefore, Your Questions Have to Be Clear and Specific. Pletcher.

4.0.1 The Keys to Working With Teens: Respect, Listening, and Recognizing Their Expertise. Kreipe.

4.1 Listen to Us: We Understand Our Lives Best. Youth.

12.3 Ensuring a Space Without Judgment or Low Expectation so Risks and Hopes and Dreams Will Be Shared. Campbell.

12.10 "Trust? What's the Point?…I Guess It's That People Kept Pushing." Adolescent-Friendly Services Never Give Up on Youth. Youth.

15.0 Body Language Conveys Respect or Judgment, Openness or Mistrust, and High or Low Expectations. Ginsburg.

18.1 Maximizing Yield From a Strength-Based Interview: Avoiding the Pitfalls of Using Only a Positive Lens. Ginsburg.

18.6 Pearls to More Effectively Elicit Psychosocial Histories. Pletcher, Campbell, Reirden, Bailer, Feit.

18.7 The Goal Is Not to Get the Most Detailed History, It Is to Get the Most Therapeutic History for the Youth at That Time: A Case of Abuse That Revealed Itself Over Time. Ginsburg.

20.0 Boundaries: Essential to Our Healthy Relationships With Youth and Our Professional Longevity. Ginsburg, Hill.

20.1 Over-empathizing Can Feel Like Judgement. Pletcher.

25.0.1 An Introduction to Behavioral Change: Youth Will Not Make Positive Choices if They Don't Believe in Their Potential to Change. Ginsburg.

25.3 Young People Speak of the Power of Being Viewed Through a Strength-Based Lens and the Harm of Low Expectation. Youth.

25.4 The Depth of Our Caring Positions Us to Enter the Lives of Youth and to Be Change Agents. Singh, Vo.

25.5 "Tell Me What You've Been Through—You've Been So Strong": A First Step of Connection. Feit.

28.0 Facilitating Adolescents to Own Their Solution: Replacing the Lecture With Youth-Driven Strategies. Ginsburg.

28.1 Teens Told What They "Should" Do Will Lose the Ability to Learn What They Can Do. Rich.

28.2 Helping a Young Person Own Her Solution: A Case of Using a Decision Tree to Prevent Violent Retaliation. Ginsburg.

29.0 Gaining a Sense of Control: One Step at a Time. Ginsburg.

31.13 The Tupperware Box: A Case Example. Ginsburg.

31.2 Stress Management and Coping/Section 1/Tackling the Problem. Ginsburg.

33.1 Asking for Help Is a Sign of Strength. Sugerman.

33.3 Seeing Youth as More Than a Label or a Disease—The First Step Toward Healing. Arrington-Sanders.

34.4 Professional and Parent: Insight From Having 2 Roles With Teens. Ford.

CHAPTER 17

Integrating the 7 Cs of Resilience Into Your Clinical Practice

Susan T. Sugerman, MD, MPH, FAAP

 Related Video Content

17.0 Integrating the 7 Cs of Resilience Into Your Clinical Practice

■ Why This Matters

A teen's best hope is the strength that young person can find in him- or herself. We can't make the world perfect for adolescents. But we have a unique opportunity to help them grow into the kinds of adults who can deal with an imperfect, stressful world. We can become the engineers of the "right place" and "right time" to challenge youth, and to support their families, toward building their competencies and confidence in their abilities to face an uncertain future.

A resilience framework focuses on what's right with a teenager and provides hope in situations that are often colored with discomfort, sadness, or despair. In this way, we avoid overfocusing on past mistakes or problems and instead build a foundation for a child and family to move forward with positive expectations.

We can include their parents and caregivers as we promote teenagers' connections to healthy individuals and communities that reinforce good character. We can inspire them to contribute to the world in ways they wouldn't have considered otherwise. We can help them understand and build on what they already do in daily life to cope with life's stresses and trauma. We can give them the vote of confidence that indeed they are in control of what happens to their future.

■ How a Resilience Framework Differs From Traditional Clinical Approaches

Adopting a resilience framework allows us to focus primarily on what's right with a child or teenager in order to understand and address what may be wrong. Using an approach that acknowledges the strengths of a child and the family helps identify positive traits and skills to empower change from within. It provides hope in situations that are often colored with discomfort, sadness, or despair. In this way, we avoid overfocusing on past mistakes or problems and instead build a foundation to move forward with positive expectations.

Setting the Tone: Proper Paperwork

Your intake forms send an important message to teens before they walk in the door. The paperwork or online information provided prior to the first appointment lets youth know what you think is important and why. Use it as an opportunity to normalize areas of questioning as standard issues for all youth. Presenting topics as matter-of-fact, appropriate areas for conversation may minimize self-consciousness or shame around sensitive issues. Even without face-to-face contact, adolescents understand they are invited to disclose areas of concern they may not have known they could ask about. Be sure to include questions about strengths as well as concerns or problems. Gather information on multiple areas of a teen's life, including satisfaction with school performance, extracurricular activities, peer relationships, family structure, stressors, etc. In addition to basic data, include questions about whether they are worried about their moods or safety. Ask if they believe whether anyone else is worried about them and why. Provide the parent or caregiver an opportunity to share their concerns and offer their perspective.

Encourage independent completion by teen and parent. This gives each of them a needed opportunity for private communication to the provider. Collecting especially sensitive information prior to the visit allows for identifying areas of concern quickly and efficiently as well as the opportunity to compare and contrast strengths and potential problems. Having even a few moments to review the "big picture" in advance of meeting with a troubled teen and family can contribute greatly to establishing context and, therefore, general orientation toward the line of questioning needed for more assessment and intervention or treatment planning (eg, a mother is worried about sexual activity in a teen who makes straight As in honors classes while volunteering in church and holding down a job). Perhaps, most importantly, this kind of advance information helps you manage the "flow" of conversation in the room without putting the parent or teen on the spot in an uncomfortable way. Finally, with skilled "reading between the lines," noting "blank" responses can be as helpful as full disclosure of problem concerns.

Face Time: Use Resilience Principles to Guide Your Interview and Assessment

 17.1

First impressions count. At your first introduction, introduce yourself by including not just your name and credentials, but also something about your background and your intentions. Let the family know what to expect at the visit, including what your approach is toward communicating with teens and their parents generally and about confidentiality specifically. Reinforce your role as a partner in facilitating positive decision-making. Ask the parent and/or child what they need or expect from the visit. Clarify intentions early to be able to use time and resources efficiently (see Chapter 14).

Lead with positives. Ask about strengths from the very beginning. Ask parents, *"What makes you proud of your child?"* Ask the young person, *"What do you like the most about yourself?"* Then follow up with questions about concerns, such as *"What is her greatest challenge?"* or *"If you could change one thing about your life, what would it be?"* This puts challenges or problems in perspective, disarms hostility, and reminds parents of their love and pride for their child. Most importantly, it clarifies the common goal of wanting the best for their child in the long term.

Make every moment count. Use every interaction and cue as data to help you understand the developmental status or mood profile of your teens. Consider the clues provided from a single question: *"What is the best thing about you?"* A young teen may say, *"My hair."* An older teen may say, *"I am a reliable friend,"* while a college student may report, *"I really know who I am and what's important to me."* If a 17-year-old struggling with school says, *"My hair,"* or a 14-year-old who has been caught cutting says *"Nothing,"* there may be good reason for concern. You may then ask, *"What would you change about your life?"* You can feel reassured if the answer is *"Nothing!"* But if instead she replies, *"I wish my sister weren't so sick all the time,"* or *"To not have to live in 2 houses,"* you have been given critically important information for directing your visit and putting clinical complaints in context.

Wrapping Up: Teach Teens and Families to Build Resilience at Home 17.2, 17.3

Once you have assessed a teen's situation with respect to his developmental status, family support, concerns, and treatment options, use the resilience principles to guide your conversation, engaging both youth and parent or caregiver in active reflection and problem-solving. By going over a structured handout you can show how to integrate the concepts of resilience into their daily lives (see Related Handouts/Supplementary Materials). In some cases, having a tangible paper in front of you to review with an adolescent gives a physical focus to the conversation that allows a reticent teen to avoid unwanted, direct eye contact but keeps him engaged (and also leaves the youth with something to take home for further reflection when he may be less stressed).

In our practice, we give "homework" assignments and readings related to the 7 Cs of resilience and then specifically follow up on their "progress" during follow-up visits (see Chapter 5). We have found this strategy to be a powerful and effective way of engaging teens and their parents in proactive, collaborative problem-solving (rather than reactive blame-seeking). Challenging families to generate concrete action steps promoting specific Cs of resilience encourages them to find the good in each other; finding what's "right" instead of "wrong" facilitates communication about what may be supporting or impeding the teen's healthy development. Even when overwhelmed by frustration, chaos, or uncertainty, coming back to the 7 Cs almost always anchors teens, parents, and professionals around something positive and provides a launching pad for building overall strength and resilience over time.

Competence

Help identify what the young person is already doing right; provide opportunity for her to consider areas of strength she could use to manage or compensate for potential problems. Help find examples of skills she has demonstrated in the past and how she could use them in new situations.

Confidence

Point out the internal self-confidence the youth has gained from successes in various areas in the past. Convey your optimism about how building on his existing strengths and developing new skills will help him to feel even more comfortable with himself and to handle situations over time.

Connection

When appropriate, reinforce the value of the love and support received from various individuals in their lives, especially parents, extended family, and community members. When a young person is struggling, brainstorm ways she can reconnect to those from whom she may have become estranged, or help her identify ways to form new connections to people and communities who may be good for her.

Character

One can find something positive to comment on in most any teen, even those that are most troubled. Help identify aspects of their character that have gotten them this far. Look for examples of positive contributions they have made to their family, friends, or community.

Help them identify ways they can continue to develop positive traits that make them feel the best about themselves. Encourage effort and tenacity.

Contribution

Remind young people that, *"There is nothing more powerful than knowing the world is a better place because you're in it."*[1] Help them to identify even one time they did something for someone else and explore how that made them feel. "Prescribe" volunteer work as the best medicine for a troubled soul. If available, point to local resources for community service opportunities. In some situations, activities in areas related to their own struggles can be very helpful (eg, working with children who may have a similar condition or disease as their own); in other cases (eg, youth with eating disorders), it may be better to direct them to activities that provide distraction and focus on something outside of their usual source of distress.

Coping

Teaching resilience provides an excellent opportunity to help young people understand what positive coping skills they already have in their "toolkit" as well as to point out the risks of maladaptive coping behaviors. By reviewing the natural cycle of stress and the implications of choosing positive or negative coping behaviors, we can engage teens in active dialogue about their behaviors in nonjudgmental ways. A guided conversation specific to developing their repertoire of positive coping skills can lead them to identify ways to find immediate relief from their stressors, if not toward insight, which may at least minimize the risk, severity, or frequency of their dangerous coping behaviors (see Chapter 31).

Control

When people achieve the first 6 Cs, they learn that they have control over their lives and what happens to them. They learn that their actions have real consequences, both positive and negative. Help young people see how they can make changes in their lives that allow them to earn more respect, freedom, and privileges over time. In this way, they avoid adopting the role of the "victim" of their circumstances and instead see how their resilience makes for a better life. Help parents to understand that when they discipline in a controlling "You'll do as I say" manner, their teens learn little about self-control. When they discipline by communicating that "the privileges you'll get are earned by the responsibility you demonstrate," they gain self-control (see Chapter 36).

Be Prepared for the "Now What?" 12.7

The problem with asking meaningful questions is that you will get meaningful answers. Provide handouts with links to Web sites or books that may be helpful, both for patients and parents. When feasible, keep recommended books in stock for parents and teens to read while waiting and for possible purchase at the end of the visit. Consider keeping a booklet of community service listings for youth to peruse as noted above. Always post or keep cards available with information for emergency resources, such as crisis hotlines, runaway shelters, suicide hotlines, etc. Have information easily available for referrals to in-house, colocated, or outside professionals as well as a system for managing these referrals (including record releases to facilitate your communication with those agencies or professionals).

■ Putting It Together: Resilience Works

Using resilience principles with adolescents makes sense. Every teenager, every family, and every story is unique. What almost always is the same is the presence of something good a young person can do to make the best of his situation. Combining a strength-based approach to assessing a young person's needs with active guidance in building resilience helps us structure our approach in productive ways, even if we don't have all the answers.

•• Group Learning and Discussion ••

Download the handouts and then discuss the following points:
1. In our practice do we use pre-visit assessments that allow us to set the tone for a visit that will address risks, but recognize, celebrate, and build on strengths?
2. Do we have a clear referral network that will allow us to efficiently uncover problems and refer for appropriate help?
3. How will the language and structure of the 7 Cs allow us to better communicate our intentions and goals to youth, to families, and between professionals (both within our group and those from different groups and disciplines)?
4. Would focusing visits on building the Cs work in our setting? If so, brainstorm strategies to do so.

■■■■■■■■ Continuing Education ■■■■■■■■■

If you are applying for continuing education credits, a test is available online. For more details, visit www.aap.org/reachingteens.

■ Reference

1. Ginsburg KR. *Building Resilience in Children and Teens: Giving Kids Roots and Wings.* 2nd ed. Elk Grove Village, IL: American Academy of Pediatrics; 2011

■ Related Video Content

17.0 Integrating the 7 Cs of Resilience Into Your Clinical Practice. Sugerman.

17.1 Using the 7 Cs as a Framework to Evaluate a Teen's Well-being. Sugerman.

17.2 Using the 7 Cs as a Framework to Offer "Homework" and a Plan to Move Forward. Sugerman.

17.3 Wrapping Up the Visit With Resilience Reporting: A Strategy to Help Parents Put Their Child's Behavior in Context. Sugerman.

17.4 How Pre-visit Surveys and Paperwork Increase the Reported History and Your Efficiency. Sugerman.

17.5 Comfortably Educating Parents and Youth in an Office About "Uncomfortable" Topics. Sugerman.

17.6 Using Resilience Principles With a Youth in Crisis. Sugerman.

17.7 Navigating Parent-Teen Relationships in a Private Practice Setting. Sugerman.

17.8 Knowing When You Should Worry About Your Child: Seeing Problems in Context. Sugerman.

12.7 A Teen-Friendly Private Practice: Resources, Referrals, and Physical Setting. Sugerman.

14.5 Setting the Stage for a Health Professional-Parent-Teen Partnership. Sugerman.

33.1 Asking for Help Is a Sign of Strength. Sugerman.

34.2 Guiding Parents and Teens to Understand the Shifting Balance Between Parental Control and Teen Decision-Making. Sugerman.

34.6 Case Example: Guiding a Parent and Teen to Work Together to Address Substance Use. Sugerman.

34.7 Helping Parents Know When to Worry and How to Initially React. Sugerman.

35.1 The Benefit of Allowing Our Children to Deal With Challenges. Sugerman.

36.6 Case Example: Supporting Balanced Parenting: Guiding a Teen to Navigate Through a Serious Internet Error. Sugerman.

39.2 Modeling Resilience for Your Children: Defining and Defending Your Priorities. Sugerman.

56.1 A Concrete Flow Sheet That Explains Healthy Versus Unhealthy Relationships to Teens. Sugerman.

56.7 Case Example: Talking About Relationships as Part of a Sexual Health Visit. Sugerman.

■ Related Handouts/Supplementary Materials

Building the 7 Cs of Resilience in Your Child

Are We Building Resilience in the Youth We Serve?

CHAPTER 18

The SSHADESS Screen: A Strength-Based Psychosocial Assessment

Kenneth R. Ginsburg, MD, MS Ed, FAAP, FSAHM

 Related Video Content

18.0 A Strength-Based Comprehensive Psychosocial Assessment: The SSHADESS Screen

■ Why This Matters

We can do our greatest good when we assess youth for risk and emotional well-being before crises present. This positions us to guide adolescents to consider safer behaviors and refer them to appropriate supports.

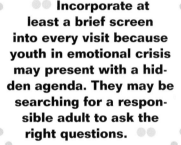

Incorporate at least a brief screen into every visit because youth in emotional crisis may present with a hidden agenda. They may be searching for a responsible adult to ask the right questions.

The SSHADESS screen offers a standard flow to the adolescent psychosocial interview that is rooted in a strength-based approach but that also explores emotional well-being and adolescent risk behaviors. The SSHADESS screen[1,2] is a modified HEADSS screen, which has been taught in adolescent medicine and pediatric training programs for many years.[3]

The rationale behind the modification includes

- **It begins with strengths.** This demonstrates that we do not only view youth in the risk context. Further, it gives us the ability to react to risk in the broader context of the youth's life, minimizing the shame associated with focusing only on risk. 18.1

- **School is addressed before home.** Home is an intimate subject that may raise sensitive issues too early. School is a "safer" subject that allows a general view of functioning. When a young person is in crisis, school usually suffers, and, therefore, can serve as a marker for stress.

- **A wider range of emotions are screened for.** Rather than just focusing on depression or suicide, additional emotions are screened for. In particular, many young people who would deny sad feelings or nervousness would readily endorse stress.

■ Screening for Strengths, Well-being, and Risks

The SSHADESS screen has been designed for direct questioning of an adolescent in a private setting after the stage has been set for a trustworthy relationship (see Chapter 14).

The SSHADESS screen can be also be used to elicit information when a parent/caregiver has accompanied an older child or younger adolescent who is not yet comfortable with a private interview. (Ideally, have a few moments of light conversation in private with these youth to normalize the experience.) When topics are broached in the presence of a parent, only the general topics should be asked directly to the youth (ie, strengths, school, and activities). Direct risk behaviors should not be elicited. Rather, use this as an opportunity to offer general guidance and model for the parent how to approach sensitive topics. Also use it as an opening to discuss whether the parents are approaching these topics at home as they prepare their child to navigate adolescence. This also presents the opportunity to explore needed supports.

Examples of key questions you might ask in a SSHADESS screen are included below. Positive or concerning responses will require a deeper level of questioning than included here. Strategies to explore each area are discussed in the chapters specific to that area.

- **Strengths:** *What do you like doing? How would you describe yourself? Tell me what you're most proud of? How would your best friends describe you?*
- **School:** *What do you enjoy most/least about school? How many days have you missed or had to be excused early or arrived late to school? How are your grades? Any different from last year? Do you feel like you are doing your best at school? (If no) Why not? What's getting in the way? Do you feel safe on the way to school and in school? Do you participate in gym class? What would you like to do when you get older?*
- **Home:** *Who do you live with? Any changes in your family? Could you talk to anyone in your family if you were stressed? Who would you go to first?*
- **Activities:** *Are your friends treating you well? Do you have a best friend or adult you can trust outside your family? Are you still involved in the activities you were doing last year? What kind of things do you do just for fun? Are you spending as much time with your friends as you used to?*
- **Drugs/substance use:** *Do any of your friends talk about smoking cigarettes, taking drugs, or drinking alcohol? Do you smoke cigarettes? Drink alcohol? Have you tried sniffing glue, smoking weed, using pills or other drugs? When/If you smoke, drink or get high, how does it make you feel or what does it do for you?*
- **Emotions/eating/depression:** *Have you been feeling stressed? Do people get on your nerves more than they used to? Are you feeling more bored than usual? Do you feel nervous a lot? Have you been having trouble sleeping lately? (If yes) What kind of trouble? Would you describe yourself as a healthy eater? Have you been trying to gain or lose weight? Tell me why? Have you been feeling down, sad, or depressed? Have you thought of hurting yourself or someone else? Have you ever tried to hurt yourself?*
- **Sexuality:** *Are you attracted to anyone? Tell me about that person? (Using gender-neutral language) Are you comfortable with your sexual feelings? Are you attracted to guys, girls, or both? What kind of things have you done sexually? Kissing? Touching? Oral sex? Have you ever had sexual intercourse? Have you enjoyed it? What kind of steps do you take to protect yourself? Have you ever been worried that you could be pregnant? Have you ever been worried about or had a sexually transmitted infection?*
- **Safety:** *Are there a lot of fights at your school? Do you feel safe at school? Is there bullying? Have you been bullied? Do you carry weapons? What kind of things makes you mad enough to fight? Has anyone ever touched you physically or sexually when you didn't want them to?* (Note that abuse is asked in the context of safey, NOT sexuality.) *Does your boyfriend/girlfriend get jealous?* (Jealousy is an early sign of controlling, potentially abusive, relationships.) *Do you ever get into*

▶ 18.9

fights with your boyfriend/girlfriend? Physical fights? Have you ever seen people in your family or home hurt each other? Say mean things? Throw things or hit each other?

■ The Brief Psychosocial Screen

Time constraints may preclude the comprehensive psychosocial screen from being completed in every encounter. However, a brief psychosocial screen can be incorporated into every visit. The rationale of incorporating this screen into even brief visits is that youth in emotional crisis may present with a hidden agenda. They may be searching for a responsible adult to ask the right questions. In particular, 50% of youth who had completed suicide were found to have presented to primary care providers in the month preceding the attempt.[4,5] Further, somatic complaints may be driven by emotional stressors. Be particularly vigilant with vague concerns or chief complaints of headache, fatigue, dizziness, abdominal pain, and chest pain (see Chapter 44).

With these points in mind, a 3-part screen is recommended.

1. *"How is school going?"* School is a proxy measure for general well-being; life's stressors are likely to adversely affect school performance. Concerning responses suggest recent changes and include, *"I had a bad quarter,"* or *"Not as well as it used to be,"* or *"I'm not going very much."* This is an invitation to ask *"Really? What's been going on?"*
2. *"Would you describe yourself as pretty happy or stressed?"* or *"How is life going for you?"*
3. No matter the response, ask, *"When you're not happy, how do you handle it and whom do you talk to?"*

The unhappy or highly stressed youth who also feels isolated and lacks anyone to talk to may be at risk. Regardless of the presenting complaint this patient deserves a more thorough evaluation. (See full SSHADESS screen demonstrations.) 18.14–18.19

■ General Tips for the Psychosocial Interview 18.6

- First, the interview should proceed from general, less intimate topics to those more personal (see Communication 101 in Chapter 16, page 121). The SSHADESS screen is designed with this flow in mind.
- Questions within sensitive topics should initially be impersonal. For example, *"Are many of the teens in your school doing drugs?"* should precede *"Are you using any drugs?"*
- Take care not to express shock or dismay to the responses. There is time later to offer guidance. A quick reaction may disrupt disclosure of the full history. Similarly, early praise makes young people want to continue to give prosocial responses to continue earning your praise.
- Be careful not to ask yes or no questions, for 2 reasons. First, they limit the depth of the responses. Second, when you ask a sensitive question and a youth does not yet fully trust you, she may lie, making her embarrassed to disclose honestly later.
- The goal is to get the most therapeutic history, not the most thorough history. Adolescents often go through a testing process before disclosing their most intimate issues, and that "test" may require several visits over time. Further, in some cases, it may not be safe to push them further than their comfort zone as the elicited shame may drive them toward risk behaviors that help them cope with stress.
- Do not assume the adolescent who offers full and rapid disclosure is not at risk. Sometimes vulnerable or isolated adolescents disclose personal information very rapidly in an effort to bond with you. Remember that monosyllabic responses can be within the range of normal for an adolescent interview; whereas sometimes excessive friendliness or revelation could be a sign that the adolescent is in crisis and unable to appropriately "edit" their disclosure.

- Above all, while listening to responses, allow time to think about what you really admire or respect about the teen. The restatement of these positive points allows you to offer guidance about risk in the broader context that also recognizes strengths (see Chapter 25). This may be particularly important for marginalized teens.
- After the interview, ask permission to address a problem or concern that may have been raised. If you don't ask teens whether they want your advice, they may be less likely to listen to it.

●● Group Learning and Discussion ●●

Prior to a discussion on SSHADESS, assign different colleagues to take a deeper dive in 1 or 2 of the specific areas (eg, mental health, sex and sexuality, substance use, violence, abuse, eating disorders, etc). On the day of the discussion, first pair up and practice routine SSHADESS screens. Then take each topic and have the colleague who focused on that area discuss the deeper level of questioning and/or office-based interventions that could be useful when screening triggers a concern. Finally, come up with a plan to create a comprehensive referral resource list so that you will have it readily available for when the SSHADESS screen raises a concern that merits further exploration or support.

◼◼◼◼◼◼◼◼ Continuing Education ◼◼◼◼◼◼◼◼◼

If you are applying for continuing education credits, a test is available online. For more details, visit www.aap.org/reachingteens.

◼ References

1. Ginsburg KR. Viewing our adolescent patients through a positive lens. *Contemp Pediatr.* 2007a;241:65–76

2. Ginsburg KR. Engaging adolescents and building on their strengths. *Adolesc Health Update.* 2007b;19(2):1–8

3. Clark LR, Ginsburg KR. How to talk to your teenaged patients. *Contemp Adolesc Gynecol.* 1995;1(4):23–27

4. Smith K, Crawford S. Suicide behavior among "normal" high school students. *Suicide Life Threat Behav.* 1986;16:313–325

5. Hawton K, O'Grady J, Osborn M, Cole D. Adolescents who take overdoses: their characteristics, problems, and contacts with helping agencies. *Br J Psychiatry.* 1982;140:118–123

◼ Related Video Content

18.0 A Strength-Based Comprehensive Psychosocial Assessment: The SSHADESS Screen. Ginsburg.

18.1 Maximizing the Yield From a Strength-Based Interview: Avoiding the Pitfalls of Using Only a Positive Lens. Ginsburg.

18.2 How a Comprehensive Assessment Positions Us to Develop and Prioritize Interventions. Ford.

18.3 A Strategy for Incorporating a Comprehensive Psychosocial Screen Into the Office Visit. Pletcher.

18.4 Using a "Self-esteem Score" to Gain Rapid Insight Into the Adolescent's Well-being. Clark.

18.5 Using Media History as a Way to Connect With and Understand Youth. Rich.

18.6 Pearls to More Effectively Elicit Psychosocial Histories. Pletcher, Campbell, Reirden, Bailer, Feit.

18.7 The Goal Is Not to Get the Most Detailed History, It Is to Get the Most Therapeutic History for the Youth at That Time: A Case of Abuse That Revealed Itself Over Time. Ginsburg.

18.8 A Change in Behavior or Emotional Status May Signal an Identity Crisis. Chaffee.

18.9 Incorporating a Screen for Abuse Into the SSHADESS Screen. Diaz.

18.10 SSHADESS Screen: Pearls on Asking About School. Diaz, Jenkins.

18.11 SSHADESS Screen: Pearls on Asking About Sexuality. Dowshen, Diaz, Pletcher, Reirden.

18.12 SSHADESS Screen: Pearls on Asking About Drugs and Substances. Diaz, Adolescent Advocates staff.

18.13 SSHADESS Screen: Pearls on Asking About Strengths. Chaffee, Diaz, Pletcher.

18.14 Case: SSHADESS Screen With Young Teen. Catallozzi.

18.15 Case: SSHADESS Screen Reveals Bullying. Lewis.

18.16 Case: SSHADESS Screen Reveals Substance Use—CRAFFT Screen Follow-up. Kinsman.

18.17 Case: SSHADESS Screen Reveals Teen Feeling Uncomfortable With Sexual Experience. Lerman.

18.18 Case: 11-Year-Old Girl With Chronic Disease and Depression. Peter.

18.19 Case: A Brief Routine SSHADESS Screen. Clark.

11.12 Avoiding Labels: Exploring Attractions, Behaviors, and Orientation. Hawkins, Arrington-Sanders.

34.0 Four Approaches to Wrapping Up the Visit: All Committed to Informing and Engaging the Parent While Maintaining Teen Confidentiality. Ford, Pletcher, Diaz, Sugerman.

34.8 Helping Parents Understand the Additive Role Professionals Can Play in Their Adolescents' Lives. Jenkins.

41.3 Peer Relationships Can Tell Us so Much if We Don't Interrupt Disclosure With Judgment. Pletcher.

CHAPTER 19

Cultural Humility

Valerie J. Lewis, MD, MPH, FAAP, FSAHM

Kenisha Campbell, MD, MPH

Angela Diaz, MD, MPH

Nadia L. Dowshen, MD, FAAP, AAHIVS

Kenneth R. Ginsburg, MD, MS Ed, FAAP, FSAHM

Renée R. Jenkins, MD, FAAP

Jarret R. Patton, MD, FAAP

Maria Trent, MD, MPH, FAAP, FSAHM

Dzung X. Vo, MD, FAAP

> ▶ **Related Video Content**
>
> 19.0 Cultural Humility: An Overview

■ Why This Matters 19.3

We must navigate our therapeutic relationships with young people in ways that are mindful of their unique differences and that embrace these characteristics in a nonjudgmental way. We must honor their diversity and recognize that each individual's unique makeup is shaped from a coalescence of their cultural, racial, ethnic, gender, religious, and sexual identities.

> **It is our responsibility to make our encounters safe and make our settings places that embrace and foster the unique differences of teens.**

How we care for young people can set the tone for their expectations in future encounters with all "systems" they may interact with. We are setting the stage and providing the tools for teens to become strong self-advocates. We can impact their trajectories—positively or negatively—based on how we treat them.

Young people come to us with assumptions and biases about how we will behave based on their prior experiences with other adults. Unfortunately, they have sometimes received negative messages from adults. As a result, adolescents may feel they lack worthiness. It is our responsibility to ensure that our settings and encounters 19.5 demonstrate that we value and foster the unique differences of teens.

■ Being Aware of Our Biases

Cultural humility is defined as a lifelong commitment to self-evaluation and self-critique, a commitment to redressing the power imbalances inherent in the patient-professional dynamic, and commitment to developing mutually beneficial and non-paternalistic clinical and advocacy partnerships with communities on behalf of individuals and defined populations. This expands on the notion of **cultural competence,** which is characterized by the acquisition of a body of knowledge and the mastery of a skill set. Both approaches ask us to be self-reflective, take note, and "check ourselves" when we interact with people from diverse or different backgrounds.[1] We begin by understanding that adolescents are attempting to find out who they are, and are in the process of solidifying their identities. Their differences may be the very basis of how they define themselves. Therefore, a key skill required to effectively work with young people is being open to their differences and being nonjudgmental, empathetic, and compassionate regarding those differences. However, in order to do this, we must have a degree of self-awareness and an intimate understanding of our own biases.

Self-awareness is a key component to providing quality care to young people. Biases are ubiquitous and are reflections of our experiences, histories, and exposures. Inherently, we are all "other" to someone. There is no blame or shame in that. However, it is our responsibility, through the process of ongoing self-evaluation and self-exploration, to overcome our biases. Having awareness of your inherent biases and working to remediate biases may strengthen the therapeutic bond you have with young people.

We All Have Biases That Impact Teens 19.1, 19.7

We (just like the young people with whom we interact) are products of our experiences. In fact, we use "mental shortcuts," or heuristics, to help us solve problems in our daily practice.[2] Another tool that we use are "schemas," which are templates of knowledge that help us to organize specific bits of information into larger categories. The schemas we use to categorize people are stereotypes. Distinct from stereotype is the concept of prejudice, which is the attitude or behavioral reaction toward people because they are members of a certain group.[3] The concept of implicit or unconscious bias suggests that our learned stereotypes, which operate automatically and beyond our conscious control, drive our social behavior and influence our interaction with others. Stereotyping is the vehicle through which our implicit bias manifests.[3] (See Chapter 21.)

Bias plays out every day in the health care setting. For example, when a 16-year-old female presents with right-sided abdominal pain, we consider the diagnoses of appendicitis, ovarian cyst or torsion, pain associated with ovulation, urinary tract infection, kidney stone, and sexually transmitted pelvic infection. In addition to our physical examination, we use the patient's medical history to guide our workup and decision-making. We may also choose one diagnosis over another, for nonclinical reasons, based on our biases about the patient's demographic. This could have unintended negative physical and emotional consequences for our patients. Many studies have demonstrated significant health disparities, resulting in differential treatment options and differential outcomes resulting from unconscious provider biases.[4]

Bias affects how we care for our teens. A provider may make a decision to offer an HIV test based on physical appearance, socioeconomic status, race/ethnicity, or sexual orientation. Regardless of whether certain populations or groups of people may be disproportionately affected by the disease, providers cannot assume any one individual's risk or protective factors. For this reason, HIV testing is now being recommended for all youth routinely. This recommendation overrides potential provider biases and provides needed care for all youth.

Our body language is as important as the decisions we make or the words we use in conveying our biases! Adolescents live up or down to our expectations, and our demeanor may communicate a sense of judgment to teenagers that our words do not. For example, when a white person is approached by a Latino teen, she may take a small step back, check to be sure her purse is closed, and then clutch her purse a bit tighter. The hidden message, *"Latinos are dangerous and one's property may be in jeopardy around them."* As a result of this interaction, the young person may assume a defensive posture, feel judged, and respond in what may be perceived as disrespectful. Teens who have experienced prejudice learn that, to reestablish the power differential, they may need to resort to using tactics of fear or intimidation. This cycle is halted when the teen is treated with respect, acceptance, and love, all of which are apparent in one's spoken word and body language (see Chapter 15). **15.0**

Bias can be expressed through microaggression. Microaggression refers to the idea that specific interactions between those of different races, cultures, or genders can be interpreted as nonphysical aggression. The term, originated by psychologist, Chester M. Pierce in the 1970s, is defined as "brief and commonplace daily verbal, behavioral, or environmental indignities, whether intentional or unintentional, that communicate hostile, derogatory, or negative racial slights and insults toward people of other races." Microaggression usually involves denigrating messages against minorities by nonminorities who may be unaware of the derogatory implications. These subtle and nonverbal exchanges may be perpetrated against members of minority groups due to gender, religion, sexual orientation, or ability status.[5] Examples of microaggression include the continued inability for a nonminority person to pronounce the name of a minority person or a teacher scheduling a mandatory test on a religious or cultural holiday. Many minority teens report being followed by a clerk as they browse in a store. The message here, *"You look like someone who should not be in this setting or who might steal."*

Learning how we inadvertently communicate bias and undermining messages strengthens each of us in our ability to overcome these entrenched patterns. Again, no shame, no blame, just a commitment to being aware and changing patterns that we may have assimilated from the broader society!

Strategies to Overcome Bias

Create an adolescent-friendly location that welcomes diversity on all levels in which young people receive care. Paying attention to the physical environment where you provide care to adolescents conveys a message of comfort, safety, and respect (see Chapter 12). Don't assume you know or understand someone else's life experiences; approach each young person as a unique individual who is developing their own identity and view of acculturation.

Invest time in learning about the "others"—their culture, religion, language, and holidays. Also, ask questions to increase understanding and clarify as necessary; use appropriate curiosity and take the stance of "teach me" to engage the young person and learn more about that individual's cultural background. At the same time, we should not expect a young person to "represent" his or her group, both because it is not fair to do so, and because it is wrong to assume any one person can represent a group. **19.6**

Role model cultural sensitivity to young children, as this is the foundation for our adolescents—set the tone and expectations regarding cultural humility from a young age, whether we are parents ourselves, care for young children in some capacity, or interact with parents or caregivers who are raising young children. Children emulate us and we have an obligation to help our young people—children and teens—understand cultural humility and promote tolerance of others, interceding in the generational cycle of passing along "-isms." Exposing children to and taking the time to learn about differences in family customs, ideals, beliefs, foods, religions, socioeconomic status, and neighborhoods all represent opportunities for the expression of cultural humility. Teach cultural humility by reading books that celebrate diversity, being understanding of and embracing differences among people, stressing that there is no "right" or "wrong" culture, and using "teachable moments" to demonstrate various aspects of culture.

■ A Lifelong Process

Cultural competence needs to be developed and nurtured in the same way as any other professional skill set. Participation in continuing education opportunities with a self-evaluative component is key. Achieving cultural competence through training is an ongoing process and requires a strong desire to be self-reflective in order to achieve proficiency.[6]

No amount of professional development can make you immune from the cultural biases that you have incorporated from a lifetime of exposure to our culture. However, an awareness of these biases and a commitment to overcome them, coupled with a desire to learn about the unique identity of each of the youth you serve, will allow you to move toward cultural competence and certainly position you to be culturally humble.

●● Group Learning and Discussion ●●

What is the experience of the youth we serve as they walk on the streets? Are they greeted with low expectations, even fear? Do they have a different experience here from the moment they walk through the door? If not, what needs to happen in our practice setting?

What are the sources from which we pick up unconscious biases? What are ours? It is nearly impossible to have no unconscious biases. If it is safe in your setting to discuss these unconscious biases, it is ideal to discuss them as a first step toward modifying them. If, however, that would be difficult in your practice setting, then allow a few moments of reflection facilitated by the following questions.

1. Close your eyes and imagine a young person from a different group walking on the street? Or perhaps he is from your own group, but you have absorbed the media messages and community biases that kids from his group are the source of many problems.
2. What is your instinctual response to him? Fear? Apprehension?
3. How might your body language reflect those feelings?
4. How might your reaction (or a cumulative total of others' reactions) affect his expectations when he comes to your office?
5. Now think about that young person. Imagine what he does for fun. Imagine him with his parents…grandmother…baby sister. Imagine what his dreams might be.
6. Imagine what you might learn from him as the expert on his own life.

■■■■■■■■ Continuing Education ■■■■■■■■■■

If you are applying for continuing education credits, a test is available online. For more details, visit www.aap.org/reachingteens.

References

1. Tervalon M, Murray-Garcia J. Cultural humility versus cultural competence: a critical distinction in defining physician training outcomes in multicultural education. *J Health Care Poor Underserved.* 1998;9(2):117–125

2. Balsa AI, Seiler N, McGuire TG, Bloche MG. Clinical uncertainty and healthcare disparities. *Am J Law Med.* 2003;29(2–3):203–219

3. Greenwald AG, Banaji MR. Implicit social cognition: attitudes, self-esteem, and stereotypes. *Psychol Rev.* 1995;102(1):4–27

4. Sue DW, Capodilupo CM, Holder A. Racial microaggressions in the life experience of Black Americans. *Professional Psychol Res Pract.* 2008;39(3):329–336

5. Green AR, Carney DR, Pallin DJ, et al. Implicit bias among physicians and its prediction of thrombolysis decisions for Black and White patients. *J Gen Intern Med.* 2007;22:1231–1238

6. Cross T, Bazron B, Dennis K, Isaacs M. *Towards a Culturally Competent System of Care.* Vol 1. Washington, DC: CASSP Technical Assistance Center, Center for Child Health and Mental Health Policy, Georgetown University Center for Child and Human Development; 1989

Suggested Reading

Balsa AI, Seiler N, McGuire TG, Bloche MG. Clinical uncertainty and healthcare disparities. *Am J Law Med.* 2003;29:203–219

Beck BJ, Gordon C. An approach to collaborative care and consultation: interviewing, cultural competence, and enhancing rapport and adherence. *Med Clin North Am.* 2010;94:1075–1088

Berger JT. The influence of physicians' demographic characteristics and their patients' demographic characteristics on physician practice: implications for education and research. *Acad Med.* 2008;83(1):100–105

Berry JW. Acculturation: living successfully in two cultures. *Int J Intercult Rel.* 2005;29(6):697–712

Berry JW, Phinney JS, Sam DL, Vedder P. Immigrant youth, acculturation, identity, and adaptation. *Appl Psychol.* 2006;55(3):303–332

Blue AV, Thiedke Chessman AW, Kern DH, Keller A. *Applying Theory to Assess Cultural Competency.* Morgantown, WV: Medical Education Online; 2005. http://www.med-ed-online.org. Accessed June 26, 2013

Chin MH, Humikowski CA. When is risk stratification by race or ethnicity justified in medical care? *Acad Med.* 2002;77(3):202–208

Cross T, Bazron B, Dennis K, Isaacs M. *Towards a Culturally Competent System of Care.* Vol 1. Washington, DC: CASSP Technical Assistance Center, Center for Child Health and Mental Health Policy, Georgetown University Child Development Center; 1989

Green AR, Carney DR, Pallin DJ, et al. Implicit bias among physicians and its prediction of thrombolysis decisions for Black and White patients. *J Gen Intern Med.* 2007;22:1231–1238

Greenwald AG, Banaji MR. Implicit social cognition: attitudes, self-esteem, and stereotypes. *Psychol Rev.* 1995;102(1):4–275

Johnson RL, Saha S, Arbelaez JJ, Beach MC, Cooper LA. Racial and ethnic difference in patient perceptions of bias and cultural competence in health care. *J Gen Intern Med.* 2004;19:101–110

Kumas-Tan, Z, Beagan B, Loppie C, MacLeod A, Blye F. Measures of cultural competence: examining hidden assumptions. *Acad Med.* 2007;82(6):548–556

Padela AI, Punekar IR. Emergency medical practice: advancing cultural competence and reducing health care disparities. *Acad Emerg Med.* 2009;16(1):69–75

Racher FE, Annis RC. Respecting culture and honoring diversity in community practice. *Res Theory Nurs Pract.* 2007;21(4):255–270

Rue DS, Xie Y. Disparities in treating culturally diverse children and adolescents. *Psychiatr Clin North Am.* 2009;32:153–163

Sue DW, Capodilupo CM, Holder A. Racial microaggressions in the life experience of Black Americans. *Professional Psychol Res Pract.* 2008;39(3):329–336

Sue DW, Capodilupo CM, Torino GC, et al. Racial microaggressions in everyday life: implications for clinical practice. *Am Psychol.* 2007;62:271–286

Tervalon M, Murray-Garcia J. Cultural humility versus cultural competence: a critical distinction in defining physician training outcomes in multicultural education. *J Health Care Poor Underserved.* 1998;9(2):117–125

■ Related Video Content

19.0 Cultural Humility: An Overview. Lewis, Trent, Jenkins, Singh, Vo, Diaz, Patton, Campbell, Ginsburg.

19.1 Unconscious Biases. Jenkins, Vo.

19.2 We Do Not Have to Be a Cultural Match to Serve Youth Well. Arrington-Sanders, Trent, Ginsburg, Singh, Lewis, Patton, Sidhu.

19.3 Every Human Interaction Is a Cross-cultural Experience. Singh.

19.4 Racial and Ethnic Identity Development. Vo.

19.5 A Diverse Workforce Generates a Sense of Safety and Security in Youth. Trent, Ginsburg, Hill, Lewis.

19.6 The Easiest Way to Be Culturally Humble: Saying, "Teach Me About You." Singh, Diaz, Bell.

19.7 We All Have Biases We Need to Bring to Awareness: Our Challenge Is to Take the Steps to Minimize Their Influence on Our Actions. Ginsburg, Jenkins, Vo, Diaz.

19.8 Racism Negatively Affects the Person Who "Benefits" From Privilege. Vo.

19.9 "Rules of Thumb" Can Be Helpful, But Generalizations Often Produce Harmful Unconscious Biases. Vo.

19.10 How Biases Can Affect Our Assumptions About Sexual Behaviors. Clark.

19.11 There Are Multiple Layers to Culture: We Must Take a Granular Approach. Diaz, Vo.

19.12 Reaffirming Self-worth for a Young Person Who Has Incorporated Society's Negative Images of His or Her Group. Lewis, Patton.

19.13 Personal Challenge: Raising African American Males in a Society That too Often Portrays Them Negatively. Lewis, Campbell.

19.14 Marginalized Youth May Make Assumptions About Us Based on Suffering They Have Endured From People Who Share Our Background. Vo.

19.15 We Must Not Assume That Well-Resourced Youth Do Not Have Problems. Campbell.

19.16 Unconditional Love and High Expectations Protect Your Child From Society's Lower Expectations. Campbell.

19.17 A Gift to Our Children: Preparing Them to Question, Rather Than Accept, Racist or Discriminatory Messages. Vo.

19.18 A Gift to Our Children: Preparing Them to Thrive in a Diverse World. Patton.

12.1 Creating an LGBTQ-Friendly Space. Dowshen, Arrington-Sanders, Hawkins.

12.3 Ensuring a Space Without Judgment or Low Expectation so Risks and Hopes and Dreams Will Be Shared. Campbell.

12.8 A Diverse Environment Is a Safe Environment. Ginsburg.

15.0 Body Language Conveys Respect or Judgment, Openness or Mistrust, and High or Low Expectations. Ginsburg.

59.7 Caring for Youth With Chronic Illness: The Importance of Understanding How They Use Traditional Healing and Complementary Medicine. Pletcher.

61.6 Your Respect and Presence Are More Important to Your Ability to Provide Care to LGBT Youth Than Your Sexual or Gender Identity. Arrington-Sanders, Garofalo.

61.16 Being LGBT Is Just One Part of a Young Person's Identity. Garofalo.

61.20 Youth Testimony: "This Is How to Address Me" (and Much More): Guidance From a Young Transgender Person. Youth.

62.0 Serving Immigrant Youth. Vo.

62.1 Serving Across Cultures. Trent.

CHAPTER 20

Boundaries

Kenneth R. Ginsburg, MD, MS Ed, FAAP, FSAHM

 Related Video Content

20.0 Boundaries: Essential to Our Healthy Relationships With Youth and Our Professional Longevity

■ Why This Matters

It is our connection that allows us to reach teens. In this text, we speak of serving youth with "absolute respect and unconditional love." * We write of engaging them in a way that listens deeply while recognizing that they are the experts in their own lives. We emphasize the importance of becoming trustworthy enough so that young people can comfortably share the details we need to know to serve them best.

The level of engagement we propose, if not carefully and thoughtfully managed, can be harmful to both you and the teens under your care. When you allow yourself to connect deeply, you become vulnerable. The exposure to others' pain and the toxic levels of stress they have endured can lead to your own traumatization and burnout. Further, for the sake of the teens with whom you make those meaningful and critical connections, you have to strive for the balance that offers absolute security without making them reliant, or even dependent, on you for their forward movement.

In order to ensure that our relationship with youth remains therapeutic for them and safe for us, we need to be thoughtful about boundaries.

> **We speak of serving youth with "absolute respect and unconditional love." The level of engagement we propose, if not carefully and thoughtfully managed, can be harmful to both you and the teens under your care.**

■ Uses and Limits of This Discussion on Boundaries

Professional organizations offer guidelines that assist us to maintain appropriate boundaries (see Code of Ethics From Key Organizations). The discussion offered here is not intended to supersede the policies and guidelines of your professional organization or institution. In fact, those guidelines should be the minimum standards to which you adhere.

The intent of this chapter is to augment existing guidelines and to engage you in a reflective process so you are better prepared to have the most effective relationships with the young people you serve. It is meant to stimulate thought, not to be prescriptive. You may find that some issues raised here can serve as starting points in discussions with colleagues about how you, as a group, can best serve youth. Further, trusted colleagues may be able to offer you valuable feedback on your own use of boundaries. Because this

---

*This phrase is a key portion of the mission statement of Covenant House, the nation's largest privately funded agency serving homeless youth.

chapter is not all-inclusive, your discussions may raise key points worthy of consideration not included here.

■ Therapeutic Connections

Absolute Respect and Unconditional Love

We are to serve youth with absolute respect. Respecting youth may involve a change in mindset, but likely does not pose any boundary issues. We offer respect when we withhold judgment and understand that even behaviors we reject likely are chosen to help one navigate through stressful situations. For example, the use of drugs may numb a young person from emotions he finds intolerable. We grant respect through thoughtful listening that elicits strengths. We act respectful when we recognize that people are the experts in their own lives and need to be in charge of determining if, and when, they are prepared to change.

We are also to serve youth with unconditional love. *Love* is more complex, and certainly raises boundary considerations. The word holds a variety of meanings, some of which imply a kind of closeness or intimacy inappropriate for a healing setting. This may limit our comfort with using the word "love" in the English-speaking world.

In other languages and cultures, there are different words for love that allow us to distinguish between sexual and other forms of love. For example, Greek clearly distinguishes between sexual love ("eros"), brotherly love ("phileo"), and the unconditional love ("agape") often referred to in Christian liturgy. Loving-kindness is a term used to convey the concept of pure compassion (eg, the Buddhist term "metta," the Hebrew word "chesed," and the Arabic word "Mahabbah").

It is the compassion we have for other humans, the commitment to loving-kindness, that is central to our mission to serve. It is this love that gives us the genuine concern and empathy that allows us to engage others in a healing process. However, because we function in a primarily English-speaking culture, we may choose to restrict use of the word "love" to avoid any miscommunications or uncomfortable feelings. Withholding use of the word, however, should not limit our use of the construct. Perhaps it may feel more comfortable to strive to be "loving." While "love" may imply a quality of deep connection or enduring devotion not applicable for our professional relationships, "loving" is to be kind, forgiving, nonjudgmental, accepting, affirming, respectful, and open.

When trainees present me with the story of a patient, their opening line needs to be "this is what I love about him/her." They need to do the hard work of seeing youth in the context of their lives and seeing their strength, their beauty, their spark. Are they compassionate despite having received very little affirmation from those who were supposed to care for them? Are they resilient in the face of repeated challenges? Do they have a sense of loyalty that arises from the need to find trust in a world that hasn't seemed so trustworthy? Once trainees view the adolescent through this lens, they have a deeper sense of genuine respect and are thus prepared to invite that youth to engage in the kind of decisions that will maximize her potential to contribute to the world. Once we have elicited stories in this context, we can reflect them back to youth in a way that takes shame away from our interaction, instills pride in the young people, and hopefully allows them to build on their inherent strengths as they continue to grow as human beings (see Chapter 25).

The love offered in a professional setting must be unidirectional. It is delivered through your empathy, respect, and deep-seated desire that the adolescent develops safely and securely. It is the lens through which you choose to care for others. It is something you give youth, requiring absolutely nothing in return. You are asking only for a youth's commitment to be her best self and permission to be part of that process. You do not require affirmation or acceptance yourself. You can rejuvenate from the energy that comes from connection and service, but it is not the adolescent's job to offer you anything. This allows the relationship to be one in which he or she can genuinely heal and grow.

The love offered in a professional setting must have boundaries. It exists so that youth can experience being valued and can know they have a space that is absolutely safe to think about who they want to be and how they will contribute to the world. It creates a safe space from which they can recover from pain and shift directions if they may be headed for trouble. The safe space should allow teens to gain confidence in their existing competencies and learn to build new ones. It must not cross the line into forging a relationship in which the teen becomes reliant on the caregiver. If it does, then the potential for harm is great because the adolescent might not develop the skills to think independently, and might be less likely to forge healthy relationships with future helping professionals.

▶ **20.3**

Sharing Your Own Experiences

We know that youth seek "friendly" caregivers to whom they relate. But to what extent does relatedness imply you need to share your personal life and experiences? Again, draw from your professional organization's guidelines and institutional regulations. I invite you to also reflect on the following points.

- If an adolescent asks you personal information consistent with typical friendly conversation, you need to determine your comfort level in responding. If that teen inquires about genuinely personal information, it is worth exploring why it feels important. If the young person persists, it is reasonable to respond that the visit must focus on him, because you are there to serve him.
- If you tend to have loose boundaries in your personal lives and with your professional colleagues, or you find that sharing is how you forge quick connections, be particularly vigilant when working with youth. Youth do not need to know your personal life to trust you or feel secure in your presence.
- Sometimes your sharing can actually be misinterpreted as if you are minimizing the teen's concerns. In some cases, it could be viewed as though you are trying to compete with their experiences or belittling what they are feeling.
- Always ask yourself about the therapeutic direction if you do choose to share something. If you feel better after sharing or relieved of a burden, the therapeutic direction is wrong. Neither the youth you serve nor their parents are supposed to be caring for you.
- Never share anything that you wouldn't want on the evening news. You are committed to upholding privacy; that is not a mutual commitment.
- Never share anything that may make you appear impaired. No one wants an impaired caregiver. This means that present struggles should never be disclosed. You have to determine whether your experience with overcoming a challenge is therapeutic for a teen. Any sharing about struggles must occur in the context of an existing solution. Each of us needs to determine what this means. In my case, I will judiciously share with a deeply depressed youth who is hopeless that I had serious depression as a 17-year-old. The context is in how treatable depression is, how it needs to be put in a "this too shall pass" category, and how lifelong lessons of sensitivity and empathy can be learned from our challenges. (For clarity, stating "this too shall pass" must not minimize the intensity of the present discomfort, instead it is intended to offer hope that the future can be brighter, to reinforce "You will get through this.")
- You may consider skillful (or judicious) self-disclosure when a teen subtly suggests he wants to see you as a real human being. This may involve sharing something that says that you are "real," but be careful not to mistakenly believe the teen cares about the details or travails of your life, lest the visit becomes more about you than about the youth. For example, you might say *"Yes, I have stress in my life as well, that is why I exercise regularly."*

Avoiding the Rescue Fantasy

It is difficult to bear witness to suffering and not want to change it. Sometimes the solutions feel so obvious to us. We care so much that we just want to "fix" the unbearable circumstances in our youths' lives. However, we can enter a "rescue fantasy" when our passion to "save" the youth we care for is so powerful that we forget that change is a process and only has staying power when a person owns that process. Further, when you dive in so deeply that you are trying to change the youth single-handedly, she might feel as if she needs to make a choice to please you. Ultimately, her fear of disappointing you might have her select an option she is not ready for or may drive her away. Perhaps as important, you will become woefully disappointed when you engage in rescue fantasies. You will view slow progress or relapses as a personal failure. This will contribute to your burnout and limit your ability to potentiate change over a long fulfilling career.

Instead, understand that you are a facilitator. The adolescent is in charge of the process. They are the experts in their lives. Their success or failure rests on their decisions. You own neither the successes nor the disappointments. You trust that your consistent presence will ultimately guide the young person in a positive direction. You give information. You believe in the potential of change. You offer affirmation. You offer options. You help her determine when change offers the best solutions.

Barriers to Forging Therapeutic Connections

Checking in With Yourself 14.1

It can be personally challenging to work with teens. In order to meet their needs, we have to have conversations about things rarely discussed in polite society, such as sexuality. We have to guide them as they try to answer the fundamental question of adolescence: "Who am I?" One of the reasons we may struggle in our work with teens is that most of us have remaining unresolved adolescent issues. First, how many of us have really fully answered the question, "Who am I?" Further, self-esteem remains an issue for many adults, but we likely remember our struggles in this area of life and development most acutely as adolescents. Were we considered attractive? Were we confused about our status in relationships?

We need to go through a reflective process to understand which "adolescent" issues remain in our adult lives. Where are we "stuck"? We also need to know which peers created particularly painful interactions or had the most powerful influences over our development. Finally, we need to think about how we were parented.

Reflecting on these questions will begin to help you understand the origin of those remaining "adolescent" issues. Only when you bring these issues to awareness will you be prepared to more objectively serve youth, leaving your past out of the equation. Only then will you be able to most skillfully work with parents to learn to effectively guide their children. This process may also help you to avoid unintended boundary issues. For purposes of illustration, let us consider a few examples.

- If you wished you were in the popular crowd, but never were quite accepted there, you might still need to prove your worthiness. A popular, athletic teen might come to you minimizing their alcoholic binges. Rather than objectively noting the warning signs he is bringing to your attention, your desire to be accepted might inadvertently have you join him in his feigned denial.
- If you were bullied, you might instinctively dislike the youth in your presence whose dress or persona reminds you of past tormentors.
- If you were parented by an authoritarian "You'll do as I say. Why? Because I said so!" parent, you might have difficulty seeing that the father in your office is drawing from the only toolbox he has to parent his son. Your judgment of him as mean or controlling may prevent you from being able to engage him to expand his skill set.

- If you did not garner the sexual attention or romantic relationships you desired as an adolescent, you might still be a bit hurt. You might resent a popular, attractive youth for having what you didn't. How can you objectively guide that teen toward healthy romantic or sexual decision-making when you are working through your own feelings of inadequacy or disappointment?

■ Overcoming Counter-Therapeutic Boundaries Incorporated During Our Training and Daily Practices 20.2

We chose to work with people so that we could make a difference in their lives. We may have held an idealistic view about the extent of our potential impact. Over time, many of us become jaded and wonder if we make any difference at all. There are multiple reasons why this may occur, but one of them may be the different lens through which we begin to view those we serve. When we view people in a negative light, judgment and shame enter our interactions, we lose our objectivity, and our ability to be change agents is diminished.

How did we begin to feel so frustrated with those we serve? How did they become "other," so different from us that we begin to see them as responsible for their own suffering, as recalcitrant to progress?

In training, as in practice, we are exposed to unimaginable pain. We see illness and death. We see the consequences of abuse. We care for people who seem to have tragedy revisit them as a constant unwelcomed, but expected, visitor. The truth is that those misfortunes and suffering could happen to us or to our family members. It is simply too painful to continuously imagine your own innate vulnerability or to see your mother's face in that of a woman worn by fate and circumstance. It is unbearable to imagine your child as you care for a young abused girl.

We cannot remain objective and feel continuously vulnerable in our professional settings just as we cannot live in constant fear as we walk the streets. When we hear of a mugging in our neighborhood, we need to convince ourselves that we remain safe. "I don't walk on that block." "I rarely go out after dark." Similarly, when we are exposed to human suffering, we need to generate a protective story that helps us not to feel personally vulnerable. In an act of self-protection, we might begin to hold people responsible for their fate. We begin to paint people as "other," someone different than me or someone I see in my photos at home. This shield may be adaptive, but it also can prevent us from seeing people accurately and can create a toxic boundary that interferes with our therapeutic interaction.

■ Creating Clear Limits

Accepting Gifts

Teens and their parents may wish to offer tokens of appreciation for your caring service. Although some institutions maintain a strict no-gift policy, many of us are left to determine our own policies. Again, there may not be clear-cut answers, but there are points to consider.

- Consider cultural context. In some cases, it may be genuinely insulting to turn down a gift.
- A teen craft or a baked item that took time and care to create, but that has little monetary value, should likely be taken with appropriate appreciation for the thoughtfulness.
- Pictures of teens or craftwork with their name on it should not be displayed in public areas. First, this is inconsistent with creating an office space that honors privacy. Second, it could be misinterpreted as favoritism; instead, say something like, "*I so*

appreciate this and I will keep it in my own area. We are not allowed to display it in public, both to guarantee your privacy and so no one else thinks we expect him or her to do this for us. Again, thank you so very much."

- If a family wishes to thank you with an item that has significant monetary value, you should graciously decline. A polite way of doing so is to say, *"I greatly appreciate your thoughtfulness, but it is so important that Ben knows I have served him as best as I could only because of how much I care about his well-being."* If the family continues to insist, you might consider suggesting they make a charitable contribution in honor of their son's well-being. Whether or not that charity can be associated with your institution is a matter for your personal consideration.

Immediacy: Central to Adolescent Care or Destructive to Preparing for Adulthood?

One of the central tenets of adolescent care is "immediacy." Adolescents aren't the best at keeping schedules. Their needs often present as crises, and even when there is no objective crisis, it may feel like one to them. Sometimes young people present with a hidden agenda and what we get is not what we expected when we walked into the room. Further, we know that when we do not offer treatment right away, we might lose a young person to an issue that feels more urgent at another time. For these reasons, many of us are committed to meeting the needs of teens in the moment.

Adult life is not about immediacy. It is about delayed gratification. It is filled with long lines and waits for appointments. This presents us with a paradox. How do we grant immediacy while preparing a teen for real life?

There are no easy answers to this question. Certainly, crises have to be met with a sense of urgency. Perhaps first and second contacts also have to be granted immediacy. But as we forge relationships, we have to also teach about how to navigate the real world. Therefore, we should approach each teen as an individual and balance their immediate need with their long-term requirement to understand responsibility. Every teen needs to receive a quick safety check to assess for the acuity of the need and for a hidden agenda. Then we offer appropriate boundaries so we can serve the needs of other waiting youth and prepare the teen to learn how best to access care over a lifetime.

24/7 Availability?

It is critical for teens to know they can reach a responsible adult if needed. However, that does not mean they have to reach each of us individually.

In today's 24/7 digital world, many youth have become accustomed to instant access. In parallel, many practices are using cell phones, texts, and e-mails to reach youth with important information. For this reason, many professionals report teens are more commonly requesting cell phone access or e-mail availability. Although most teens will likely be respectful of that privilege, the reality of how teens use communication today is that some may begin using these available means of contact liberally and at all hours.

It is critical that we maintain some personal boundaries that allow us space and time to recharge. You will have to determine whether the specific needs of your professional services require you to give teens immediate contact. However, even if you do, consider a policy that ensures a teen can connect with a caring adult immediately who will assess the situation, refer if immediate care is required, and report to you as you become available during routine hours. This self-protective strategy will also reinforce to youth that you are a professional, not a friend.

■ Personal Limits and Burnout Prevention

How Much Do I Give? 66.1

We all have only so much time and energy. This text offers a variety of intervention strategies and techniques. We certainly cannot offer every adolescent each strategy. Rather, we draw from our repertoire to meet the immediate needs of youth. If each teen received hours of your time, you would serve very few. If each received all of your energy, you would have no reserves to take home with you. We must choose how much to give in each situation. As you think about the boundaries around how you offer service, here are a few thoughts for reflection.

- All youth and families deserve respectful, thoughtful, competent service.
- All youth deserve an assessment at every encounter to consider whether their presenting concerns mask hidden agendas or underlying crises.
- Some youth have a concern that will require a long-term therapeutic alliance. You may not be the one who will offer that long-term care. In these cases, your role is to reinforce that effective treatment is available and that seeking help is an act of great strength. By helping the adolescent understand that he deserves to feel better and that you admire him for seeking guidance, you reduce the shame or stigma that serves as a barrier to forward movement (see Chapter 33). In these cases, you do not want to delve too deeply beyond an assessment for safety because you want the teen's connection to be with the person with whom they will forge a long-term relationship rather than with you. If a young person needs more than you can offer, it would be counterproductive if he believed you were the most effective caregiver he could have.
- On the other hand, when youth are not in need of a different level of service than the one that you can offer, you should do everything to fulfill their needs. In practical terms, this means that you might offer more personal attention to the youth who does not have the greatest needs because you will refer those with the most urgent or complex issues to more specialized services.
- Every teen you encounter needs to know the breadth of services you offer and to form a trustworthy relationship so they know how to access care in times of greater need.
- All youth need to know that you have colleagues. You will not be universally available. They need to know that other trustworthy adults can also serve their needs. In fact, they should learn that they can get second opinions and respectfully disagree with what you may recommend.

The Safety of a Toolbox 67.1

How do you feel deeply and have genuine empathy without losing yourself? How do you expose yourself to others' pain and have strong enough boundaries that you can leave work behind and go home to tend to your own needs?

Again, no easy answers. But please allow me to share my journey. I have long understood that my caring is precisely the ingredient that allows me to enter teens' lives. In my earlier years, my caring was mediated through the emotional impact their stories held over me. (They still do.) In my younger years, I experienced the vulnerability fully and reflected back how I was moved. It worked, but it was a drain of energy and was moving me toward burnout. In a matter of time, I would have grown numb to the pain if only to protect myself.

Many of the brief intervention techniques offered in this work allow me to feel without experiencing pain. With eliciting and reflecting, I listen genuinely for strengths and share my perceptions, hopefully empowering the patient (see Chapter 25). With techniques that make youth own their solutions, I facilitate while granting ownership to the youth (see Chapter 28). With motivational interviewing techniques, I use my empathy to create a safe space for youth to determine the pace of change (see Chapter 26). When I guide youth to manage stress, I know that ultimately their decisional balance will change and they will more comfortably choose prosocial behaviors over quick, easy fixes (see Chapter 31).

I care. I feel. I reflect those feelings. I draw from my toolbox and trust that I have given all that I could. I no longer bleed. I have abandoned the rescue fantasy and know that youth empowerment is far more effective. I go home and recharge.

Handling Others' Pain While Avoiding Burnout

Boundaries are needed to protect us from repeated exposure to pain. But those boundaries need to be managed in a way that still allows us to process our experiences and reactions.

The strongest among us cannot endure unlimited contact to pain. One of my mentors, Dr Stephen Ludwig, metaphorically describes witnessing others' trauma and suffering as being similar to radiation exposure. In sharp contrast to the belief that repeated exposure immunizes us, he states that there is only so much pain a person can absorb. Just as a person who works with radioactive materials wears a counter on their protective vest that both measures acute and long-term exposure, we need to check in with ourselves to see how cumulative contact with toxic stress is affecting our own well-being.

Our challenge is to try to handle and transform the pain, instead of simply allowing it to build to a toxic level. It is critical to know our own capacity for absorbing pain in any particular moment. But the capacity may be somewhat dynamic. If we can recognize and skillfully transform our pain, perhaps we can heal ourselves and build our capacity to continue to serve others.

Many of us try to protect ourselves from our painful experiences and contacts by tucking them away "safely" into a container. Our intent is to process the situation later, when we have the safety of time and space. We move to our next encounter with a false confidence, believing that our experience has been contained. The problem is that too often we do not process our emotions as we had planned. As more content is downloaded into the temporary safety of our containers, the walls of that container need to become stronger and thicker to hold the content. The container figuratively transforms into a leaden box; lead is toxic to our systems, impossible to see through, and too heavy to lift. When our passion and pain are trapped inside of a leaden box, we become numb. We have inadvertently created a toxic boundary; one that closes ourselves off from our emotions and that may limit our ability to access the very passions that support our ability to be a healer. When we are numb, our ability to be fully present with the youth we serve, to listen with kindness, curiosity, and without judgment, is limited.

Instead, we need to create a safe repository for our emotions and experiences, one in which we can both safely deposit and easily access material. If we can create a "Tupperware box," we can plan to store what we cannot immediately digest. Rather than having randomly placed our experiences and emotions into an impermeable container, we remain cognizant of the vessel's content. We decide which portion we would like to digest at any moment. We then can "ladle" that content out while retaining the rest safely inside for later processing. We figuratively "burp" the box knowing the ▶ **67.2** remaining contents remain safely stored inside for a later day.

In order to feel comfortable "ladling" out these experiences and stories, we have to possess the emotional tools that can safely process the content. These emotional tools can include talking, writing, journaling, praying, crying, laughing, and creative expression. Most critically, we all benefit from colleagues with whom we can debrief and process. As long as we pretend that it is brave to ignore how personally exhausting and challenging it can be to bear witness to these issues, we will feel ashamed of our internal struggles.

Together we can stem burnout and consistently remind each other that we need to care for ourselves with the same level of compassion as we care for others (see Chapter 67).

■ Final Thought

Never think of boundaries as something that gets in the way of your service. Think of them as something adolescents need to gain a personal sense of empowerment and something you need so you can offer compassionate, caring service over a lifetime.

•• Group Learning and Discussion ••

Boundaries are something that have to be reflected on throughout our careers. Our challenge is to create a safe space where we can address the issues that challenge our boundaries.

First, conduct a thoughtful conversation about the challenges to safe and appropriate boundaries that have occurred in your setting. This conversation will likely reveal that all professionals sometimes struggle with boundaries. Hopefully, that process will make it easier to move toward the next step: consideration of how to create both planned and spontaneous opportunities to address boundaries on an ongoing basis. One such model is "supervision," where each of us, no matter how senior, has the opportunity to debrief with colleagues about experiences we find challenging as well as to proactively prepare for challenging interactions. "Supervision" has to feel safe enough that it is not viewed as criticism but rather as an opportunity for growth and reflection. Further, it has to be valued as a key strategy in burnout prevention and professional self-care. Supervision is only one model.

Use this opportunity to discuss as a group what model would work best to allow each of you to continue to address boundaries within your practice.

■■■■■■■■ Continuing Education ■■■■■■■■

If you are applying for continuing education credits, a test is available online. For more details, visit www.aap.org/reachingteens.

■ Suggested Reading

American Academy of Pediatrics Committee on Bioethics. Pediatrician-family-patient relationships: managing the boundaries. *Pediatrics.* 2009;124:1685–1688

Good Medical Practice. *Maintaining Boundaries—Guidance for Doctors.* http://www.gmc-uk.org/guidance/ethical_guidance/maintaining_boundaries.asp. Accessed June 25, 2013

Jain S, Roberts LW. Ethics in psychotherapy: a focus on professional boundaries and confidentiality practices. *Psychiatr Clin N Am.* 2009;32(2):299–314

National Council of State Boards of Nursing. *A Nurse's Guide to Professional Boundaries.* Chicago, IL: National Council of State Board of Nursing; 2009. https://www.ncsbn.org/2906.htm?iframe=true&width=500&height=270. Accessed June 25, 2013

Pope KS. *Dual Relationships, Multiple Relationships, & Boundary Decisions.* http://kspope.com/dual. Accessed June 25, 2013

van Dernoot Lipsky L. *Trauma Stewardship: An Everyday Guide to Caring for Self While Caring for Others.* San Francisco, CA: Berrett-Koehler Publishers; 2009

■ Related Video Content

20.0 Boundaries: Essential to Our Healthy Relationships With Youth and Our Professional Longevity. Ginsburg, Hill

20.1 Over-empathizing Can Feel Like Judgment. Pletcher.

20.2 Toxic Boundaries: How Seeing People as "Other" Disrupts Our Connections and Diminishes Us. Ginsburg.

20.3 Professionals Offer Healing "Love," But for Youth Who Have Been Mistreated or Let Down, It Is Only Safe With Clear Boundaries. Hill, McAndrews.

14.1 Checking in on Yourself: What About Your Own Adolescence Might Flavor Your Interactions With Youth? Ginsburg.

34.5 Addressing Worrisome Behaviors and Addictions: Partnering With Parents to Create Safe and Appropriate Boundaries. McAndrews.

34.8 Helping Parents Understand the Additive Role Professionals Can Play in Their Adolescents' Lives. Jenkins.

36.1 Offering Boundaries and Being Role Models: Adults' Critical Role in the Lives of Adolescents. Ginsburg.

66.11 Never Make Promises to Homeless and Marginalized Youth That You Cannot Keep. Hill

66.12 Homeless Teens: Boundaries, Rules, and High Expectations Can Be Welcomed by Underparented Youth. Hill, Covenant House PA staff.

66.13 The Importance of Understanding Boundaries (and Your Own Buttons) When Working With Marginalized Youth. Hill.

67.1 How "Choreographed Conversations" Can Prevent Burnout While We Still Give Youth What They Need. Ginsburg.

67.2 The Tupperware Box: A Model for Releasing Trapped Emotions. Ginsburg.

67.5 Deep Boundaried Connections Restore Our Own Energy. Singh.

■ Code of Ethics From Key Organizations

American Medical Association: AMA's Code of Medical Ethics (1995–2012)
www.ama-assn.org/ama/pub/physician-resources/medical-ethics/code-medical-ethics.page

American Association for Marriage and Family Therapy (AAMFT) Code of Ethics (2012)
www.aamft.org/imis15/Content/Legal_Ethics/Code_of_Ethics.aspx

American Association of Pastoral Counselors: Code of Ethics (2010)
www.aapc.org/about-us/code-of-ethics.aspx

American Association of Sex Educators, Counselors and Therapists: Code of Ethics (2004–2008)
www.aasect.org/codeofethics.asp

American Counseling Association: Code of Ethics and Standards of Practice (2005)
www.counseling.org/Resources/CodeOfEthics/TP/Home/CT2.aspx

American Mental Health Counselors Association: Code of Ethics (2010)
https://www.amhca.org/assets/news/AMHCA_Code_of_Ethics_2010_w_pagination_cxd_51110.pdf

American Music Therapy Association: Code of Ethics (2008)
www.musictherapy.org/about/ethics

American Psychoanalytic Association: Principles and Standards of Ethics for Psychoanalysts (2009–2012)

www.apsa.org/About_APsaA/Ethics_Code.aspx

American Psychological Association: Ethical Principles of Psychologists and Code of Conduct (2010)

www.apa.org/ethics/code/index.aspx

American School Counselor Association: Ethical Standards for School Counselors (2010)

www.schoolcounselor.org/files/EthicalStandards2010.pdf

CHAPTER 21

Examining Our Unconscious Biases

Amanda Lerman, MD

■ Why This Matters

To provide the best service to adolescents, we must be open to their individual needs and expectations and deliver information and services in a developmentally and culturally appropriate manner. Only if we offer a safe and open-minded environment will youth engage in a collaborative process to improve their health and well-being. To ensure that the advice we give or the diagnoses we make are the most beneficial, it is critical to be receptive listeners or we may miss the full story. A first step is to bring to awareness unconscious biases present in all of us that, if unchecked, can limit our capacity to connect with youth, interfere with our ability to make accurate assessments and plans, and ultimately hinder our power to help.

Because adolescents evoke strong emotional responses, they are particularly vulnerable to our unconscious biases, faulty reasoning, and resultant errors. In fact, since the teenage years are a formative and emotional time for most people, interacting with adolescents may evoke our own memories and feelings. The feelings elicited within us, combined with the heavy emotional content of their stories, may alter our listening experience and influence the way we process information.

Unconscious biases cause cognitive errors (mistakes in our thinking patterns or conclusions) that impede our efforts to provide optimal care. Adolescents may be particularly vulnerable to receiving substandard care due to these phenomena because they are often judged quickly based on their age, their environmental context, or their visible external characteristics. Recognizing our unconscious biases is a critical first step toward preventing them from harming the relationships we build with adolescents and lowering the quality of care we deliver.

■ Background

Much of the research on the phenomenon of unconscious biases currently resides in the medical literature and focuses on how these biases affect health professionals' ability to make diagnoses. Some of the best illustrations of the effects of unconscious biases focus largely on patient safety and the effect of biases on medical diagnosis. Many of the lessons, however, likely apply to all decision-making interactions with youth and, therefore, may resonate with all professionals who serve adolescents. Each of us, regardless of discipline, can go through a reflective process to consider our own biases and their effect on the conclusions we draw and treatment plans we make. Specific types of biases, therefore, will be described here in terms that apply to all of our interactions with youth, including those that occur in a health care setting.

As the patient safety movement has drawn increasing attention to the prevalence of medical mistakes and their impact on the health of large numbers of patients, a new field dedicated to characterizing, understanding, and minimizing medical errors has emerged. Initial investigation focused on simple human errors, such as administering the wrong dose of a medication or performing surgery at the wrong site,[1] and medicine has made strides toward minimizing these missteps. Systems-level interventions, such as read-back protocols and procedural checklists have successfully reduced these errors.[2]

Cognitive errors are more difficult both to understand and to prevent.[1] An erroneous medication administration has numerous potential underlying causes: the ordering physician may have insufficient knowledge of correct dosing; the nurse may mishear a verbal order; the doctor, the nurse, or a pharmacist may mistype the digits on a computer or dispenser, but dissecting causes of such an event is easily achievable with review practices, such as root cause analyses (a common health care practice of convening the people involved after a negative patient outcome to uncover underlying causes and formulate potential solutions to prevent future errors). It is much more challenging, however, to disentangle the underlying thought processes that may cause a health professional to miss a diagnosis or select the wrong treatment for a patient.

Leaders in this field hope that considering the ways in which mistakes of cognition can lead to misdiagnoses and flawed decisions will allow medical professionals to recognize their faulty mental habits, adjust their reasoning processes, and prevent future blunders that could lead to patient harm. There may, however, be additional benefits to the effort: New focus on unconscious biases can help professionals be more open, connect better with patients, fight burnout, and reduce prejudices. (Note: "Prejudices" here refers to prejudgments or biased thinking, it does not necessarily relate to ethnic or racial biases.)

In attempting to deconstruct clinical reasoning—how doctors and other health professionals think and make decisions—and the ways in which it can fail, researchers have examined the *heuristics*—mental shortcuts—medical providers use and identified situations in which they can cause providers to have blind spots when they assess patients. Heuristics are strategies used to make decisions quickly, and they are based on pattern recognition. Students learn a systematic process to evaluate a patient, but in practice professionals often lack the time to execute a comprehensive deductive procedure for each patient. Instead they rely on mental shortcuts when making diagnoses, often citing "clinical intuition" as their guide. Sometimes these processes are based on experience or objective knowledge, and they frequently work well. Studies show that experienced clinicians can make many correct diagnoses without going through an exhaustive cognitive process.[3]

Other times, though, heuristics fail. When providers rely on shortcuts, they cannot verify the patterns on which they are depending. Their quick, instinctive assessments may be based on stereotypes or other erroneous patterns, and their thinking may be biased. This distortion of thinking explains why doctors are more likely to diagnose heart attacks in white men than in African Americans or in women. It could explain why African American girls presenting to the emergency department with abdominal pain may be more likely to receive a diagnosis of pelvic inflammatory disease (PID), a complication of sexual transmitted infection, while white girls with the same presentation may be more likely to be diagnosed with constipation or viral illness. Since PID can harm fertility, especially if not treated in a timely manner, guidelines recommend a conservative approach that "overcalls" the diagnosis. In this case, it would be the white girls suffering harm if they are denied this protective approach because providers do not think of sexually related causes of their pain.

Debate is active in the literature about the value of heuristics in decision-making. Some believe mental shortcuts increase cognitive errors by creating blind spots that could be eliminated with more deliberate, systematized reasoning and have argued that we should minimize reliance on heuristics. Others, especially those in the field of psychology, defend intuition-based reasoning; they contend that evidence suggests the results of such thinking may be *more* accurate than those derived through systematic analysis.[4-6]

Despite such disagreement, it is clear that underlying, unconscious preconceptions can warp professionals' reasoning. Whether rapid, automatic thinking is especially vulnerable to this corruption or not, confronting our patterns of thought and striving to keep an open mind can help us intercept cognitive errors.

■ Biases to Consider

Many cognitive biases stem from subconscious emotional responses. For example, in a medical setting, a preliminary diagnosis likely guides testing and care decisions, so medical providers may feel attached to that first diagnosis and fail to consider others out of fear that an early misstep led to the wrong initial care. (See anchoring bias.) Similarly, medical professionals caring for a patient whose condition is worsening may blame the disease process and neglect to consider treatment side effects, since it is emotionally difficult for clinicians to acknowledge that their attempts to heal may be causing harm to the patient. A clinician who missed a diagnosis and felt responsible for a poor patient outcome may feel so guilty that she will test nearly every similar patient for that disease, no matter how unlikely it may be in each case. This practice could result in both unnecessary testing and insufficient consideration of alternate diagnoses. (See availability bias.)

There are many types of unconscious biases that have been identified. Examples include the following[7,8]:

Anchoring bias: If a diagnosis or decision is made, we can lock onto this explanation and fail to consider other options. This can be true even when new data are presented that do not fit.

Premature closure: If our reasoning stops after a putative conclusion emerges, we may not ask all pertinent questions and may miss a true underlying cause. In the medical context, this error can happen if a health professional recognizes a likely diagnosis in the case's first impressions, inherits a diagnosis from another provider who evaluated the patient, or is swayed by the patient's beliefs about what is causing her symptoms (about which patients are increasingly vocal in the Internet age). In the case of a troubled teen, we may miss an underlying case of abuse by accepting the "excuses" offered rather than noticing a repetitive pattern of "accidents."

Confirmation bias: Similarly, when we have drawn a conclusion, we may preferentially hunt for clues to support this hypothesis and unwittingly ignore or pay less attention to evidence inconsistent with it.

Availability bias: Our recent memory is always the easiest to access. Additionally, an event or experience that was traumatic, shocking, or upsetting will likely be recalled first. For example, diseases that clinicians have recently seen or with which they have had a memorable experience may stick out in their minds and cause them to consider those diagnoses even if they are relatively rare. Similarly, a school counselor who recently cared for a young person who committed suicide after reporting an extreme fear of failure may start to assume that every young person with school-related anxiety is in grave danger.

Omission bias: The imperative to "first do no harm" can bias us toward inaction and prompt us to overestimate the appropriateness of a conservative approach.

Commission bias: Conversely, we may be compelled by a desire to "at least do something" for the teen and may overvalue a course of treatment involving more action.

Order effect: As we listen to a story, we may pay different attention to the various facts depending on the order in which they are relayed. In particular, studies show listeners pay more attention to the information at the beginning or the end of the story.[9] This could pose a serious problem caring for teens, because youth often test the waters, choosing not to share something significant until the listener's reaction to less important disclosures proves to be sufficiently nonjudgmental. Moreover, order bias could prevent us from noting the serious concerns that are often "slipped in" between other thoughts.

Framing effect: The context in which we encounter an adolescent (eg, inner city emergency department vs private suburban clinic, school vs homeless shelter) or the way another professional tells us the teen's story may color our interpretation of the information. Other circumstantial cues, such as a young person's attire, may lead us to make assumptions about youth, their behaviors, and their environments, which can skew our assessments and decisions.

Visceral bias: Our emotional responses can impair our objective assessment. For example, a professional who is frustrated by frequent experiences with narcotic-seeking street youth may feel immediate distaste toward a homeless adolescent complaining of pain, mistrust the story, and be more liable to miss a serious concern than he would in another teen presenting similarly. Conversely, when a young person engenders positive feelings, we may dismiss ominous conclusions too readily. A physician may, for example, disregard the possibility of cancer in her favorite patient. A counselor highly engaged by an adolescent's passion and intensity may ignore that the story she is telling may be false and fail to dig deeper for the truth.

■ Adolescent-Specific Bias

Because adolescents evoke strong emotional responses, they are particularly vulnerable to our unconscious biases, faulty reasoning, and resultant errors. Unlike younger children, they do not appear helpless or innocent, but they cannot yet express their feelings or communicate their needs as effectively as adults. As a population, they are an extremely healthy group, so providers may be quick to disregard symptoms, even though serious illness certainly occurs in some young people. Furthermore, since teenagers are widely viewed as reckless, self-centered, and foolish, some professionals may be more likely to mistrust them and to assume that their symptoms or life circumstances are a result of some risky behavior. Some may tend to minimize severe symptoms or serious complaints because teens are often viewed as overly dramatic or histrionic. In addition, since the teenage years are a formative and emotional time for most people, interacting with adolescents may evoke our own memories and feelings. The feelings elicited within us, combined with the heavy emotional content of their stories, may alter our listening experience and influence the way we process information (see Chapter 20).

We must remember that all patterns have exceptions and that all youth are individuals who may or may not fit into any schema. When caring for adolescents, we must recall that not every patient with weight loss has anorexia nervosa or else we will miss diagnosing some cases of cancer, lupus, thyroid disorder, and other diseases. Since not every change in a teenager's mental status is caused by drug use or a psychotic break, we must consider all possibilities so we do not miss other treatable conditions. We certainly must consider that the teen with bloodshot eyes and a distant gaze might be high on marijuana, but we must not overlook the possibility that he is depressed and had been crying.

As we work with youth, we need to resist the urge to place them in circumscribed boxes so that we stay ever mindful of their individuality.

■ Personal Reflection as a First Step

There is growing literature exploring means to combat cognitive errors due to unconscious biases, but the verdict is not yet in on how to do so most effectively. As previously stated, there are conflicting views on which type of reasoning is better—quick, intuitive thinking or more thoughtful, systematic analysis. Certainly there is a role for both; our goal cannot be to eliminate heuristics. Routinely recognizing our thoughts, however, can allow us to examine existing biases and potentially flawed thinking patterns.

There is no place for shame or blame in this reflective process. We are all human, and each of us has a unique set of biases. Acknowledging that reality and considering our own individual prejudices and assumptions is the first step toward eliminating their harmful effects. This endeavor can make our work more rewarding and increase the longevity of our service.

Professionals in the helping fields face high rates of burnout. Even as we witness wrongdoing and suffering, though, staying cognizant of the individuality of each person can protect us from cynicism and hopelessness. Assessing the subconscious biases and thought patterns we may have acquired can enhance our ability to see youth as they truly are and form meaningful connections—and that may promote our own resilience and career satisfaction.

■ Stop, Ask, and Reconsider

It might seem daunting to excavate deep-seated beliefs or assumptions, but we can make it a routine part of forming an assessment and plan. We can learn to stop, reflect, and ask ourselves, *"What are my assumptions?" "How might those judgments cause me to draw an incorrect conclusion?"* and *"What else could be going on?"* Asking ourselves these questions is particularly essential when an adolescent causes a strong emotional response or seems to fit a stereotyped picture. When in doubt, we open our minds, reconsider, and ask more questions, recognizing that young people know their lives better than anyone else and that they can offer the clarity we need to best serve them.

•• Group Learning and Discussion ••

This chapter presents 9 different types of unconscious biases that may lead us toward faulty decision-making.

1. Anchoring bias
2. Premature closure
3. Confirmation bias
4. Availability bias
5. Omission bias
6. Commission bias
7. Order effect
8. Framing effect
9. Visceral bias

This list may not encompass every type of bias your group believes influences the care you give teenagers. Take a few moments to review each of these biases and then to consider unconscious biases not captured in this list.

Pick a recent complicated case or 2 that has come through your office, whether or not the conclusions you reached were accurate. As you present the case, pause at key decision points and allow the group to consider what assumptions—or shortcuts—each of you is using to formulate an assessment. Discuss how these shortcuts may bias your assessment and take note of how many different biases can come into play in one case.

The content of this chapter will best enhance your practice if it becomes a routine part of your group's culture and your personal approach to thinking. We recommend that as your group debriefs cases on an ongoing basis, you consider what assumptions either helped you reach conclusions or led you astray.

We recommend that as you make assessments, you learn to habitually stop, reflect, and ask yourself, *"What are my assumptions? How might those judgments cause me to draw an incorrect conclusion? What else could be going on?"* We predict you will learn to better trust your conclusions after going through this thoughtful process.

We recommend that, during professional handoffs, the receiving caregiver always reflects on what biases the previous clinician may have held. Furthermore, the receiving caregiver must determine if she has blindly accepted any conclusions drawn by her colleague and must consider the possibility that a cognitive error was made.

■■■■■■■■ Continuing Education ■■■■■■■■■

If you are applying for continuing education credits, a test is available online. For more details, visit www.aap.org/reachingteens.

■ References

1. Graber M, Gordon R, Franklin N. Reducing diagnostic errors in medicine: what's the goal? *Acad Med.* 2002;77(10):981–92
2. Ely JW, Graber ML, Croskerry P. Checklists to reduce diagnostic errors. *Acad Med.* 2011;86(3):307
3. Hobus P, Schmidt H, Boshuizen H, Patel V. Contextual factors in the activation of first diagnostic hypotheses: expert-novice differences. *Medl Ed.* 1987;21(6):471–476
4. Norman G. Dual processing and diagnostic errors. *Adv Health Sci Ed Theory Pract.* 2009;14:37–49
5. De Vries M, Witteman CLM, Holland RW, Dijksterhuis A. The unconscious thought effect in clinical decision making: an example in diagnosis. *Med Decis Making.* 2010;30(5):578–81

6. Coderre S, Mandin H, Harasym P, Fick G. Diagnostic reasoning strategies and diagnostic success. *Med Ed.* 2003;37(8):695–703

7. Croskerry P. Achieving quality in clinical decision making: cognitive strategies and detection of bias. *Acad Emerg Med.* 2002;9(11):1184–1204

8. Croskerry P. The importance of cognitive errors in diagnosis and strategies to minimize them. *Acad Med.* 2003;78(8):775–780

9. Murdock BB Jr. Serial order effects in short-term memory. *J Exp Psychol.* 1968;76(4):1–15

■ Related Video Content

There are no films specifically made for this chapter; however there are several found in Chapter 19, "Cultural Humility," that cover how to address those unconscious biases that may affect our ability to work across cultures.

■ Related Web Site

Society to Improve Diagnosis in Medicine
www.improvediagnosis.org

173

CHAPTER 22: TRAUMA-INFORMED PRACTICE: WORKING WITH YOUTH WHO HAVE SUFFERED ADVERSE CHILDHOOD (OR ADOLESCENT) EXPERIENCES

CHAPTER 22

Trauma-Informed Practice: Working With Youth Who Have Suffered Adverse Childhood (or Adolescent) Experiences

Sandra L. Bloom, MD

Zeelyna Wise

Joseph Lively

Marcos O. Almonte, MDiv

Stephanie Contreras

Kenneth R. Ginsburg, MD, MS Ed, FAAP, FSAHM

 Related Video Content

22.0 Trauma-Informed Practice: Working With Youth Who Have Suffered Adverse Experiences

■ Why This Matters

Youth who have experienced trauma have learned to be reactive. In fact, their brain, stress hormones, and even the expression of their DNA have been altered by their adverse experiences. As a matter of survival, some youth may have needed to act reflexively before thinking, to take an offensive stance rather than leave themselves vulnerable. Others may have learned to dissociate themselves from the horrors they experienced—to zone out or disconnect from reality when they were powerless to change it.

Adverse childhood experiences can affect people in every racial and ethnic group, and occurs across all economic strata. Therefore, we must consistently practice in a trauma-informed manner that assumes the young person we serve has endured severe adversity. This assumption reminds us to ask the right questions, interact

> **We introduce a radical calmness in their chaotic realities. We acknowledge trauma. We name it to address it, we address it to resolve it, and we resolve it by empowering youth to define themselves outside of their past traumas.**

with young people in a way that will not trigger their reactivity or cause them to dissociate, and structure our practices in a way that will not re-traumatize youth by reinforcing their sense of powerlessness or shame.

■ The Effects of Toxic Stress and Trauma on Development and Well-being

The immediate and long-term effects of stress and trauma are discussed in detail in Chapter 6. The following points represent a brief summary:

- *Positive stress* produces short-lived physiological responses that promote growth and change necessary for healthy development.
- *Tolerable stress* occurs as the result of more severe, longer-lasting difficulty. If it is time-limited and there are sufficient social supports, there can be recovery without long-term negative effects.
- *Toxic or traumatic stress* can change the brain's architecture with long-term physical, emotional, and psychological consequences. Research demonstrates that adverse childhood experiences (ACEs) affect health over the life span.
- In response to adversity, we prepare for fight or flight. When this is a response to real danger, is time-limited, and is effective, it is life-saving and adaptive. Problems arise when this reaction is evoked in the absence of any threat, when the threat is prolonged, or when nothing can be done to protect oneself from the threat.
- Under conditions of chronic stress, something goes wrong as the body attempts to cope with a chronic overload of physiological responses. The system can become dysregulated, resulting in dysfunctional and maladaptive brain activities. People who have been severely or repeatedly traumatized are in a state of chronic hyperarousal and may lose the capacity to modulate their level of arousal.
- Under normal conditions, the brain is constantly integrating every component of experience—behavior, emotions, sensations, and knowledge. Under extreme stress, the brain stops properly integrating experience, leading to *dissociation*. As an acutely adaptive state, dissociation prevents a vulnerable and frightened person from needing to process an unimaginable reality. In the longer term, the loss of integration creates significant problems.
- Putting all of this together, we might note the following in teens who have experienced trauma:
  — It may be harder to forge a trusting relationship, because the young person has not experienced adults as consistently safe.
  — Parents and teachers may describe the youth as easily upset, easily provoked, or highly reactive.
  — The youth may display what others consider inappropriate emotions and behavior.
  — The young person may be triggered by traumatic reminders, and emotional responses may be occurring during an altered state during which the youth experiences flashbacks.
  — The youth may be diagnosed as hyperactive, oppositional, or conduct disordered.
  — The teen may appear inattentive as he is focused on internal stimuli or hyperattentive to "danger signals" of which adults are not aware.
  — A common post-traumatic presentation is dissociation. This may be reported as "lying," which actually represents a confabulated reality produced to replace actual events difficult to recall, or "zoning out," which has proven adaptive during traumatic moments.

175

CHAPTER 22: TRAUMA-INFORMED PRACTICE: WORKING WITH YOUTH WHO HAVE SUFFERED ADVERSE CHILDHOOD (OR ADOLESCENT) EXPERIENCES

■ The Protective Force of Connection With Caring Adults

Substantial research demonstrates the protective nature of caring connections with adults. Children exposed to trauma or toxic stress who also have a nurturing parent are far less likely to suffer long-term consequences from ACEs.

A person's repertoire of responses to high levels of stress is often described as fight–flight–freeze. However, the data that prove how protective connection is in early childhood supports the work of Taylor et al[1] that suggests "tend and befriend" is also part of the stress response. The question, of course, is whether others will be there to care for children in need of attentive care.

Although there is not yet a parallel body of evidence that proves the powerful protective nature of connection against trauma during adolescence, it remains our most important tool. This chapter, at its core, is about how to connect with traumatized youth to offer them the needed support to move forward.

■ Behavioral and Emotional Manifestations of Trauma

Many kinds of symptoms become intertwined with development over the course of time, making the symptom picture complex and sometimes perplexing. There is no classic picture to which all traumatized youth adhere; however, certain behavioral constellations are common and may raise concern that a history of trauma drives the behavior. Bear in mind, however, pain and trauma can also result in resilience and a deep commitment to repair the world.

In some cases, the young person's life becomes organized around unintegrated fragments of experience. They remain stuck in time, unable to move ahead, haunted by an unspoken and unresolved past. The most significant and recurrent problems will arise in young people who have been exposed to high levels of toxic stress, traumatic stress, and allostatic load (the wear-and-tear on the body and brain resulting from forces such as poverty, bigotry, chronic hunger, and lowered socioeconomic status). If we summarize what actually shows up differently in every youth, what do we see?

They may have a fundamental mistrust of others, especially adults because adults have not proven trustworthy and have often betrayed their trust. They have developed a protective shell around their emotions; they are numb and want to stay that way. They are most likely to become aggressive toward themselves or others as a way of warding off disturbing feelings, memories, or traumatic reminders, but they cannot openly talk about any of this. Instead, they communicate largely nonverbally, through behavioral reactions. They are unable to remember the worst aspects of their experiences, have difficulty learning from new experiences, and tend to repeat relational patterns from the past. They often do not recognize danger until it is too late and are unlikely to make meaningful connections between their previous experiences and the problems they are having in the present. They are likely to have very uneasy relationships to authority. They seem unable to anticipate the consequences of their behavior. They feel helpless and hopeless about being able to solve their problems, even while denying they have any. They are likely to have a very confused, injudicious, and erratic sense of justice and fair play. Real and imagined loss of any sort is likely to be a trigger for negative emotional reactions.

In brief, (1) they have difficulty maintaining safety in interpersonal relationships largely due to disrupted attachment experiences and the erosion of trust that accompanies such experiences; (2) they have significant challenges in adequately managing distressful emotions in ways that are not self-destructive, including exercising the capacities for self-discipline, self-control, and willpower; (3) cognitive problems beset them, particularly when stress occurs and the development of essential higher-level brain functions has not

The Sanctuary Model: Healing = Integration

Over time and after working with many survivors of terrible life events, we recognized that their past experiences had produced symptoms of post-traumatic stress and the chronic hyperarousal that accompanies it, but often with no memory. The symptoms were the remnants of attempts to cope with overwhelming stress and had become firmly entrenched bad habits, severely compromising their capacity to create and sustain interpersonal trust. The challenges presented to us as helpers were significant and, without this new understanding, incomprehensible.

Understanding that most of the symptoms we were seeing were secondary to a failure to fully integrate past experiences, we began to see how we could meaningfully facilitate recovery. We had to teach safety skills so they could build their capacity for trust. They had to learn how to manage intense emotion in safe and secure ways and to learn to use reason and judgment even in the face of emotional arousal. We had to teach communication skills so they could clearly assert their needs, create safe boundaries, and exercise self-control and self-discipline. We had to help people mourn for what was lost, prepare for the losses associated with change, and imagine a future that would make all of this new learning and habit change worthwhile.

This then was what we came to understand as "trauma-informed" treatment. As we saw it unfolding, developing these cognitive-emotional-behavior skills set the stage for trauma-specific treatment approaches that had a cathartic effect and helped people integrate fragmented bits of experience into a cohesive whole that allowed the past to reside safely in the past rather than continuing to haunt the present. This was RECOVERY.

Experience in creating healing environments taught us that we had to have a very broad definition of what it means to be safe and secure. Our clients reacted to a multitude of toxins, some from their families, some from others, and some from dysfunctional systems that were supposed to help them. All of this represented a loss of social support, which is the only barrier any of us have against the cruelties of life.

In order to create safe environments for healing, we needed to concern ourselves not just with physical safety, but with psychological, social, and moral safety as well. That meant staff had to "walk the talk" if we were to be trusted. When we grasped the enormous power behind the reenactment dynamic (the powerful inclination to repeat the past that is so typical of human behavior), we realized interpersonal trust was vital. If our clients were to change, they would have to make significant decisions to go against their own "instincts" and listen to us instead. But, we recognized that we were not always trustworthy. Things had happened to us as well, and those injuries had shaped who we had become as helping professionals. If we wanted our clients to change, then we had to change as well.

In the context of the treatment/intervention setting, much is demanded of anyone associated with young people. We must model and support the development of (1) safety skills and significant improvements in the capacity for interpersonal trust; (2) emotional management skills, including self-control, self-discipline, and the exercise of willpower; (3) cognitive skills, including identifying triggers and problematic patterns while still being able to think in the presence of strong emotion; (4) communication skills that include rehearsals in what to say and how to say it; (5) participatory and leadership skills; (6) judgment skills, including socially acceptable and fair behavioral schemas; and (7) skills to manage grief and plan for the future.

What characteristics best describe people able to do this complex, demanding work? They need to be secure, reasonably healthy adults who have good emotional management skills themselves. They must be emotionally intelligent and able to teach new skills and routines while serving as role models. There are constant demands on them for patience and for empathy so they must be able to endure intense emotional labor. To balance the demands of home and work, managers and supervisors, children and their families, they must be self-disciplined, self-controlled, and never abuse their own personal power.

That means that the place in which you serve youth, the practice context, must be a safe and healthy environment for everyone, including staff. Young people can sense immediately if an environment is hostile, even without any overt visible behavior. It must have a *commitment to open communication;* how else could it become a place that is (ultimately, when the youth is ready) safe enough to discuss the "undiscussables"?

The sanctuary model is described fully in Bloom SL, Farragher B. *Restoring Sanctuary: A New Operating System for Trauma-Informed Systems of Care.* New York, NY: Oxford University Press; 2013.

gone as smoothly as it should; (4) as a result, open and direct communication at home, at work, and at school pose significant challenges and they frequently communicate through behavior, not directly, openly, or in words; (5) they feel helpless and powerless in the face of a world they perceive has been unjust and cruel and, as a result, may be repeatedly bullied or become bullies themselves; (6) living under adverse conditions, these youth frequently do not develop a clear sense of social responsibility even into adulthood, and moral development may have been affected by disrupted attachment experiences and inadequate role models; (7) they are likely to have experienced significant loss while lacking the capacity to grieve secondary to emotional management problems, may repeat the experiences that are a part of their past, and often lack any hope that the future will be any better; and (8) their emotional and cognitive challenges interfere with the capacity to plan ahead and tolerate delayed gratification (Figure 22.1).

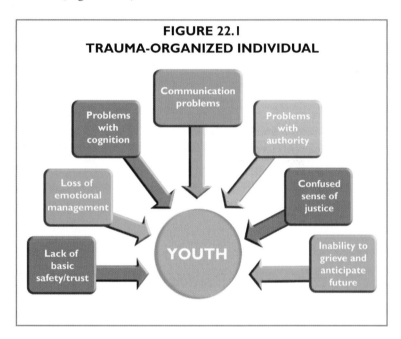

FIGURE 22.1
TRAUMA-ORGANIZED INDIVIDUAL

■ How Might Youth Be Described?

"It doesn't take anything to set this kid off!" This is a good description of chronic hyperarousal as a result of which the teen is easily provoked, highly reactive, and displays what others consider to be inappropriate emotions and behavior. Unrecognized by others, the youth may be triggered by traumatic reminders in the environment, and the emotional responses may be occurring during an altered state during which the teen is experiencing flashbacks.

"This kid cannot keep still and he won't pay attention." Some hyperactivity may actually be secondary to chronic hyperarousal and the physical agitation that accompanies it. Remember, under normal conditions, the stress response is preparing our minds and bodies to physically *react*, not to sit quietly and listen. The chemistry of a chronically hyperaroused young person is set to attend and respond to *danger*, not to geography or geometry. You may also hear something like, *"with this kid, things go in one ear and out the other."* Again, this may represent the cognitive problems associated with chronic hyperarousal since only things tagged with danger are cognitively attended to and retained.

"This kid is really going to hurt someone." Aggression can get people to distance themselves from you, an especially important response if someone is getting a little too close to you and to the memories you cannot process. But it is important to recognize

177

CHAPTER 22: TRAUMA-INFORMED PRACTICE: WORKING WITH YOUTH WHO HAVE SUFFERED ADVERSE CHILDHOOD (OR ADOLESCENT) EXPERIENCES that aggression is a normal part of the human stress response—the *fight* part. The more frightened or startled we are, the more likely we are to respond aggressively and our body responds with aggression long before our brain has time to make a judgment about whether or not fighting is a good idea.

"This girl is a pathological liar—she lies all the time, even when it's obvious she'll get caught." No one is likely to come to you with the complaint that a youth is dissociative. You may hear accusations of lying, but the behavior may be confabulation. A person who has gaps in time where she does not remember what happened or who she was with will fill in the gaps with whatever seems like it might fit. Young people who do this are often very poor liars; their lies are frequently glaringly obvious and without underlying motivation.

"This kid is looking for trouble." Parents or teachers may complain about a teen who causes trouble wherever he goes and who takes unnecessary risks. Traumatized youth can become physiologically "addicted to trauma" and unwittingly hooked on the internal physical changes associated with the stress response.

"He's a loner." The difficulties that chronically traumatized youth have in trusting others can lead to severe deficits in age-appropriate social skills.

"Nothing bothers him. He has enough to handle just managing his pain." Many young people will internalize their pain and present with somatic symptoms (fatigue, dizziness, pain syndromes). They are not "faking"; their pain is real. They are unlikely to grasp the connection between the trauma and their pain, but may be guided toward understanding that their pain worsens with stress. Over time, therapy is an important part of the healing process.

"He's got oppositional defiant disorder/conduct disorder/bipolar disorder/attention-deficit disorder." Trauma generates volatility, moodiness, and reactivity. Always consider that a young person diagnosed with one of the psychiatric disorders that also manifests with unstable behavior or mood actually has a history of trauma.

■ Tips for Youth-Serving Professionals

Interview and Assessment

Youth-serving professionals are on the front lines in identifying and responding to young people who have already experienced adversity as well as those at risk. In light of this, accurate screening and assessment becomes essential. Because we may be unlikely to have the time or knowledge to do in-depth assessment, it is important to work with colleagues and have a referral network. Regardless of the depth of involvement your position allows, remember that every time a youth interacts with an adult there is an opportunity for a trustworthy interaction.

- Ask about the trauma history like you would any other part of the history—it doesn't mean you have to fix it. It does, however, mean you need a sound and reliable referral network so that you can make whatever effort you can to provide integrative body-mind-spirit care. You may say, *"At some point in their lives, many people have experienced extremely distressing events, such as the death of a loved one, physical or sexual abuse, or a bad accident. Have you ever had any experiences like that?"* You don't have to go into details but be matter of fact, direct, supportive, and encouraging. Use language that is concrete and specific to behaviors. Not, *"Were you ever sexually abused?"* but, *"Did anyone ever force you to have sex with them, including unwanted touching, against your will?"* Not, *"Are you being physically abused?"* but, *"Is anyone now hitting you repeatedly or physically harming you?"* *"Has anyone ever hit you repeatedly or physically harmed you?"*
- Make no assumptions about how the young person has been affected—ask him.

How Do We Work With Our Traumatized Youth?

Unconditional LOVE

1. Because our youth come from a place of mistrust/distrust toward adults, we stress relationship building as the foundation that holds the rest of our work and progress with each student. We reach out to youth through casual conversations, a game of ping-pong and, generally, through relating on a human level. The optimal atmosphere when working with trauma is one in which youth and staff are unafraid of having or discussing healthy human experiences. We affirm our roles as professionals while still making ourselves relatable and approachable.

2. We give them the opposite of what they are used to. They are used to abusive relationships and we give them a safe place of compassion and love, and one that is free of judgment.

3. We don't undermine their acuity/perceptiveness in picking up on triggers and responding to their perceived/real threats. If it's real to them, it is real and worthy of a space to be heard and processed.

4. We are honest and hold them to the standard of staying honest with themselves and us.

5. We empower them to break abusive patterns in their lives. We advocate wholeheartedly.

6. We are active listeners who play back their stories with an outsider's voice.

7. We are unafraid of showing them what is both right and wrong in how they deal with conflict. We hold them accountable when negative behaviors become comfortable coping mechanisms.

8. We cannot react back to their behaviors.

9. We stay mindful of the big picture and their point of reference when we see inappropriate behaviors.

10. We do not speak over them. If they are in an escalated state, we provide a safe space for them to take a time-out and pass the reactive state. We work to get them into a reflective and thoughtful state, thereafter using calm, respectful tones.

11. We introduce a radical calmness in their chaotic realities.

12. We let them be their own teachers by learning from their patterns in their lives or in their family and friends' histories. We let them be the authors of their own stories.

13. We acknowledge trauma. We name it to address it, we address it to resolve it, and we resolve it by empowering youth to define themselves outside of their past trauma(s).

14. We focus on what is right rather than what is wrong in them. We take a strength-based approach instead of a fix-it approach.

15. We encourage a high emotional base with youth to allow them to feel and express suppressed emotions or those others have invalidated.

16. We choose our words carefully; we use words that construct versus destruct. We don't generalize negative behaviors by making global judgments on youth (for example, "You are bad because you act like this."). Instead we work to have them replace negative self-image with a positive and confident self-esteem.

17. We allow and encourage the necessary meltdowns or breakdowns to reach the breakthroughs. We are prepared to see and handle high-intensity situations.

18. We are conscientious of our body language, tones, and word choice.

19. We reinforce that relationship-building, in and outside of the school, is foundational to their recovery.

20. Sometimes in order to focus on academics, we have to first address trauma.

21. Stay innovative and creative. We are inventive in how we approach nuanced situations without imposing an inflexible predetermined approach to youth.

22. We keep a dignified space/energy that is inviting but demanding of a high level of respect, both to self and others.

—Wisdom from resilience specialists at El Centro de Estudiantes

- If a teen discloses something that reveals her experience of past trauma, listen. Don't pressure her and don't falsely reassure her. You are a mandated reporter, so there is only so much you can promise. Never promise what you cannot deliver. Follow her lead—if she clams up, ask her if it would be easier to write it down.
- Sexual victimization of children is appallingly common, so know the signs, such as early substance abuse, chronic running away, self-harming behavior, eating disorders, abrupt personality changes, and sexual promiscuity. Alone, none of these prove sexual abuse occurred, but, combined with the history and with each other, they can be strong indicators.
- Adolescents are often embarrassed by their bodies and any kind of physical examination. Be on the lookout for young people who react strongly in 1 of 3 ways to physical examination. Strongly consider the possibility of past or present physical maltreatment or abuse if the youth is nonchalant or brazen in their disregard for what you are doing, is hypersensitive to or repelled by touch, or behaves in a sexually provocative manner.

Interpersonal Interactions

- Many who have experienced trauma have a harder time distinguishing between healthy and unhealthy relationships. Therefore, the issue of trust and betrayed trust will be a major ongoing issue. Relationships worthy of trust are the foundation of progress.
- Appropriate boundaries are key underpinnings of relationships. Because traumatized youth have so little experience with trust, breaking their trust or not following through on a perceived commitment can cause great harm.
- Think about the possibility of past adversity as an underlying problem when you are up against something you don't understand. If you cannot understand why someone does or doesn't do something that seems to be common sense, be curious and ask, *"What happened?"*
- Offer youth the absolute respect and unconditional love they may never have experienced.
- Do not speak over them. If they are in an escalated state, provide a safe space for them to take a time-out and pass the reactive state. Use calm tones and space to guide them out of their altered state
- Be an active listener; play back their stories with an outsider's voice. Be unafraid of showing them what is both right and wrong in how to deal with conflict. Hold them accountable when negative behaviors become comfortable coping mechanisms.
- Don't belittle their sensitivity. If it feels real to them, it is real and worthy of a space to be heard and processed.
- Allow psychiatric diagnoses to inform your approach, but not to define the teen. Remember, traumatized youth are often misdiagnosed.

Support and Treatment

- Psychoeducation can change a person's view of themselves, and that is often enough to increase adherence to other strategies. Handouts, books, movies, and Web sites are available and cover a wide range of relevant topics.
- Write everything down that you want them to retain. Assume that, under stress, people are not taking in all the information they need
- Encourage activities that are self-soothing—meditation, mindfulness, prayer, yoga, etc. If you can, offer opportunities for young people to learn to practice these skills individually or in groups.
- Encourage creative activities—writing, art, music, dance, theater—anything that offers the young person an opportunity for self-expression and possibly opens the door to healing experiences.
- Promote as much mastery and self-help as possible—involve people in their own care.

181

CHAPTER 22: TRAUMA-INFORMED PRACTICE: WORKING WITH YOUTH WHO HAVE SUFFERED ADVERSE CHILDHOOD (OR ADOLESCENT) EXPERIENCES

- A calm environment is a safe environment. No matter how stressed you become, lower the tension in the room to avoid triggering a traumatic memory or creating a perceived threat to safety.
- A traumatized individual may need more physical space. Any sudden moves can be misinterpreted as an attack; an encroachment on personal space can trigger a memory of being trapped.
- Body language is critical to maintaining a sense of safety. Traumatized youth will react to being judged and are hypervigilant to any perceived threat.
- Traumatized youth will often react before thinking about consequences, largely because the part of their brain that fires in response to threat reacts instantly. Activation of the reasoning, judging, and evaluating parts of the brain happens later and only then may the young person be able to inhibit their instantaneous reactions, but by that time it may be too late. In any situation where the young person is frightened, upset, or angry, it is better to create a safe space where the youth can retreat and take the time needed to calm down.

Preventing Re-traumatization

We must look at our practices and consider whether our actions could inadvertently trigger youth to become "reactive." Remember, this reactivity was hardwired as a survival mechanism in response to past trauma; triggers can occur any time an interaction reminds a youth of loss of control, shame, or powerlessness. The reactivity is triggered because the teen is hypervigilant to danger.

Triggers can include
- Invasion of body space
- Behaviors perceived as rude, dismissive, or aggressive
- Inflexible rules that can be overinterpreted as attempts at control
- Questions that can be viewed as intrusive, or that are asked before trust is established

When looking at these triggers, it becomes clearer why a staff that treats ALL youth uniformly in a respectful, calm, welcoming manner sets the tone for a trauma-informed setting.

Case 1

Sixteen-year-old Lisa states that guys have noticed her for quite some time. She has had many boyfriends, but does not stay in a relationship very long; perhaps because she has a difficult time forgiving and an even more difficult time controlling her anger. Behind the attitude, we find a young woman who skipped her childhood. Life dealt her some traumatic blows.

She is bright and could excel at any school, but she has bounced between schools because of altercations with students or faculty. Despite anger-management classes, psychotherapy, and medication, she remains volatile. She has insight and verbalizes when she is angrier than usual so people can leave her alone.

After being expelled from her previous school, she came to a second-chance school to get her diploma. She tends to be on edge most of the time and is easily set off. She has shared that she has a hard time controlling her emotions when "irked." She defined "irk" as someone standing over you or continually "nagging" without giving you needed space. While the details of Lisa's life are not known, it is evident she has major struggles with her emotions and respect for authority.

One day she stormed out of her classroom after her advisor (teacher) expressed frustration with her inattention and asked her to regain focus. Lisa went to the resilience specialist's office. She was given space and silence, letting her vent for a minute until she sat down, signaling that her emotional burst was subsiding. The resilience specialist knelt down, taking a "one down" position, and told her she was in a safe space and that no one would harm or bother her. She had the freedom to be silent or speak. When asked if she wanted to talk about what was going on, she said no. At this point she uncrossed her arms and relaxed her shoulders a bit and her leg stopped shaking. The resilience specialist reaffirmed that she could be silent, but suggested that he ask her questions to which she could nod yes or no.

"Are you upset about something relating to your friends?" She said no. The resilience specialist asked a few similar questions, and then asked a question he knew would get a verbal response. "Are you pregnant?" She said resoundingly, "Hell NO!" and they both laughed.

At that point she opened up and shared what set her off in her classroom. The resilience specialist worked through that situation and rephrased it back to her to reinforce that she was really heard. She was calmly told that her anger and her reactions went beyond the norm, being angry is not bad but what we do when we are angry can cause problems. She nodded in approval. She was told that it appeared her anger was deeply seated and that she needed to find the source because no matter how much therapy or anger management she received, without dealing with the source she would not overcome or properly manage it. She was told that he would be there when she was ready. She gave a longing look that suggested she was ready then and confirmed it with a nod.

The resilience specialist gently proceeded using trial and error. "Was the source a recent experience?" She shook her head no. "Is it your relationship with your mother?" She was silent. "Could it be your father?" Tears began to roll down her cheek. The resilience specialist stated, "It seems to me, Lisa, that your tears confirm that you don't have the relationship with him you desire. Has he ever hurt you?" "No." "Are you angry at him for not being around, miss him, and wish things were different?" She cried inconsolably, ran out of the office and out of the school.

Sometimes pain is a by-product of the process of finding the source of emotional anguish. The resilience specialist later spoke with her and her stepfather to confirm she was all right. When the resilience specialist met with Lisa and her mother the next week, Lisa stated, "Mom, no one has done what he did. He helped me identify the source of my anger. Now I can deal with it."

Since then, Lisa has had some ups and downs, but has proven to be an engaged student. Her trauma is not healed, but the foundation has been set for the recovery process to begin. It began with discussing what had been "undiscussable." This can only work when trust is in place and the youth is empowered to set the pace.

Case 2

I am a resilience specialist in a school. One day I was walking up a flight of stairs in the school when I heard loud, angry voices. As I got to the top of the steps, I looked up and saw a young man, Rodney, whom I have known to be playful, easy to talk with, and energetic, walking toward me while, at the same time, turning back to the classroom he had just exited, yelling at someone. I heard his advisor telling him to lower his voice and instructing him to walk away while, at the same time, trying to control other students who had gathered around the entrance to her class, eager to witness the fireworks.

I could tell that Rodney needed a way of getting away from the scene without losing face, since he was still being taunted by the other students standing behind the advisor. Using the excuse that I needed his help with something, I quickly walked him into my office and closed the door. He was still breathing hard when we arrived in the room, his head hung low, shoulders slumped, fists clenched. He looked defeated but ready to fight. His thoughts seemed to be flying around faster than he could get them out.

He said, "Mr Jones, I don't know what happened. That girl Carol came at me and I didn't start anything, but I'm not going to stay shut!"

His speech was high and fast and his breathing rapid. *"It's okay,"* I responded, keeping my voice even while making sure to give him space. *"Let's take a couple of really deep, slow breaths and then we can talk about this."*

He leaned back against my door his body was loosened, but his gaze was still focused on the floor. A moment or 2 passed, then he began again. *"I'm gonna leave, Mr Jones. I didn't do anything wrong. She came at me in group and she came in snapping. I was just standing off to the side where I always do."*

His voice this time was more even, his breathing had calmed, he raised his head, and our eyes met. *"I hear you,"* I started, *"so when she came back in what happened next?"*

"We were finishing group when she came back," he said.

Then she said, *"All I know is, you need to sit down with your fake shoes."*

"I was stunned," Rodney said, *"and then everyone in the class started adding their two cents."*

"Okay," I said, *"then what happened?"*

Rodney cracked a smile. *"I might have said a few bad words in there."* We both smiled.

Suspecting that there might be a little more between these 2 students than he had told me about thus far, I asked if they had any past issues.

"No, I mean we don't talk to each other," Rodney declared. *"I try to stay basically to myself. I'm just here to get my education and that's it."*

Again sadness entered into his words, *"I'm gonna go, Mr Jones."*

"Why would you do that?" I asked. He looked up. I said, *"You said yourself you are here to get your education, your diploma, and all the positive things that both will bring. If you leave, you put that at risk; if you choose to stay, we can work through this and nothing is lost."*

At this point, another student who I had worked with, Bill, entered and began explaining how he had gone through similar problems. *"You can't let other people take your future away,"* Bill told Rodney. *"If you're about getting your education, then you can't let small things stand in your way."* Rodney stood with his head up, his eyes moving back and forth from me to Bill, nodding in agreement.

I began again, *"You said she came in when group was ending. Where had she been?"*

He responded, *"She was meeting with the teacher for like a half hour, and she came back looking mad as ever."*

"Do you think she got bad news?" I asked.

"Yeah probably, because when she came in she slammed her stuff down and everybody looked up."

"Do you think she might have been taking out her anger on you because you were standing and probably caught her attention first?"

He nodded and said, *"Yeah, you're probably right. She might have been upset about something else."* He paused for a moment. *"If I could do it over again, I would have just talked to her later, like one on one."*

Bing! It was like a light went on in his head and he understood it was never about him or his shoes.

"How do you feel? Would you like to join your class?" I asked.

"Yeah. I wanna go back."

The 3 of us started walking back toward his classroom. There were some last-minute words of encouragement from his schoolmate. *"Don't let the little things stop you. You're here for a reason!"* Bill said. Peers can be powerful forces of healing.

183

CHAPTER 22: TRAUMA-INFORMED PRACTICE: WORKING WITH YOUTH WHO HAVE SUFFERED ADVERSE CHILDHOOD (OR ADOLESCENT) EXPERIENCES

■ Trauma-Informed Strategies

The techniques presented throughout *Reaching Teens* are presented as strength-based or resilience-building strategies, but are also trauma-informed. The following chapters are a representative, but not exhaustive, sample of those that include trauma-informed communication or behavioral-change techniques.

"Who's the Expert? Terms of Engagement in Adolescent Care" (Chapter 4) reinforces that youth need to have relationships with adults who understand that teens must maintain control over their decisions.

"Setting the Stage for a Trustworthy Relationship" (Chapter 14) reinforces that trust needs to be earned. This is a critical point for youth who have not experienced adults as trustworthy.

"Body Language" (Chapter 15) speaks to how low expectations and aggressive versus helpful intention can be conveyed through body language.

"Boundaries" (Chapter 20) covers the importance of not overpromising. Youth who have a history of being let down by adults are particularly vulnerable to broken expectations.

"De-escalation and Crisis Management When a Youth Is 'Acting Out'" (Chapter 23) discusses how to lower the temperature during rising conflicts. **23.0** The importance of giving space and respectful listening is emphasized.

"Addressing Demoralization: Eliciting and Reflecting Strengths" (Chapter 25) covers how to listen deeply so that youth are able to display their better sides. When existing strengths are reflected back to the teen, it can be a pivotal step to **25.0.2** breaking the cycle of disempowerment and hopelessness.

"Health Realization—Accessing a Higher State of Mind No Matter What" (Chapter 27) is rooted in the belief that all people, no matter how traumatized, have the inherent ability to self-right and heal.

"Gaining a Sense of Control—One Step at a Time" (Chapter 29) allows an individual to move past the sense of disempowerment associated with seeing problems as insurmountable. It helps youth break problems into manageable components.

"Helping Adolescents Own Their Solutions" (Chapter 28) discusses how to empower youth to reach their own conclusions. Specifically, it recognizes that, because youth in crisis cannot think abstractly, a lecture can be experienced as condescending, even offensive. The chapter offers alternative communications strategies.

"Stress Management and Coping" (Chapter 31) offers strategies for healing, including safe emotional expression and healthy disengagement strategies.

"Mindfulness Practice for Resilience and Managing Stress and Pain" (Chapter 32) offers techniques that allow an individual to live in the present rather than being trapped in the past.

"Somatic Symptoms" (Chapter 44) discusses how to work with youth whose stress has been internalized into physical symptoms.

"Grief" (Chapter 45) discusses how to help young people recover from pain and loss.

"Emotional, Physical, and Sexual Abuse" (Chapter 57) covers assessing and supporting youth who have experienced these profound traumas.

"Healer, Heal Thyself: Self-care for the Caregiver" (Chapter 67) recognizes that, as we are exposed to others' unimaginable pain, we must stem the forces that create a "protective" shell between us and youth, and us and our emotions. To remain emotionally intelligent, we must first care for ourselves.

Authors Zeelyna Wise, Joseph Lively, Marcos Almonte, and Stephanie Contreras are resilience specialists at El Centro de Estudiantes, a Philadelphia school whose mission includes "providing transformative educational experiences for under-served high school youth."

•• Group Learning and Discussion ••

1. Discuss some of the adverse childhood experiences you have seen in your practice. Then discuss how youth with those experiences generally behave.
2. Reflect on how you respond to the reactivity of traumatized youth. Are youth given the calm space to regain their footing? Might they feel controlled? Shamed?
3. Reflect on whether you routinely accept diagnoses and labels of youth who often "act out." How might these labels create unconscious biases in the way you serve these adolescents? (See Chapter 21.)
4. Reflect on whether anything in your setting might inadvertently re-traumatize adolescents. If so, what action steps could be taken in your practice setting?
5. Recognizing your own human limitations, what steps can you take to control your own reactions so that you can be "radically calm" amidst chaos?
6. Read Chapter 23. Break into pairs and apply those strategies to a case your practice has recently seen.

▪▪▪▪▪▪▪▪ Continuing Education ▪▪▪▪▪▪▪▪

If you are applying for continuing education credits, a test is available online. For more details, visit www.aap.org/reachingteens.

▪ Reference

1. Taylor SE, Klein LC, Lewis BP, Gruenewald TL, Gurung RAR, Updegraff JA. Biobehavioral responses to stress in females: tend-and-befriend, not fight-or-flight. *Psychol Rev.* 2000;107:441–429

▪ Suggested Reading

Bloom SL, Farragher B. *Restoring Sanctuary: A New Operating System for Trauma-Informed Systems of Care*. New York, NY: Oxford University Press; 2013

Bradley R, Heim A, Westen D. Personality constellations in patients with a history of childhood sexual abuse. *J Trauma Stress.* 2005;18(6):769–780

Dube SR, Anda RF, Felitti VJ, Chapman DP, Williamson DF, Giles WH. Childhood abuse, household dysfunction, and the risk of attempted suicide throughout the life span: findings from the Adverse Childhood Experiences Study. *JAMA.* 2001;286(24):3089–3096

Edwards VJ, Holden GW, Felitti VJ, Anda RF. Relationship between multiple forms of childhood maltreatment and adult mental health in community respondents: results from the Adverse Childhood Experiences Study. *Am J Psychiatry.* 2003;160(8):1453–1460

Felitti VJ, Anda RF, Nordenberg DF, et al. Relationship of childhood abuse and household dysfunction to many of the leading causes of death in adults: the Adverse Childhood Experiences (ACE) Study. *Am J Prev Med.* 1998;14(4):245–258

Garner AS, Shonkoff JP; American Academy of Pediatrics Committee on Psychosocial Aspects of Child and Family Health, Committee on Early Childhood, Adoption and Dependent Care, Section on Developmental and Behavioral Pediatrics. Early childhood adversity, toxic stress, and the role of the pediatrician: translating developmental science into lifelong health. *Pediatrics.* 2012;129:e224–e231

Groves B, Zuckerman B, Marans S, Cohen DJ. Silent victims: children who witness violence. *JAMA.* 1993;269:262–264

McEwen BS, Gianaros PJ. Central role of the brain in stress and adaptation: links to socioeconomic status, health, and disease. *Ann N Y Acad Sci.* 2010;1186:190–222

Osofsky JD, Wewers S, Hann DM, Fick AC. Chronic community violence: what is happening to our children? *Psychiatry.* 1993;56:36–45

Pitman RK, Orr SP. The black hole of trauma. *Biol Psychiatry.* 1990;27:469–479

Putnam F. *Dissociation in Children and Adolescents: A Developmental Perspective.* New York, NY: Guilford; 1997

Richters JE, Martinez P. The NIMH community violence project: I. Children as victims of and witnesses to violence. *Psychiatry.* 1993;56:7–21

Shonkoff JP, Boyce WT, McEwen BS. Neuroscience, molecular biology, and the childhood roots of health disparities: building a new framework for health promotion and disease prevention. *JAMA.* 2009;301(21):2252–2259

Shonkoff JP, Garner AS; American Academy of Pediatrics Committee on Psychosocial Aspects of Child and Family Health, Committee on Early Childhood, Adoption and Dependent Care, Section on Developmental and Behavioral Pediatrics. The lifelong effects of early childhood adversity and toxic stress. *Pediatrics.* 2012;129:e232–e246

Taylor SE, Klein LC, Lewis BP, Gruenewald TL, Gurung RAR, Updegraff JA. Biobehavioral responses to stress in females: tend-and-befriend, not fight-or-flight. *Psychol Rev.* 2000;107:441–429

■ Related Video Content

22.0 Trauma-Informed Practice: Working With Youth Who Have Suffered Adverse Experiences. El Centro staff, Covenant House staff.

22.0.1 Trauma-Informed Practice Part 1: What Happens to Youth From Traumatizing Environments? El Centro staff, Covenant House staff.

22.0.2 Trauma-Informed Practice Part 2: The Positive Force That Traumatized Youth Bring to the World. El Centro staff, Covenant House staff.

22.0.3 Trauma-Informed Practice Part 3: Essential Elements of a Healing Environment. El Centro staff, Covenant House staff.

23.0 De-escalation and Crisis Management: Wisdom and Strategies From Professionals Who Serve Youth Who Often Act Out Their Frustrations. Youth-serving agencies.

23.2 Why Youth Act Out...and What They Really Need. YouthBuild youth.

25.0.2 Addressing Demoralization: Eliciting and Reflecting Strengths. Ginsburg.

25.9 Behaviors Must Be Seen in the Context of the Lives Youth Have Needed to Navigate. Auerswald.

57.2 The Making of a Girl. The GEMS Project.

■ Related Handout/Supplementary Material

Hidden Among Us: Sexually Exploited and Trafficked Youth

CHAPTER 23

De-escalation and Crisis Management When a Youth Is "Acting Out"

Cordella Hill, MSW
Hugh Organ, MS
Kenneth R. Ginsburg, MD, MS Ed, FAAP, FSAHM

 Related Video Content

23.0 De-escalation and Crisis Management: Wisdom and Strategies From Professionals Who Serve Youth Who Often Act Out Their Frustrations

■ Why This Matters

This text focuses on connecting with youth and reasoning with them in a shared decision-making process while engaging them to consider positive behavioral changes. In sharp contrast, during an acute crisis that may involve acting out, the only goals are safety and de-escalation. In fact, attempts at reasoning may be counter-productive because expecting an irrational youth to consider long-range outcomes or abstract concepts may enhance his feelings of incompetence and frustration, inadvertently magnifying the crisis.

> **The actions necessary to de-escalate a rising crisis run counter to the fight or flight instincts we have to respond to stressful or threatening situations. Therefore, it is especially important to draw from a well thought out, practiced skill set.**

The actions necessary to de-escalate a rising crisis run counter to the fight or flight instincts we have to respond to stressful or threatening situations. Therefore, it is especially important to draw from a well thought out, practiced skill set.

The overall goals of acute crisis management are to
1. Ensure immediate safety for the teen and others in the setting, including yourself.
2. Deescalate the situation.
3. Assess for the potential of ongoing harm to self or others.
4. Refer to appropriate resources.
5. Debrief with your colleagues to process emotions and learn from the episode.

■ Limitations of This Chapter

If you work in a youth crisis center or facility that serves youth with mental health challenges, you deserve an intensive training in crisis management. This chapter is designed to introduce concepts and broaden your repertoire; it does not substitute for formal professional development.

■ Safety First

Safety always comes first. It is optimal to be able to communicate with a person in acute crisis and resolve any outstanding issues. However, if there is any potential for physical harm, security or the police need to be involved, and you might have to consider physical and/or medical restraints. Appropriate use of restraints is beyond the scope of this chapter.

When considering safety, the following points may be helpful:

- Inform colleagues that you are entering a difficult situation before you enter the room, and have someone monitor the evolving scenario.
- Prior to entering the room, remove any necklaces, ties, or other objects from around your neck. (If someone cuts off your air supply, you cannot summon help.)
- Remove any religious or political symbols, as it is difficult to predict a reaction they might trigger.
- Keep the door open.
- Do not allow anything to be between you and the door.
- Do not stand between the youth and the door so that he does not feel trapped.
- Consider going in with another person. Depending on the situation, this may interfere with or enhance optimal communication, but it can be critical if there is a serious concern about safety.
- Never turn your back for any reason.

Quickly Assessing for Drug Use or Psychosis

It is important to quickly assess whether verbal de-escalation may help you address a crisis.

- If a person is psychotic, as indicated by his behavior being disconnected to reality, it is especially important to be calming and to use nonconfrontational body language. It is also especially important to remain nonjudgmental, but it may not be helpful to enter a verbal discussion.
- Similarly, if a person appears to be hallucinating, it may be dangerous to attempt to reach him, as his distorted sense of reality may paint you as antagonistic. Although youth under the influence of most drugs can be calmed, youth on PCP as well as some other hallucinogens, such as bath salts, may become more agitated with any attempts at communication. One telltale sign of PCP is horizontal, vertical, and rotatory nystagmus, as indicated by eyes making quick involuntary movements in all directions as they attempt to track an object.

Getting Rid of the Audience

A critical first step to de-escalation is to clear the area of any audience. Especially in the case of a conflict or a fight, a young person's need to perform for onlookers will make it much harder for her to back down or return to calm. Further, youth in crowds can intentionally inflame a situation.

Breaking Up a Fight

It is beyond the scope of this chapter to offer physical maneuvers that may help you to safely separate 2 aggressive parties. The wisest strategy is to remember that safety comes first and to involve police or security right away.

Below are some general rules.

1. First, attempt to stop the fight using a clear, stern, loud voice to demand the fight stop immediately.
2. Remove the crowd immediately.
3. Do not step into the middle of the fight.
4. If you have a prior relationship with either combatant, verbally redirect that combatant to leave the situation. If no prior relationship exists, then identify the least aggressive combatant and verbally redirect that person away from the situation.
5. If the combatants are not separating, create a loud distraction. When you gain their eye contact, demand that they separate.
6. Move combatants into 2 separate areas.
7. Do not ask, "Who started this?"
8. Do very little talking until the adrenalin surge appears to be subsiding, as judged by breathing returning to normal and the youth seeming less physically agitated.
9. Follow de-escalation strategies discussed elsewhere.

■ De-escalation

Absolute Respect

An irritable or agitated teen is acutely sensitive to being disrespected or feeling shamed. He needs to know that, even as we set limits, it comes from our caring and desire to protect him. Our challenge is to remain deeply respectful throughout our intervention and to treat him with full dignity, even in the extreme case where physical restraints are needed.

Anticipating a Problem

Your practice group should devise a plan to deal with adolescent crises before one is needed. Your decisions are more likely to be thoughtful than those made when on the receiving end of anger or emotional outbursts. Think about those issues likely to arise in your setting and develop strategies as a group ahead of time.

On any given day, the best de-escalation plans occur before a crisis strikes. If a youth seems angry at something that you did, apologize. If a youth feels frustrated and powerless, give a choice that allows her to regain a sense of power. If a teen feels frightened, reassure her that you will keep her safe. Notice signs of increasing anxiety, such as pacing, fidgeting, hand wringing, or withdrawal, and share that the young person seems upset or worried. Ask if there is anything you can do to be supportive. If stress is building, listen to the teen's concerns until she feels as if she has been fully heard. If it is clear that a crisis is at hand, consider referral to a crisis center or psychiatric emergency department in advance of escalation.

The Body Language of De-escalation

The young person in acute crisis is likely to be experiencing anxiety or anger, and may feel vulnerable to attack. Therefore, she is likely to be hypervigilant of any movement perceived to be potentially hostile. The first step of de-escalation is to reassure the youth that there is no imminent threat and, indeed, that your presence supports, rather than challenges, safety. Calming body language is critical in combination with verbal reassurance.

Your natural reaction to an impending challenge or threat is to have anxiety or to feel personally endangered. Therefore, your instincts will be telling you to either flee or take an offensive position yourself. First, control your breathing with deep slow breaths so that you will reverse the "fight or flight" response (see Chapter 31). Then, use reassuring "self-talk" to gain confidence that you are well prepared and are best able to handle the situation with your skill, rather than your physical power. Remind yourself that the hostility or fear is likely not directed at you. Even if it is directed toward you, then you are especially well positioned to de-escalate the situation with an apology for anything you might have done to cause offense. These thoughts and actions will control your instinctual biological reactions and may better allow your body to display the calm, yet controlled, demeanor needed to reassure the young person of safety.

It is important to give the agitated young person plenty of physical space. His or her "personal space" will be greater than normal. A hostile or frightened youth will be sensitive to any threat; therefore, movement into personal space can trigger alarm. This is particularly true if the youth has a history of trauma. It is best not to have any physical contact while the youth is agitated. If you extend a hand, make sure that your hands are clearly open. That will help the teen see that there is no weapon present and prevent your movement from being interpreted as if you are planning to grasp and control the arm. Similarly, keep your hands out of your pockets both to signal that you have no weapon and so that they are available for self-protection. A palms-up position illustrates that your desire is to serve rather than dominate (see Chapter 15).

Try to communicate reassurance and concern with your facial expression. Hopefully, your reassuring self-talk will allow you to avoid a countenance of fear. A smile may be viewed as insincere or can be misinterpreted as nervousness, a grimace, or as if you are minimizing the irritable youth's concerns. Eye contact is a sign of respect in most cultures. Remain at the same eye level as the youth. Try to stay seated, but if he needs to stand, rise to meet his eyes. Although eye contact is respectful, allow him to break his gaze and look away.

Next, position your body at an angle to the youth. A chest-to-chest position can send subconscious hostile messages and trigger instinctual expectations of an imminent attack. An angled position diminishes this sense while actually better positioning you to escape if necessary (see Chapter 58).

It is important to also watch the pace of your movements. Slow, methodical movements reinforce calm. Quick movements may give away your own anxiety. Further, any rapid movements can trigger anxiety or a defensive hostile reaction in a young person acutely sensitive to danger.

Listening

It is hard to find the perfect words to say when a person is frantic or acting out. The good news is that listening—the relative absence of words—is the key to de-escalation. Start by telling the young person that your goal is to listen to their feelings and concerns. Sit down or use other body language cues to demonstrate that you are not in a hurry. Silence can be an effective tool because it reinforces your intention to listen. If the young person continues to yell, you might consider saying in a calm even tone, *"I really want to hear you, and I'm having trouble hearing what you're telling me when you are talking this way. I am really here to listen, and I'm going to listen until you're done talking."*

A Few Words to Say...and What Not to Say

An acute crisis is not the time to help someone resolve multiple issues. It is not a time to argue or try to convince a teen of your viewpoint. Therefore, keep conversations simple and concrete, while avoiding any abstract complexity or lectures. A person in crisis cannot think abstractly. When your discussion is complex, you can inadvertently reinforce a sense of shame because of the teen's inability to grasp your points while she is in crisis mode. Once she has been calmed, you can consider facilitating her to develop and own her own solutions (see Chapter 28). Until she has reached that state of calm, which you can sense by the rate of her breathing, the cadence of her speech, and her posture, your words should be few, simple, reassuring, and calming. Avoid language that implies you understand what she is feeling or that belittles or negates her emotions. Don't say too much; instead focus on listening and use silence judiciously. Silence can trigger discussion as people tend to fill the void. Never interrupt while the youth is talking. When the teen is done talking, ask *"Is there anything else you'd like to tell me?"*

DON'T SAY	SAY INSTEAD
I understand.	Help me to understand.
I know how you feel.	I can't imagine how you feel.
Just calm down.	You seem angry. I'm here to listen so you can get your feelings out.
Just get over it.	After you work out your feelings, you're going to get through this.
You're making a big deal out of nothing.	This seems so important to you.
You're always causing trouble here and that's not acceptable.	This place has to feel safe for everyone, including you.
I agree.	I hear you.
It sounds like he was totally wrong.	I hear what you are saying. I'll get to the bottom of this.
Don't have an attitude with me, I'm here to help you.	You really seem frustrated. I definitely want to hear everything you have to say, and we're going to figure this out together.
You're always causing trouble.	You've come so far. I've been so proud of you because _____. You're having a tough day. I have confidence you'll get through this.

Tone of Voice

Verbal communication is more than about what you say; it is also about how you say it. Your tone and cadence easily give away your anxiety or anger. Your volume suggests whether you wish to dominate or control. A loud volume can be interpreted as an attempt to dampen another's voice. Softer speech suggests you are listening with no intent of diminishing the other's ability to express their thoughts and feelings. In fact, as a person raises their voice, lower yours. As their cadence increases, slow yours. This way you can show with your body language, your words, and how those words are expressed that your goal is to listen. A young person who feels heard will often be able to return to a state of calm.

Offering an Apology

If a young person is angry with you, an apology can go a long way. If you may have done something wrong, a heartfelt apology is warranted. Ideally, an apology should be spontaneously given prior to escalation, because it can prevent the cycle of anger from the beginning. An apologetic statement does not have to be an admission of guilt, rather it is used to acknowledge someone's feelings and begin to redress a perceived wrong. You can always choose to apologize for someone's experience: *"I am sorry for how that felt to you"* or *"I am sorry for how my words made you angry."*

Avoid Defensiveness and Answer All Questions Respectfully

Even if the anger or insults are directed at you, it is critical to remember they are rarely really about you. Do not feel the need to defend yourself or any of your colleagues from insults, curses, or denigration about their roles. Answer all questions that are genuinely seeking information no matter the tone in which they are asked, because the information may defuse the crisis. Do not feel the need to respond to questions that feel abusive, and that are not really calling for information (eg, *"Why does everyone here suck?"*). Such a question needs neither a response nor defensiveness.

Giving Something

A person in crisis may make unreasonable or irrational demands. Even if their request is appropriate, you still may not be able to fulfill it. In order to avoid escalation, it can be strategic to offer something else. You might say, *"I'm sorry but I don't think I'll be able to _____, but I think I will be able to _____."* Even if the young person does not make a request, it is still nice to offer something because it places you in the role of caregiver. Consider saying, *"Do you want me to get you some water/juice/a snack while we talk?"* (Only offer a physical object, even a snack, as the situation is calming. Otherwise, it can be thrown at you.) Depending on the circumstance, you might consider stating, *"I'm wondering if I was able to _____, whether that would help. What do you think?"* It can also be effective to offer the youth the opportunity to choose between different appropriate choices because choices give teens a sense of control, and few things can restore calm like a sense of control.

Offering Clear Boundaries

Even amidst a crisis, do not be afraid to explain limits and rules in an authoritative, firm tone. It actually may make the teen feel safer to know that you need to maintain safety for everyone and that he will be contained. It also offers him a face-saving way to de-escalate when you respectfully, but clearly, demand appropriate behavior. Offer choices in which both alternatives are reasonable (eg, *"Would you like to continue our discussion now or would you prefer to come back later when you have had a chance to think things through?"*). It is possible to empathize fully with a feeling without validating a behavior (eg, *"I understand that you have a really good reason to feel frustrated, even angry, but it is not okay for you to threaten me or any of the other youth."*).

■ Assessing Ongoing Risk

After de-escalating the acute crisis, you need to determine the young person's risk for harm to self or others. If the youth does express suicidal or homicidal intent, it becomes both your ethical and legal obligation to protect the teen, and you may not keep the information confidential.

Tell the young person that you are glad that she was able to express herself and that although she seems to feel better, you want to make sure she remains safe. Then ask directly whether you have to worry about the possibility of her hurting herself or someone else. Explore the degree of likelihood of a further incident by asking whether a plan exists and ascertaining the details of that plan. Always err toward caution, and do not assume the teen is just blowing off steam.

■ Referral

The immediacy and type of referral depends on whether the situation was able to be calmed and whether your assessment revealed an imminent risk. If you were not able to de-escalate the episode, you may need to involve the police or a mobile crisis team. If the crisis is de-escalated, but the teen remains at imminent risk, then he or she requires immediate psychiatric evaluation. If there is no imminent risk, then your challenge is to persuade the young person that he is deserving of further ongoing support (see Chapter 33). It may be that the youth will not be prepared to transition to mental health care, in which case your goal should be to maintain a relationship so you can continue to guide him, reassess his need in the future, and continue to build trust so that you can readdress the need for mental health care later.

■ Debrief

It is important to debrief with colleagues or a supervisor after a major episode. First, it is important to process your own emotions to relieve some of your stress. Don't be surprised, even if you were the model of collection in the midst of a crisis, if your fears come out after calm is restored. A debrief is also a good time to consider quality improvement: What was done well? What could have been handled better? How could the response be improved the next time a crisis presents? Perhaps most importantly, when we debrief as a group, it allows the entire team to learn from a situation that may only have involved 1 or 2 people.

●● Group Learning and Discussion ●●

Preparing a Practice for a Potential Episode
- What are the kinds of crises likely to present in our setting?
- What plans do we have in place to ensure the safety of our staff and teens in crisis, as well as other teens and families?
- Is security easily accessible? Could we easily signal distress to our colleagues such that a staff member not directly involved would know when and how to summon security?
- Does everyone know to eliminate the audience first, to ensure their safety and decrease the likelihood they will inflame the situation?
- What steps does a staff member need to take before entering a room to ensure his or her own safety?
- Review key elements of a nonconfrontational body language.
- Review key points about what to say and what not to say in a potentially explosive situation.
- Discuss the strategic reasons to apologize to an angry youth.

The Debrief: Discussion Questions for After an Episode
- Were there any indications that the teen was moving toward a crisis?
- Is there anything that we could have done to have prevented the escalation?
- Is there anything we did that upset the teen? Was it avoidable?
- Assuming that we were verbally attacked or insulted, or one of our colleagues was defamed, how did that affect us emotionally?
- How did it feel to see a youth in that much pain?
- Did we do everything we could to ensure safety first? Let's review those steps.
- Did the issue get resolved adequately? If not, where do we stand now? If yes, what seemed to have made the difference? What allowed the young person to calm down?
- Are there any lessons learned that we have to put into place to make us better prepared for the next incident?

▪▪▪▪▪▪▪▪ Continuing Education ▪▪▪▪▪▪▪▪

If you are applying for continuing education credits, a test is available online. For more details, visit www.aap.org/reachingteens.

■ Suggested Reading

Couvillon M, Peterson RL, Ryan JB, Scheuermann B, Stegall J. A review of crisis intervention training programs for schools. TEACHING Except Child. 2010;42(5):6–17

Crisis Prevention Institute. CPI Nonviolent Crisis Intervention Training Program. De-escalation Techniques. http://www.crisisprevention.com/Resources/Knowledge-Base/De-escalation-Tips/De-escalation-Techniques. Accessed June 25, 2013

Skolnik-Acker E, Committee for the Study and Prevention of Violence Against Social Workers, National Association of Social Workers, Massachusetts Chapter. Verbal De-escalation Techniques for Defusing or Talking Down an Explosive Situation. http://www.naswma.org/displaycommon. cfm?an=1&subarticlenbr=520. Accessed June 25, 2013

■ Related Video Content

23.0 De-escalation and Crisis Management: Wisdom and Strategies From Professionals Who Serve Youth Who Often Act Out Their Frustrations. Youth-serving agencies.

23.1 De-escalation if Someone Wants to Leave to "Get Even." Covenant House.

23.2 Why Youth Act Out…and What They Really Need. YouthBuild youth.

22.0 Trauma-Informed Practice: Working With Youth Who Have Suffered Adverse Experiences. El Centro staff, Covenant House staff.

■ Related Web Sites

If your group is interested in formal training in nonviolent de-escalation, below are reputable programs that offer staff professional development sessions.

CPI Nonviolent Crisis Intervention Training
www.crisisprevention.com

Handle With Care Behavior Management System
http://handlewithcare.com

CHAPTER 24

Delivering Bad News to Adolescents

Daniel H. Reirden, MD, FAAP, AAHIVMS

Kenneth R. Ginsburg, MD, MS Ed, FAAP, FSAHM

 Related Video Content

24.0 Among the Hardest Things We Do—Delivering Bad News

■ Why This Matters

As we care for adolescents, we often have to share news that they would rather not hear. There is no way to make these disclosures pleasant, but we can make a difference in the adolescents' experience. How they experience receiving the news may make a large difference in the next steps they take (or don't take) to address the issue. If they experience shame or stigma, they may reject further services. If they are left feeling without hope, they may catastrophize the situation and move into denial, or, worse, entertain self-harm. On the other hand, if they feel cared for and about, they may engage in a relationship that will enable you to guide them toward the best outcome.

> As important as it is to make yourself available for follow-up, it is even more vital not to overpromise. Many youth have experience with adults who have been inconsistent and unavailable; you do not want to be added to that list. Be clear and honest about your service and limitations.

■ Tips for Breaking Bad News

The following tips are not meant to feel formulaic or to constitute a recipe. Rather they are general thoughts for your consideration.

1. *Consider your own reaction prior to working with the youth or family.* It is normal, even desirable, to be genuinely saddened by news that you know will alter a teen's life direction. In some cases, you might be particularly shocked if, for some reason, you related closely to the youth. In other cases, you may need to work through a sense of guilt or responsibility for not having prevented the problem. All of these feelings are reasonable and normal, but have to be resolved before you interact with the youth because he or she will read your affect and that will alter the experience. The youth should not feel as though he or she needs to care for you.

2. *Decide if you are the best person to break the news.* It is okay to determine that a colleague has a better relationship with the youth or more expertise in a specific area. However, this can only be done in a setting where the colleague would naturally be exposed to the information; confidentiality remains a paramount issue. Further, a teen may experience another caregiver delivering the news as being passed off or may conclude that you consider the issue stigmatizing. Depending on your assessment of

these considerations, you can have the colleague with the longstanding relationship be available for partnering with you if the youth requests it.

3. *Practice what you will say*. This is especially important if this is a difficult topic for you or the news raises strong feelings in you. Stumbling with the news will raise the youth's anxiety about the gravity of the situation.

4. *Consider who should be present*. Is there someone that the youth would like to be there for emotional support? Are there key members of the care team who should be present?

5. *Assess the physical space*. Select a space that is as quiet and private as possible. Arrange to have adequate time to spend with the teen, and make every attempt to limit interruptions during this period. Making sure that you're prepared with items, such as tissues, conveys a message that you have thought about the youth's emotional needs beforehand. Sit down when you deliver the news. Do not block an exit from the room, as people who receive concerning news often have a need to flee. Although people almost universally control this instinctual impulse, if an exit is blocked, it can reinforce the sense of being trapped.

6. *Be prepared for escalations*. If the news is likely to create an angry response, (eg, a murder of a friend) or if the youth has a history of volatile reactions, have a safety plan in place. A colleague, or security if appropriate, should know the timing and location of the disclosure and you should be certain that the exit is not blocked for you. Be prepared to de-escalate the situation, with the initial step always being listening without judgment (see Chapter 23).

7. *Be conscious of your body language*. Remember that about 80% of what we communicate is conveyed nonverbally. All of your preparation and practice in finding the right words to say can be undermined by your body language. Take deep breaths or practice mindfulness techniques to stabilize your emotions before entering the room. Then be conscious of your body language as youth, particularly marginalized adolescents, are acutely sensitive to body language that conveys fear or judgment. Your body language, which may actually be associated with your own discomfort or sadness, may be misinterpreted as being judgmental. It is important, therefore, to maintain an open, calm body posture (see Chapter 15). **32.3**

8. *Be direct*. Beating around the bush or engaging in prolonged small talk will increase anxiety and generate confusion. Be calm and gentle, but come to the point quickly. Avoid retreating to the professional comfort zone of offering technical details rather than attending to the youth's emotional needs. If you are providing bad news related to a medical condition, it can be extremely helpful to assess what the teen's understanding of the situation is prior to disclosing the news. You might say something like, *"I want to get a sense of what you remember about why we got this particular medical test."* You may have a sentence that emotionally prepares the youth to listen carefully. *"I have some bad/upsetting news to share with you today."* Then, share the news gently and directly. *"I am sorry to have to tell you that there was a terrible crash today, and _____ was killed."* *"I am sorry to tell you that your HIV test was positive, meaning that you are infected with HIV."* *"I am so sorry to tell you that there was a gang shooting earlier in the day, and _____ was killed."* If the bad news is related to a medical diagnosis, asking about how much detail/information the youth wants in that moment can be helpful. In the case of test results, have written proof available, as youth often request to see it.

9. *Allow time for initial reaction*. The emotions may be shock, anger, or denial. None of them are wrong. This is the time to listen. If the teen doesn't respond immediately, the importance of allowing a period of silence to occur cannot be overemphasized. During this time, maintain an open, calm body posture and remain connected to the teen by not looking away. After a suitable period of silence, an open-ended question, such

as, *"Tell me how you're feeling right now,"* or *"What's going on in your head?"* can help facilitate further conversation.

Never minimize an emotion by saying, *"I understand,"* or *"It isn't that bad."* Just listen. When you do say something, make the connection between the reaction and the news. This will validate the emotions and make it clear that you see their reaction as connected to the news and are not judging it. *"This is clearly shocking news, and I see how angry you are."* Do not be shocked, yourself, if the news does not seem to shake the youth. Sometimes in the context of a hectic life, a youth may not view a situation in the same catastrophic manner that you would in the same situation. One of the reasons it is so important that you control your own verbal and nonverbal messages is that otherwise you can convey a sense of catastrophe that a youth may not have experienced.

10. *Appropriate touching.* Touch needs to be used judiciously, leaving absolutely no room for misinterpretation, because we need to assume the possibility that the young person has been exposed to inappropriate touch. If an adolescent is weeping silently, a hand on the youth's shoulder or hand can be an appropriate way to reinforce that you are fully present. In the case of a young person receiving news of a condition that is stigmatizing (eg, HIV or other sexually transmitted infection), touch can contribute to healing because it conveys that you do not see the young person as somehow tainted.

11. *Convey messages of hope whenever possible.* Sometimes the most hopeful message you can convey is that *"You'll get through this."* But even that message may not feel helpful in the case of the news of a death. On the other hand, in the case of news about illness like HIV or cancer, it is important to convey hope. However, it is also important to be accurate. In the case of diseases, learn as much as you can about prognosis prior to the discussion and offer as much hope as possible. If there is any degree of uncertainty about the prognosis, don't make promises or offer unrealistic expectations. Even when delivering news about potentially life-ending illnesses, a caring statement such as, *"No matter what happens, we'll do everything we can to keep you comfortable"* is more authentic than promising false hope. In the case of HIV, it is critical to address prevailing myths about the virus. HIV is not a death sentence and can be well managed. Whenever possible, offer a reassuring statement that suggests that the teen is not alone and that you believe he will get through this: *"I have cared for [many/several] other youth with X and I have seen them get through this. I believe that you will also."*

12. *Continue to listen.* As the moments proceed, the youth will often reveal what he needs through his words or actions. Listening may be more important than anything you say. Listening reinforces that you are present. Listening conveys that you respect the youth as the expert on his own life. Listening allows you to serve as a sounding board as the adolescent facilitates his own progress.

13. *Explore how best to get ongoing support.* It is important before the youth leaves your presence that he has thought through who else can offer ongoing support. Ask directly, *"Who in your life can be most helpful now?"* That person does not have to be a parent, but ideally will be a supportive adult. If there is no accessible or responsible adult, then your continued presence becomes particularly important. In the case of bad news, particularly the kind that may (sadly) have stigma attached (eg, HIV), you should not push toward disclosure before the young person is ready.

14. *Assess for safety.* It is imperative that you ask directly if the young person feels safe. In the case of bad personal news, he may be considering self-harm. In the case of bad news about a friend or family members, particularly if it involved violence, the teen may be considering retaliation. In either case, safety becomes the top priority and, after a more thorough assessment, you might need to heighten the level of protection for the young person or report a threat to authorities. Privacy is no longer protected when a life is threatened.

15. *Create a follow-up plan.* In some case*s, you might refer* to a person more adept at the level of care the youth needs. Even in these cases, the adolescent should still have a follow-up plan to see you in a few days. This will reinforce that you are committed to the teen getting through this and not feeling alone. In a crisis situation, let the adolescent know that someone in your practice or agency is available at all times if the youth needs added support. If this is not the case, then make sure the young person has a hotline number to call if for some reason he cannot wait until morning. As important as it is to make yourself available for follow-up, it is even more vital not to overpromise. Many youth have experience with adults who have been inconsistent and unavailable; you do not want to be added to that list. Be clear and honest about your service and limitations. When you will try to make something happen but cannot guarantee the result, say just that. 66.1

The Debrief as a Standard Part of the Process

Witnessing pain takes a toll on us. No matter how many times you will shepherd young people through difficult times, it will continue to affect you. Debrief with colleagues both to process your own emotions and to incorporate "lessons learned" to be able to handle similar situations in the future.

Parents as Critical Allies

Ideally, parents will be the most supportive figures in their children's lives. However, they also experience grief, shock, and stigma. Those emotions may prevent them from giving their best performance. In addition, they may experience anger and guilt. The combination of anger and guilt are a toxic mixture, because, to alleviate their own sense of guilt, they may intensify their anger toward their teen. This may be particularly true in your presence because they are trying to communicate to you, the authority figure, *"This is not my fault."*

It is important, therefore, to break bad news to parents in a way that diminishes their guilt. Their presence alone enables you to do this. A full discussion is offered on breaking bad news to parents in Chapter 37.

Contributing to the World as a Healing Exercise

The following strategies are not recommended on the first day that bad news is delivered. Then, your goals are conveying accurate information, providing emotional support, and crisis management, if necessary. However, the follow-up visit may be the time to help the youth think about how to move forward in a way that allows them to improve the situation for someone else. In some cases, it may be something you suggest long after a teen has progressed on their own healing journey.

The technique may be helpful when the bad news involved loss of someone who the youth cared deeply about. People who experience grief often have no place to channel it, and can sometimes come up with very negative responses such as, *"I'll kill myself to be closer with my grandma,"* or *"They killed my brother; he's not around to get even, I will."* Instead, help the youth to take on a good deed or activity to honor the life of the loved one. *"Tell me about your grandma." "What were her dreams for you?" "Could you imagine making them come true to honor her life?"* or *"Tell me about your brother." What are the good things he brought to the world?" "How can you make his memory live on in a positive way?"* This technique is particularly useful when someone leaves behind a child or elderly relative to be cared for. *"Let's make sure your niece knows about your brother's sense of humor and how much he loved her. Could you imagine making her a storybook about him? Do you think you can watch out for her?"*

In the cases of teens whose bad news is about themselves, they may eventually benefit from sharing lessons learned with peers. It may help them to make more sense of why something happened to them. *"I guess it is my job to make sure this doesn't happen to other kids."* This strategy is not something to be pushed; it needs to follow disclosure. Rather, it remains an option that some youth may find healing. A sense of contribution is a core element of resilience. **31.5, 45.1**

●● Group Learning and Discussion ●●

Break into pairs and choose scenarios that match your professional settings from among the following and practice breaking the news to the young person. Alternatively, pick an actual situation and share it with your partner. Before you role-play, discuss how you might feel as the professional in each situation. That process will parallel the recommendation that in an actual situation you first consider your own reaction.

1. You are in a group home. Tyler is a 14-year-old boy who was removed from his home for parental neglect and school truancy. You just received a call that his 18-year-old brother was shot and killed.
2. You are a nurse practitioner who just received biopsy results on Lisa, a 16-year-old patient who reminds you of your niece. She had a long-standing enlarged lymph node, and, although you were very reassuring, you sent her to have it biopsied. She has cancer. After a preliminary discussion with an oncologist, you are reassured that her prognosis is good.
3. You work in a testing center, and Felipe, a 15-year-old boy, has tested positive for HIV.
4. You work in a residential setting that serves youth. You receive a call that 13-year-old Marita's mother was in a car crash and died. There is not a family member available nearby.

▮▮▮▮▮▮▮▮ Continuing Education ▮▮▮▮▮▮▮▮

If you are applying for continuing education credits, a test is available online. For more details, visit www.aap.org/reachingteens.

▮ Suggested Reading

Leventown M; American Academy of Pediatrics Committee on Bioethics. Communicating with children and families: from everyday interactions to skill in conveying distressing information. *Pediatrics.* 2008;121(5):e1441–e1460. http://pediatrics.aappublications.org/content/121/5/e1441.full.html. Accessed June 25, 2013

▮ Related Video Content

24.0 Among the Hardest Things We Do—Delivering Bad News. Ginsburg, Reirden, Arrington-Sanders, Garofalo, Hawkins, Pletcher.

31.5 Stress Management and Coping/Section 4/Making the World Better/Point 10: Contribute. Ginsburg.

32.3 Mindful Walking. Vo.

45.1 Dealing With Grief by Living Life More Purposefully. Ginsburg.

66.11 Never Make Promises to Homeless and Marginalized Youth That You Cannot Keep. Hill.

Empowering Adolescents to Change

This section offers approaches and strategies that support adolescents to make wise behavioral decisions. "Addressing Demoralization: Eliciting and Reflecting Strengths" (Chapter 25) is an approach that allows the interviewer to see risk in the context of existing strengths, and then reflect those assets back to the teen. That strategy can be useful with all young people, but may be key to engaging demoralized youth who may not even be receptive to contemplating change because they have internalized disempowering messages. "Motivational Interviewing" (Chapter 26) is a strategy rooted in the transtheoretical model of behavioral change that facilitates youth to consider advancing to the next stage of change. "Health Realization—Accessing a Higher State of Mind No Matter What" (Chapter 27) assumes that humans have a natural predisposition to be healthy, and that professionals can be more effective when we assume the role of facilitating youth back to that state of equilibrium. "Helping Adolescents Own Their Solutions" (Chapter 28) offers

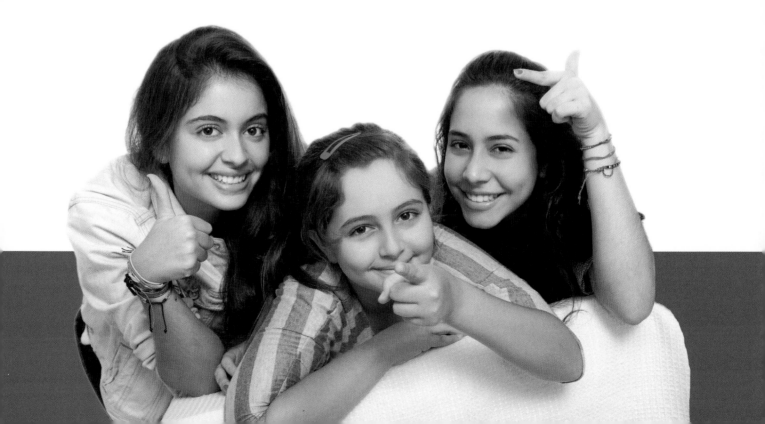

an approach to facilitate youth to make their own decisions. It offers concrete strategies to use in lieu of the dreaded lecture. Lecturing too often backfires because it disempowers youth by delivering guidance in a style that makes them feel incompetent. "Gaining a Sense of Control—One Step at a Time" (Chapter 29) offers a useful strategy for working with youth with an external locus of control who have grown to view themselves as powerless in their ability to move away from worrisome behaviors. It allows them to contemplate alternate futures and take simple steps toward desirable behaviors. "Strength-Based Interviewing: The Circle of Courage" (Chapter 30) is an interview technique that elicits and reinforces existing strengths by focusing on 4 assets—belonging, mastery, independence, and generosity. It allows the interviewer to also have a focused discussion on building strengths in those areas that need further development. "Stress Management and Coping" (Chapter 31) will allow you to move beyond telling youth what not to do, and instead will prepare you to suggest positive coping strategies that will also alleviate stress. The comprehensive coping strategy presented will aid youth to choose healthy means to deal with discomfort rather than reaching for potentially dangerous quick fixes. "Mindfulness Practice for Resilience and Managing Stress and Pain" (Chapter 32) helps youth live fully in the moment while forgetting the past and not worrying about the future. It relieves stress and allows focused thinking. Finally, strategies are offered in "Helping Youth Overcome Shame and Stigma (and Doing Our Best to Not Be a Part of the Problem)" (Chapter 33) for guiding youth to overcome some of the key barriers that may prevent them from seeking needed support.

CHAPTER 25

Addressing Demoralization: Eliciting and Reflecting Strengths

Kenneth R. Ginsburg, MD, MS Ed, FAAP, FSAHM

 Related Video Content

25.0.1 An Introduction to Behavioral Change: Youth Will Not Make Positive Choices if They Don't Believe in Their Potential to Change
25.0.2 Addressing Demoralization: Eliciting and Reflecting Strengths

■ Why This Matters

A fundamental aspect of contemplating change is consideration of whether change is even possible.[1] If a person does not believe she is capable of change, she will stifle consideration of progress, or perhaps deny the existence of the problem altogether to avoid the frustration that accompanies powerlessness. It is easier to deny a problem exists than to meet with failure, especially if a person has repeated experience of having failed. For this reason, the first step toward behavioral change may be attaining confidence that one can change.

> **Young adults who have changed their life path often recall a pivotal moment when a caring professional made them realize they had potential.**

Confidence is rooted in competence.[2] A person gains confidence partially through receiving and believing feedback from others that he has demonstrated capabilities. He solidifies confidence when further actions demonstrate the experience of success.

A person's confidence is undermined when he receives and internalizes messages that he is incapable. Even typical adolescents absorb messages that they are the source of problems and prone to impulsive rather than reasoned action.[3] However, some adolescents have heard undermining messages consistently that have not been counterbalanced by supportive relationships. These youth have learned to see themselves as undeserving and have grown to see their destiny as out of their control. Still other youth have made repeated efforts to change their life circumstances and have met with failure. These latter 2 groups may become demoralized and, therefore, particularly resistant to the possibility of change. They are deserving of a strength-based approach that helps them recognize they can control their destiny. A first step toward this goal is facilitating them to recognize they possess skill sets they can use to change their life circumstances.

■ How to Combat Demoralization

A professional using a problem- or risk-focused approach may begin with a statement of the problem and offer reasons why current behaviors will cause harm or lead to a feared outcome. This approach does not recognize the context of a young person's life and may leave him thinking he is seen only as "a problem." If this occurs, it can reinforce a sense of shame, undermining both the potential for change and the forging of a therapeutic relationship. On the other hand, if after a comprehensive SSHADESS screen (see Chapter 18), which included close attention to existing strengths, you can place the problem amidst a sea of strengths, the young person is less likely to feel ashamed and more likely to be receptive to guidance. This may be even more effective if the **25.0.1** existing strengths can be tightly linked to the desired behavior.

Several examples help to illustrate this point.

- A young person who is smoking marijuana to relieve stress, to chill, may possess tremendous sensitivity and a real desire to improve the challenges at home. He may be smoking precisely because he is the kind of person who cares deeply.
- A young woman who wants to become a mother has the desire to be nurturing.
- The 15-year-old drug dealer is also an entrepreneur who may be driven to contribute to his family.
- The gang member has a deep sense of loyalty and a desire to belong and to feel protected from a dangerous environment.

Recognizing the positive contexts that drive a negative behavior neither condones the behavior nor diminishes our desire to address it. Rather, it allows us to see youth in a way that will prevent shame from being inadvertently communicated through our interaction. The goal is to build on the point of strength and hope for a ripple effect that will diminish the teen's need to continue engaging in the maladaptive behavior. For example, a young person who uses drugs but who is also recognized for her sensitivity may be more receptive to other means to diminish stress as well as strategies to creatively and safely express sensitivity.

An approach to intervention that both recognizes strength and invites a collaborative approach follows: **25.0.2**

Step 1: **Elicit.** Listen for context and strengths.

Step 2: **Reflect.** Tell the young person what you admire about her and what you see as her strengths.

Step 3: **Pause.** Take a breath for a moment and allow the youth to absorb the genuineness of your reflection. It may be a rare or singular experience for the teen to be noticed for what she is doing right.

Step 4: **Share** what you may be worried about. Ideally, tell the teen why you are concerned that the current behavior may get in the way of achieving her stated goals.

Step 5: **Ask permission** to discuss the issue further. This may be an unusual experience for the adolescent, as young people are not usually asked whether they want to engage in a conversation.

If the youth does suggest she wants to engage in further discussion, consider using motivational interviewing techniques to further increase motivation to change (see Chapter 26).

■ Case 1

Lisa is a 14-year-old girl who tells her doctor that her grades have been dropping and that she is worried that they will prevent her from becoming the pediatric nurse practitioner she has dreamed of becoming. The doctor refrains from launching into a talk about the importance of good grades, and simply asks her why she thinks her grades have declined.

Lisa explains that her mother relies on her pretty heavily to take care of her 3 younger siblings. She describes how much she loves her mother and understands she is overburdened, especially because she is working extra hours to make sure she will have enough money to send everyone to college.

Lisa quickly jumps in, *"I really love taking care of my little brothers and sister!"* She helps them with homework, picks out their clothes for the next day, makes sure they take their baths, and even does bedtime prayers with them. *"They are my heart."* It's just that after she spends so much time helping them, there is very little time for her own homework, and she is worried about herself.

The doctor comments that it sounds stressful and asks her how she manages that stress. *"To chill,"* she said, she smokes marijuana, *"only after they go to bed. I never smoke in front of my brothers and sister."*

Lisa could be reprimanded or given 40 reasons not to smoke marijuana, but that would shame her and likely have no yield other than increasing her stress level, perhaps leading directly to increased marijuana use.

Instead, the doctor listened silently to her story without interruption or criticism. By listening to her intently, all that she is doing right becomes clear. When she finishes talking, the doctor says, *"We need you to be a pediatric nurse. Look how good you are with little kids. You get your brothers and sister dinner. You make sure they're safe. You bathe them and put them to bed. You're really responsible. You've already proven how good you are at caring for people and how much you love children."* After a short pause, he states, *"I'm feeling worried, though, about how much marijuana you are smoking and am concerned that may interfere with your future plans. Can we talk about this?"*

It is so much easier for young people to deal with why we are worried if we first note their successes. When we get their permission to address the problem, we get buy-in and offer them the kind of control and self-confidence they need to be willing to consider taking steps to change.

Listening and reflecting takes on even greater importance for the demoralized youth who may have little experience with a person seeing the best in them. Central to both the resilience and youth development frameworks is the notion that youth live up or down to people's expectations of them. Young people who have internalized low expectations do not always see their potential to change. For them, it may be transformative for someone to notice positive traits.

In this author's experience, it is common for older teens or young adults who have changed their life path to recall a pivotal moment when a caring professional made them realize they had potential.

For these youth, listen silently and with full attention as their story unfolds. Rather than considering your next counseling steps, allow yourself to view the youth through a different prism; think only of what you admire about the young person. Even a patient whose history concerns you deeply is being honest. Many youth with the most traumatic histories have displayed tremendous resilience. They have been survivors; doing the best they can to deal with a world that wasn't fair to them. Older teens who "have been there and done that" are often able to display great insight into their behaviors. It is common for these very same youth who have had the roughest lives thus far to ▶ 25.8 dream of becoming helping professionals so they can help other children have smoother lives.

■ Case 2

Shawn is a 17-year-old young man who has just been released from a youth detention facility after a short stay. He grew up in a highly stressed household where abuse was pervasive. He recalls witnessing his father beating his mother when he was as young as 3 years. He recalls trying to stand between them to protect his mother. His jaws clench as he tells you how his father would throw him against a wall and would reprimand him for his interference. Shawn learned not to cry because, when he did, he was told, *"Men don't cry,"* and *"You want to be a man, I'll show you how to be a man,"* as his father would proceed with the beating. His mother turned to drugs to forget about the pain and died when Shawn was 11 years old. His father has been in jail since Shawn was 12 and he was sent to live with his grandmother. When he was too "disrespectful" to her he was put into foster care. He has been through 6 placements and was maltreated in 2 of them. He turned to drugs himself and was arrested for possession when he was 15. Most recently, he was arrested for dealing, but that was found to be a case of mistaken identity.

Shawn is an artist who uses paper to release his feelings. He hasn't used drugs since he was 15 years old, except for one brief period when he was particularly stressed. He has a girlfriend who he cares about deeply and whom he would, *"never put my hands on."* He dreams of being a youth services worker who could help abused children. His eyes redden as he shares the fact that someone like him doesn't have a chance to have that dream come true, he really isn't good at school and only made it to the ninth grade.

The social worker listens and notes how bright this young man is. He notices his sincerity and his genuine desire to become a youth services worker. However, he also notes that the teen does not believe in his potential and likely lacks the confidence to take even the first steps necessary to return to get his education. He also has no support structure in place to facilitate him through the administrative steps necessary for him to follow through on his vision. In essence, he lacks the confidence and the skills to move his dreams from contemplation to action.

He retells the young man his story, perhaps in a way that the teen has never experienced previously: *"Wow. You have been through a lot. More than anyone your age deserves to have been through. I wish I could say that your story shocks me, that I've never heard anything like it before. That you were the first young man who has had to suffer through abuse and see the tragedy of your mother being hurt and turning to drugs. But the truth is that I've seen it too often. But you know what? Most of those kids are seething with anger. I know you've been there and that's probably why you acted out earlier. Many of those kids turn to drugs themselves to deal with the pain. I know you've "been there, done that" for a little while too, but you figured out on your own to stop. Instead, you turned to art to deal with your feelings rather than just letting them cloud over. Many of those kids take out their anger on women, but you know how to care for women. Many of those kids have given up hope and just dwell in anger, but you want to help kids. You want to take your experience and make the world better. Teach me about you. Teach me about how despite all that you've been through, you've come out as a caring man committed to protecting children."*

After a brief discussion where the young person becomes emotional and shares his insights, the social worker continues one step at a time allowing the teen to determine his readiness for each option: *"You deserve to have your dreams come true. Many children will benefit from your experience. You also deserve healing first, to help you get past some of the pain that happened to you. Do you have any ideas about what will work for you? May I suggest some healthy ways that help people cope?* (See Chapter 31.) *You are so good at talking. May I arrange for you to have your own counselor who will listen to you, and perhaps guide you as you take next steps? Does now feel like the right time to think about getting the education you need? If so, I would love to connect you to a community resource that helps young people return to school. Can we schedule a check-in for 2 weeks from today to follow the progress you've made?"*

•• Group Learning and Discussion ••

It is so easy to see risk. It is much harder to look beneath the surface to see strengths, yet it is key to positioning you as a change agent. It is an active choice to decide to see youth through a positive prism, and it may take practice before it comes routinely. It begins with a SSHADESS screen that starts with teens describing their positive attributes. Then, it is about listening for strength. For example, it may involve allowing yourself to be surprised by the compassion some people possess despite the fact they were offered little. It may be respecting the resilience they demonstrate. It may be admiring their plans to repair the world, so that it looks more like they wished it had looked for them.

Exercise

(1) Share stories about some of the youth who you have cared for who maintained a positive outlook despite dire circumstances. (2) Practice the eliciting and reflecting approach in pairs, with one of you taking on the role of professional and the other that of the youth.

Ongoing Practice

Make a point of sharing inspirational stories within your practice. Share especially those stories of youth that surprise you. This will lead to different expectations for all youth.

- Especially when you are struggling to find the positive in a young person, debrief with a colleague whose role will be to elicit the strengths the youth may be exhibiting in that situation.
- Share with each other how the tone and demeanor of your interactions with demoralized youth changes when using this strength-based approach.
- Share with each other how the experience of seeing marginalized youth through a positive lens changes your work experience, and why it may diminish your likelihood of burnout.

Continuing Education

If you are applying for continuing education credits, a test is available online. For more details, visit www.aap.org/reachingteens.

References

1. Prochaska JO. Decision making in the transtheoretical model of behavior change. *Med Decis Mak.* 2008;28(6):845–849
2. Schwarzer R, Fuchs R. Changing risk behaviors and adopting health behaviors: the role of self-efficacy beliefs. In: Bandura A, ed. *Self-efficacy in Changing Societies*. Cambridge, United Kingdom: Cambridge University Press; 1997
3. Hein K. Framing and reframing. *J Adolesc Health*. 1997;21:214–217

Related Video Content

25.0.1 An Introduction to Behavioral Change: Youth Will Not Make Positive Choices if They Don't Believe in Their Potential to Change. Ginsburg.

25.0.2 Addressing Demoralization: Eliciting and Reflecting Strengths. Ginsburg.

25.1 Covenant House Staff Share How Recognizing Strengths Positions Them to Support Progress. Covenant House PA.

25.2 YouthBuild Staff Share How Recognizing Strengths Positions Them to Support Progress. YouthBuild Philadelphia.

25.3 Young People Speak of the Power of Being Viewed Through a Strength-Based Lens and the Harm of Low Expectation. Youth.

25.4 The Depth of Our Caring Positions Us to Enter the Lives of Youth and to Be Change Agents. Singh, Vo.

25.5 "Tell Me What You've Been Through—You've Been So Strong": A First Step of Connection. Feit.

25.6 Helping Youth With Chronic Disease Own How Adversity Has Built Their Resilience. Pletcher.

25.7 Substance Users Often Possess the Gift of Sensitivity. Pletcher.

25.8 Sometimes Youth Who Have Survived Adversities Have the Biggest Hearts and Largest Dreams. Diaz.

25.9 Behaviors Must Be Seen in the Context of the Lives Youth Have Needed to Navigate. Auerswald.

18.1 Maximizing the Yield From a Strength-Based Interview: Avoiding the Pitfalls of Using Only a Positive Lens. Ginsburg.

42.2 Teen Testimonial: Survival, Resilience, and Overcoming Depression. Youth, Ginsburg.

50.2 Sensitivity: A Common Trait of Youth Who Use Substances—A Blessing and a Curse. McAndrews.

CHAPTER 26

Motivational Interviewing

Nimi Singh, MD, MPH, MA

 Related Video Content

26.0 Motivational Interviewing With Adolescents

■ Why This Matters

Adolescents' health and well-being are tightly linked to the behavioral choices they make. These choices, although made in the teen years, can have a lifelong impact. Therefore, it is imperative that youth-serving professionals become adept at supporting adolescents in choosing to adopt healthier lifestyle behaviors. Motivational interviewing (MI) has been shown to be an effective counseling style that promotes healthy behavioral change, both in adults and in adolescents.

> **Motivational interviewing is an empathetic, person-centered counseling style. It is based on the recognition that the most powerful motivations for changing our behaviors don't come from others, but from us.**

■ What Is Motivational Interviewing?

Motivational interviewing is more than a set of techniques. It is an empathetic, person-centered counseling style. It is based on the recognition that the most powerful motivations for changing our behaviors don't come from others, but from ourselves. This approach creates the conditions for positive behavioral change by gently guiding youth into articulating their own reasons for change, and identifying how they hope to achieve it. It is well-suited for brief clinical encounters; evidenced-based (>200 clinical trials in both adults and adolescents); grounded in health behavior theory; verifiable and generalizable; and can be delivered by a wide range of professionals who are addressing a variety of behaviors.

Motivational interviewing is based on 2 assumptions. First, a person's motivation to change his or her behavior can be elicited by a conversation with someone skilled to draw out the person's own reasons for changing. Simply telling someone why they need to change is experienced as confrontational and, as such almost always creates resistance to the suggestion. Alternately, empathy, understanding, and exploration of the young person's experience creates a space for self-reflection and the desire for change. The second assumption is that ambivalence toward the possibility of change is normal and to be expected. In contemplating a change, there are always competing positive and negative feelings, a weighing of pros and cons.

What is unique in MI is that it is the *youth* who articulates arguments for change and the treatment plan. The role of the professional is *not* to provide reasons for behavior change, but rather to act as a facilitator, guiding the adolescent through questions and reflections, listening for ambivalence in the teen's own words, and reflecting back negative and positive aspects of both the current behavior and of the desired behavior change. The professional also needs to be able to support self-efficacy (that is, the confidence that one can achieve what one sets out to do). This is done by pointing out strengths and previous successes, and acknowledging the difficulties of making the behavioral change. The practitioner also needs to, above all, avoid resistance by refraining from lecturing and arguing with the adolescent. Finally, the practitioner asks teens what *they* want to do/are willing to do; their answers often become the starting point or goal for the treatment plan.

■ Underlying Theoretical Framework: Stages of Change

Prochaska and DiClemente[1] articulated the stages of change model, in which they hypothesized that behavioral change doesn't happen in one stage, but rather that a person goes through several stages before adopting and maintaining a new behavior. These stages are (1) pre-contemplation, (2) contemplation, (3) action, (4) maintenance, and (5) relapse. Pre-contemplation means that the person isn't even thinking about changing her behavior, and if asked if they were considering it, they would say "no." Contemplation is the stage where the person is waxing and waning toward the idea of change, and wrestling with the reasons for and against changing their behavior or habit. This is the stage of ambivalence. The action stage occurs when ambivalence is subsiding, and the person is ready and motivated to implement the change. Maintenance is the stage when the person continues to exert effort to continue the new behavior. Of note, this stage is also often the time when services and support are withdrawn. This is highly unfortunate because this stage is an especially vulnerable time, and life stressors may cause the person to relapse back into the old behavior. For this reason, it is critical to have frequent follow-up to reinforce the benefits of the changes while youth are in the "maintenance" stage. Relapse represents a return to the previous behavior, is common, and should be expected for most long-term behavioral changes.

Ideally, we hope to avoid relapse, but, if it occurs, it is critical to support return to the desired behavior afterward. Once there has been a lapse or relapse, the individual reenters the process at either pre-contemplation (becoming discouraged or convinced that they can't change after all), contemplation (begins the weighing of pros and cons again), or action (jumps back on track and picks up the new behavior once again with little hesitation). One of the most important points to remember is that it is the professional who plays a *key* role in influencing a person's reentry point into the process! Youth will experience guilt and shame even when there is no one blaming them. This often causes an adolescent to be defensive from the get-go. It is critical, therefore, for the professional to shift the conversation from "relapse" to "success": this is done by focusing on the period prior to the relapse as a success and asking how that success was possible for that long. Then have the young person identify what stressor triggered the relapse. Following this, have her brainstorm what would help avoid a future relapse, should the stressors recur. We will give an example of this later in the chapter.

When first articulated by Prochaska and DiClemente,[1] a stage between contemplation and action was termed preparation. For the purposes of this discussion, preparation is incorporated into the contemplation stage. Here, the pros and cons of behavior change are explored, and potential supports and barriers are identified and addressed, in order to prepare the individual for taking action.

■ Rethinking Conventional Training

Why doesn't our conventional training work optimally in counseling youth? Most of us were trained in a directive counseling style that looks (or at least feels) something like the following admittedly simplified approach:

I'll ask you close-ended questions.

I'll tell you what's wrong with you.

I'll tell you what you need to do.

I'll assume that you're going to do it.

This approach is often adequate for simple, short-term behaviors and interventions, such as taking a medication for a short time. This approach also works well for motivated youth/families (those in the action stage).

Motivational interviewing, alternatively, is a combination of 3 counseling styles: (1) following (establish rapport, have youth expand story), (2) guiding (asking questions that support self-reflection), and (3) gently directing (asking permission before giving information first, checking in after). These styles rely heavily on open-ended questions, reflecting back what a teen says, and waiting for further elaboration before offering information. This approach works well for youth ambivalent about behavioral change (in contemplation stage).

We like working with young people in the action stage because our conventional tools fit well with their stage of change; they cooperate and typically do what we suggest; we tend not to experience anger, frustration, and impatience; and they make us feel competent. We may not like working with youth in the contemplation (ambivalence) stage because our tools *don't* fit with their stage of change, and they don't do what we suggest. We then experience anger and frustration when we see them again, and may even feel relief when they don't show up. We "pathologize" ambivalence when it's, in fact, the norm when it comes to behavioral change. In the end, we may become disheartened and give up on the youth we serve (and ourselves), saying:

"I can't help someone who doesn't want to be helped."

"I can't help someone who doesn't admit to having a problem."

We don't realize we're inadvertently perpetuating the resistance.

■ Who Are the Youth We See?

Studies estimate that, in the case of health care, only 30% of patients who present to clinic are actually in action stage! This means that a full 70% are in pre-contemplation or contemplation stages. We, therefore, *over*estimate the motivation of those who say they're ready to change (we give them information without exploring possible ambivalence/barriers to change). At the same time, we *under*estimate the motivation of those who indicate no interest in change. We don't realize that reluctance is often due to underlying values, beliefs, and fears associated with changing the behavior. When we understand these, we can help reconnect adolescents to their own values, and help them see how certain behaviors are incongruent with what they care about the most in their lives. In other words, MI may be *the* treatment of choice for ambivalence to change for roughly 70% of our population!

■ Philosophical Approach

The approach to the adolescent, instead of simply imparting information, is exploratory. It is respectful, nonjudgmental, reflective, and compassionate. We are asked to shift our goal from "fixing it" to "listening for understanding." In doing so, we are then able to create the environment in which "change talk" can be elicited.

■ Principles

The foundation for successful implementation of MI is based on the following guiding principles:

1. Establish rapport, and meet youth where they are. A very effective way to achieve this is to start with a broad psychosocial interview.

   "How are things going? What's going well? Tell me about life...."

2. Listen for understanding (as opposed to listening briefly and then offering information right away).

3. Elicit their story: It's important to elicit not only what's going on in adolescents' lives, but also their values and beliefs, even their future goals for themselves.

4. Express empathy. When they discuss the difficulties of behavioral change, it's critical that we acknowledge these.

   "Given that smoking is your only way of relieving stress, I can see why it would be hard to give it up."

5. Develop discrepancy. Reflect back the teen's own ambivalence about change.

   "So on the one hand...but on the other hand...."

6. Resist the "righting reflex." Don't argue why the teen should do something. Remember, this naturally creates resistance, making adolescents feel compelled to say why they can't. Remember, it's *their* job to present argument for change, not ours!

7. Reflect back resistance. If a teen doesn't seem to want to engage in the conversation at all, name what you see.

   "It looks like you really don't want to be here today."
   "It sounds like it's impossible for you to check your sugars four times a day."

8. Allow silence. Elaborate on their resistance.

   "What makes it so hard?"
   "What would help?"

9. Support self-efficacy. This is done by pointing out successes.

   "Wow. You quit smoking for 2 whole weeks...that's tremendous."

10. Explore self-efficacy:

    "So how did you resist the urge to light up a cigarette when it happened? What did you do instead?"

    Have the youth brainstorm with you about overcoming triggers in the future.

11. Explore triggers for relapse (either past or future).

    "When did you have that first cigarette again? What pushed you over? If that were to occur again, what do you think you could you do in the future to resist the urge?"

12. Support the teen in defining a treatment plan and commitment to change.

    "What do you think about trying again? When do you want to try? When would you like to check in again?"

■ Evoking "Change Talk" (Specific Tools)

There are several interviewing "tools" that have been developed over the years to assist in getting youth to identify their desire and ability to change the target behavior. A few of these are explored as follows, using some of the principles described above:

Elaborating

Understand the teen's world view. As mentioned above, it's very helpful to start with a general psychosocial screen before asking specifics about the issue at hand. Then explore the issue using open-ended questions.

"Tell me about your diabetes. How does it affect the rest of your life?"

"Tell me about your (behavior). When did it start?"

"How do you feel about it?"

"What do you get out of (problem behavior)?"

"How do you think it causes difficulties for you?"

Express Empathy

"I can see why it must be hard for you…."

Develop discrepancy between the polarized urges (summarize ambivalence by reflecting back pros and cons).

"So on one hand…and on the other…."

"Part of you wants…and the other part…."

Using the "Importance" Ruler

There are 3 parts to using the importance ruler (see Figure 26-1). The first part is as follows:

"On a scale of 1 to 10, 10 being 'absolutely yes' and 1 being 'not at all,' how motivated are you to ____(check your sugars at school)?"

Ten is always the direction in which you want the change to go.

The second part is to then explore whatever number the teen gives you. If she picked "5," elect 1 or 2 numbers *below* and ask: *"Why a 5? Why not a 3?"* By choosing a number below the one she picked, you are eliciting "change talk" (getting her to describe what her reasons are for changing).

The third part is to then take a number or 2 above what she gave you and ask, *"What would it take to move you to a 6 (not actually changing the behavior, but a little more comfortable with the idea)?"* Be sure to elicit something the teen has control over. Whatever the adolescent tells you may become the treatment plan. Remember, it is critical to make sure the plan is something that can actually be accomplished. Work with the youth to explore potential barriers to the plan and appropriate solutions:

"What do you think might get in the way?"

"What could you do to ensure that it doesn't?"

Have the teen set an appropriate timeline for implementing the plan.

Sometimes the issue is not importance or motivation, but confidence that she will be able to make the change. An example of this might be weight loss. Use the same strategy, only as a "confidence" ruler:

"On a scale from 1 to 10, how confident are you that you could…?"

If you don't distinguish between these 2 (importance vs confidence), you may inadvertently explore the wrong idea with the youth, who will consequently disengage from the conversation. One strategy is to explore both.

FIGURE 26.1
READINESS, IMPORTANCE, AND
CONFIDENCE RULERS

Readiness, Importance and Confidence Rulers

READINESS: On a scale from 1 to 10, with 10 being very ready, how ready are you to make a change?

1	2	3	4	5	6	7	8	9	10
Not at all				Somewhat					Very

IMPORTANCE: On a scale of 1 to 10, with 10 being very important, how important is it for you to change?

1	2	3	4	5	6	7	8	9	10
Not at all				Somewhat					Very

CONFIDENCE: On a scale of 1 to 10, with 10 begin very interested, how interested are you in changing?

1	2	3	4	5	6	7	8	9	10
Not at all				Somewhat					Very

Adapted with permission from Gold MA, Kokotailo PK. Motivational interviewing strategies to facilitate adolescent behavior change. *Adolescent Health Update.* 2007;20(1)

Similar rulers can be found at the listed reference above.

Querying Extremes

Always start by exploring the youth's feelings about the *current* behavior.

If the behavior is undesired or a "problem", start by asking, *"What's the best thing about it?"* Then ask *"What's the worst thing about it?"* That way, the youth feels understood as to why the behavior change is difficult at the beginning of the conversation before exploring what might be advantages and benefits to changing their behavior.

If the behavior is desired or the "solution," start by asking, *"What's the worst thing about it?"*

Hopefully, that will help the youth also be able to discuss what is good about the desired behavior.

Exploring Goals and Values

There are 2 parts to this tool: exploring goals and values, and exploring how the current behavior fits with those goals and values:

1. *"What things are most important to you in your life right now?"* (You may want to do a general psychosocial screen, such as **SSHADESS**.) (See Chapter 18.) Then reflect back what is said: *"It sounds like being able to do what your friends do is important to you."*

2. The second part is to then explore how the current behavior is affecting this value or goal.

   "How do you think (diagnosis/current behavior) fits with these goals/values?"

   "How can you minimize (the problem) so it doesn't get in the way of living your life the way you want/fully?"

Your tone of voice must be gentle and exploratory, and not critical, in order for this approach to be successful. This technique alone has been most highly correlated with behavioral change; understandable since the youth begins to realize that his current behavior is not in alignment with his *own* values and beliefs.

Elicit-Provide-Elicit

Sometimes we still need to give information and advice. How do we do this without creating resistance? A very powerful way of maintaining openness while receiving information is to simply *ask* for permission before giving advice. This supports the young person's sense of autonomy.

"Of course, while I can only suggest, you're ultimately the one to decide...."

It is also helpful to first elicit what the youth knows about the topic to be discussed, and offer praise for whatever is known **(Elicit).**

"What do you know about (health condition/problem behavior, etc)"? "It sounds like you know quite a bit about...."

Next, you ask for permission to share further information **(Provide).**

"There is some other information that might be helpful to you...may I share that with you?"

Finally, you explore how the information you provided was received **(Elicit).**

"What are your thoughts about that? How might you use that information? Is there anything that might be relevant for you?"

When given permission to offer suggestions, it's often helpful to offer several strategies. If you offer only one suggestion, it looks like the "right" answer, and it will create resistance. It might inadvertently drive the young person to offer reasons why it won't work.

"Here are some ideas...which one do you think might work best for you? Tell me more."

In the case of weight loss,

"Which would you like to work on first: healthy food choices, moving your body more, or reducing your stress levels?"

"How would you like to achieve this?"

"When would you like to start?"

"When would you like to come back and see me?"

If you offer solutions one at a time, it too creates resistance, and the young person may be more likely to offer reasons why each one won't work.

■ FRAMES

A mnemonic that may be particularly useful for those new to motivational interviewing is FRAMES. This brief adaptation of MI may be useful for helping a young person move into action and make a needed change, especially when time is limited.

1. **Feedback:** Offer personalized information about a behavior. For example, *"You told me that you are drinking alcohol almost every weekend at parties and that you are worried that it is too much for someone your age. You are right that drinking alcohol is not the safest thing for a teenager to be doing because it impairs your thinking and can lead to some unsafe decisions."*

2. **Responsibility:** Emphasize the young person's autonomy. *"Of course, in the end, it's up to you to decide if you are going to stop drinking alcohol."*

3. **Advice:** Ask permission and then offer clear recommendations based on your own experience. For example, after gaining permission to share ideas, you can say, *"In my experience it is most helpful for people your age to stop drinking altogether because even small amounts of alcohol can be problematic. Sometimes people find it helpful to not be around alcohol for a while, say a few weeks, until they feel confident in their ability not to drink. What do you think about that? Is that something you might be interested in trying?"*

4. **Menu:** Elicit options for change and help the young person develop a list of potential methods for change. By eliciting suggestions from her and by identifying several options you support the young person's autonomy to make a decision about the strategy she feels is best for her. For example, *"So we talked about ways to help you stop drinking alcohol. You can ask your friends not to drink around you. You can stay at home and watch movies with your sister when you know there will be drinking at a party. Or you can bring a soda with you to drink instead."*

5. **Empathy:** Remain nonjudgmental and show your support for the young person regardless of how ready she is to change. For example, *"It must be really hard to choose not to drink when all of your friends are doing it."*

6. **Self-efficacy:** Support the young person's strengths and reinforce her ability to make changes. For example, you might ask, *"Let's talk about times in the past where you had to do something that was hard, like learning to play a new sport or musical instrument. Maybe together we can figure out how you were successful and how you can use those same skills to help you reach your goal of not drinking so much."*

◼ OARES

Another mnemonic that incorporates key MI communication components is OARES: **o**pen-ended questions, **a**ffirmation, **r**eflective listening, **e**licit change talk, and **s**ummarizing. This technique may be especially useful in initial encounters, when developing rapport and attempting to demonstrate support of the young person's autonomy and self-efficacy.

26.3

◼ Motivational Interviewing and Adolescent Development

Using MI with adolescents is particularly important, since it is *critical* to engage them in decision-making and treatment planning for developmental reasons.

1. Adolescents begin to shift from the concrete thinking of childhood to the more abstract, sophisticated thinking of adulthood, causing them to want to be seen as part of the solution, not just the problem.

2. Their sense of self (identity formation) becomes front and center, as do the development of their personal values and beliefs.

3. A desire for autonomy/individuation and resistance to being told what to do emerges during adolescence. (It doesn't necessarily resolve later in life, explaining why adults, too, are often resistant to advice about changing behaviors!)

◼ Remember

Stress physiology and subsequent distorted cognition are often driving the "problem behavior" (see Chapter 27).

When stress is managed in a healthier, prosocial way, the need to use problem behavior as a coping strategy diminishes (see chapters 31 and 50).

•• Group Learning and Discussion ••

In the following scenarios, how might each of the following techniques be used to explore behavior change in young people: Elaborating? Confidence ruler? Querying extremes? Elicit-provide-elicit? FRAMES? Break into pairs and work through these scenarios.

1. A 16-year-old comes to see you for a sports physical examination. During the conversation, when asked if she smokes cigarettes, she states, *"Only at parties."* How could you explore her smoking behavior further using open-ended questions?

2. A 17-year-old shares that he wishes he could lose weight, but doesn't think he can. How might you explore this issue further using open-ended questions?

3. A 15-year-old is struggling with managing her time more efficiently so that she can get to sleep early enough so that she's not so tired "all the time." How might an adult in her life help her understand what the barriers are to her getting to bed on time?

■■■■■■■■ Continuing Education ■■■■■■■■

If you are applying for continuing education credits, a test is available online. For more details, visit www.aap.org/reachingteens.

■ Reference

1. Prochaska JO, DiClemente CC. Stages of change in the modification of problem behaviors. *Prog Behav Modif.* 1992;28:183

■ Suggested Reading

Levy S, Knight JR. Office-based management of adolescent substance use and abuse. In: Neinstein LS, Gordon CM, Katzman DK, Rosen DS, Woods ER, eds. *Adolescent Health Care: A Practical Guide.* 5th ed. Philadelphia, PA: Lippincott, Williams and Wilkins; 2007

Miller WR, Rollnick S. *Motivational Interviewing: Preparing People to Change.* New York, NY: Guilford Press; 2002

Miller WR, Rollnick S. *What's New Since MI-2?* Stockholm, Sweden, June 2010. http://www.motivationalinterview.org/Documents/Miller-and-Rollnick-june6-pre-conference-workshop.pdf. Accessed June 25, 2013

Miller WR, Sanches VC. Motivating young adults for treatment and lifestyle change. In: Howard GS, Nathan PE, eds. *Alcohol Use and Misuse by Young Adults.* Notre Dame, IN: University of Notre Dame Press; 1994

Naar-King S, Suarez M. *Motivational Interviewing With Adolescents and Young Adults.* New York, NY: The Guilford Press; 2011

Rollnick S, Miller WR, Butler CC. *Motivational Interviewing in Health Care: Helping Patients Change Behavior.* New York, NY: The Guilford Press; 2008

■ Related Video Content

26.0 Motivational Interviewing With Adolescents. Singh.

26.1 Motivational Interviewing With a Young Woman With an Eating Disorder. Kreipe.

26.2 Motivational Interviewing: Making Sure to Uncover the Teen's Perspective. Singh.

26.3 Motivational Interviewing: OARES. Kinsman.

26.4 Using Motivational Interviewing to Help Substance-Using Youth Consider Change. Pletcher.

26.5 Case: Motivational Interviewing in Substance-Using Youth. Singh.

■ Related Web Site

Motivational Interviewing
www.motivationalinterview.org

CHAPTER 27

Health Realization— Accessing a Higher State of Mind No Matter What

Nimi Singh, MD, MPH, MA

 Related Video Content

27.0 Achieving a State of Optimal Health: Stress and the Health Realization Model

■ Why This Matters

Teaching adolescents to increase their ability to cope with stress optimizes physical and psychological well-being, strengthens decision-making, and leads to positive social interactions and improved school performance.

■ Stress Response and Its Effect on the Mind

The stress response allows us to perceive a potential environmental threat to our survival. It triggers a physiological response that allows us to get ourselves to safety quickly, by either fighting a potential predator, fleeing, or freezing and blending unnoticed into the environment. Each of these actions requires providing those parts of the body critical for fighting, fleeing, or even freezing with a sudden burst of energy. This is achieved by the shunting of blood to vital organs so oxygen and nutrients are delivered to the heart, lungs, muscles, and our brain stem, the part of the brain that controls heart rate, breathing rate, and temperature. As blood shunts to these organs and tissues, it shunts away from those organs *not* critical for survival, namely the digestive system, the reproductive system, the immune system, and the prefrontal cortex, that part of the brain that provides "executive functioning," including abstract thinking and creative problem-solving, that allows us to see the "big picture." In other words, our highest cognitive functioning is impaired as those bodily systems not critical for survival-in-the-moment become relatively compromised. In parallel, our bodies don't function well when the stress response is chronically firing in response to real or perceived challenges.

We are most prepared to deal with life's challenges when our bodies and minds are functioning in a healthy, integrated manner.

> By becoming aware of the quality of our thinking and disengaging from negative thoughts, we can learn to shut off our stress response and think more clearly.

Unfortunately, the stress response gets triggered just as easily in the face of a mis-perceived threat to our survival as it does to a true threat. Even remembering negative thoughts about the past, as well as having worries about the future can trigger this survival mechanism. These thoughts are not true threats to our survival, but our body doesn't know this!

Stress causes our minds to perceive the world through a lens of increased arousal, alertness, and vigilance, where every stimulus in the environment is misperceived as a potential threat to our survival. While this can be life-saving in truly dangerous circum-stances, it hinders our ability to think clearly in other situations. As blood flow shunts away from the higher-functioning areas of our brains to our brain stems (also called the "reptilian" brain), we can experience our minds going "blank" when we try to retrieve stored information. In this state, we also become unable to take in and easily process new information. This can lead to distorted or "negative thinking." Chronic repetitive, negative thoughts about the future can increase anxiety. Negative thoughts about the past (eg, anger, sadness, shame, regret, guilt) can contribute to depression. Harmful coping mechanisms or addictive behaviors (eg, substance use or cutting) can be understood as attempts to mini-mize stress and "quiet the mind" of negative thoughts (see Chapter 31).

What's extraordinary about our consciousness is the fact that the mind has an innate ability to *self-right;* that is, disengage from negative thoughts and return to present-moment thinking. When this occurs, it allows the blood flow to shunt back to the prefrontal cortex, the seat of higher cognitive functioning. Most of the time this happens automatically, but sometimes we get stuck in "stress mode." In order to facilitate the mind's ability to self-right, we need to understand what helps to shut off the stress response.

■ Shutting Off the Stress Response

Critical first steps in optimizing our ability to let go of negative thoughts, and, therefore, shut off the stress response, include good sleep hygiene, optimal nutrition, and adequate physical activity (see Chapter 40). Learning self-regulatory techniques, such as progressive muscle relaxation, deep breathing, and mental imagery (also known as self-hypnosis), is also helpful, as are other forms of biobehavioral training, such as using biofeedback machines and programs. Inviting adolescents struggling with stress to reconnect with recreational activities that they enjoy also helps reduce baseline stress levels over time.

Body movement therapies, such as yoga, have been shown in clinical studies to reduce stress and improve mental and physical functioning. Finally, psychotherapies that fall under the category of "cognitive behavioral therapies" teach people struggling with anxiety and depression that stress-based thinking is faulty thinking, and that they can learn to notice their own negative thoughts and choose to ignore or override them. Health realiza-tion, one form of this type of therapy, focuses on the mind's innate capacity to self-right simply by noticing the quality of one's thinking.

■ Health Realization

Health realization explores healthy psychological functioning: what it looks like, what gets in its way, and what we can do about it. We can train ourselves to get into the habit of noticing our own negative thoughts, disengaging from them, and thus shifting to a higher state of functioning. It reminds us that
- We are the creators of our own thoughts.
- The quality of our thinking (positive, negative, or neutral) creates our perception of reality in the moment.
- Negative thoughts trigger our stress response, which distorts our perceptions and yields unreliable and inaccurate information.

By becoming aware of the quality of our thinking and disengaging from negative thoughts, we can learn to shut off our stress response and think more clearly.

Understanding Our Thoughts Better

Estimates of how many individual thoughts the average person has in a given day range from 40,000 to 60,000. Most are old thoughts we've had over and over again. Furthermore, these repetitive thoughts tend to be either worries about the future or anger/sadness/regret/shame/guilt about the past. If we allow ourselves to repeat these thoughts, we trigger our stress physiology and impair our physical and psychological functioning.

Physical stresses, such as being tired, hungry, or ill, increase our awareness of these old thoughts. One way to mitigate this is to be aware of what is needed to restore optimal functioning (eg, restful sleep, healthy nutrition, exercise, and focusing on self-care).

Two Modes of Thought

We can consider 2 modes of thought. The first is "left-brain" or "conditioned mode," which is associated with accessing stored information, computation, and comparison, and can be likened to being in "computer" mode. Our state of mind in this mode tends to be busy and mechanical. This is useful when we're exploring situations that have only one right answer. The second mode is "right-brain" or "exploratory" thinking, which is associated with creativity, insight, inspiration, and accessing one's own wisdom and common sense, and can be likened to being in "receiver mode." In this "exploratory mode," our state of mind tends to be more calm and peaceful, and this is useful in situations when there is no one "right" answer. We get into trouble when we're in "conditioned mode" when we should be in "exploratory mode." "Exploratory mode" helps us interact positively with others, understand new or different points of view, or expand our thinking beyond what we already know. When we find ourselves interacting ineffectively with others, we can learn to notice if we're accidentally seeing the person through "old thoughts" about who we think they are. We are likely to find these old thoughts are keeping us from interacting in a fresh, unbiased, and exploratory manner. This realization can ultimately create a new dynamic of interaction.

Moods

Moods, like thoughts, come and go. It's helpful to think of moods as being "high" or "low," rather than "good" or "bad." This takes the judgment out of our observations. Our moods can affect the quality of our thinking (eg, low moods cause stress and distorted thoughts) and can themselves be created by the thoughts we're entertaining (eg, negative thoughts create a low mood). Just like thoughts, moods can be affected by one's physical state. Fatigue, illness, or a stressful event can bring on a "low" mood. Some people's moods can be affected by what they eat, what chemicals they're exposed to in the environment, even the weather.

We can't always change the mood we're in, but we can learn to notice our mood and try and support ourselves to minimize the effects of the mood on our functioning. Being aware of moods can help one understand others. Others may behave poorly at times due to a low mood or negative thinking, which distorts how they're seeing and interacting with the world. If their mood were higher, they'd see the world more clearly and make better choices.

This allows us, as professionals, to see the blamelessness and innocence of others. When communicating with someone in a stressful situation, try to notice your own mood, quiet your own thinking, and just observe. Listen carefully and with understanding.

Remember that you can project feelings of warmth and safety, which will help the other person feel more secure, shut off their stress response, and, therefore, raise the quality of their thinking.

Guidelines Around Moods

Recognize Moods

- Assess your mood level and that of others.
- Recognize how thoughts can create moods (and let negative thoughts go!).
- Remember: *You* create/sustain moods (inside-out process).
- Be easy on yourself and others.
- "See the innocence!"

Managing a Low Mood

- Develop a way to recognize this in yourself.
- Suspend major decisions until you are coming from a place of calm and security.
- Don't always trust your own thinking.
- Be careful about taking yourself/others too seriously.
- Be cautious of verbal/behavioral interactions.
- Don't commiserate—moods can be infectious!
- Let others know what you need.
- Slow down your thinking (drop, distract, dismiss, and ignore)—**drop** negative thoughts, **distract** yourself away from those thoughts, **dismiss** them as you notice them arise in your mind, and train yourself to **ignore** them when they reappear.
- Pamper yourself.
- Give yourself a time-out.

Separate Realities

Thoughts, along with our past experience, shape our sense of reality. Our view of reality changes moment to moment depending on our emotional state. The "lower" our mood, the more attached we are to our view of reality. The "higher" our mood, the more comfort and tolerance we experience with respect to different realities and points of view. People unknowingly create their reality based on the quality of their moment-to-moment thinking. Further, most people are often unaware how their mood is affecting their thinking. In other words, our thoughts at any given moment *are* what creates our experience and view of reality.

■ When More Is Needed

When supporting someone who is struggling with stress and low moods, there may be signs that they need to be referred to a professional, either for formal cognitive behavioral therapy, medication, or both. These signs include excessive irritability, loss of pleasure in activities, marked weight loss or weight gain, marked change in sleeping habits, difficulty concentrating, low energy, feelings of low self-worth, excessive guilt, or hopelessness. In this situation, assisting the young person in getting a formal mental health evaluation is critical.

•• Group Learning and Discussion ••

In order to most effectively convey the benefits of the health realization model to teens, it may be helpful for you to first experience how it can control your reactions to your own thoughts.

1. Listening exercise

    In order to become more aware of how our minds stay active with intrusive thoughts, even when our role is to simply listen, engage in the following exercise:

    a. Sit in pairs. Each person will spend 3 minutes telling a childhood story to the other person. It can be a happy, sad, or neutral story. The role of the listener is to simply listen. Even if the other person says something that elicits an emotional response in the listener, the listener can notice it but should not act on it. There should be no comments made, conversation, or even gestures made to the other in response to the content, other than simply listening deeply.

    b. After the 3 minutes are done, the storyteller and listener switch roles.

    c. At the end of the exercise, the facilitator asks people to share what it was like to be the storyteller. Then the facilitator asks what it was like to be the listener. The facilitator should acknowledge and validate all responses, since there is a wide range of human reactions to being listened to deeply and to listening deeply.

    d. After the respondents are finished sharing their experiences, the facilitator can gently point out the extent to which we all get caught up in our own thoughts and how that takes us out of being fully present to the other person when we interact with them. The facilitator may also point out how powerful (and sometimes even healing) it is to have someone simply listen to our stories.

2. Separate realities

    a. Have a bath towel available and ask the group if someone is willing to come up and show the group the "proper way" to fold a bath towel. Next ask someone else to show their way if it's different. After 3 or 4 people have shown how they fold bath towels, ask each of them to explain why their way "makes the most sense." The facilitator can then review with the group how we, as human beings, all have our own reasons for doing things the way we do, and they seem "right" to us, even if they seem "wrong" to others. The facilitator may then point out that no one is "right" or "wrong," we simply all have our own "separate realities" based on our life experiences.

▪▪▪▪▪▪▪▪ Continuing Education ▪▪▪▪▪▪▪▪

If you are applying for continuing education credits, a test is available online. For more details, visit www.aap.org/reachingteens.

■ Suggested Reading

Claypatch C. Articulating health realization in a nutshell (monograph). Minneapolis, MN: Glenwood-Lyndale Health Realization Training Center; 2005

Folkman S. Positive psychological states and coping with severe stress. *Soc Sci Med.* 2006;45:1207

Halcon L, Robertson CL, Monsen KA, Claypatch CC. A theoretical framework for using health realization to reduce stress and improve coping in refugee communities. *J Holis Nurs.* 2007;25:186–194

Pransky J. *Parenting from the Heart: A Common Sense Approach to Parenting.* Moretown, VT: NEHRI Publications; 2001

■ **Related Video Content**

27.0 Achieving a State of Optimal Health: Stress and the Health Realization Model. Singh.

CHAPTER 28

Helping Adolescents Own Their Solutions

Kenneth R. Ginsburg, MD, MS Ed, FAAP, FSAHM

 Related Video Content

28.0 Facilitating Adolescents to Own Their Solution: Replacing the Lecture With Youth-Driven Strategies

■ Why This Matters

Young people have repeated experiences being told what to do. In their quest for independence, they become resentful toward adults informing them of their unwise decision-making skills and can be reflexively resistant, if not rebellious, against the guidance. To steer youth away from risk behaviors and toward healthier behaviors, we have to be able to deliver information in an engaging and informative, rather than alienating, manner.

The ultimate goal of any information exchange is for teens to reach their own healthy conclusions. When teens "own" the solution, they have nothing to be resistant against. In contrast, when we impose our solutions on them, we undermine their sense of competence by communicating, *"I don't think you can handle this."*

There is another reason young people resist adult guidance: They don't understand it and naturally reject advice that makes them feel stupid or incapable. This is because most adult guidance is offered through a lecture. The intentions are good, but lectures backfire because youth cannot absorb their content.

> **Young people reject adult guidance they don't understand and rebel against advice that makes them feel incapable. When they own their solutions, they want to follow through on *their* plans.**

■ Helping Youth Arrive at Their Own Conclusions

To appreciate why youth may not get reasonable cause-and-effect lectures, we must consider how they think. Children and early adolescents think concretely; as they grow, they become more capable of understanding abstract concepts.[1,2] Then, they become capable of imagining the future and recognize how choices they make in the present lead to different future outcomes. Most teens in mid- to late adolescence are abstract thinkers, but some teens of below average intelligence will never get there. It is also critical to understand that *all* people think concretely during times of extreme stress,[3] and, in our professional settings, we are often dealing with people under acute stress.

Now let's break down a typical lecture.

- *"What you are doing now, let's call it behavior A, will very likely lead to consequence B. And then consequence B will go on to consequence C, which almost always ends up with D happening! At this point, you'll likely lose control, making you much more vulnerable to consequence E. [If it is a parent doing the lecturing, add here, "Look at me when I'm talking to you, I'm not talking for my own good!!"] Then, depending on several factors likely out of your control, consequence F, G, or H will happen. I may even happen. Do you know what happens if I happens? You might die!"*

We lecture to spare youth the fate of learning through painful life lessons. But, the typical lecture has an algebraic pattern—variables affect outcomes in mysterious ways. Algebra isn't taught to pre- or early adolescents because their brains aren't ready for abstract thinking. And a person in crisis wants to be running; they really shouldn't be contemplating algebra. When we lecture young people, they become frustrated because they're not yet capable of following our thoughts. They hear our concern but not the content of our message.

Our challenge is to deliver information so that youth can figure things out themselves. If they do, the lesson is more likely to be long lasting and to reinforce their motivation.

Early adolescents (and people in crisis) can grasp information if it is delivered in a more concrete, mathematical cadence—like 2 plus 2 equals 4. They can better follow our reasoning if instead of a string of abstract possibilities (A to B to C to D), the lesson is broken down into separate steps. *"I appreciate your desire to do A, but I am worried A might lead to B. Do you have any experience with something like that? Tell me about that experience. What might you do to make sure that doesn't happen to you? Do you see how B might lead to C? Have you ever seen that happen? What are your plans to avoid that happening here?"* We congratulate them and reinforce their existing plans to be safe and healthy. We pause at each step as they figure things out that they had not previously considered. They are the experts in their own lives. We are only the facilitators.

This approach increases competence because we're asking youth to consider possible consequences step by step with their own thoughts, based on their own experiences, rather than through scenarios we dictate. They may better learn the lessons because they have figured them out.

Here are some specific techniques you might use to guide adolescents to recognize consequences and generate their own solutions.

■ Choreographed Conversations

This is the most casual way to teach problem-solving and build competence. Like choreography, it should appear spontaneous but be thoughtfully planned. This technique was described above.

Role-playing

Role-playing allows youth to arrive at their own conclusions. This strategy also allows them to explore hypothetical situations and grasp how their decisions or actions determine outcomes. It is important to set up role-playing casually. If you suggest, *"Let's role-play,"* they may quickly seek an exit. Instead, be subtle and work *"what if..."* and *"what'll happen when..."* scenarios into your conversations. Keep the tone light and avoid confrontational dialogue. Don't jump in with answers. Role-playing is an ideal way to teach social skills.

- For example, you have just done a SSHADESS screen (see Chapter 18) and learned that older kids have approached Yael, a 12-year-old, to try marijuana. Rather than telling her, *"Lets role-play what you should say,"* you might start with, *"Well, older kids do sometimes try to influence younger kids, but you can be well prepared."* An eighth grader might come up to you and say, *"All the cooler kids are already smoking weed, you seem pretty cool for a sixth grader, have you tried it yet?"* What might you say?

Decision Trees

A decision tree allows you to transform the choreographed conversation onto paper (Figure 28.1). It makes the lesson even more concrete and allows the young person to leave the office with lesson in hand.

The decision tree can be used with a variety of scenarios including, *"What will happen to you if you become pregnant?" "Where does using drugs lead you?" "Where does putting in a really good effort in school now lead you to?"* and *"I know you're angry, but what will happen if you fight?"*

The ladder diagram described in Chapter 29 is one form of a decision tree.

Case Example 28.2

A 14-year-old female presented with blood on her eye to a school-based clinic. She had been in a fight the day before with a classmate who insulted her mother.

When asked what was going to happen next, she responded, *"I'm going to kill her, that's why I brought this knife* [which she had in her pocket] *to school."*

- A lecture may have backfired and possibly created a hostile exchange between the doctor and this knife-wielding patient. Instead, it was calmly requested that the girl keep the knife in her pocket and role-play the possible scenarios with a marker substituting as a knife. At each point the doctor wrote down her response into an evolving decision tree. He asked short questions and allowed her to respond thoughtfully and at her own pace.
- At first, she was guided to walk through various scenarios to grasp the fact that the knife could be turned on her with serious consequences.

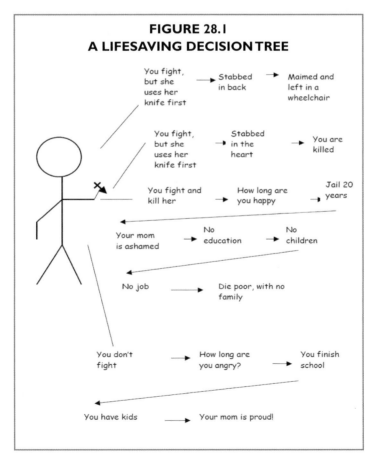

FIGURE 28.1
A LIFESAVING DECISION TREE

- Then she was allowed to imagine that she had successfully killed the intended victim. When asked how that would make her feel. She responded, *"Good!"* When asked how long she would feel good she responded, *"All day!"* She was then guided to consider how her actions would affect her mother, since she was getting into this fight to protect her mother's honor. The next steps in this path are illustrated on the accompanying decision tree.
- Finally, the girl was asked to consider how she would feel if she did not get into the fight. She responded, *"Angry!"* When asked how long she would feel angry she responded, *"All day!"* When she realized that this path led to children, an education, and making her mother proud, the choice became clear.

This girl needed a technique that would allow her to contemplate future consequences in the safety of an office, rather than the realities of the street. It convinced her to engage in a process of conflict resolution. She owned the solution and wanted to follow through on her plans.

■ Final Thought

You don't have to learn anything new to begin implementing these strategies and help adolescents own their own solutions. You already have the wisdom that connects their actions to long term consequences. The only thing you may need to do is change the cadence with which you deliver the information from an abstract lecture to a concrete step-by-step technique.

●● Group Learning and Discussion ●●

You do not have to learn new content to improve on the wisdom and advice you have been sharing. Your challenge is to change the delivery style so that young people figure things out by themselves (aided with your facilitation) so that they own the solutions.

In a group setting, recall some cases where you needed to guide a young person toward safer behaviors. Then break into pairs and practice using choreographed conversations, role-playing, or decision trees to facilitate youth thinking. If you prefer, you can use the following cases.

1. Emily is a 16-year-old who wants to get pregnant. She states, *"I am so ready to love my baby. My boyfriend will make the best father. My mother had me at 17 and she may have struggled, but she is a great mom and has given me everything I ever needed."*
2. LaVon was in a fight yesterday. He got jumped by 3 guys. He knows that they will get him again until he proves he's not a punk. He is thinking about getting even. But, he's not going to be unprepared. He knows where to get a switchblade. (Consider reading Chapter 58.)
3. Nathan is 15 and hates school. He can't wait until he turns 16 so he can drop out. He'll just get a job. No one at school cares about teaching. They don't teach what he needs anyway. He wants to be a car mechanic and he's great with his hands and can take things apart and put them back together easily. (FYI, you live in a mid-sized city with 6 high schools, including one that focuses on vocational technical education.)

▪▪▪▪▪▪▪▪ Continuing Education ▪▪▪▪▪▪▪▪

If you are applying for continuing education credits, a test is available online. For more details, visit www.aap.org/reachingteens.

■ References

1. Piaget J. *The Child's Conception of the World.* London, United Kingdom: Routledge and Kegan Paul; 1951
2. Pandit A, Archana, Raman V, Ashok MV. Developmental pediatrics. In: Bhat SR, ed. *Achar's Textbook of Pediatrics.* 4th ed. Andhra Pradesh, India: University Press; 2009
3. Horowitz MJ. Cognitive response to stress and experimental demand. *J Abnorm Psychol.* 1971;78(1):86–92

■ Related Video Content

28.0 Facilitating Adolescents to Own Their Solution: Replacing the Lecture With Youth-Driven Strategies. Ginsburg.

28.1 Teens Told What They "Should" Do Will Lose the Ability to Learn What They Can Do. Rich.

28.2 Helping a Young Person Own Her Solution: A Case of Using a Decision Tree to Prevent Violent Retaliation. Ginsburg.

34.2 Guiding Parents and Teens to Understand the Shifting Balance Between Parental Control and Teen Decision-Making. Sugerman.

■ Related Handout/Supplementary Material

Stop Lecturing: Guiding Adolescents to Make Their Own Wise Decisions

CHAPTER 29

Gaining a Sense of Control—One Step at a Time

Kenneth R. Ginsburg, MD, MS Ed, FAAP, FSAHM

 Related Video Content

29.0 Gaining a Sense of Control: One Step at a Time

■ Why This Matters

Sometimes a decision to move toward a new positive behavior seems so overwhelming or a goal so elusive that young people don't even consider trying.[1] They feel frightened and frustrated by their powerlessness. They convince themselves that they have no choices. They believe they're controlled by outside forces that determine their destiny—they have an external locus of control.[2–4]

When young people feel incapable of changing, we can offer a relatively brief intervention that may help them get past the mental block that serves as a major barrier to contemplating change. This technique is designed to help a young person revisualize a problem into manageable steps and then, perhaps, even to experience a moment of competence in their decision to consider action. Even the brief experience with success may give a youth enough of a sense of control to consider further steps.

> We can help a young person revisualize a problem into manageable steps and then, perhaps, even to experience a moment of competence in their decision to consider action. Even a brief experience with success may give a youth enough of a sense of control to consider further steps.

■ It Is Stressful to Feel Powerless

A sense of powerlessness increases one's stress. Some of the most effective stress reduction strategies are those that are problem-focused, because they help an individual to address, manage, and hopefully diminish a problem.

In the 10-point stress reduction plan offered in Chapter 31, point 1 is to identify and then address the problem. A key to using this strategy is to clarify the problem and then divide it into smaller pieces, committing to work on only one piece at a time. This decreases the sense of being overwhelmed and increases efficacy. ▶ **31.2**

Metaphorically, this is about helping teens revisualize problems from being mountains too high to be scaled into hills situated on top of each other. As they stand atop each hill, the summit appears more attainable.

The ladder technique is one strategy that can be used to help teens approach larger crises or emotional issues by breaking them into manageable steps. Consequently, it may also increase one's internal locus of control.

■ The Ladder Technique

The ladder technique can be used with adolescents who never thought they could succeed in school or never considered that they could become healthier by losing weight or exercising. It's been used with young people burdened with drug addiction or trapped in gangs. All of these groups have in common the sense of being so "stuck" that they don't believe they have control over their lives. It is about focusing on one step at a time so that a teen can revisualize a problem from being too large to manage into one that can be tackled.

Many teens can only consider one step at a time and may need to return another day to consider next steps. In fact, a teen who is steeped in a sense of powerlessness may not even be able to come up with the very first step. Invite him to come back anyway. Even if he returns still unable to imagine the first step, you can reinforce that just the act of returning *is* a step. The acknowledgment that he is choosing to move forward can be powerful in itself and may "unblock" his creative juices and, therefore, facilitate further action.

- **Step 1:** When you sense the adolescent is too stuck to even consider the possibility of change, explain that all people get overwhelmed and have moments when they can't imagine taking any steps that would actually make a difference.
- **Step 2:** Help the teen to think about where he is presently. Draw that present state as the base of a diagram; it can even just be called "Today."
- **Step 3:** Tell the teen that you certainly don't have the answers but hope he can find them himself.
- **Step 4:** Tell him that after listening to him you do know there are a couple of different possible futures for him. Write them at the top ends of 2 separate ladders leading to 2 distant but real destinations. One is the positive, hopeful future and the other is the future he hopes to avoid. This is not a threat; in fact, the positive future should reflect precisely his stated goals. Use all of the strengths you have elicited about him to make him know that you sincerely believe in his potential to reach that goal.
- **Step 5:** Repeat that, while you don't have the solutions, you do know that each ladder has several rungs along the way, and that everyone climbs a ladder one step at a time before they reach the top. Sometimes people don't even look to the top, they just know that if they hold on and find their balance they can take one step at a time.
- **Step 6:** Ask the teen to suggest what steps will lead to the less desirable end. Because he's feeling overwhelmed and helpless, he may know precisely which steps lead to the negative outcome. Unfortunately, he may feel he has mastered those decisions and actions.
- **Step 7:** Challenge him to visualize even the first step on the positive path and ideally help him achieve mastery over that first step.
- **Step 8:** As he attempts to write the steps toward the positive endpoint, remind him how much easier it is to divide difficult tasks into many small steps. Guide him to keep his eye on the future dream to stay motivated, but focus on only one step at a time to avoid feeling overwhelmed.

■ Cases

Case 1

Felipe is an 11-year-old morbidly obese boy who is unable to participate in sports because he is unable to keep up with his peers. His parents are obese but nag him to lose weight, and his peers tease him. He desperately wants to lose weight, but can only admit that while looking at the floor. Until his conversation in the office, he has never even talked about how much he wanted to lose weight. Instead, he became hostile when people brought up weight: *"I don't care. Why should you?"* He confides that he's failed every time he's tried to lose weight in the past. He doesn't even want to try again; he knows he will fail.

- The clinician sketched out the 2 ladders and asked what steps Felipe had to take to continue gaining weight. He knew exactly the unhealthy habits that were leading to his obesity. These habits were written on different rungs.
- Then he was asked to name only one step he could take toward a healthier path. He was assured that once he just mastered one step, each successive step would seem easier. Felipe struggled at first to come up with a single step, explaining with each option what would get in the way, why he would fail. He eventually decided that he could stop drinking sugary drinks and replace them with water and diet drinks.
- When he returned to the clinician's office a month later, he had lost 3 pounds! More importantly, he realized that food did not control him; rather, he controlled what he ate. He realized he could follow through on a decision. This experience of self-control gave him the confidence to contemplate his next step and then to put it into action. He began taking walks.

Case 2

Tori is a 14-year-old girl trapped in a gang run by her 16-year-old female cousin. She is a bright, engaging girl who was too overwhelmed to escape her dangerous circumstances. She wants to become an architect when she gets older because she hopes to build buildings in her community to keep neighborhood children off the streets. Every effort at counseling from the clinician was met with resistance. She repeatedly stated, *"You don't know what you are talking about. That's family!"* She didn't say this with hostility, just with a pervasive sense of hopelessness.

- The ladder diagram (Figure 29.1) allowed Tori to visualize her different futures. She knew precisely which steps would continue to lead her toward trouble and maybe even death.
- The ladder technique allowed the abstract concept of *"you need to turn your life around"* to be divided into much smaller concrete steps. Nevertheless, on her first visit she was unable to even name the first steps on the positive ladder. She did agree, however, to return for a check-in the next week.
- She returned and voiced her embarrassment that she couldn't even think of one right step. She told the clinician, *"I failed you. I took this out every night and all I could see was me headed down the wrong path."* She was told that just returning was a very positive step. This simple realization allowed her to realize that she did have some control over her decisions. This instantly belied her belief that she was powerless, trapped by her fellow gang members.

The same girl who spent the week unable to come up with any possibilities immediately began generating ideas. She needed her mother to help her navigate her away from the gang. Her cousin loved and respected her mother (that was family too!) and ▶ **37.0** would allow Tori to have that relationship. Tori's mother was engaged in the plan using a strength-based approach (see Chapter 37). In a *"just blame me"* conspiracy,

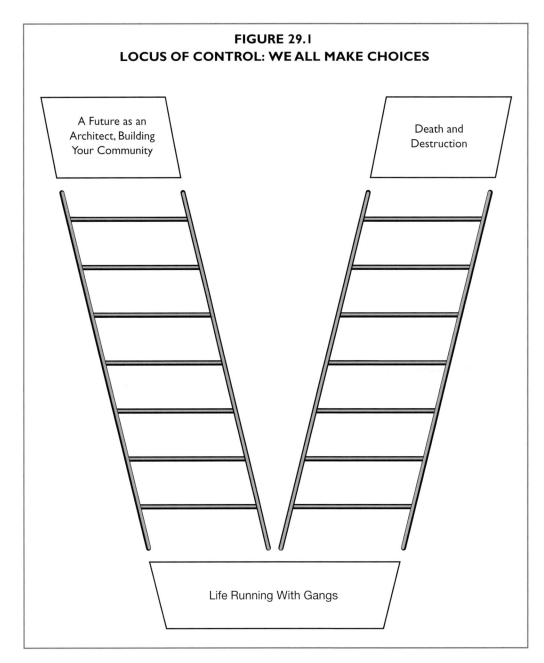

**FIGURE 29.1
LOCUS OF CONTROL: WE ALL MAKE CHOICES**

A Future as an Architect, Building Your Community

Death and Destruction

Life Running With Gangs

Tori would call her mother when she was in a potentially dangerous gang scenario. Her mother would recognize the "code word" and then demand that she come home (see Chapter 41, page 335). Ultimately, they moved a couple of miles away, enough of a distance to be out of gang territory. Tori was able to leave the gang and later attended college.

■ Final Thoughts

This brief office-based intervention facilitates adolescents to overcome their sense of powerlessness, their lack of control, and their belief that only fate determines their futures. A pattern of repeated failures that stifles contemplation toward change can sometimes be broken when even a small success is experienced.

•• Group Learning and Discussion ••

Discuss cases in which teens felt powerless and strategies you have used to help them gain a sense of control. Either use those cases or choose from those below to practice creating a ladder diagram so youth can learn to achieve success a step at a time. Feel free to assume that your conversation occurs over several weeks.

Case 1: Aamina is a 14-year-old young woman who has tried "everything" to lose weight, but has never succeeded. She has even gained weight after every effort. She thinks that is because she eats more when she is frustrated.

Case 2: Grayson has never done well in school. When he was 16 years old, he dropped out as soon as it became legal to do so. He "lived the life" for a while, but wants to be able to have a family one day and have kids who would be proud of him. He would love to be a mechanic. He can't imagine going through the applications or even getting started. He had one teacher who said that he had attention-deficit/hyperactivity disorder, but he never told his mom.

Case 3: Dalia was always a very good student. She got straight As, volunteered in a neighborhood animal shelter, and had dreamed of going to a top college. Her parents are immigrants and want her to get her education, but were never able to receive theirs. They push her at home, but have never gone into a school meeting. Dalia is in 11th grade and her friends are applying to colleges. She has a meeting with her school counselor in 6 weeks. She says it is "all stupid" and tells you that her cousins are doing fine in the family business. Her grades are dropping.

Continuing Education

If you are applying for continuing education credits, a test is available online. For more details, visit www.aap.org/reachingteens.

■ References

1. Schwarzer R, Fuchs R. Changing risk behaviors and adopting health behaviors: the role of self-efficacy beliefs. In: Bandura A, ed. *Self-Efficacy in Changing Societies*. Cambridge, United Kingdom: Cambridge University Press; 1997

2. Rotter, JB. *Social Learning and Clinical Psychology*. Upper Saddle River, NJ: Prentice-Hall; 1954

3. Rotter JB. Generalized expectancies of internal versus external control of reinforcements. *Psychol Monogr.* 1966;80:609

4. Lefcourt HM. Internal versus external control of reinforcement: a review. *Psychol Bull.* 1966;65(4):206–220

■ Related Video Content

29.0 Gaining a Sense of Control: One Step at a Time. Ginsburg.

31.2 Stress Management and Coping/Section 1/Tackling the Problem. Ginsburg.

37.0 Delivering Upsetting News to Parents: Recognizing Their Strengths First. Ginsburg.

CHAPTER 30

Strength-Based Interviewing: The Circle of Courage

Barbara L. Frankowski, MD, MPH, FAAP

Larry K. Brendtro, PhD, LP

Stephen Van Bockern, EdD, MA

Paula M. Duncan, MD, FAAP

 Related Video Content

30.0 The Circle of Courage: A Strategy for Eliciting Strengths and Addressing Risks

■ Why This Matters

Incorporating strengths in our interviews is not an "add-on" to the visit but, rather, a rethinking of the way we work with adolescents, a way to efficiently reorganize and prioritize the content of our guidance.[1] The goals of a strength-based approach are to raise adolescents' awareness of their developing strengths and to motivate them to take responsibility for the role they can play in their own well-being. Brendtro and colleague's[2] Circle of Courage offers an easy-to-use and effective framework to elicit, reflect, and build on the strengths of our adolescents.

> **Many talented youth do not recognize their own strengths until they are pointed out to them.**

■ How to Incorporate the Circle of Courage Into Practice

The Interview

The Circle of Courage asks about strengths in 4 essential areas (see Figure 30.1 and Table 30.1).[2] You would not use all the questions in one visit and may want to adapt the questions based on the adolescent's age and what you already know about her strengths and challenges.

Using the Circle of Courage in Practice

After eliciting strengths, there are several things you can do with the information. First, you can identify or reflect back the adolescent's strengths as a teaching tool about strengths and youth development (much as we encourage parents to identify or put into words a younger child's emotions). Many talented youth do not recognize their own strengths until they are pointed out to them. Second, you can make suggestions to boost strength areas that may be lacking or deficient, because adolescents need strengths in

FIGURE 30.1
CIRCLE OF COURAGE

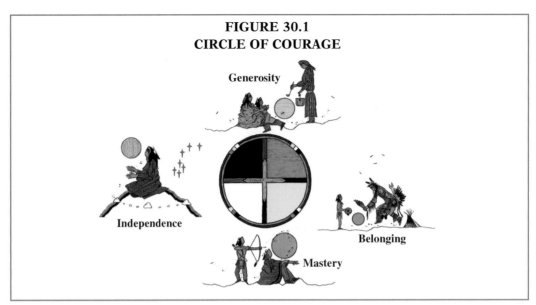

Circle of Courage™ image painted by George Blue Bird Sr; used with permission of Starr Global Learning Network through its corporate division, Reclaiming Youth International; see www.reclaiming.com for additional information.

TABLE 30.1
IDENTIFYING STRENGTHS

Belonging (connection)	How do you get along with the different people in your household? What do you like to do together as a family? Do you eat meals together? Do you feel you have at least 1 friend or a group of friends with whom you are comfortable? What do you and your friends like to do together after school? On weekends? How do you feel you fit in at school? In your neighborhood? Do you feel like you matter in your community? Do you have at least 1 adult in your life who cares about you and to whom you can go if you need help? When you're stressed out, who do you go to?
Mastery (competence)	What do you do to stay healthy? What are you good at? How are you doing in school? What do you like to do after school with your free time? Do you feel you are particularly good at doing a certain thing like math, soccer, theater, cooking, hunting or anything else? What are your responsibilities at home? At school?
Independence (confidence)	Do you feel that your have been allowed to become more independent or make more of your own decisions as you have become older? Do you feel you have a say in family rules and decisions? Are you able to take responsibility for your actions even when things don't work out perfectly or as you planned? Have you figured out a way to control your actions when you're angry or upset? Everyone has stress in their lives. Have you figured out to how to handle stress? How confident are you that you can make a needed change in your life?
Generosity (contribution, character)	What makes your parents proud of you? What do your friends like about you the most? What do you like about yourself? What do you do to help others (at home, or by working with a group at school, church, or community)? What do you do to show your parents or siblings that you care about them? How do you support your friends when they are trying to do the right thing, like quitting smoking or avoiding alcohol and other substances?

Reprinted with permission from Frankowski BL, Leader IC, Duncan PM. Strength-based interviewing. *Adolesc Med State Art Rev.* 2009;20:22–40 all areas to become healthy, happy, productive adults. See Table 30.2 for some examples of how you and parents can boost needed strengths. Third, you can use strengths as an engagement strategy to lead into a discussion about a needed behavior change. Fourth, you can bring strengths into a structured discussion about behavior change, such as shared decision-making or motivational interviewing.[3]

The following case illustrates the practical application of the Circle of Courage:

Rochelle, who is 12½ years old, comes in with her mother for her checkup. She continues to live at home with both parents and her younger brother. Rochelle gets along "fine" with everyone in the house, although her mother comments that they "clash" over things more than they have in the past. When asked what they disagree on, Rochelle shrugs, and her mother expresses concern about Rochelle's weight. She does mention that Rochelle continues to get along with her younger brother, aged 10, and has a lot of patience with him and helps him with his math homework.

Rochelle just started the sixth grade 2 months ago; this is her first year in middle school. She expresses disappointment that most of her friends from last year are not in her classes, and she occasionally eats lunch by herself. She continues to do well in her classes and got all As in her first-quarter report card. She did not join the soccer team this year because she wanted to focus on her schoolwork. In addition, her mother had been finding it difficult to drive Rochelle to practice with her new job. Rochelle now has to babysit her brother after school. She does not mind, because they watch television together. Her father has a demanding job in sales that requires him to work 10-hour days and travel a lot, but the family manages to eat dinner together 4 nights per week.

Her diet is "okay," with fruits and vegetables, 2% milk, lots of cheese, and mostly chicken and fish. She usually buys soda at school; there is a new vending machine in the cafeteria. She admits to snacking a lot after school with her brother. She denies the use of tobacco, alcohol, marijuana, and other drugs. Her parents do not smoke, and neither do her friends. She is not interested in any "romantic relationships" at this time, although she does have some friends who are boys, mostly ones with whom she played soccer last year. She has never had sex. She always wears a seatbelt in the car and a helmet on her bike. She used to ride her bike more often but now stays home after school.

TABLE 30.2
PROMOTING STRENGTHS THAT ARE LACKING

Generosity

  Ask "What are you doing to help out at home?" "How can you contribute to your community?"

    Suggest a volunteering commitment that takes advantage of something the youth is good at or interested in. Parents can help steer towards a volunteer experience.

Independence

  Ask "How do you make a decision about something important?" "How do you control your feelings when you are angry?"

    Suggest writing down pros and cons the next time they are struggling with a decision, or point out ways to alleviate stress with deep breathing, etc. Parents can help by discussing how they make decisions (about saving money for a needed item, for whom to vote in an election).

Mastery

  Ask "What are you getting good at?" "What are you interested in outside of school?"

    Suggest joining a club or sport. Parents can help by providing transportation to or from after-school or weekend meetings or events.

Belonging

  Ask "Who do you go to for help?" "Who are the adults you trust?"

    Suggest getting involved in a mentoring program. Parents can help by pointing out relatives or neighbors who can be trusted to go to for help and advice.

Reprinted with permission from Frankowski BL, Leader IC, Duncan PM. Strength-based interviewing. *Adolesc Med State Art Rev.* 2009;20:22–40

Rochelle says that things are "fine," but she is disappointed that school is not as fun as it was in the fifth grade. Her mom has been "getting on her" about her weight, but she thinks it is not her fault, because both her parents are overweight. She says she feels "kind of down" a lot of days but not really bad, and she would never consider harming herself.

Rochelle's risks are

- Poor nutrition (more snacking, soda at school)
- Inadequate physical activity (not playing soccer this year, more television time)
- Sadness or depressed mood (misses friends from soccer, school not as fun)

Her strengths are

- Generosity (takes care of her brother after school, helps him with his homework)
- Independence (knows how to keep herself and brother safe when parents are not home)
- Mastery (good at school, all As)
- Belonging (family, but not as much with friends now)

Use a written change plan.[4]

- *"Rochelle, you are showing a lot of strengths in your life now. You've successfully transitioned to middle school and are keeping up your excellent grades. You are demonstrating independence and maturity by watching your brother after school, and you are very generous to be spending the time helping him with his homework. But, it seems that you are not as active and not eating as well as you were last year, and you seem not as happy with things. Can we talk about that today?"* (Rochelle indicates that she really wanted to talk about her weight, because she does not like the way she is looking these days. She wants some help deciding what to do.)
- *"Rochelle, on a scale of 1 to 10, with 1 being not ready and 10 being very ready, how ready are you to start making a change?"* (Rochelle says 10!) (See Chapter 26.)
- *"Some people find it helpful to write down their ideas about change. Would you like to fill out this change plan with me today while you are here?"*
- Fill out the change plan together and give her a copy to take home.

Engaging Parents to Reinforce the 4 Core Elements of the Circle of Courage

The 4 core elements offer a nice framework to discuss how parents can effectively support their children's healthy development.

Mastery

"What am I good at?" Parents need to help their adolescent figure this out, especially if he or she is not a great student.

- Encourage your adolescent to try sports, clubs, a musical instrument, etc.
- Make him an expert on something in the family (eg, research driving directions online before a family trip).
- Model problem-solving behaviors when something does not go well.
- Help the adolescent to be persistent when he does not succeed at something the first time around (or second).
- Make him feel competent in more than one area.

Belonging

"Who do I fit in with? Who do I feel connected to?" Parents are often disappointed as friends become more important, but peer relations are vital to adolescents.

- Keeping your adolescent attached to your family as she develops friendly and romantic relationships is tricky. Get to know your adolescent's friends and make your home a welcome place for them.

- Encourage appropriate relationships with other adults you trust.
- Be sure your child knows to whom she can go if there is a problem that she does not feel can be shared with you (her health professional/coach/clergy/teacher could be one of these people).
- Help your adolescent figure out how she "fits in" with your extended family *("Your little cousins sure look up to you and love to play soccer with you!"),* your neighbors *("If I wasn't home and you had a problem, you could get help from Mrs X or Y." "Let's help Mr Z shovel his driveway/mow his lawn."),* her school *("Who are the teachers/students you get along with the best?"),* and her community (attend neighborhood events together, or encourage your adolescent to go with her friends), including faith-based organizations.

Independence

This is scary for parents of early adolescents, but we all want our children to grow up and be able to function independently (yet remain attached). For many adolescents, this means starting to make healthy independent decisions for themselves, especially decisions to avoid unhealthy risks.

- Guide your adolescent in healthy decision-making; let him work out the solution to a problem and then run it by you for final approval.
- Independence also means being responsible; as time goes by, this should happen more and more with less and less reminding from you. Some adolescents have a harder time gaining independent control of their behavior and showing self-discipline. Point out to your adolescent that every time he makes a healthy decision and controls his behavior without reminders from you, he is exercising independence.
- Encourage confidence in your adolescent by putting your trust in him when you assign a task to do. Good teachers will try to do the same thing. Let your adolescent take a leadership role in something he is good at.

Generosity

This can be the most difficult strength for some adolescents to develop, because most of them go through a stage when they are naturally self-centered as they try to figure out who they are.

- Point out and name qualities, such as caring, sharing, loyalty, and empathy, when you see your adolescent displaying them with her friends.
- Encourage the adolescent to practice these qualities when it is more difficult (eg, with a younger brother or an unpopular classmate).
- The broadest definition of this strength is the sense of giving back to one's community. This can start with parents involving adolescents in volunteering in their neighborhood, school, or faith-based community. Many older adolescents who have not developed this strength feel like they do not "matter" in their family, school, or community. The ability to feel like what you do matters—that the world (or at least your family, school, or community) is a little better because you are there—is very empowering, gives adolescents confidence and hope, and keeps them engaged.

Armed with these strengths, adolescents can be encouraged to take "healthy" risks. As youth advocate Matt Morton[5] has noted, *"If you don't give us healthy risks to take, we'll take unhealthy ones."* Remember, it is the taking of risks and failing, then having the strength, confidence, and hope to try again, that helps adolescents become resilient adults.

This chapter is adapted with permission from Frankowski BL, Leader IC, Duncan PM. Strength-based interviewing. *Adolesc Med State Art Rev.* 2009;20:22–40.

•• Group Learning and Discussion ••

1. Discuss as a group 2 recent cases of young people who had risks that merited attention. Fill in the details of both the risks and the strengths you believe they may have had even if you did not elicit them. Then pick one of the cases and break into pairs with one of you taking the role of professional and the other of teen. First gather the history using the Circle of Courage and then reflect your findings back to the young person. Be sure to include both areas of strength and areas that require further development. Finally, bring in a third person to act as a parent or guardian. Report your findings back to the adult caretaker.

2. Discuss as a group how this strategy could be incorporated into your practice setting. [Note: We found that practitioners were more likely to implement this strategy when they added a prompt for strengths assessment to their electronic or paper records. It both reminded them to do it and gave them a place to write down their findings for future reference and follow-through.[6]]

3. Discuss the potential benefits of using a strength-based interview in terms of your own well-being and job satisfaction.

■■■■■■■■ Continuing Education ■■■■■■■■■

If you are applying for continuing education credits, a test is available online. For more details, visit www.aap.org/reachingteens.

■ References

1. Ozer EM, Adams SH, Lustig JL, et al. Can it be done? Implementing adolescent clinical preventive services. *Health Serv Res.* 2001;36(6 pt 2):150–165

2. Brendtro LK, Brokenleg M, Van Bockern S. *Reclaiming Youth at Risk: Our Hope for the Future.* Bloomington, IN: National Education Service; 2002

3. Comprehensive Health Education Foundation. C.H.E.F. http://www.chef.org. Accessed July 22, 2013

4. Miller WR, Rolnick S. *Motivational Interviewing: Preparing People to Change Addictive Behaviour.* New York, NY: Guilford; 1991

5. Morton M. Lunch key note speech. Presented at: the 2nd Annual Vermont Working With Youth Conference; May 18, 2007; Burlington, VT

6. Duncan P, Garcia A, Frankowski B, et al. Inspiring healthy adolescent choices: a rationale for and guide to strength promotion in primary care. *J Adolesc Health.* 2007;41:525–535; editorial, 519–520

■ Related Video Content

30.0 The Circle of Courage: A Strategy for Eliciting Strengths and Addressing Risks. Frankowski.

30.1 Case Example: Circle of Courage as a Strategy to Reflect on Strengths After a Full Psychosocial Screen. Frankowski.

30.2 Case Example: Circle of Courage as a Strategy to First Reflect on Strengths Prior to Addressing Risks. Duncan.

CHAPTER 31

Stress Management and Coping

Kenneth R. Ginsburg, MD, MS Ed, FAAP, FSAHM

 Related Video Content

31.0 Stress Management and Coping

■ Why This Matters

The ability to cope with life's stressors in a positive way is key to overcoming adversity.[1] Figure 31.1 illustrates how stress can lead to a variety of outcomes. A life stressor creates discomfort that is reduced by employing a coping strategy. If equipped with positive adaptive strategies, the individual will gain some degree of relief, but maladaptive strategies also offer relief. In fact, many negative coping strategies are quick and easy fixes that offer near-instant relief.[2]

> **Rather than condemning negative behavior, which may only increase stress, we invite youth to join with us in a healing process to build positive coping strategies.**

These quick fixes might be the social morbidities we worry about the most—drinking, drug use, sensation seeking, self-mutilation, sex out of the context of a healthy relationship, truancy, gang affiliation, violence, and running away, among others. All of these strategies offer fleeting relief but lead to troubling patterns. First, stress leads to an unhealthy action that, in turn, may lead to increased tension within the individual, conflict with parents, educational underperformance, or social failures. These added pressures lead to more stress that leads to ever more reliance on the unhealthy fix.

■ Assessing the Stressor

A first step is to accurately assess the stressor. Stress is an adaptive tool that transforms our minds and bodies to react to potentially life-threatening emergencies. A small amount of stress increases our vigilance and prepares us to react. A large amount of stress prepares our body to fight or escape. The problem is that our stress-response system was not designed for the modern world. When a person reacts to a stressor with the same full-blown response he would to a true life or death emergency, it can be maladaptive. When a stressor is experienced out of proportion to its real potential effect, it is known as "catastrophic thinking." If a person is stuck in a pattern of catastrophic thinking, it can lead to ongoing anxiety and hyperreactivity. The first step of accurately assessing the stressor is determining if it is a "real tiger" or a "paper tiger." A worry is not a "real tiger." The next step to avert catastrophic thought is to remember that bad things are often temporary. Once a person considers how he will feel in a week or 2, he can remind himself that he can get through this. Equally as important is to grasp that good things might just be well deserved and can be permanent. Otherwise, people can experience stress even during good

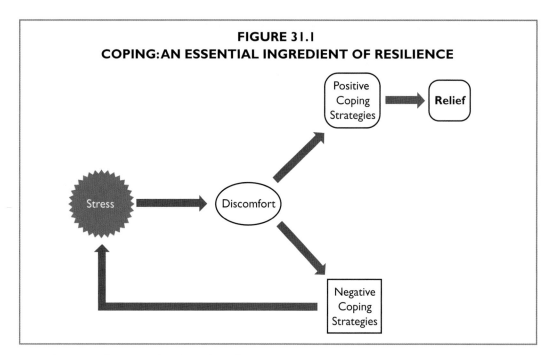

FIGURE 31.1
COPING: AN ESSENTIAL INGREDIENT OF RESILIENCE

times because they wait for the other shoe to drop.[3,4] The best strategy to help coping in those cases where simple reflections will not suffice may be to work on adjusting thinking patterns through cognitive behavioral therapy.[5–7] Healthy thinking patterns are important for reframing negative thoughts that interfere with forward progress.

The coping plan to be presented here is designed to build a repertoire of positive coping strategies so that, in times of inevitable stress, a person will naturally turn to these healthy strategies rather than to the quick, but dangerous, fixes that are termed "negative coping strategies" in this model.

■ Coping: An Essential Component of the Behavioral Change Process

One of the key concepts within Prochaska's[8] transtheoretical model of behavioral change is decisional balance. This involves an individual weighing the costs and benefits or pros and cons of any behavior.[9] The relative weighing of the pros or cons helps determine readiness for forward movement. Motivational interviewing uses this concept when it facilitates adolescents to consider the pros and cons of a given behavior to develop discrepancy between current behaviors and goals.[10]

If the perceived benefits (pros) of a behavior outweigh the perceived costs (cons), it may make no sense to consider thinking about change (ie, they will not move beyond pre-contemplation). For example, a teenager who finds that cigarettes offer the only respite she knows from a stressful home life will not be motivated to quit by being told of health risks that may affect her many years away, long after she has moved out of the challenging environment ("I'll quit then."). She will consider quitting cigarettes when she has other strategies to manage her current stress *and* she recognizes risks that affect her currently (such as high cost, reputation, yellow teeth, etc).

Because many worrisome behaviors reduce stress, it is critical that the adolescent has alternative existing positive strategies that also mitigate stress. Otherwise, the social morbidities will continue to offer present benefits that outweigh the costs. One could hypothesize that a teen would be less likely to reach toward a negative behavior in the first place (eg, using marijuana to "chill") if he already had a repertoire of effective positive strategies in place (eg, *"When I get stressed I just escape into a book."*). For this reason, time spent teaching about healthy coping can be seen both as primary and secondary prevention. In primary prevention, we reinforce a wide repertoire of activities and skill sets that serve as positive stress-reduction strategies.[11] In secondary prevention, we work with an adolescent already engaging in a negative behavior.[12] Rather than condemning his behavior, which may increase his stress, we invite him in a healing process to build positive coping strategies.

■ Coping Style

People respond to challenges differently. Researchers describe coping styles as problem-focused or emotion-focused[13] and engagement or disengagement coping.[14,15] People who use problem-focused engagement coping tend to choose 1 of 2 approaches—either they make an active effort to change the stressor itself or they change themselves enough to adapt to the stressor.[16] A major advantage of problem-focused strategies is that they either eliminate the source of the stress or help a person change enough so that the stressor has less of an effect. People who use emotion-focused disengagement coping focus on the emotions and discomfort the problem generates. People who disengage from problems can do so passively (eg, withdrawal) or actively (eg, alcohol).

Research has explored the relative benefits of problem-focused versus emotion-focused strategies.[16–19] Those who use problem-focused coping strategies tend to fare better than those who use emotion-focused coping because, if only emotions are addressed, the problem remains unresolved and can resurface. Nevertheless, emotion-focused strategies often involve seeking support from others, thereby allowing people to forge supportive connections. There is agreement that people who engage problems (via problem- or emotion-focused strategies) do better than those who disengage from problems altogether. However, disengagement may also be adaptive. Avoidance allows a person to choose the timing of when to confront an issue. It might be wise to delay a response to a problem until safety is ensured, skills are developed, and strategies are formed. Further, although we might assume disengagement strategies are unhealthy (substance use, running away), there are also healthy disengagement strategies (reading a book, working on a hobby).

■ Deriving a Comprehensive Coping Plan for Adolescents

A comprehensive stress-reduction plan should include a wide array of strategies that would prepare youth to
• Accurately assess the stressor.
• Effectively problem-solve.
• Maintain a state of health optimal for managing stress.
• Manage emotions in a healthy way.
• Use safe, healthy strategies to avoid other problems.

A stress-management plan needs to be presented quite differently for different ages both because coping strategies change across the life span[20] and because children's cognitive capacity to implement a plan varies substantially by developmental stage.[21]
• **Children.** They should be offered opportunities to learn how to feel emotionally healthy and physically strong. They will learn that they feel better after exercise and happier after they have expressed themselves creatively. Blowing bubbles can teach them about controlled and relaxing breathing. Even the youngest child can learn how much better it feels to talk if she is consistently offered a lap and a listening ear. She can learn about escape (healthy disengagement) through play, fantasy, and reading.

- **Preadolescents and early adolescents** will listen attentively as they are taught stress-reduction strategies. They will appreciate parental guidance and an acknowledgment that their lives are becoming more complex. They should be offered opportunities to practice what they have learned.
- **Mid- and late adolescents** likely will not want to hear about stress reduction from parents but may still be responsive to professionals. They can learn from written or Web-based materials and should be given opportunities to design their own plans.

All children and adolescents will learn from what their parents model. This offers a real opportunity to talk to parents about the importance of self-care. Many parents that will normally reject taking the steps to care for themselves will consider action when they are reminded how closely their children and adolescents are watching them (see Chapter 39).

A Stress Reduction Plan for Children and Teens

(The following plan is published in full by the American Academy of Pediatrics in *Building Resilience in Children and Teens: Giving Kids Roots and Wings*.[22])

First, it is important that young people learn to assess the stressor as a first step of coping. Then, the plan includes problem-focused engagement strategies, emotion-focused engagement strategies, and healthy disengagement strategies. It also includes basic wellness strategies that build a strong body capable of enduring stress (exercise, relaxation, nutrition, and proper sleep).

The plan has 4 broad categories and 10 points. It is not a 10-step plan; there is no designated order to approach stress. Rather, it offers a repertoire to draw from at appropriate times. For example, some strategies are cognitively based, making them unhelpful at times of severe stress. During extremely stressful moments, it may make more sense to exercise to use the stress hormones before attempting to thoughtfully resolve an issue.

Each of the points includes a variety of activities and actions to handle stress. No one should expect to use all of the techniques. Rather, they should pick an item or 2 from each point to see which best meets their needs, while remembering that the most suitable strategies change with circumstances and over time.

The stress-reduction plan includes 4 categories.

1. Tackling the problem
2. Taking care of my body
3. Dealing with emotions
4. Making the world better

Category 1: Tackling the Problem

- ***Point 1: Identify and then address the problem.*** (This point offers problem-focused engagement strategies.) Action that addresses the problem diminishes the source of stress. A key to using this strategy is to clarify the problem and then divide it into smaller pieces, committing to work on only one piece at a time. This decreases the sense of being overwhelmed and increases efficacy. Strategies to implement this point include making lists and timelines followed by a plan to address each component of the problem. Metaphorically, this is about helping teens revisualize problems from being mountains too high to be scaled into hills situated on top of each other. As they stand atop each hill, the summit appears more attainable. ▶ 31.2.1

  Strategies can be used in counseling to help teens approach larger crises or emotional issues by breaking them into manageable steps. For an example of strategies, see the "Ladder Diagram" in video 29.0, the "Tupperware Box" in video 31.13, and the "Decision Tree" in video 28.2. ▶ 28.2, 29.0, 31.13

- *Point 2: Avoid stress when possible.* (This point is a problem-focused strategy that leads to thoughtful disengagement.) This avoidance strategy teaches all young people to consider their triggers to stress and to realize that some of them can be avoided entirely. It teaches that avoiding trouble is an act of strength. A central theme of addictions treatment is to avoid the triggers that perpetuate cigarette smoking or drug use. For example, thoughtfully avoiding people, places, and things that set off stress can open the door to healthier ways of coping. This strategy should not be reserved for people in recovery and can be taught on a preventive basis. **31.2.2**

- *Point 3: Let some things go.* (This is another thoughtful, problem-focused, disengagement strategy.) While it can be useful to try to fix some problems, people who waste energy worrying about things they can't change don't have enough energy conserved to address problems they can fix. The serenity prayer, a mainstay of recovery programs, summarizes this point:

    "Grant me the serenity to accept the things I cannot change; the courage to change the things I can; and the wisdom to know the difference." **31.2.3**

Category 2: Taking Care of My Body: **40.0**

- *Point 4: The power of exercise.* Exercise may be the single most important part of the plan, and it is certainly the starting point for someone whose stress hormones prevent them from addressing any other problem or having insight into how to address a problem. When a stressed person does not exercise, their body is left feeling as if they haven't run from the "tiger." Therefore, their body senses it is still lurking and they remain hypervigilant (nervous) and their chronic stress hormones keep their blood pressure raised in preparation for the need to leap at any moment. It is not surprising, therefore, that exercise is so tightly linked to increased health and has been shown to contribute to emotional well-being and to positively affect stress, anxiety, depression, and attention-deficit/hyperactivity disorder.[23] Young people can be taught

    — *"When you are stressed, your body is saying, 'Run!' So do it."*

    — *"You may think you don't have time to exercise when you are most stressed, but that is exactly when you need it the most."*

    — *"You will be able to think better after you have used up those stress hormones."* **31.3.1**

- *Point 5: Active relaxation.* Because the parasympathetic (relaxed) and sympathetic (emergency/stressed) systems do not operate simultaneously, a key to relaxation is to stimulate the parasympathetic system. Deep methodical breathing, therefore, is the portal to relaxation. This is a mainstay of Eastern medicine techniques, yoga, and meditation, and it is even used to gain focus in the martial arts. Young people can be taught

    — *"You can flip the switch from being stressed to relaxed if you know how to turn on the relaxed system."* One technique is 4 to 8 breathing: *"Breathe deeply and slowly. Try to take a full breath. First, fill your stomach and then your chest while counting to 4. Hold that breath as long as it feels comfortable, let the breath out while counting to 8. This requires your full concentration. If your mind wanders, as it will, remind yourself to refocus on your counting and breathing. Over time, your mind will be more able to stay focused on how you are feeling now rather than past or future worries."*

    Mindfulness is a powerful technique that achieves a state of relaxation by living fully in the present while actively reminding you to let go of worries from the past and fears of the future (see Chapter 32). **31.3.2**

- *Point 6: Eat well.* Proper nutrition is essential to a healthy body and clear mind (see Chapter 40). Young people can be taught
  — *"Everyone knows good nutrition makes you healthier. Only some people realize that it also keeps you alert through the day and your mood steady. People who eat mostly junk food have highs and lows in their energy level, which harms their ability to reduce stress. Eating more fruits, vegetables, and whole grains can keep you focused for a longer time."* ▶ **31.3.3, 31.14**

- *Point 7: Sleep well.* Proper sleep is key to stress management. Some people do not sleep well because of poor sleep hygiene, including having too much stimulation in their bedrooms and keeping irregular hours. Another source of lost sleep is stress itself; people use the bed as a place to resolve their problems. The basics of sleep hygiene include
  — *"Go to sleep about the same time every night."*
  — *"Exercise 4 to 6 hours before bedtime. Your body falls asleep most easily when it has cooled down. If you exercise right before bed, you will be overheated and won't sleep well."*
  — *"A hot shower 1 hour before bedtime also helps your body relax to fall asleep."*
  — *"About half of an hour before bed, go somewhere other than your bed and do something to set your worries aside (see Point 9). Do this in dim light. If you are the kind of person who thinks about all the stuff you have to do tomorrow, make a list before you go to bed and set it aside (see Point 1). If you wake up in the middle of the night thinking, move to another spot to do your worrying. You'll get tired soon, then go back to bed."*
  — *"If you have trouble falling asleep, try 4 to 8 meditative breathing."* ▶ **31.3.4**

Category 3: Dealing With Emotions

- *Point 8: Take instant vacations.* (This point offers healthy disengagement strategies.) Sometimes the best way to de-stress is to take your mind away to a more relaxing place. Young people can be taught to take advantage of their imagination and ability to focus on other interests. Young people can be reminded to take breaks from stress.
  — **Visualization:** *"Have a favorite place where you can imagine yourself relaxing."*
  — **Enjoy your interests or hobby:** *"Get into whatever you enjoy doing that is fun and creative."* (This might include playing an instrument, drawing or writing—activities that focus and use a more creative part of a young person's brain.)
  — **Change your venue:** *"Take a walk outside."*
  — **Read:** *"Read a good book, even one you have read before."* (It may be that reading is the best diversion because it uses all of the senses—one has to imagine the sounds, sights, and smells and one also feels the emotions; there is little room left for your own worries. You are on a real vacation.)
  — **Music:** *"Listening to music can be a great break from stress and it can "reset" your emotions."* ▶ **31.4.1**

- *Point 9: Release emotional tension.* (This point offers emotion-focused engagement strategies.) A person needs to be able to express emotions rather than letting them build inside. The ideas in this category include connecting to others and letting go of feelings with verbal, written, nonverbal, and creative expression. There are a wide variety of options available to meet someone's temperament and talents.
  — **Talking to someone who is worthy of your trust:** *"Talking to a good friend, parent, teacher, or a professional, like a doctor, nurse, or counselor, can really help you get worries off your mind. Find an adult who will listen and whom you can ask for advice."*
  — **Creativity:** *"Things like art, music, poetry, singing, dance, and rap are powerful ways to let your feelings out."*
  — **Journaling:** *"Write it out!"*

— **Prayer or meditation:** *"Some people find that praying or meditation alone or with family or friends can ease their problems."*

— **Crying or laughing:** *"Some people feel so much better inside after they cry hard or laugh hard by themselves or with other people."* **31.4.2**

Category 4: Helping a Little Can Make Your World Better and Help You Feel Better

- *Point 10: Contribute.* Children and adolescents who consider how to serve their family, community, school, and nation will feel good about themselves, have a sense of purpose, and benefit from making a difference in other people's lives. First, they will learn that it feels good to serve, and that may reduce their sense of shame or stigma when they need to reach out for help themselves. Second, children and adolescents who serve others become surrounded by gratitude, and that can be a powerful reinforcement to continued positive behaviors. It is particularly important to adolescents who often are recipients of low expectations. Finally, people who serve others may be better able **31.5** to put their own problems in perspective.

■ Final Thoughts

We cannot take away all exposure to risk. We can, however, acknowledge that much of risk represents a young person's attempt to deal with uncomfortable feelings. Most importantly, we can make sure that young people possess a wide repertoire of positive coping strategies. When they do, the path of least resistance, during stressful times, may be the one that leads to healthy, adaptive behaviors.

•• Group Learning and Discussion ••

Healthy stress-management strategies represent both primary and secondary prevention. Primary prevention offers children and teens the tools and strategies to manage stress on a purely preventive basis to promote general wellness. In secondary prevention, these strategies offer an opportunity to shift from telling a young person what not to do toward guiding her in what she can do to both relieve stress and be healthier. The first step is to recognize that existing worrisome behaviors fill a need. In some cases, you can elicit that from young people. In other cases, they are not able to safely arrive at this insight. It is reasonable to simply ask, *"Tell me what _____ does for you."* Then, rather than condemning youths' actions, we invite them to consider healthy alternatives. Recognizing they are the experts on their own lives, it is critical to explore what already works and invite them to consider what other strategies might also work.

Break into pairs, and practice shifting young people toward healthier coping strategies. (Assume that your earlier assessment leaves you concerned, but that you have no worries of imminent self-harm.)

- A 16-year-old boy, Tony, smokes marijuana 2 to 3 times a day. His father is in prison and his mother works a double shift every day. He used to be on the track team, but now does not have time because he cares for his 3 younger siblings.
- A mother brings in her 14-year-old son, Travis, because she can't get him off of the computer. He is gaming until the early morning each night. His grades are dropping. His father is an airman who is deployed overseas. He draws cartoons for fun.
- A 15-year-old girl, Jade, is brought in by her father to discuss "laziness." She used to do well in school and now tells you that she just doesn't care anymore. She has a term paper due in 2 weeks in what used to be her favorite subject. She has had 3 months to get started. She tells you the subject is "lame." (Hint: See Point 1.)
- Lydia is a 17-year-old girl who is a straight A student. She only sleeps about 5 to 6 hours per night, because she studies until 1:00 am nightly to maintain her GPA. She plans on attending an Ivy League university. You notice that her fingernails are bitten and that she has a spot of very thin hair on her left temple. She is a wonderful writer, but stopped writing for pleasure because she has no time.

■■■■■■■■ Continuing Education ■■■■■■■■■

If you are applying for continuing education credits, a test is available online. For more details, visit www.aap.org/reachingteens.

■ References

1. Masten A. Ordinary magic: resilience processes in development. *Am Psychol.* 2001;56:227–238
2. Wills TA, Shiffman S. Coping and substance abuse: a conceptual framework. In: Shiffman S, Wills TA, eds. *Coping and Substance Use.* Orlando, FL: Academic Press; 1985
3. Brunwasser SM, Gillham JE, Kim ES. A meta-analytic review of the Penn Resiliency Program's effect on depressive symptoms. *J Consult Clin Psychol.* 2009;77(6):1042–1054
4. Reivich K, Shatté A. *The Resilience Factor.* New York, NY: Broadway Books; 2002
5. Abrahamson LY, Seligman M, Teasdale M. Learned helplessness in humans: critique and reformulation. *J Abnorm Psychol.* 1978;87:49–74
6. Beck AT. *Cognitive Therapy and the Emotional Disorders.* New York, NY: Penguin Books; 1976
7. Ellis A. *Reason and Emotion in Psychotherapy.* Carol Publishing Group; 1962
8. Prochaska JO. Decision making in the transtheoretical model of behavior change. *Med Decis Making.* 2008;28(6):845–849

9. Velicer WF, Prochaska JO, Fava JL, et al. Smoking cessation and stress management: applications of the transtheoretical model of behavior change. *Homeost.* 1998;38:216–233

10. Miller WR, Rollnick S. *Motivational Interviewing: Preparing People to Change Addictive Behavior.* New York, NY: Guilford;1991:191–202

11. Prochaska JO, Velicer WF, Rossi JS, et al. Stages of change and decisional balance for problem behaviors. *Health Psychol.* 1994;13:39–46

12. Brady SS, Tschann JM, Pasch LA, et al. Cognitive coping moderates the association between violent victimization by peers and substance use among adolescents. *J Pediatr Psychol.* 2008;34(3):304–310

13. Lazarus RS, Folkman S. *Stress, Appraisal, and Coping.* New York, NY: Springer; 1984

14. Ebata A, Moos R. Coping and adjustment in distressed and healthy adolescents. *J Appl Dev Psychol.* 1991;12:33–54

15. Tobin DL, Holroyd KA, Reynolds RV, Wigal JK. The hierarchical factor structure of the coping strategies inventory. *Cognit Ther Res.* 1989;13:343–361

16. Compas BE, Connor-Smith JK, Saltzman H, et al. Coping with stress during childhood and adolescence: problems, progress and potential in theory and research. *Psychol Bull.* 2001;127:87–127

17. Hampel P, Petermann F. Perceived stress, coping, and adjustment in adolescents. *J Adolesc Health.* 2006;38(4):409–415

18. Clark AT. Coping with interpersonal stress and psychosocial health among children and adolescents: a meta-analysis. *J Youth Adolesc.* 2006;35(1):11–24

19. Fields L, Prinz R. Coping and adjustment during childhood and adolescence. *Clin Psychol Rev.*1997;17(8):937–976

20. Diehl M, Coyle N, Labouvie-Vief G. Age and sex differences in strategies of coping and defense across the life span. *Psychol Aging.* 1996;11(1):127–139

21. Compas BE, Worsham NL, Ey S. Conceptual and developmental issues in children's coping with stress. In: La Greca AM, et al. eds. *Stress and Coping in Child Health.* New York, NY: Guilford Press; 1992

22. Ginsburg KR, Jablow MM. *Building Resilience in Children and Teens: Giving Kids Roots and Wings.* 2nd ed. Elk Grove Village, IL: American Academy of Pediatrics; 2011

23. Ratey JJ, Hagerman E. *Spark: The Revolutionary New Science of Exercise and the Brain.* New York, NY: Little, Brown and Company; 2008

■ Related Video Content

31.0 Stress Management and Coping. Ginsburg.

31.1 Stress Management and Coping/Introduction. Ginsburg.

31.2 Stress Management and Coping/Section 1/Tackling the Problem. Ginsburg.

31.2.1 Stress Management and Coping/Section 1/Tackling the Problem/Point 1: Identify and Then Address the Problem. Ginsburg.

31.2.2 Stress Management and Coping/Section 1/Tackling the Problem/Point 2: Avoid Stress When Possible. Ginsburg.

31.2.3 Stress Management and Coping/Section 1/Tackling the Problem/Point 3: Let Some Things Go. Ginsburg.

31.3 Stress Management and Coping/Section 2/Taking Care of My Body. Ginsburg.

31.3.1 Stress Management and Coping/Section 2/Taking Care of My Body/Point 4: The Power of Exercise. Ginsburg.

31.3.2 Stress Management and Coping/Section 2/Taking Care of My Body/Point 5: Active Relaxation. Ginsburg.

31.3.3 Stress Management and Coping/Section 2/Taking Care of My Body/Point 6: Eat Well. Ginsburg.

31.3.4 Stress Management and Coping/Section 2/Taking Care of My Body/Point 7: Sleep Well. Ginsburg.

31.4 Stress Management and Coping/Section 3/Dealing With Emotions. Ginsburg.

31.4.1 Stress Management and Coping/Section 3/Dealing With Emotions/Point 8: Take Instant Vacations. Ginsburg.

31.4.2 Stress Management and Coping/Section 3/Dealing With Emotions/Point 9: Release Emotional Tension. Ginsburg.

31.5 Stress Management and Coping/Section 4/Making the World Better/Point 10: Contribute. Ginsburg.

31.6 A Simple Explanation of How Stress Affects the Teen Brain. Vo.

31.7 The Forces in Teens' Lives That Produce Stress. Vo.

31.8 Brain Hygiene: The Very Basics of Stress Management. Vo.

31.9 Youth Professionals Speak of How Environmental Stressors Produce Worrisome Behaviors. Covenant House, YouthBuild, El Centro.

31.10 Youth Speak of the Forces That Create Stress in Their Lives. Youth.

31.11 Youth Speak of How Stress Drives Behavior. Youth.

31.12 Define and Defend Your Priorities: Critical to Managing Stress. Sugerman.

31.13 The Tupperware Box: A Case Example. Ginsburg.

31.14 Limiting Empty Calories From Drinks: A Small Step Toward Better Nutrition. Ginsburg.

28.2 Helping a Young Person Own Her Solution: A Case of Using a Decision Tree to Prevent Violent Retaliation. Ginsburg.

29.0 Gaining a Sense of Control: One Step at a Time. Ginsburg.

32.0 Mindfulness in Practice. Vo.

39.1 Our Feelings Are Contagious: We Help Our Children When We Care for Ourselves. Vo.

39.4 Parents Model Healthy Versus Unhealthy Coping. Ginsburg.

40.0 The Role of Lifestyle and Healthy Thinking in Mental Health Promotion. Singh.

67.2 The Tupperware Box: A Model for Releasing Trapped Emotions. Ginsburg.

■ Related Handout/Supplementary Material

Just for Teens: A Personal Plan for Managing Stress

CHAPTER 32

Mindfulness Practice for Resilience and Managing Stress and Pain

Dzung X. Vo, MD, FAAP

> **Related Video Content**
>
> 32.0 Mindfulness in Practice

■ Why This Matters

Mindfulness simply means, "paying attention in a particular way: on purpose, in the present moment, and nonjudgmentally".[1] Clinical mindfulness-based interventions train participants in formal and informal meditation skills to promote coping and resilience. Mindfulness-based interventions are emerging as a feasible and effective method to promote resilience and coping among adolescents with chronic stress, mood symptoms, chronic illness, and pain. 32.8

> ●● **Much of our stress and suffering comes from being pulled away from the present moment. Our minds may be caught in regrets about the past, worries about the future, or judgments about the present. Mindfulness is practiced with a sense of loving-kindness, being fully present with whatever is inside and around you in the present moment, and meeting it with kindness and without judgment.** ●●

■ Case: 17-Year-Old Female With Back Pain

Susan is a 17-year-old female who suffered a serious injury several years ago. Since that time, she has suffered from severe, chronic back pain. The pain profoundly disrupted her functioning at school and at home, and significantly impacted her stress and mood. Susan had seen multiple medical and surgical specialists over several years, and had not experienced significant relief with standard therapies. She was beginning to lose hope, feeling, *"I can't have a future"* and *"This will never get better."*

Through the course of our initial discussions, Susan was able to identify relationships between her mind state and her body state, observing that when she was feeling stressed and depressed, her back pain worsened and was more difficult to cope with, and vice versa (her back pain worsened her stress and mood). I verbally reinforced this insight, and used this strength as a starting point to discuss the potential role of mindfulness training as a mind-body intervention to help her cope with pain and improve her functioning and her quality of life. Susan agreed to try an 8-week individual mindfulness training program, adapted from mindfulness-based stress reduction (MBSR).

Together with Susan's mother, every week we learned and practiced formal mindfulness practices such as sitting meditation and body scan meditation, as well as informal mindfulness practices such as eating meditation and walking meditation. We discussed and explored Susan's experiences, successes, and challenges with mindfulness practice at home. Ultimately, I encouraged Susan to develop her capacity, as much as possible, to be mindful in every moment and every activity of her everyday life, training herself to continually bring awareness to the present moment without judgment, and with kindness and compassion.

After 8 weeks of mindfulness training and practice, Susan reported that her pain had improved somewhat but, more importantly, her relationship with her pain and with her body had transformed profoundly. *"I'm fine with having the pain now…as opposed to learning how to ignore my pain, I've learned how to accept my pain. What makes me really happy is not being stressed about the pain."* Susan's mother agreed with her observations, and, as a side benefit, reported that the whole family benefited from the mindfulness training. Susan's newfound sense of hope helped her to complete high school, and she is now planning to enter the health care field.

■ Mindfulness: Background

Mindfulness practice has its historic origins in Eastern meditation and traditions, and can also be found in wisdom traditions worldwide. Jon Kabat-Zinn and others[2,3] have developed secular (nonreligious) mindfulness-based training programs such as MBSR, adapting mindfulness practices for application in clinical and community settings. Other evidence-based mindfulness-based interventions include mindfulness-based cognitive therapy for depression, mindfulness-based relapse prevention for substance abuse, and mindfulness-based childbirth and parenting.

A large body of literature in adult populations demonstrates benefits of mindfulness-based clinical interventions in heterogeneous disorders and populations, including chronic pain, mood disorders, substance abuse, and coping with chronic illness.[4] Recent studies suggest that mindfulness training may alter physiological parameters, including immune function, brain gray matter concentrations visible on magnetic resonance imaging scans, and even cellular telomeres associated with aging.[5-7]

Mindfulness-based interventions are now being developed and offered to children and youth in medical and mental health settings, as well as schools, community-based settings, and juvenile justice settings. Research on mindfulness with youth is in its infancy and is developing rapidly. Early studies on mindfulness with youth show promise for potential improvements in emotional regulation, attention, learning, and mental health symptoms.[8,9]

Mindfulness practice is based on the observation that much of our stress and suffering comes from being pulled away from the present moment. We spend much of our time in "autopilot" mode, going through the motions of life without being fully present in the here and now. Our body may be in one place, and our mind may be somewhere else entirely. Often our minds may be caught in regrets about the past, worries about the future, or judgments about the present. In this ruminative or "mindless" state, we are vulnerable to "reacting" to stressful and painful situations from a state of fear, with our higher cortical brain function (our prefrontal cortex, or "human brain") overwhelmed by the fight, flight, or freeze stress response (sometimes described as the "reptile brain"). We may lose regulation and integration of our brain and emotions, and get caught in negative mood states and/or reactive behaviors that can make the situation worse.

Dr Daniel Siegel's "hand model of the brain" is a concrete and simple way of teaching what happens in our brains and bodies, when we become overwhelmed with stress and "lose it."[10] Children as young as 5 years can understand the hand model of the brain. Fortunately, we can learn how to reengage the "human" part of our brain using mindfulness and other practices, thereby reestablishing integration and healthy regulation. From this state of present-moment awareness, we can see and respond to situations with more wisdom and clarity, and access our innate capacity for healing.

31.6

For example, in the case study, Susan's chronic pain led to recurrent thoughts like, *"I wish that injury had never happened," "My pain is always terrible and will never get better,"* and *"I won't be able to have a future."* Every time she experienced physical pain, these thoughts were repeatedly reinforced, which, in turn, amplified the suffering caused by her physical sensations. The thoughts pulled her away from her actual present moment experiences. She became caught in ruminative judgments, regrets, and worries, which triggered and reinforced her stress response in a vicious cycle. Mindfulness training helped Susan to free herself from this cycle, and change her relationship with her thoughts, emotions, and physical sensations. Susan rediscovered and strengthened her capacity to be awake to the present moment, deeply in touch with what was happening in the here and now, with an open heart and without judging. All youth have this innate capacity, and systematic mindfulness training helps them to employ this capacity more consistently and effectively.

Adolescence is a particularly critical window both to the vulnerability to stress and the opportunity for intervention to promote stress management and resilience. Adults expect adolescents to be able to regulate their emotions, manage stress, plan for the future, act with empathy and compassion, and think abstractly. However, adolescent brains do not fully mature until the mid-20s, especially in the prefrontal areas responsible for executive functioning, integration, and regulation. Mindfulness practice is a concrete tool to stimulate and promote neural circuits associated with resilience and emotional regulation, and may promote healthier adolescent brain development[10] (see "The Teen Brain" on page 57). Teaching mindfulness to youth has the potential to help them develop lifelong coping habits and profoundly affect their life trajectory.

■ Here's How It Works: Office-Based Mindfulness Training

- **Step 1: Psychoeducation on brain, body, stress, and coping.** Provide background on stress, mind, body, and coping (see chapters 31 and 40). The key messages are
  — Everyone has stress and pain. Stress is inevitable. Suffering may be, at least to some degree, optional. What matters is how you manage stress and pain.
  — You can cope with stress and pain in a positive (healthy) or negative (unhealthy) direction. (This message should avoid the implication of judgment.)
  — Symptoms of stress and pain can be experienced in both the body and the mind, and the body and mind are interconnected in complex ways. Practices that integrate the mind and body can promote health and resilience.
  — Consider teaching teens and families the "hand model of the brain" to illustrate what happens under stress.
  — You can learn tools to engage your whole brain and innate strength to manage stress and pain in a healthy way.
- **Step 2: Setting the stage for mindfulness.** Adapt the information in the text above to offer a definition of mindfulness and brief background on the clinical application and potential benefits of mindfulness practice. Use motivational interviewing techniques to explore and promote engagement and motivation. If the teen is somewhat open-minded

or motivated to try mindfulness, then set the stage for mindfulness training. Key messages to convey include

— Encourage an attitude of "beginner's mind": letting go of preconceived ideas, expectations, and judgments.

— Tell the teen, *"As long as you are breathing, there is more right with you than there is wrong with you."* Mindfulness is a deeply strength-based approach, based on the insight that if you can learn to allow yourself to be present with whatever you are experiencing, you will rediscover your innate strength and capacity to more skillfully handle any situation, any feeling, any emotion you might encounter. You do not need to keep running away, covering up, fighting, or denying anything.

— One of the most important "mindful qualities" is loving kindness (or compassion, friendliness, or heartfulness). When you practice mindfulness with a sense of loving-kindness, it means you are being fully present with whatever is inside you and around you in the present moment, and meeting it with kindness and without judgment.

— Another mindful quality is an attitude of curiosity: experiencing each moment with the question, *"What is happening right now?"*—just posing the question with an open heart and mind, and without necessarily trying to find or get attached to an "answer."

— Mindfulness means becoming aware of, and then letting go of, judgments about yourself. This includes judgments about whether or not you are doing mindfulness "correctly."

— Relaxation and calmness are common side effects of mindfulness practice, but relaxation is not the explicit goal of mindfulness practice. Mindfulness means to become aware of whatever you are experiencing, whether it is pleasant or unpleasant. So, in some cases, you may feel relaxed, but, in other cases, you may not. Either way is OK. The important thing is the awareness, with an attitude of kindness and curiosity.

- **Step 3: Introducing a formal mindfulness practice.** Mindfulness of breathing is a simple practice that forms the foundation of other mindfulness practices. The body scan is useful for patients with insomnia, chronic pain, and other mind-body syndromes. Formal mindfulness practices can be practiced in as little as 3 to 5 minutes, or up to 30 minutes or longer. Other mindfulness practices include walking meditation, loving-kindness meditation, and eating meditation. Formal practices can be guided by voice or by an audio recording, or self-guided (silent). Encourage the teen to set aside time in her day for a formal mindfulness practice every day (for example, in the morning or before bedtime). Remind her that short periods (even 3 to 5 minutes) of frequent practice are more likely to be beneficial than longer infrequent practices. See the handouts at the end of this chapter for details on mindfulness of breathing and body scan. Visit the Kelty Mental Health Resource Centre Web site (http://keltymentalhealth.ca/healthy-living/mindfulness) for free audio recordings of guided mindfulness meditations.[11] **32.1, 32.2**

- **Step 4: Introducing informal mindfulness practices.** Formal mindfulness practices are practices that you set aside time to do. Informal mindfulness practices, on the other hand, bring that same mindful, present-moment, and nonjudgmental awareness to all activities of daily living. Concrete mindfulness practices that can be done formally or informally are walking meditation and eating meditation. After **32.3** demonstrating and practicing an informal mindfulness practice with the teen, encourage her to use her creativity and intelligence to bring present-moment, nonjudgmental awareness to activities that she already does during the day, such as walking, eating, talking to a friend, or riding the bus. Encourage her to find and use reminders in the environment (such as phones or school bells ringing) as virtual "bells of mindfulness," reminding her to come back to the present moment, breathe 3 mindful breaths, and carry on in mindfulness. Remind her that the mindful qualities of kindness and curiosity are available in every moment, and that, by practicing coming back to the present moment over and over again, she can train herself to live life more fully and handle her stress and pain more effectively.

Office-based teaching and practice can be performed in a few repeated brief weekly office visits, and subsequently reinforced periodically. For teens who may benefit from or need more intensive mindfulness training, consider referring to a provider with expertise in mindfulness-based interventions, and/or referring to a formal group mindfulness training program (see Related Web Sites). Teens in our formal mindfulness programs often report that after 8 weeks of mindfulness training, they have learned more than just a "technique" to apply in specific situations. They have learned a new way of being and a healthier way of looking at the world, and have regained hope and courage that they thought was lost.

The most important aspect in teaching mindfulness to teens—more important than what words you say or what format or techniques you apply—is the quality of your own mindfulness practice.

■ Here's How It Works: Mindfulness for Providers

There is growing interest and literature in mindfulness training for providers as a tool to promote stress management, decrease burnout, and increase empathy and effective clinical communication skills.[12] Moreover, having a personal mindfulness practice can be very useful for teaching mindfulness effectively to teens. When you teach mindfulness directly from your own experience and practice, you role-model and embody mindfulness with an authenticity that is critical to teaching this practice. If you are interested in teaching mindfulness to teens, first begin to develop your own mindfulness practice. You can start by enrolling in an 8-week MBSR course or other mindfulness training program in your local area (see Related Web Sites). Once you begin to experience mindfulness practice and its benefits for yourself, you can slowly start to teach the practices that you have found useful in your own life.

▶ **32.5, 67.6**

●● Group Learning and Discussion ●●

Discuss
1. Who among our youth would benefit from the practice of mindfulness?
2. How might it help us better serve youth and their families?
3. How could we make it feasible to incorporate mindfulness into our practice? Should we consider group mindfulness sessions for select youth? Should we investigate mindfulness training referral resources for our youth? Could we at least make Dr Vo's explanations available for our youth and their families?
4. How might we benefit as providers from personal mindfulness practice?

Practice
Mindfulness is far better practiced than discussed. Use the supplementary tools as well as the videos to prepare yourself to incorporate mindfulness into your practice and, perhaps, your own self-care regimen.

■■■■■■■■ Continuing Education ■■■■■■■■

If you are applying for continuing education credits, a test is available online. For more details, visit www.aap.org/reachingteens.

■ References

1. Kabat-Zinn J. *Wherever You Go, There You Are: Mindfulness Meditation in Everyday Life*. New York, NY: Hyperion; 1994
2. Kabat-Zinn, J. *Full Catastrophe Living: Using the Wisdom of Your Body and Mind to Face Stress, Pain, and Illness*. 5th ed. New York, NY: Delta; 1990
3. Stahl B, Goldstein E. *A Mindfulness-Based Stress Reduction Workbook*. Oakland, CA: New Harbinger Publications; 2010
4. Baer R. Mindfulness training as a clinical intervention: a conceptual and empirical review. *Clin Psychol Sci Pract*. 2003;10:125–143
5. Davidson RJ, Kabat-Zinn J, Schumacher J, et al. Alterations in brain and immune function produced by mindfulness meditation. *Psychosom Med*. 2003;65(4):564–570
6. Holzel BK, Carmody J, Vangel M, et al. Mindfulness practice leads to increases in regional brain gray matter density. *Psychiatry Res*. 2011;191(1):36–43
7. Jacobs TL, Epel ES, Lin J, et al. Intensive meditation training, immune cell telomerase activity, and psychological mediators. *Psychoneuroendocrinology*. 2011;36(5):664–681
8. Burke CA. Mindfulness-based approaches with children and adolescents: a preliminary review of current research in an emerging field. *J Child Fam Stud*. 2010;19:133–144
9. Harnett PH, Dawe S. Review: the contribution of mindfulness-based therapies for children and families and proposed integration. *Child Adolesc Ment Health*. 2012. DOI: 10.1111/j.1475-3588.2011.00643.x
10. Siegel, Daniel J. *Mindsight: The New Science of Personal Transformation*. New York, NY: Bantam; 2010
11. BC Children's Hospital. Kelty Mental Health Resource Centre, BC Children's Hospital. http://keltymentalhealth.ca/healthy-living/mindfulness. Accessed June 25, 2013
12. Krasner MS, et al. Association of an educational program in mindful communication with burnout, empathy, and attitudes among primary care physicians. *JAMA*. 2009;302(12):1284–1293

■ Suggested Reading

Vo DX, Park MJ. Stress and stress management among youth and young men. *Am J Mens Health*. 2008;2(4):353–366

Willard C. *Child's Mind: Mindfulness Practices to Help Our Children Become More Focused, Calm, and Relaxed*. Berkeley, CA: Parallax Press; 2010

■ Related Video Content

32.0 Mindfulness in Practice. Vo.

32.1 The Body Scan. Vo.

32.2 Awareness of Breathing. Vo.

32.3 Mindful Walking. Vo.

32.4 Getting Practical: Bringing Mindfulness Into Your Life. Vo.

32.5 Mindfulness as a Tool to Increase Your Clinical Effectiveness. Vo.

32.6 Planting the Seeds…Trusting the Flower Might Bloom. Vo.

32.7 Mindfulness as a Means to Increase Self-acceptance, Diminish Shame, and Defeat Self-hatred. Vo.

32.8 Mindfulness: Youth Voices (Kelty Mental Health Resource Centre). Vo, Youth.

67.6 Mindfulness Allows Us to Remain Fully Present Even Amidst Our Exposure to Suffering. Vo.

■ Related Handouts/Supplementary Materials

Sample Guided Mindfulness of Breathing Meditation

The Body Scan

■ Related Web Sites

Greater Good Guide to Mindfulness, University of California, Berkeley

http://educ.ubc.ca/research/ksr/docs/mindfulnessguide_may2010.pdf

Short articles written for non-specialist audience, on mindfulness background, mindful parenting, and teaching mindfulness in prisons, schools, and with veterans.

Kelty Mental Health Resource Centre, BC Children's Hospital

http://keltymentalhealth.ca/healthy-living/mindfulness

This Web site offers free audio recordings of guided mindfulness meditations that we use in our mindfulness for teens programs at BC Children's Hospital.

Mindfulness in Education Network

www.mindfuled.org

A network of professionals interested in mindfulness with children and youth. Resources include an e-mail listserv and professional conferences.

University of Massachusetts Center for Mindfulness in Medicine, Health Care, and Society

www.umassmed.edu/content.aspx?id=41252

Mindfulness-Based Stress Reduction (MBSR) was developed here, and this Web site offers numerous resources for clinicians, patients, and researchers.

CHAPTER 33

Helping Youth Overcome Shame and Stigma (and Doing Our Best to Not Be a Part of the Problem)

Kenneth R. Ginsburg, MD, MS Ed, FAAP, FSAHM

 Related Video Content

33.0 Helping Youth Overcome Shame and Stigma (and Doing Our Best to Not Be a Part of the Problem)

■ Why This Matters

We can best serve youth when we have the opportunity to assess them for risk and then engage them in a positive change process that may include referral to appropriate behavioral specialists and supports. Our potential impact is affected by youths' decision to disclose their concerns to us, and ultimately by whether they allow us to guide them. Whether or not they choose to share their feelings and behaviors may be related to how stigmatized they perceive their issues to be. Then their decision to join with us in a healing partnership may be affected by how deeply they have internalized shame.

> When we approach youth from a positive lens and with the desire to build on existing strengths, our interactions are inherently less likely to induce shame.

Stigma (negative societal attitudes) and shame (negative personal feelings) can serve as a barrier to seeking treatment for a variety of issues, including substance use, sexually transmitted infections, emotional and mental health, and obesity.[1–10] In fact, efforts to use stigma in order to generate motivation for change have backfired. A clear example is that obesity campaigns that have depicted overweight individuals as unattractive, slovenly, or lazy have increased shame and hopelessness, which has led to forgone care and contributed to health disparities.[7]

We can challenge society to take a hard look at how stigma affects the already demoralized, but we must not allow our frustration with the pace of change to limit our ability to take immediate action to minimize shame in our practices and help youth feel empowered to seek the services they deserve.

■ Reducing Shame for the Youth We Serve

We are ideally situated to advocate for changing the way society stigmatizes some of the challenges youth need to overcome. As we do so, we need to illuminate both pervasive attitudes and how structural issues within the care system perpetuate stigma. As long as mental, emotional, and behavioral health do not enjoy true parity of resources with physical health, the implicit message is that they are of lesser value.

Regardless of whether you become involved in advocacy, you can reduce the potential for shame in your office by addressing (1) professional development needs of office staff and structural factors that may prevent all youth from feeling safe, (2) your own perceptions of problem behaviors that may directly affect delivery of care or be inadvertently or subliminally communicated to youth, (3) parents' attitudes and beliefs about problems as well as the feelings of inadequacy raised when their children are struggling, and (4) youth views both of their problems and of help-seeking.

When we approach youth from a positive lens and with the desire to build on existing strengths, our interactions are inherently less likely to induce shame. As a strength-based body of work, strategies are offered throughout this text that serve to mitigate stigma and reduce the potential for shame.

■ Structural and Interpersonal Issues in Our Offices

The first steps to take involve looking at the structure of the office and considering how to minimize discomfort. These steps include creating a teen-friendly space and creating spaces where all teens are welcomed and are not labeled merely by walking in the door. For example, a program that serves HIV-infected or substance-using youth can be imbedded in a larger center that welcomes all youth (see Chapter 12).

Far more important than the décor on the walls or the structure of the center are the people who work there. The adolescent's experience begins well before they see the helping professional. It begins with the telephone receptionist and continues with the front desk and other support staff (see Chapter 12).

We can offer professional development opportunities that reinforce the importance of being uniformly respectful and consistently sensitive to all aspects of diversity. Include mental illness in discussions about acceptance of diversity. The offerings have to pay particular attention to body language, privacy, and labeling. All members of the service team need to be reminded to refer to people by name rather than by their conditions (see chapters 15 and 19).

We need to remind youth that no one in our offices except for team members who care for them directly know any of their private information (see Chapter 14).

■ Our Own Attitudes and Interactions

We can reduce the potential for a teen feeling shamed or stigmatized in our office when we

1. Earn their trust, ensure that we serve without judgment, and guarantee privacy.
2. Work to recognize our unconscious biases.
3. View risk in the context of existing strengths.
4. Avoid labeling.
5. Refrain from separating the mind from the body.

Making Ourselves Trustworthy

Youth, especially those with experiences of marginalization, may not easily trust an adult. They may assume that a professional will judge them or reinforce negative messages they have previously received about their emotions or behaviors. Before we can reasonably expect youth to disclose their private information, we need to earn their trust through our words, body language and, most importantly, actions (see chapters 14 and 15).

Recognizing Our Unconscious Biases

We all have unconscious biases. They exist to simplify our lives, and, in some cases, to protect us from imminent harm. They allow us to navigate dangerous environments without needing to formally process or analyze. The challenge is that this type of thinking can form the basis of prejudices (ie, prejudgments) that can harm our relationships with people and perpetuate shame and stigma.

We sometimes use heuristic (intuitive, automatic, implicit) reasoning in order to create quick judgments. When the use of intuition alone (even if it is based on epidemiologic data or past experiences) dominates problem-solving, it may preclude the analytic, innovative, or creative thinking required to make clear diagnoses and accurate decisions.[11] (See Chapter 21.)

Youth who have ample experience with judgments may quickly grasp when a professional is avoiding thorough consideration because of predrawn conclusions and may interpret it as being dismissive of their concerns. This may prevent full disclosure and interrupt the engagement process. Further, it may reinforce shame or even generate hostility.

Ask yourself without self-condemnation how you might react differently to each of the pairs of scenarios.[12]

> A 16-year-old boy is using marijuana regularly. His mother is wearing a knit sweater and has well-groomed hair.
>
> A 16-year-old boy is using marijuana regularly. His mother is wearing a long sleeved tee shirt with a large motorcycle logo and is missing several teeth.

Might you make different intuitive conclusions about why the teen is using drugs?

> A 15-year-old girl from an urban area of concentrated poverty has lower abdominal pain.
>
> A 15-year-old girl from a suburban area has lower abdominal pain.

Might they receive different evaluations?

> A 12-year-old white girl has a black eye. She nervously explains that she fell down the steps. She is present with both parents.
>
> A 12-year-old African American girl has a black eye. She nervously explains that she fell down the steps. She is present with both parents.

Might you consider the possibility of abuse differently?[12]

It may not be possible, or uniformly beneficial, to remove all of our unconscious biases. But it is necessary to be aware of them so that they do not interrupt the delivery of outstanding service delivered without shame (see Chapter 19).

■ Addressing Risk While Recognizing Strengths

One of the strongest rationales for shifting toward a strength-based model is that it decreases the potential for shame in our interactions. Rather than focusing on risk, it sees risk in its context. It understands that much of risk is, in fact, a person's effort to navigate stress and the complexities of life. It strives to learn how to maximize the opportunity for each teen to contribute to the world. It sees risk, therefore, as something that needs to be addressed so that the person can meet their full potential. It sees emotional distress as something that needs to be managed so that the person can fulfill their promise.

The technique described in Chapter 25 can be particularly helpful in setting the tone of your interactions. First, it ensures that you put the problem in context and that the young person knows you also recognize her strengths. Perhaps more importantly, it asks you to reframe how you see risk-takers. You can reject drug use entirely as terribly dangerous, but know that drug users tend to be among our most sensitive youth who use substances to numb their acute ability to feel. You can abhor gang affiliation, but know that gang members are seeking safety and have a tremendous capacity for loyalty. You can grasp how destructive teen pregnancy can be to the chances that a young girl will break the cycle of poverty and still be moved by her desire to share her love.

It is not just that these positive perspectives allow you to initiate an intervention from a different lens; these strength-based outlooks will subconsciously flavor your interaction style with youth. It may serve to modify your unconscious biases. When a young person knows that a professional genuinely holds him with positive regard, there is less reason to feel ashamed or stigmatized. In turn, he may feel less demoralized and be more likely to join in a positive change process (see Chapter 25).

■ Who's the Expert?

When we recognize that each teen is the expert on her own life, we implicitly recognize her strength and minimize the shame that comes from feeling as if she is being "fixed." This does not mean that we believe that teens hold all of the solutions, or are blind to their struggles and the poor decisions they sometimes make, rather it positions us as facilitators who support them as they consider how best to navigate their world (see Chapter 4). It means that we see youth as problem-solvers rather than as problems to be solved (R. Little, personal communication, March 5, 2012).

Motivational interviewing is one technique that recognizes that the behavioral change process is most successful when driven by the teen. The teen determines her readiness to change and makes her own decisions to move forward after considering the benefits of current behaviors versus those of potential changes.[2-4] In sharp contrast to experiencing shame, when she arrives at a solution she can take pride in owning the path forward.[13] (See Chapter 26.)

■ A Person-Centered Approach That Avoids Labels

Generally, we must refrain from using labels to categorize people. When diagnoses are needed to get appropriate medication or services, we must help teens understand that the diagnosis represents only a small description of who they are. They are individuals who have problems; they are not problems. All staff need to consistently call people by names rather than use shorthand diagnoses.

Labels can have a lasting impact on individuals' self-perception and on the manner in which adults, other youth, institutions, and communities interact with a teen. Think for a moment of how you respond to a teen labeled with conduct disorder versus if you were told that he had been traumatized and can sometimes be reactive. You need to protect yourself from the teen with a conduct disorder, whereas you likely would want to be supportive to the traumatized youth and choose to have a particularly empathetic, sensitive, and calm demeanor (see Chapter 22).

▶ **33.2, 33.3**

> I cared for a homeless young woman, who I will call "Teresa" here. Teresa hoped to be a counselor one day. She reported that at one time or another she had been diagnosed with depression, bipolar disorder, obsessive compulsive disorder, conduct disorder, schizophrenia, multiple personality disorder, and post-traumatic stress disorder. She also listed more than 10 medical disorders, all of which caused different types of pain. She shared a history of abuse too horrific to describe here. She had been off of her multiple medicines for months and was sad, but engaging.
>
> I asked for permission to give her one more label. She was hesitant, but reluctantly agreed. *"You are Teresa. That's all, you are Teresa."*
>
> She wept for 20 minutes.
>
> After she collected herself, we were able to together describe who Teresa was— A survivor of terrible abuse who was wise enough to learn how to remove her thoughts from her daily realities. A strong young woman who wanted to heal others. A woman whose emotional pain was running through her body—the pain was real, but her body was healthy. Teresa was a woman who could be whole. She was a young woman who deserved the kind of emotional treatment that would allow her to heal from a past no child should have endured. She was Teresa. Nothing more. And being Teresa was a good thing, because the very pain she had endured was going to position her to help others. First, she would commit to healing herself so that she could more comfortably serve others.

■ Recognizing That the Body and Mind Are Part of an Integrated Whole

The body often manifests stress. This has been understood for millennia, and different cultures and healing practices have often explained many physical symptoms in the context of the body and emotions being out of balance. A healing approach that recognizes that the body and mind are connected can explain symptoms without needing any explanation that could be misinterpreted as the caregiver believing the teen is "faking" or that her symptoms are "in her head." A paradigm that integrates the body with the mind is inherently less shameful and allows a teen to join in a healing process that attends to both psychological and physical care (see Chapter 44).

It may also be worth framing emotional and mental health issues, when reasonable, as biochemical or biological conditions. For example, substance use, many mental health conditions, and eating disorders during times of starvation can be framed as biochemical issues. It can be helpful to explain to youth that they have a treatable condition. Our goal in treatment, whether we use medication, therapy, exercise, or a combination of the 3, is to restore chemical balance.

However, because these conditions may have begun as a choice (eg, substance use) it is important not to take a purely biochemical approach. Youth have to understand they do have choices and their actions can make a difference. Explain that the brain is very complex and that, even with a chemical condition, the power of the mind can be pivotal in restoring other parts of the brain to balance. Therapy, for example, is known to help even in many mental health conditions known to be biochemically mediated. Intensive group support strategies, such as Alcoholics Anonymous or Narcotics

Anonymous, can be highly effective even though substance use is known to be a chemical condition.

33.4

■ Addressing Parents Attitudes and Concerns

Parental attitudes about emotional struggles or behavioral problems can contribute to stigma. Following are some key points that may serve as conversation starters:

- Negative parental attitudes about an issue (eg, substance use, homosexuality) might serve as a barrier to teens getting needed support.
  — If you have any mixed feelings about an issue your child is struggling with or about seeking professional help, I strongly suggest you try to resolve them before talking to your teen. He will pick up on your emotions easily and become even more ashamed or resistant to getting help. If you genuinely believe that seeking professional help is a positive move, your adolescent is more likely to see it that way.

- Parents need to be supported to understand that though they may strongly disapprove of a behavior, their children must never feel rejected.

- Parents need to understand to never lower their expectations for their children because core to resilience theory is that youth live up or down to our expectations. The worst outcome of a parental reaction may be a teen feeling she has nothing to lose if she spirals further into negative behaviors.

- We need to help parents continue to see what is going well in their child's life so they do not lower their expectations.

- If parents begin to see their teen's problem as defining her, the teen will incorporate that as her self-image and begin relating to the parent through that persona. This process may make the teen learn that in order to get parental attention, she needs to behave in this "expected" manner.

- It may be helpful for you to support parents to see problems in the contexts of strengths. The classic example here is that some of the most sensitive, thoughtful young people mask their emotions through drugs. We must address drug use, while recognizing how the youth's sensitivity will serve her well later.

You have a role in diminishing parental shame and guilt as well. It is important to take an "agnostic" approach when you serve families. For too long, parents were held responsible for a wide range of conditions, including autism, that we now know conveyed humiliating and damaging messages to parents. The truth is that we often do not know whether or not parents contributed to a problem, but we do know that (with rare exceptions) they can be a vital part of the solution. Further, when a teen does reach the limits of her resilience, she has to deal with a sense of inadequacy. It is important that she not also have to deal with the feeling that she is somehow letting her parents down. Following are some conversation starters:

- Parents need to understand that we must never believe resilience means invulnerability. All people, even the most stable, reach their limits sometimes. It is not a sign of weakness on the teens' part, nor is it a sign of poor parenting, when children show their human limitations.

- Parents need to let go of the fantasy that their teens will be able to handle everything if they parent effectively. If they view their adolescent's problems as a reflection of them, they won't be able to help them through tough times because they will have to work through their own feelings of failure.

- Specifically, parents do not need to feel guilty for missing their child's depression. Many parents are very attentive to signs of depression but make the mistake of believing that adolescent depression appears the same in teens as it does in adults. Adults who are particularly sad or depressed tend to have sleep disturbances, become withdrawn, lack energy, seem to have a lower capacity to experience pleasure, and often express hopelessness. This is true of some adolescents, but nearly half are irritable instead of withdrawn. They may have boundless energy and are likely to act out with rage. It is sometimes difficult for parents to tell a normal teenager from a depressed one because most teenagers have phases where they're irritable at home and have occasional outrageous outbursts. Because parents may have adjusted to this moodiness, they can miss a teen whose rage and irritability are signals of emotional turmoil or depression.

- Rather than feeling ashamed of needing help, parents need to become comfortable with their role. They need to reinforce that they are there to be fully supportive, listen, be a sounding board, and perhaps even offer advice. They need their children to know that their most important source of security remains constant. Then, with no sense of failure, they need to understand that it may be time to turn to professional help. Many parents have to work through their own disappointment that their child needs something more than they can give. They may need help reframing it as an act of love, not of failure. They love their child so much that they will get whatever help she needs to be able to thrive.

- Parents will often be angry that their teen did not include them earlier. Remind parents that sometimes precisely because of fear of disappointing them, teens often mistakenly shield them from their realities. Reinforce that their involvement now is critical and that their child desires that involvement; and that speaks highly of their relationship (see Chapter 37).

Perhaps most importantly, parents have a critical role in modeling help-seeking and healthy coping mechanisms. They need to understand that during this trying time, the most important thing they can do is remain strong. Their teen will need them over the long term, and self-care is both strategic and critical (see Chapter 39).

■ Communicate With Youth About Seeking Further Help

We've focused on how aspects of our interactions can mitigate stigma and avoid shame (Box 33.1). The focus here is on guiding youth to take the next steps in seeking help.

It can be tough to guide a teenager to agree to seek professional guidance. Adolescents may feel ashamed that they can't handle their own problems and worry that going for help confirms they are weak or "crazy." It is important for adolescents to understand a few key points about help-seeking.

1. Emotional distress is treatable, and we know how to support teens so that they can feel better.
2. Seeking help is an act of strength because strong people know they are capable of feeling better, deserve to feel better, and will take the steps to feel better.
3. Professionals do not pity the youth they serve; they serve because they want to.
4. Professionals honor privacy and strive to serve without judgment.
5. Professionals do not give answers or solve problems, but instead try to find the strengths of each person and build on them. They will solve their own problems, but will have the support to do so.

Treatment Can Work

"What good will it do? It's just gonna waste my time."

A major barrier to seeking help can be a youth's perception that *"It wouldn't help anyway."* Remember that hopelessness can be an element of depression. It may be hard for a young person to see the light at the end of the tunnel. Or she may have seen others

Box 33.1. Strategies to Reduce Shame and Stigma

Structural and Interpersonal Issues in Our Offices
- Create a teen-friendly space.
- Imbed services for special groups within larger teen-serving centers.
- Prepare staff to sensitively honor all aspects of diversity.
- Refer to all youth by name; never use diagnoses for shorthand.

Reflect on and Adjust Our Own Attitudes and Interactions
- Ensure attention to privacy and commitment to serve without judgment.
- Recognize your unconscious biases.
- Always view risk in the context of existing strengths.
- Recognize that teens are the experts in their own lives.
- Avoid labeling.
- Use an approach that integrates the body and mind.

Work Effectively With Parents
- Use an agnostic approach that does not assume they are the problem.
- Reassure them you see them as important parts of the solution.
- Help them to gain insight on their own attitudes about the problem.
- Help them understand the importance of seeing help-seeking as a positive step forward.
- Remind them of the importance of continued high expectations.
- Help them to focus on their teen's strengths.
- Guide them to model positive coping strategies.

Communicate With Youth About Seeking Further Help
Help youth understand
- Treatment works.
- Seeking help is an act of strength.
- Privacy is ensured.
- Professionals do not have pity; they wish to serve.
- Professionals do not solve problems; they facilitate teens to become better problem-solvers.

fail repeatedly. It may be that the most important thing you can do on an initial visit is to reinforce that treatment can work and is worth investing in.

Seeking Treatment Is an Act of Strength, Not of Weakness

 33.1, 63.5

"I can handle it."

Here it is critical that friends, family, and community do not undermine the change process by framing help-seeking as a sign of weakness. A first step is for the young person to know that she deserves to feel better. It can be an act of tremendous bravery and conviction to clearly state, *"I don't feel like everything is right, and I deserve to feel better."* Here, it can also be helpful to state why you so deeply want her to feel better. This can be much easier when you have recognized her strengths and know how she is poised to contribute. For example, you might state that the very sensitivity that plagues her now is what positions her to have a full life later.

Empathy Is Not Pity

"I don't need any pity."

No one wants to be pitied, and teens may make assumptions that professionals will look down on them. They need to understand that we choose to work with youth because we care for and respect youth.

It may be that the most effective thing you can do is suggest the young person experience service herself. Youth experiencing problems may benefit from service opportunities because it will help them put their problems in perspective and reinforce for them that despite their problems they can still make contributions. Further, the ultimate act of resilience is to turn to another human being in times of extreme need and say, *"Brother or sister, I need a hand."* This is never easy, but may be necessary. When young people experience service, they will learn that it feels good to give. People who contribute to others' well-being don't feel burdened or put upon, they feel honored to have been in the right place at the right time, perhaps with the right training. They often get more than they give. People with this experience may be able to turn to others more freely because they're equipped with the understanding that the person guiding them through troubled times is there because he or she wants to be there, not out of pity. ▶ **31.5**

Privacy Is Guaranteed

"I don't want to tell someone my business."

Youth need to be reminded that honoring privacy is central to the care of adolescents. They also need to understand the limits of privacy. Finally, they need to know that our goal is to put together the best team to support them, and that we'll find someone who is respectful and will honor their privacy (see Chapter 14).

Counseling Is About Guidance, Not Being Repaired

"I'll figure it out. I can solve my own problems. No one else knows what I've been through anyway."

Adolescents should understand they will only be guided to become stronger by using skills they already have and new ones that they will be taught to put into place for themselves. They should understand that counseling is a learning process that offers new information that will empower them to make good decisions.

Counselors can

- Help restore trust.
- Help you learn how to better communicate your thoughts and feelings.
- Help you learn forgiveness.
- Help you to free yourself of guilt and feel better about yourself.
- Help you find ways to begin to repair or improve your relationships.
- Help you take control of thoughts that can produce anxiety or other uncomfortable feelings.

Counselors are there to support you, but you do the heavy lifting.

•• Group Learning and Discussion ••

Many of the concepts included in this chapter (see Box 33.1) are covered in greater depth elsewhere. Therefore, the group learning process here will focus on guiding youth to seek help without shame or stigma. First, share as a group what "pearls" have worked for you in supporting youth to seek further help. Also, discuss cases that have gone awry and debrief on what you think may have gone wrong. Then break into pairs and use the following cases to practice helping youth be receptive to your suggestion that they seek further support.

Use the following key points as well as some of the "pearls" generated by your group:

- Treatment works.
- Seeking help is an act of strength.
- Privacy is ensured.
- Professionals do not have pity; they wish to serve.
- Professionals do not solve problems; they facilitate teens to become better problem-solvers.

The following cases are offered with few contextual details. This is so you can fill in the details based on your experience with the population you serve. Alternatively, use your own cases.

Case 1: A 16-year-old boy, Noah, is brought in by his father because he has been acting out at home and his father is at the end of his rope. The boy has always been a good student, but his grades have been dropping sharply. He says he just doesn't care about school. He has been having frequent headaches in the last couple of months.

Case 2: A 14-year-old girl, Phoebe, is brought in by her mother. She says that she has no problems at all, everything is fine. She gets straight As, is the captain of her travel soccer team, and plays the violin. Her mother is worried that she is getting lazy and that will interfere with her success. She notes that her daughter almost got a B in biology and just doesn't seem to practice her violin enough to make the high school orchestra. She is worried Phoebe will never get into college. In a private conversation, Phoebe admits that she is sleeping poorly, especially the night before tests. She worries about going blank on her tests, so she stays up very late studying every night. She has belly pain almost every day. She knows that she is smart, she has been told she is brilliant from the time she was very young. She worries she won't do as well in high school, and she doesn't want to disappoint her mother.

Case 3: A 15-year-old girl, Taylor, is brought in by her mother and grandmother. She has been cyberbullied by a group of girls who have focused on her weight and have said that she was "available" to any guy who was willing to have her. She has been staying home from school for the last week because she hasn't been feeling well. In your interview you learn the bullying has been going on for a year, but that Taylor forgets about it all when she self-mutilates.

Case 4: A 15-year-old boy, Jameel, comes in for a routine visit. His mother dropped him off and has no concerns. In a SSHADESS screen, he seems very uncomfortable around questions about sexuality. At first, he smiles nervously, but then becomes tearful. He is worried he might be gay. He does not know anyone at school or in the neighborhood who is gay. He feels alone. He could not imagine sharing his confusion at this time with anybody.

Case 5: A 13-year-old girl, Lin, lost her grandmother 4 months ago. Her grandmother lived 2 blocks away and was a tremendous source of strength to her. She cried for 2 days and then her parents and friends told her that she just had to get past it. She admits that she still thinks about her grandmother every day. Her biggest problem now is that she and her mother just aren't getting along. She said her mother's not the same anymore. Her mother says that she is moody and angry most of the time.

▪▪▪▪▪▪▪ Continuing Education ▪▪▪▪▪▪▪

If you are applying for continuing education credits, a test is available online. For more details, visit www.aap.org/reachingteens.

References

1. Weiss MG, Ramakrishna J, Somma D. Health-related stigma: rethinking concepts and interventions. *Psychol Health Med*. 2006;11:277–287

2. Livingston JD, Milne T, Fang ML, Amari E. The effectiveness of interventions for reducing stigma related to substance use disorders: a systematic review. *Addiction*. 2012;107(1):39–50

3. Heflinger CA, Hinshaw SP. Stigma in child and adolescent mental health services research: understanding professional and institutional stigmatization of youth with mental health problems and their families. *Admin Policy Ment Health*. 2010;37(1-2):61–70

4. Pescosolido BA, Martin JK, Lang A, Olafsdottir S. Rethinking theoretical approaches to stigma: a framework integrating normative influences on stigma (FINIS). *Soc Sci Med*. 2008;67:431–440

5. Mukolo A, Heflinger CA, Wallston KA. The stigma of childhood mental disorders: a conceptual framework. *J Am Acad* Child *Adolesc Psychiatry*. 2010;49(2):92–103

6. Cunningham SD, Kerrigan DL, Jennings JM, Ellen JM. Relationships between perceived STD-related stigma, STD-related shame and STD screening among a household sample of adolescents. *Perspect Sex Reprod Health*. 2009;41(4):225–230

7. Puhl RM, Heuer CA. Obesity stigma: important considerations for public health. *Am J Public Health*. 2010;100(6):1019–1028

8. Dalky HF. Mental illness stigma reduction interventions: review of intervention trials. *West J Nurs Res*. 2012;34(4):520–547

9. Schachter HM, Girardi A, Ly M, et al. Effects of school-based interventions on mental health stigmatization: a systematic review. *Child Adolesc Psychiatry Ment Health*. 2008;2(1):18

10. Heijnders M, Van Der Meij S. The fight against stigma: an overview of stigma-reduction strategies and interventions. *Psychol Health Med*. 2006;11:353–363

11. Hicks EP, Kluemper GT. Heuristic reasoning and cognitive biases: are they hindrances to judgments and decision making in orthodontics? *Am J Ortod Dentofacial Orthop*. 2011;139(3):297–304

12. Lane WG, Rubin DM, Monteith R, Christian CW. Racial differences in the evaluation of pediatric fractures for physical abuse. *JAMA*. 2002;288(13):1603–1609

13. Miller WR, Rollnick S. *Motivational Interviewing: Preparing People to Change*. New York, NY: Guilford Press; 2002

▪ Related Video Content

33.0 Helping Youth Overcome Shame and Stigma (and Doing Our Best to Not Be a Part of the Problem). Ginsburg, Feit.

33.1 Asking for Help Is a Sign of Strength. Sugerman.

33.2 Psychiatric Labels Can Reinforce Stigma. Chafee.

33.3 Seeing Youth as More Than a Label or a Disease—The First Step Toward Healing. Arrington-Sanders.

33.4 Helping Youth Understand That Talking Literally Makes Them Feel Better. Kinsman.

14.9 Making Inroads With Youth Who Put Up Barriers. Arrington-Sanders.

24.0 Among the Hardest Things We Do—Delivering Bad News. Ginsburg, Reirden, Arrington-Sanders, Garofalo, Hawkins, Pletcher.

31.5 Stress Management and Coping/Section 4/Making the World Better/Point 10: Contribute. Ginsburg.

34.3 Preparing Youth to Disclose Difficult Personal Information to Parents. Reirden, Hawkins.

37.0 Delivering Upsetting News to Parents: Recognizing Their Strengths First. Ginsburg.

63.5 Seeking Help Can Be an Act of Strength. Lemmon.

65.8 Shame and Stigma as a Toxic and Persistent Force in Serving HIV-Positive Youth. Reirden, Hawkins, Dowshen, Arrington-Sanders.

Supporting Effective Parenting

It is likely the connection to responsible adults who believe in youth unconditionally and hold them to high expectations is the pivotal determinant of whether a youth will thrive. Ideally, that connection is to parents. When it is, then we professionals add an extra layer of protection. When it is not, then our role takes on even greater importance.

Despite the popular assumption that teens reject their parents' views entirely, it is parents who have the greatest influence on teens. We professionals may do our greatest good by supporting the parent-adolescent connection and by guiding parents on how to most effectively make use of that connection.

Reaching Teens offers a wide variety of communication strategies that are directed to professionals but that can certainly be passed along to parents. Further, the importance of building trustworthy

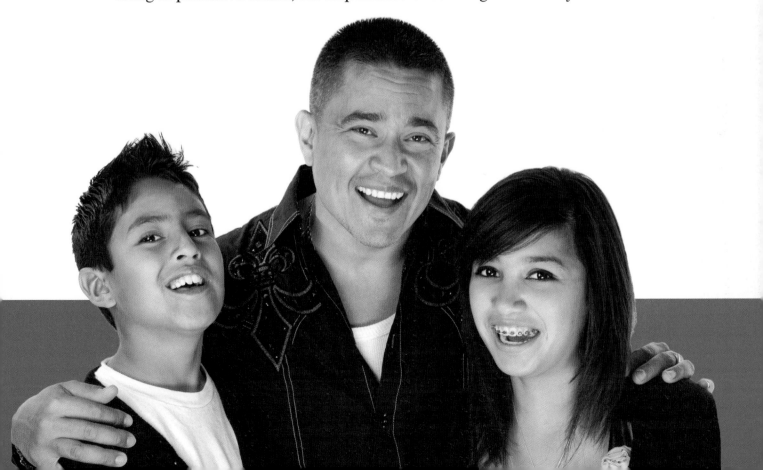

partnerships with parents is highlighted in many chapters. However, this section focuses specifically on how you might consider communicating with parents about (1) raising healthy teens; (2) maintaining strong, nurturant connections with their adolescents; and (3) caring for themselves while they care for others.

In the first chapter in this section (Chapter 34), Dr Ford sets the tone by reinforcing the importance of a professional-parent-teen partnership. "Preparing Parents for Their Children's Adolescence" (Chapter 35) suggests that looking forward to adolescence with a sense of dread will create a self-fulfilling downward spiral. It also outlines a strategy that will help parents learn to honor adolescents' growing independence, and, therefore, hopefully prevent part of the rebellion associated with the teen years. Next, "Promoting Balanced Parenting: Warmth, Clear Boundaries, and Effective Monitoring" (Chapter 36) will help you guide parents toward a parenting style that has been demonstrated to be associated with greater academic success and lower risk among a wide spectrum of behaviors. "Delivering Upsetting News to Parents: Recognizing Their Strengths First" (Chapter 37) offers a strategy to engage parents so they can support their children to navigate through challenges. It focuses on doing so without shame or stigma, and while recognizing the parents' strengths and their critical role in their teen being able to move forward. "When Parents' Resilience Reaches Its Limits" (Chapter 38) recognizes that parenting a teen can be difficult, and that moments of anger and exhaustion are expected. It emphasizes that especially during those times, parents need to make the effort to renew strong connections with their teen. Finally, "The Importance of Self-care for Parents" (Chapter 39) reminds us that parents of this generation often sacrifice themselves in order to give to their children. We professionals have a critical role in reminding parents that they need to put their oxygen masks on first. They are the role models of healthy adults, and the greatest gift they can give their child is demonstrating wise decision-making, healthy coping strategies, and living a balanced life that cares for others along with self.

CHAPTER 34

The Professional-Parent-Teen Partnership

Carol A. Ford, MD, FSAHM

 Related Video Content

34.0 Four Approaches to Wrapping Up the Visit: All Committed to Informing and Engaging the Parent While Maintaining Teen Confidentiality

■ Why This Matters

Parents sometimes feel that they are raising their teenagers alone. The relationship between a parent and adolescent child is absolutely unique, and the strength that an adolescent gains from this relationship is fundamental to healthy growth and development. Nonetheless, particularly when adolescents are going through difficult times, or when communication between parents and adolescents becomes challenging, or when—quite simply—parents are worried, it is important for them to realize that they are not alone in the work of raising healthy, resilient adolescents. Professionals can often play a critical role in helping parents to keep their teenagers on track in life and thriving. These professionals may include teachers, coaches, clergy, social workers, police, health care professionals, and a variety of other adults who routinely come into contact with teenagers in the course of their life and work. Sometimes the "professional" is a parent of one of their adolescent child's best friends.

> **The relationship between a parent and adolescent child is absolutely unique, and the strength that an adolescent gains from this relationship is fundamental to healthy growth and development. It is important for them to realize that they are not alone in the work of raising healthy, resilient adolescents.**

▶ 34.8

This chapter will describe a model for how professionals can work with parents to support the healthy development of their adolescents and minimize the risk of negative health and behavioral outcomes. This model was developed based on research focused on parents, adolescents, and health care professionals, with this group of professionals broadly defined as physicians, psychologists, nurses, and social workers. It is a model that may be useful to the wide range of professionals who regularly interact with teenagers and parents outside of the world of health care and traditional clinic settings.

■ Background

Before the age of 10, the vast majority of communication in clinic settings typically occurs between health care professionals and parents on behalf of the child's health. As children enter adolescence, health care professionals are encouraged to start spending at least part of each visit privately with adolescent patients to help them learn about and take increasing responsibility for their own health and health care needs in preparation for adulthood.[1] This is also the decade during which competent adolescents gain increasing legal authority to obtain health care on their own.[2] The challenge for health care professionals is to provide respectful and developmentally appropriate care, which sometimes includes providing confidential services, without losing the extraordinary potential of parents to influence favorable adolescent health outcomes. How can we best work with parents to improve adolescent health without betraying the trust of our adolescent patients or clients as they grow up? This is a general question that will resonate with many professionals who work with adolescents outside of health care settings.

To better understand how health care professionals might meet this challenge, a formative research project was conducted that involved interviews with a diverse group of parents, experienced adolescent health care professionals (physicians, nurses, social workers, and front desk receptionists), and adolescents.[3,4] The study was designed to learn parents' perspectives on what health care professionals do, or could be doing, to support them in their role as parents who are, of course, highly invested in the health of their own adolescents. It was also designed to learn the perspectives of experienced adolescent health care professionals regarding what they do, or could be doing, to more closely work with parents to support healthy adolescent development and health. Finally, we presented the perspectives of parents and clinicians to groups of adolescents who were asked to reflect and comment on the perspectives of parents and clinicians, and to provide their ideas about how parents and clinicians can best work together to help adolescents stay healthy and get the care they need. The major themes that we heard and strategies that may help to increase alliances between parents and professionals to reach the shared goal of adolescent health are summarized in Figure 34.1.

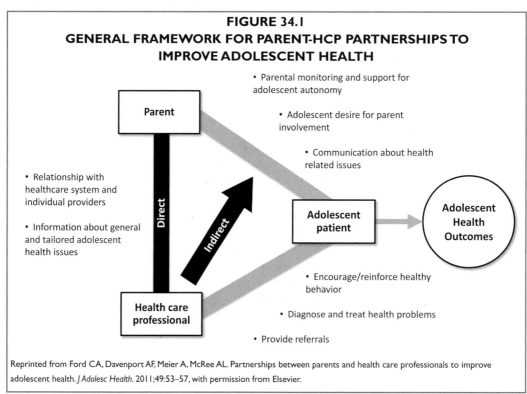

FIGURE 34.1
GENERAL FRAMEWORK FOR PARENT-HCP PARTNERSHIPS TO IMPROVE ADOLESCENT HEALTH

- Parental monitoring and support for adolescent autonomy
- Adolescent desire for parent involvement
- Communication about health related issues
- Relationship with healthcare system and individual providers
- Information about general and tailored adolescent health issues
- Encourage/reinforce healthy behavior
- Diagnose and treat health problems
- Provide referrals

Parent
Direct
Indirect
Health care professional
Adolescent patient
Adolescent Health Outcomes

Reprinted from Ford CA, Davenport AF, Meier A, McRee AL. Partnerships between parents and health care professionals to improve adolescent health. *J Adolesc Health.* 2011;49:53–57, with permission from Elsevier.

What Parents Do to Keep Their Adolescents Healthy

When asked what parents can do to keep teens healthy and address health problems, the most common themes we heard from parents were monitoring and keeping their teens busy. One parent reported, *"We try to monitor their friends. We know how they look, and who they're going out with. We try to pay attention to the way they act. If it doesn't seem right, we have to pay attention."* Parents also discussed the value of keeping teens busy, involved in activities, and making sure that they have enough things scheduled to avoid excessive boredom. Many parents discussed the importance of parent-teen communication, such as making sure they take the time to really listen to their adolescent, talk "with them" rather than "at them," and give them encouragement. Parents also reported that the work parents do for adolescents, such as providing nutritious food, opportunities for sports, and health insurance all influence adolescent health. They discussed the importance of parents being a good example for a wide variety of behaviors that influence adolescent health. One-third discussed the importance of parents being able to ask for and accept help from a health care professional when they needed it.

It seemed clear that the parents in this study recognized that a wide range of activities typically considered the "work of parenting" is important in protecting adolescent health and well-being. Some of these activities are strongly correlated with adolescent health in the research literature (eg, parental monitoring, providing a positive role model, parent-teen communication, health insurance). The value of professionals explicitly acknowledging and encouraging parenting activities shown by research to improve adolescent health outcomes may be one important strategy for strengthening parent-professional partnerships to build adolescent resilience and improve health. For parents struggling with feelings of guilt or stigma because their adolescents are engaging in "bad behaviors," it may be especially useful for professionals to acknowledge the hard work parents do to try to keep their adolescents "on track" and to also remember to congratulate them for seeking help (see Chapter 37).

What Professionals Do to Keep Adolescents Healthy—From Parents' Perspective

When asked what health care professionals can do to keep teens healthy and address health problems, the most common theme reported by parents focused on the importance of teenagers being able to openly communicate so that professionals can get an accurate assessment of an adolescent's behaviors and health. For example, one parent reported, *"My daughter might be able to talk to a doctor or a nurse, if she can't talk to me. She might be able to talk to a doctor about anything and not feel stupid. They (doctors) have to be respectful, open to discussing rather than just discounting things. You run into doctors that won't listen, or they just want to write a teenager off. They can't have that kind of attitude. They need to see beyond the obvious. They have to be sure that they don't shame the child or make them feel uneasy or bad. I don't think at this point I have to worry about the sexual issues and stuff, but they (doctors) should be open, try not to be judgmental, but to guide the teen."* A few parents explicitly commented that they thought it was helpful for professionals to learn about things that parents might not know about, but which might impact their child's health. Parents also discussed the importance of professionals *"telling teenagers what they are doing right, and when they are doing a good job."* Other themes were consistent with making diagnoses, providing treatment, and making appropriate referrals.

34.1

■ Strategies to Increase Parent-Professional Partnerships to Improve Adolescent Health

Parents were able to describe the developmental complexities of parent-clinician communication during the second decade of a patient's life. One parent described this complexity, but also how a health care professional can directly or indirectly partner with a parent to work toward the shared goal of adolescent health:

> *Keep an open line of communication with me as the parent as much as possible without breaking confidentiality. If the child wants confidentiality, keep it, but if it's not a confidential issue, then the doctor and parent should let each other know what's going on. Keep an open door there. Or encourage the child to talk to the parent if there is an issue. Basically, communication within reason, and if the child does want confidentiality, encourage the child to talk to the parent.* ▶ **34.0**

Building Direct Professional-Parent Partnerships Within Clinical Settings

When children have been taken care of within a primary care home, there is often an existing relationship between health care professionals and a parent by the time the child reaches adolescence. There are, however, many other situations where an adolescent will be seen by a professional who may not have an existing relationship with the parent, such as in emergency departments, school-based health centers, specialized adolescent clinics, family planning or sexually transmitted infections clinics, and nontraditional community sites targeting high-risk youth. Regardless, to the extent possible, it is often useful to involve parents in supporting your efforts to address the adolescents' health and behavioral issues, and one way to do this is to try to build a bond with the parent. You share common ground, which is an alliance to promote the health and well-being of one specific adolescent.

Parents described strategies to strengthen relationships between parents and professionals with comments such as, *"Recognize that I know something about my child, and listen to me and tell me about how to help my child. Doctors and nurses can give written material to me and my child. Parents and health care providers can keep in contact with each other."* Adolescents reported that, *"Doctors and nurses can tell parents to get kids checked regularly. Education is key, not just of teens but parents too. If parents know more and are more comfortable, teens would be more likely to go to them for help."*

Building Indirect Professional-Parent Partnerships Within Clinical Settings

There are times when health care professionals will need to keep sensitive information disclosed by adolescent patients confidential because of professional recommendations, laws, and ethical standards of care.[2,5–7] This is important to increase the likelihood that adolescents will seek health care and will openly communicate with professionals in a position to address their needs. Although these scenarios may preclude direct communication between a clinician and a parent, when clinicians use their unique relationship with adolescents to reinforce the contribution parents make to promoting adolescent health, and encourage parent-teen communication, they are indirectly partnering with parents in an effort to improve adolescent health even when the parents are not present.

For example, within the context of private visits, professionals can discuss and help adolescents see the value of parental support, involvement, and monitoring, and they can also encourage and facilitate parent-adolescent communication. Professionals may also be able to develop strategies to convey messages about adolescent health issues to parents in a way that provides tailored parental guidance while also respecting adolescents' desires for confidential care when appropriate. For example, a professional can generally encourage parent-adolescent communication about dating and romantic relationships, without disclosing confidential information about adolescent sexual behaviors.

Professionals, parents, and adolescents all provided examples of how clinicians can build partnerships with parents, even when they are seeing adolescents alone.

- Professional: *"I try to teach the child good communication skills and I encourage them to experiment with that at home and see what happens with their parent as a result."*
- Professional: *"If it helps for that patient to be able to talk with their parent with us in the room, we'll do that. We'll set up a meeting with the parents and bring them on in and then discuss what the kids want to discuss, but they just kind of need that little, I guess, increased comfort to be able to take that leap with their parents."*
- Parent: *"Doctors should encourage the child to talk to the parent. For example, if a child gets pregnant, I know there are restrictions with confidentiality, but it would be good if they could offer to have the parent come in and talk together. They could act as a buffer."*
- Adolescent: *"Doctors should let parents know that it is okay for teens to get checked regularly and that it is okay for them to do some of that on their own."*
- Adolescent: *"They can encourage teens to have other adult support as well, people they can relate to if not their parent, just so there is somebody."*

Building Community-Level Professional-Parent Partnerships

Professionals can also develop partnerships with parents outside of clinic settings that focus on improving adolescent health and well-being. Parents, professionals, or health care systems can work together to increase general community awareness of adolescent health issues, advocate for effective prevention strategies, and improve relationships between parents and systems providing adolescent health care or other services. One clinician reported, *"Parents say 'I need help' and help is available, but they don't know how to link to that help. And I think, as health care professionals, one of our goals is to make help in the community more visible and assist parents to navigate the system to get it."* One parent described an example of parent-professional partnerships at the community level as follows: *"Doctors and nurses and parents should go to the school board and let them know there should be more in-depth training and health education in schools."* An adolescent provided the following example: *"Kids' doctors should have educational sessions for parents about health topics and parenting teenagers. Maybe even community support groups."*

■ Final Thoughts

Although the research project described focused on health care professionals and clinic settings, the model and themes that emerged highlight the importance of all professionals considering how we can better align with parents to support adolescent resilience and health. For many professionals, the question will be, *"How can I do this?"* The following chapters offer concrete strategies to forge this essential partnership, including a focus on supporting parents through these sometimes challenging times.

The opportunity to influence professional-parent-adolescent partnerships in a way that leads to improved adolescent resilience and health is extraordinary, and this is an opportunity we do not want to miss.

•• Group Learning and Discussion ••

This chapter focuses on the potential benefit of a real partnership between professionals, parents, and teens. Other chapters will build just a few of the strategies that may make that partnership most effective. Here, however, is an opportunity for your group to discuss whether or not it will take a philosophical shift to build this partnership.

To benefit from the potential power of this partnership, the expertise of each member must be valued. Some practice settings may be so adolescent-focused that a parent might feel marginalized. Conversely, some practice groups are primarily child-focused, and teens might feel limited in expressing their autonomy. The principle of adolescents being the experts in their own lives may be a novel one in some settings. (If this is the case in your setting, see Chapter 4.)

Your group should reflect on the "culture" of your setting and discuss what steps might need to be taken to more actively engage either parents or teens as partners. If your group thinks that it already has a culture that promotes this partnership, you might spend your professional development session building some of the specific strategies discussed in the next chapters.

■■■■■■■ Continuing Education ■■■■■■■

If you are applying for continuing education credits, a test is available online. For more details, visit www.aap.org/reachingteens.

■ References

1. Hagan J, Shaw J, Duncan P. *Bright Futures: Guidelines for Health Supervision of Infants, Children, and Adolescents*. 3rd ed. Elk Grove Village, IL: American Academy of Pediatrics; 2008

2. English A, Bass L, Boyle AD, Eshragh F. *State Minor Consent Laws: A Summary*. 3rd ed. Chapel Hill, NC: Center for Adolescent Health & the Law; 2010

3. Ford CA, Davenport AF, Meier A, McRee AL. Parents and health care professionals working together to improve adolescent health: the perspectives of parents. *J Adolesc Health*. 2009;44(2):191–194

4. Ford CA, Davenport AF, Meier A, McRee AL. Partnerships between parents and health care professionals to improve adolescent health. *J Adolesc Health*. 2011;49(1):53–57

5. Ford C, English A, Sigman G. Confidential health care for adolescents: position paper of the Society for Adolescent Medicine. *J Adolesc Health*. 2004;35(1)

6. Gans J. *Policy Compendium on Confidential Health Services for Adolescents*. Chicago, IL: American Medical Association; 1993

7. American Medical Association Council on Scientific Affairs. Confidential health services for adolescents. *JAMA*. 1993;269(11):1420–1424

■ Related Video Content

34.0 Four Approaches to Wrapping Up the Visit: All Committed to Informing and Engaging the Parent While Maintaining Teen Confidentiality. Ford, Pletcher, Diaz, Sugerman.

34.1 Professionals Support Parents by Creating a Space Where Teens Can Receive Caring, Objective Guidance Without Fear of Judgment or Punishment. Diaz.

34.2 Guiding Parents and Teens to Understand the Shifting Balance Between Parental Control and Teen Decision-Making. Sugerman.

34.3 Preparing Youth to Disclose Difficult Personal Information to Parents. Reirden, Hawkins.

34.4 Professional and Parent: Insight From Having 2 Roles With Teens. Ford.

34.5 Addressing Worrisome Behaviors and Addictions: Partnering With Parents to Create Safe and Appropriate Boundaries. McAndrews.

34.6 Case Example: Guiding a Parent and Teen to Work Together to Address Substance Use. Sugerman.

34.7 Helping Parents Know When to Worry and How to Initially React. Sugerman.

34.8 Helping Parents Understand the Additive Role Professionals Can Play in Their Adolescents' Lives. Jenkins.

36.6 Case Example: Supporting Balanced Parenting: Guiding a Teen to Navigate Through a Serious Internet Error. Sugerman.

37.0 Delivering Upsetting News to Parents: Recognizing Their Strengths First. Ginsburg.

37.1 Parental Involvement Is Critical to Helping Teens Navigate Through Crises. Ford.

56.2 Case Example: Helping a Teen Navigate an Unhealthy Relationship. Sugerman.

CHAPTER 35

Preparing Parents for Their Children's Adolescence

Kenneth R. Ginsburg, MD, MS Ed, FAAP, FSAHM

 Related Video Content

35.1 The Benefit of Allowing Our Children to Deal With Challenges

■ Why This Matters

Some parents approach their children's adolescence with a sense of foreboding. Because young people live up or down to the expectations set for them, assumptions that adolescence is a time of "storm and stress" can be undermining to teens' healthy development and to the critical connection between parent and child.

Professionals can play an important role in reinforcing that adolescence is, in fact, a time of great potential. By reframing this stage as a time when growth and increasing independence should be celebrated, we can alleviate some parental anxiety and position parents to more effectively guide their children.

> **Assumptions that adolescence is a time of "storm and stress" can be undermining to teens' healthy development and to the critical connection between parent and child. By reframing this stage as a time when growth and increasing independence should be celebrated, we can alleviate some parental anxiety and position parents to more effectively guide their children.**

■ Preparing Parents

Many topics may merit discussion with parents as they prepare for their children's adolescence. Following are some key areas you might consider covering either in person or through making resources available. Some of these topics are covered in depth elsewhere and will be presented very briefly here, while others will receive full attention in this chapter.

Adolescent Development

Adolescence is a time of rapid physical, psychological, emotional, moral, and social growth. That makes it an exciting time filled with great possibilities. However, it is also a time when parents may experience insecurity as the child they have known rapidly changes. Parents equipped with an understanding of adolescent development may feel better prepared to meet the challenges and to celebrate the changes.

Core to parents being able to support their child through moments of angst and confusion is their understanding of the 2 fundamental questions of adolescence: *"Who am I?"* and *"Am I normal?"* When they grasp the magnitude of these 2 questions, they may better be able to empathize with why adolescence can sometimes be so challenging to navigate. Further, when they understand adolescent development, they will better be able to proactively answer their children's ever-present, but usually unasked, questions and to communicate with them in a way that their adolescents will understand (see Chapter 8).

Helping Parents Understand the Core Principles of Resilience

Every parent wants his or her child to thrive and to be able to handle adversity. If parents understand the core principles of resilience, they will grasp how much parents matter. Three essential themes describe how adults can build children's resilience: (1) unconditional love is the bedrock of resilience because it generates security; (2) teens meet adult expectations, for better or worse; and (3) youth watch what we do more than they listen to what we say.

Let's look at these themes more closely.

- Unconditional love gives youth the deep-seated security that allows them to take chances when they need to adapt to new circumstances and the knowledge that in the long run they will be okay. Teens must never worry that their parents have diminished their love or concern, even when they dislike or disapprove of their behaviors. Unconditional love doesn't mean unconditional approval. The young person is not the behavior. Love is never withdrawn or threatened to be withheld based on a behavior. Teens need to know that their parents are not going anywhere, no matter what. Parents need to be clear that they love the child they have, rather than somehow communicating that their adolescent has to be fixed or improved. Hopefully parents will be the source of this essential ingredient of resilience, but others can also fill that role. The more supportive adults there are in a young person's life, the more firmly rooted and unshakeable is his or her security. **35.5**

- Teens live up or down to their parents' expectations. If parents expect the best, kids tend to live up to those standards. High standards really matter, but, by high standards, we are not focusing on achievements. These standards refer to being a good human being—considerate, respectful, honest, fair, generous, and responsible. When parents expect their teens to be lazy, argumentative, thoughtless, selfish, or dependent, kids sense those negatives. *"Why,"* they figure, *"should I try to be any different?"*

- Young people also absorb messages from peers and the media and change their behavior to meet those expectations. Sometimes these messages support a positive image. Other times parents must shield their teens from harmful portrayals of youth and low expectations and consistently advocate for more positive portrayals so that teens have a prosocial sense of what is "normal."

- As adolescents' most powerful models, parents are in the best position to teach them about stress and resilience. Teens observe parents closely, particularly how they manage and navigate through difficulties.

Maintaining Control of Their View of Adolescents: Ignoring Popular Images…the Media…and Even Friends and Neighbors

It is not surprising that parents have a sense of dread about their children's adolescence. The media is filled with popular images of teenagers at risk. The news rarely has feel-good stories about the contributions young people are making to our communities. The talk shows don't have discussions on the pleasures of parenting adolescents. Even friendly conversations on the sidelines of soccer games tend not to focus on the simple joys of parenting. Instead, they naturally gravitate to more "interesting" conversations on the challenges adolescence offers. As a result, the parents of tweens begin to assume their children will also be trouble and begin to mourn the loss of childhood and fear the advent of adolescence. Children pick up on this anxiety and may begin to paint a distorted picture of what a "normal" adolescent looks like and thereby live down to those expectations. For this reason, it becomes imperative that parents of tweens receive positive messages about adolescence and are even told to ignore the parents of teens who are blowing off steam and to instead engage in serious conversations with families who have well-functioning, contributing teens. Advise parents that the next time a friend tells them, *"Uh-oh, she's 12, put on your safety belt,"* to smile and say, *"I'm ready for the ride. There will be some bumps, but I expect her to come through just fine. She has already shown me what a fine person she is."*

35.7

Helping Parents Understand How Much They Matter

Although there are popular notions that parents become relatively insignificant during adolescence compared to peers and media, they remain the most important force in their children's lives. The following is written to remind parents of their critical role and to reassure them that, although adolescents may reject them, they are still highly valued. I use the same metaphor in a practice setting.

But Do We Matter?

To begin to grasp the challenging developmental work your teen is facing, imagine a table covered with 10,000 pieces of a jigsaw puzzle. The puzzle is titled "Who Am I?"—the fundamental question of adolescence. Not realizing he has a lifetime to complete the puzzle, he ferociously tackles it because he believes he needs to get it done by the time he graduates from high school or even by the time he writes his college essay.

How does someone put together a puzzle? One begins with the corners and then creates the borders. Only once the borders are in place does a person have the confidence to work out all of the pieces in the middle—occasionally trying to force together those that don't quite seem like a natural fit.

It is the boundaries you create and the monitoring you insist on that creates those trustworthy borders that your teen can push against as he tries to manipulate the harder inner pieces on his own.

Once the borders are securely in place, what is the next step of putting together an impossibly complex puzzle? One looks for matching pieces and imagines how the patterns might fit together. A wise person looks at the picture on the lid—over and over again.

You are the picture on the cover your child compares himself against. When teens have a role model of what healthy adults looks like, it becomes easier for them to complete their own puzzles.

The good news is that our teens can be so darned loveable and cuddly moments after they are, well...not quite so endearing. Remind yourself, especially during those moments when you are feeling less than fully appreciated, that you are critical to your child completing his "puzzle." How can he be expected to answer the question *"Who am I?"* if he doesn't have you serving as a role model and offering those boundaries from within which he can safely stumble.

36.3

Occasional Rejection Is to Be Expected—Take It as a Backward Compliment

It is challenging to parent an adolescent. It is easy for parents to feel pushed away by their teenagers. After all, it's not uncommon for them to tell parents that they can't stand their presence.

We need to remind parents that their children sometimes hate them precisely because of how deeply they really do love them and resent how much they know they need them. They need to fly from the nest. Who would want to fly from a warm, cozy, and comfortable nest? They have to imagine it as prickly at best, maybe even uninhabitable. They have to figure out who they are—identity development is the task of adolescence. The first step of teens figuring out their own identities is to prove themselves different from their parents. In order to know how different they are from parents, they sometimes have to see them as offensive, as hopelessly embarrassing at the very least. Adolescents need parents to be invisible with their friends because kids see themselves in their parents' faces and mannerisms and have enough trouble managing their own behavior without also having to worry about how their parents' actions reflect on them.

Knowing How to Listen So Teens Will Talk

So many parents will start questions with, *"What do I say when…?"* This positions you to respond, *"It is less important what you say, and more important that you listen."* Then cover 3 key topics.

1. Turn off the "parent alarm." Listen without judgment and reaction. When your son says, *"Mom, I met this girl"* and you react by saying, *"You're too young to date,"* that instinctual alarm prevented you from being able to hold a meaningful discussion on healthy sexuality. **35.2, 35.6**

2. Don't catastrophize. When teens come to their parents with concerns, they need a calming, rational presence that will create a safe space for them to figure things out. When parents make it seem worse than they had imagined, they leave more anxious and won't return.

3. Don't over empathize. Adolescents need a sounding board. Sometimes they exaggerate; sometimes they express fleeting feelings. When you over empathize, it can heighten their emotions and make you look naïve or overly involved. Imagine your empathizing by condemning their friend who your daughter had a fight with. You'll look "wrong" the next day when your daughter is best friends again with the girl she hated yesterday. **35.8**

Knowing How to Talk So Their Children Will Hear

Teens are happy to hear their parents' values and opinions, but these opinions should not be shared in a way that feels judgmental or condescending and should try to avoid personal territory that will position a teen to need to become defensive of friends or self.

Parents who lecture are not heard. The lecture is often condescending or hostile, and is delivered with an abstract string of possibilities loosely tied together. Young adolescents are still not thinking abstractly, and all teens who are upset or in crisis mode will not absorb lessons delivered abstractly. Parents may increase their yield if they are able to convey their wisdom in a more concrete manner that adolescents can follow. This topic is covered fully in Chapter 28.

Knowing Their Importance in Teaching Values

Parents may shy away from talking about the "big" topics like sex and drugs. It is important that they understand that they can be the very best teachers. They might benefit from your referral to credible resources both for their own education and for their teen's use. If they remain uncomfortable with specific content, reinforce that they are the most credible and important sources of values education. For example, the mechanics of sex can be taught in health class or through a book, but only they can best teach the values that inform healthy, respectful relationships. Remind them that when they choose not to do so, they abdicate this role to peers, the media, and the Internet.

Finally, reassure them that raising a topic, such as drugs or birth control, does not give tacit approval. To the contrary, it allows their children to learn about something under their safe guidance and to be reminded that they are the source of information and are consistently available to help them navigate through challenges.

Parents' Role as Guide and Monitor

Ultimately, the parents' job is to launch their children into adulthood safely and headed toward a future where they can earn a living and contribute to society. A large body of evidence demonstrates that an authoritative (or balanced) style of parenting decreases risk behaviors and positions youth to be more successful in school. This style balances warmth, support, and responsiveness with effective discipline and monitoring. It is also known that the key to monitoring is not asking young people what they are doing but having the kind of relationship, communication style, and discipline strategies that make teens choose to disclose to their parents. This topic is covered fully in Chapter 36.

Success

Our goal has to be to raise children who will be successful 35-year-olds. That means we want them to have those traits they will need to thrive in the workplace and in relationships. We need them and others in their generation to be prepared to lead us into the future. This means we need our young people to be hard working, to be compassionate and generous, to be socially and emotionally intelligent, to be receptive and responsive to constructive criticism, to be creative and innovative…and to be resilient.

Hard work and tenacity drive success, because effort is what brings ideas to fruition.

Compassion and generosity is what it will take to repair the world and serve others.

Social and emotional intelligence are what foster empathy and collaboration, and collaboration breeds success.

The ability to respond to constructive criticism with self-improvement and without defensiveness fosters personal and career growth.

Creativity and innovation are what it will take to generate the best ideas, especially those that only people who can think outside of the box will produce.

Resilience is what it takes to navigate life's bumps and bruises and to thrive 48.1 through good times and bad.

Preparing Parents to Teach Peer-Navigation Tools

Young people may know the right thing to do and still do what their friends are doing. Although this can be maddening for parents, it makes more sense when teens are understood in the context of trying to figure out if they are "normal"—a key question central to identity development. Teens may be more likely to do the right thing when they have the skills to both make safe decisions *and* save face with their friends. Therefore, parents may increase the yield of their guidance if they also teach their children peer negotiation and navigation skills. These strategies are covered in Chapter 41. Parents may increase their empathy toward the complex world their adolescents are trying to navigate if they are reminded of what that environment looks like (see Chapter 9). 41.1

Joining With Other Parents

Because youth want to be "normal," they tend to casually accept rules that others also need to adhere to and reject those that seem unique to them because they view them as overly restrictive or controlling. Professionals can encourage parents to join with the parents of their teen's friends and the broader community so that more young people have the rules and boundaries they set for their teen. Adolescents who see these boundaries as normal have no reason to rebel against them.

Role as Disciplinarian

The word *discipline* means to teach or guide. It doesn't mean to punish or control. Parents who discipline successfully see discipline as an ongoing responsibility to teach. The best disciplinarians (or teachers) hold high expectations for children and give appropriate consequences, or allow them to occur naturally, rather than dole out arbitrary punishments when children fall short of those expectations.

Parents can be guided, *"The key to achieving this balance is to honor her growing independence by giving her freedoms in a measured way. You'll keep your eye out for safety, but always with the goal of giving her increased privileges that match her growing displays of responsibility. She'll demonstrate the responsibility you insist on both to please you and to gain privileges. She'll appreciate your guidance when it is clear that its goal is to help her develop the skills and strategies to ultimately navigate the world on her own."* (See Chapter 36.)

Honoring Growing Independence

We can remind parents of the following:

It is an adolescent's job to gain the confidence to be able to stand on his or her own. As challenging as it is to watch our children grow up, it is critical to their well-being and to the health of our relationships that we honor their growing independence. When we hold them back, they rebel against us. When we monitor their safety while guiding them toward independence—sometimes actively and sometimes by getting out of the way—they appreciate us. When our children know that we supported them to become independent, they will soon return to us for that *inter*dependence that defines loving families well beyond childhood.

It is everyday issues, even seemingly mundane ones, that trigger most parent-child struggles and offer opportunities for fostering independence. Teens might think they should be allowed a new privilege just because they're a certain age or because their friends are doing it, but they might lack the skills needed to manage the situation. When parents focus on preparing their adolescents, they can turn potential sources of conflict and rebellion into opportunities for their children to master new skills and demonstrate responsibility.

Adolescence is naturally filled with opportunities for trial and error and ultimately success. Our challenge is to make sure adolescents learn from day-to-day mistakes rather than view them as catastrophes. At the same time, parents need to be vigilant in helping teens avoid those errors that could cause irreparable harm. On the other hand, if they are overprotective, it will limit opportunities to gain valuable positive life experiences and to make those mistakes that offer the chance to learn how to rebound, recover, and move on. Parents should want teens to make errors while still under their watchful eye when they can offer the life lessons that build enduring resilience.

The answer to when a teen is ready to meet a new challenge is when there are enough pieces in place so the chances for success are enhanced. A request by a 14-year-old to spend the afternoon at the mall won't hinge on answering on the spot, *"Is she old enough?"* if she has been taught, in part through example, about spending wisely and treating clerks with respect. The day teens begin to drive won't be so nerve-wracking if parents have modeled safe driving behaviors and made it clear they will monitor their teen's progress even after licensure. Parents won't have to hold their breath on their child's first date if they have raised him or her to have self-respect, the skills to recognize and respond to pressure, and the knowledge of self-protection.

Parents should start by doing some observing. *"Think back to when you baby-proofed your home. If you just guessed what needed safeguarding, you might have missed some opportunities to protect your baby. The first step was to walk around on your knees and see the surroundings at the same level as your toddler. Once you saw the world from his vantage point, you knew to turn that pot handle inward. That same sort of observing—getting a 'kid's eye view' of the mall or the route to school—will heighten your senses about the challenges your teen is likely to encounter. You'll be better prepared to think of how best to phase in new privileges and what kinds of emotional support as well as monitoring need to be in place to help things go smoothly."*

It is important to use a step-by-step approach to allow teens to succeed, sometimes recover from failure, and then demonstrate they're ready to assume more responsibility. It starts by understanding the environment they will need to navigate. Parents will be so much better prepared to offer practical guidance if they have observed the reality their children will face, rather than have only a fantasy of what it might look like. Next, their ability to individualize guidance rests on their considering their adolescent's temperament and unique developmental needs. The next step involves listening. When parents listen respectfully to what their adolescents think they can handle, they are better prepared to develop a plan. We must guide parents to approach these conversations with the attitude that, even though their teens remain young, they are still the greatest expert on themselves.

Finally, guide parents to generate a roadmap with their adolescents of each step that needs to be mastered to gain the skills and confidence that will prepare the teen to meet the overall challenge. Teens need to understand that they will continue to gain more independence and privileges as long as they continue to demonstrate responsibility. When they know that their parents' goal is to help them ultimately get to their goal, ▶ **35.3** they'll be much less likely to complain about monitoring.

Practicing a No-Nag Zone

Parents' resilience will reach their limits at times, and even the best parents may have moments when they don't like their children very much. It is at these moments that they need to give themselves the opportunity to fall back in love with their children, this means leaving the stagnant and destructive cycle of efficiency so many parents have developed during the teen years when they focus their increasingly limited time on "high-yield" conversations like school and behaviors and forget to just "be" with their children and enjoy them as they did in earlier years. Remind parents that their son who might smell quite badly and talk back to them is the same person who used to make them laugh when he burped out loud and who gave them endless joy when he ran to them as they arrived home. Invite parents to create instant vacations where their kids have nag-free zones where they can reconnect—no high-yield discussions, just fun, moments at the park or around dinnertime where defensiveness is never raised and everyone's better selves are evident. For a deeper discussion, see Chapter 38.

■ Model Coping and Self-care

Parents need to be prepared for the fact that there may be moments that their adolescents just don't seem to be listening to what they are saying. It is our job to remind parents that teens never stop watching what they do. In fact, sometimes kids can't hear the words we say because our actions are deafening. For this reason, if no other, parents need to model healthy coping strategies, positive behaviors, help-seeking when appropriate, and self-care. Further, they need to do so to maintain the strength to care for others. Further still, they need to do so to model what a healthy adult looks like, to be the picture on the box. Of course, they also need to care for themselves because they are humans who deserve to feel good, but, if they can't hear that message, stay focused on the fact that self-care is a selfless act. See Chapter 39 for a richer discussion.

Many of these concepts are adapted or excerpted from Dr Ginsburg's recent books for parents. Ginsburg KR, Jablow MM. *Building Resilience in Children and Teens: Giving Kids Roots and Wings.* 2nd ed. Elk Grove Village, IL: American Academy of Pediatrics; 2011 and Ginsburg KR, Fitzgerald S. *Letting Go With Love and Confidence: Raising Responsible, Resilient, Self-Sufficient Teens.* New York, NY: Avery Press, Penguin Books; 2011.

•• Group Learning and Discussion ••

This chapter serves as a "landing page" for many other topics covered in greater depth elsewhere. The concepts uniquely covered here involve the parent grieving the loss of childhood and the importance of them understanding that, even when being actively pushed away, they continue to matter.

The importance of each of us reflecting on our own adolescence to understand why we react to certain youth or circumstances was discussed in the chapter on boundaries (see Chapter 20). Here, for those among you who are parents of preteens or teens, it may be worth reflecting on our own occasional, but real, feelings of inadequacy. It is likely that even though we are professionals who work with adolescents we sometimes wonder whether we matter. It is common for adolescent-professionals with their own adolescents to sometimes feel like "imposters" because they struggle with their own teens.

If your group has members with their own adolescents, use this opportunity to discuss these feelings. Otherwise, you can be nearly certain that they will flavor the interactions you have with teens and families. If your group does not have parents of adolescents, then consider practicing how you can best help the parents you serve know how much they will continue to matter.

■■■■■■■■ Continuing Education ■■■■■■■■

If you are applying for continuing education credits, a test is available online. For more details, visit www.aap.org/reachingteens.

■ Suggested Reading

Ginsburg KR, Jablow MM. *Building Resilience in Children and Teens: Giving Kids Roots and Wings.* 2nd ed. Elk Grove Village, IL: American Academy of Pediatrics; 2011

Ginsburg KR, FitzGerald S. *Letting Go With Love and Confidence: Raising Responsible, Resilient, Self-Sufficient Teens.* New York, NY: Avery Press, Penguin Books; 2011

■ Related Video Content

35.1 The Benefit of Allowing Our Children to Deal With Challenges. Sugerman.

35.2 Even During Your Toughest Parent-Teen Moments, Remember That Your Teen Loves You so Much, It Hurts. Sugerman.

35.3 Raising Independent Children Who Will Choose to Be Interdependent With Us. Ginsburg.

35.4 The Teen Brain: A Balancing Act Between Thoughts and Emotions. Catallozzi.

35.5 The Power of Unconditional Parental Love to Help Teens Get Through Even the Hardest of Times. Vo.

35.6 Why Teens Push Us Away: "I May Not Know Who I Am, But I Sure Know I'm Not You!" Sugerman.

35.7 Ignore the Negative Hype About Teenagers: Expecting the Best From Adolescence Will Pay Off. Ginsburg.

35.8 Listening: The Key to Guiding Your Child. Ginsburg.

35.9 Thoughts on Parenting: The Voice of Adolescents. Youth.

36.2 Parental Involvement: Balancing Consistency and Flexibility. Campbell.

36.3 The Critical Role of Continued Parental Involvement During the Teen Years. Campbell.

41.1 Peer Negotiation Strategies: Empowering Teens AND Parents. Ginsburg.

48.1 Raising Children Prepared for Authentic Success. Ginsburg.

48.2 Using Praise Appropriately: The Key to Raising Children With a Growth Mind-set. Ginsburg.

48.4 Because We Need to Learn How to Recover From Failure, Adolescence Needs to Be a Safe Time to Make Mistakes. Ginsburg.

■ Related Handouts/Supplementary Materials

Avoiding Conflict: The Use of "I" Statements in Parenting Adolescents

Building the 7 Cs of Resilience in Your Child

Listening: The Key to Effective Communication between Parent and Child

Parent Involvement: The Key to Helping Teens Make Wise Choices

Stop Lecturing: Guiding Adolescents to Make Their Own Wise Decisions

CHAPTER 36

Promoting Balanced Parenting: Warmth, Clear Boundaries, and Effective Monitoring

Kenneth R. Ginsburg, MD, MS Ed, FAAP, FSAHM

 Related Video Content

36.0 Balanced Parenting: A Key to Adolescent Success and Healthy Behaviors

■ Why This Matters

Although parents of adolescents sometimes mistakenly adopt the belief that only peers matter to adolescent behavior, they are key to promoting positive behaviors in youth. Research clearly demonstrates that youth who have warm, supportive parents that set and monitor clear boundaries have better educational and behavioral outcomes. Professionals can play an important role in reinforcing the benefits of engaged parenting throughout adolescence.

> **Youth given clear boundaries and parental supervision are less likely to engage in violence, substance use, and early initiation and engagement in sexual activity. They are more likely to wear seatbelts and less likely to use substances while driving, to speed, and to crash. Finally, they are less likely to be delinquent and more likely to do well in school.**

■ Background

One framework used to study the effect of engaged parents is the "parenting style" model based on the work of Baumrind[1] and Steinberg and colleagues.[2] It creates 4 categories from the interplay of control (monitoring and rules) and support (warmth and responsiveness). Responsiveness refers to engaging youth in back-and-forth discussion and reacting with flexibility to their needs and concerns. Parents are described as (1) authoritarian (low support and high control), (2) permissive (high support and low control), (3) uninvolved (low support and low control), or (4) authoritative (high support and high control).[3]

Parents have the best interest of their children in mind and may be repeating the style they were raised with or that they believe produces children most prepared to meet challenges. Therefore, it is important not to label any style as right or wrong, and instead to guide parents toward a balanced approach to parenting—one that both gives support and ensures appropriate control through effective monitoring. ▶ **36.0**

- **Authoritarian parents** set high expectations for their children, but may expect conformity and reject questioning authority. A typical response of an authoritarian parent may be, *"Why? Because I said so."* Authoritarian parents may be highly involved and view rules as the expression of parental love. They are less likely to communicate warmth or caring. Their teens may miss the opportunity to learn how to problem-solve and take ownership of decisions. They may become rebellious to confront their parents' hard-line approach.
- **Permissive parents** are generous with affection and eager to please their children. They teach values, but often fail to make demands or establish boundaries. They instead communicate, *"I trust you to make good decisions."* Permissive parents sometimes believe being friends with their children will ensure ongoing communication. Children of permissive parents often have to create their own boundaries. They generally want to please their parents by behaving well but are motivated largely by a fear of disappointing their parents. This can lead them to withhold information from their parents.[4]
- **Uninvolved (or disengaged) parents** provide their children with few rules, little monitoring, and inconsistent emotional support. In some cases, a parent's lack of involvement is due to overwhelming demands in other areas of their life. Some adopt the attitude, *"Kids will be kids; they need to learn through their own mistakes."* They may enforce new rules and punishments when their children get into severe trouble. Because they get the most attention when in trouble, children of uninvolved parents might behave poorly to get desired attention.
- **Authoritative (or balanced) parents** offer a balance of warmth, support, and monitoring. These parents support movement toward independence while setting reasonable boundaries with clear expectations and consequences. Authoritative parents are flexible and responsive, they listen to their teen's viewpoint and encourage them to make choices and solve problems. But, when safety is involved, they have clear rules. *"I care about you, and I'll give you the freedoms you earn, but for safety-related issues you'll need to do as I say."*

Research demonstrates balanced parenting promotes positive behaviors and psychosocial well-being in youth.[3,5] Youth given clear boundaries and parental supervision are less likely to engage in high-risk, worrisome behaviors,[6] including violence,[7] substance use,[1,8,9] and early initiation and engagement in sexual activity.[10] They are more likely to wear seatbelts and less likely to use substances while driving, to speed, and to crash.[11] Finally, they are less likely to be delinquent[12] and more likely to do well in school.[2,13] Adults raised by authoritative parents report greater psychological well-being and fewer depressive symptoms.[14]

■ Promoting Engaged and Effective Parenting

You can encourage authoritative parenting in a way that does not alienate parents with different styles. The goals should be to (1) help parents understand how much their involvement matters, (2) encourage effective monitoring, and (3) support parent-child relationships that minimize rebellion and encourage disclosure and open communication.

Starting the Conversation

Because validated parenting style assessment tools may be too long for routine office use, consider open-ended questions that allow you to get a feel for a parents approach.

- *"A lot of people think that as children approach adolescence parents have very little power because kids only care what their friends think. Others think that kids continue to care very deeply about what parents think. What are your thoughts about how much influence parents have over their kids as they get older?"*

- *"Do you talk at home about things like school performance, drug use, and sexuality? What are those conversations like? What are your thoughts about rules and boundaries for kids?"*

You can then share that, despite what it may feel like sometimes, research demonstrates that teens do care about their parents' opinions and actually crave boundaries.[15] Boundaries give them opportunities to test their own limits while still knowing a safety net is in place. Adolescents that perceive parental warmth, support, and monitoring are more likely to approve parental authority, to call on parents for advice and support, and to obey parental commands.[16,17] ▶ **36.3**

Inviting Parents to Consider Learning About Next Steps: Effective Monitoring and Communication Strategies

- **To a parent you suspect is authoritarian:** *"It is wonderful that you give clear rules and boundaries. Kids crave boundaries, even when they pretend they don't. You know kids often think we make rules just to control them, so it is important they know that you make rules because you care about their safety and well-being. Would you like to learn about some strategies research has shown actually make it more likely for kids to follow your rules?"*
- **To a parent you suspect is authoritarian:** *"It is good that your child knows exactly where you stand. I want him to continue to follow your rules. A lot of times, children hide from parents when they sneak around those rules. One of the most important things you can do is bend the rules or make an exception when your son makes a really good case and has demonstrated responsibility. That way, he'll learn to keep discussing things with you because he'll have the experience that proves to him that you are fair and only have safety in mind. Would you like to talk more about this?"*
- **To a parent you suspect is permissive:** *"It is nice to see how much you value a close relationship. It is clear that trust is an important part of your relationship. How do you feel about still setting and monitoring clear boundaries? That way, he'll be clear about exactly what you expect of him. Would you like to learn a little more about this?"*
- **To a parent you suspect is permissive:** *"I admire how much the 2 of you value your ability to talk with each other. Would you like to talk about some strategies that have been proven to actually keep kids and parents talking even through some tough times?"*
- **To a parent you suspect is disengaged:** *"I'll bet your child really benefits sometimes from your philosophy that life is full of lessons and sometimes he has to learn them for himself. At the same time, though, it is important that he is clear that you set limits to protect him from anything that might actually affect his safety. Do you agree? Would you like to talk a little bit more about this?"*
- **To a parent you suspect is disengaged:** *"As much as life teaches lessons, sometimes the best lessons are taught when parents share their thoughts/wisdom/experience. I hear how much you've been through. Have you ever been able to take the time to set aside your worries and just be together as a family?"*
- **To a parent you suspect is authoritative:** *"It sounds like you are pretty committed to both supporting your child emotionally and to making sure she is protected with clear boundaries. This balanced approach to parenting is really protective to kids. Does your spouse agree with your philosophy? Do you want to talk a bit more about strategies to make sure your daughter is even more likely to tell you about what is going on in her life?"*

■ Monitoring Strategies That Work

Parents have been told for many years about the importance of consistently asking where their teens are, who they're with, and when they will be home. These questions remain important. However, our understanding of monitoring has expanded in recent years to reveal that it is less about what parents ask and more about what rules adolescents choose to follow and which behaviors they decide to disclose to their parents.[18–20] Further, research offers a better understanding on how to frame limits, rules, and boundaries so they will be more acceptable and, therefore, presumably more likely to be followed.[4] Similarly, we have an expanded understanding of what makes it more likely adolescents will disclose their whereabouts and actions.[4,21]

Making It About Safety, Not About Control (and *Not* About Friends)

The first challenge is to give clearly defined rules and boundaries in a way that is acceptable to children. Judith Smetana and colleagues[20,21] have explored what adolescents consider "legitimate authority" of parents and substantiate that parents really only know what their teens choose to tell them. In general, adolescents believe parents are obligated to be involved with their safety and have a responsibility to guide them how to interact with society, including respecting others' rights and following the law. However, they do not believe parents should transcend on personal territory. They may see issues about their friendships or personal behavior that doesn't affect their safety as out of bounds.[21]

This informs us how parents should consider presenting rules and boundaries. It must be clear that rules exist to preserve safety—they are neither "random" nor created to "control" them.[17] Ideally, they will know that the caring adults in their lives honor their growing independence and recognize their developing skills and competencies. They also need to understand that while some rules are "always" or "never" rules, most exist until teens' demonstrated experience and responsibility indicate they need less supervision.

Parents can be guided to frame rules and boundaries about safety whenever possible. If they condemn their teen's friends, they transcend into personal territory and may make their company more enticing.

- Parents shouldn't say, *"I don't want you to go to Sophie's house because I think she's a bad influence on you."* But they can say, *"I worry about you going to a house where parents aren't home—it's a safety issue for me."* Parents can be guided to listen with minimal reaction when information about friends is shared. After careful listening and thought, parents can then reframe their concern to be about safety rather than connecting it directly to the friend.

Teen driving serves as a useful example of how to frame a situation to be about safety instead of about control or friendships. Peer passengers in the car make a new driver much more likely to crash because they create a heightened emotional environment where teens lose focus and, therefore, are distractions.[11,22] This is not about misbehavior but rather about the undivided focus young drivers need.

- If a parent says, *"You can't have any friends in the car while you're driving,"* the teen may react, *"My friends are my business, why do you hate them so much?"* and determine to secretly take them regardless of their parents' wishes. The alternative statement for parents is, *"I care about your safety, and teen passengers distract new drivers, so you can't drive with passengers until you've had at least 6 months' driving experience."* This way, the conversation is in legitimate territory—safety—and stays away from the personal domain.

- Parents can go further to explain that boundaries are flexible and will change as responsibility is demonstrated. A teen may respond, *"That might be because other kids act wild; my friends just sit there and we talk."* The parent could respond, *"Actually, you know I like your friends, but everyone gets excited when they're having a good time. New drivers can't keep their focus on the road, control the car, and have friends in the car. This is a firm, nonnegotiable rule, but it's also temporary. When you get more experience driving, and you've proven you're responsible in the car, you can drive your friends. For now, you're going to continue building your driving skills, and when you want to go somewhere with friends, I'm glad to drive all of you."*

Keeping Teens Talking—The Keys to Disclosure

Effective monitoring depends on back-and-forth communication. Parents can ask the where, when, and who questions, but they actually only *know* what is going on when their teens tell them. The first key to keeping teens talking is for parents to learn to be effective listeners. When parents react with quick judgment or condemnation, teens stop talking. Further, when every roadblock is solved by parents, adolescents that have a strong desire to arrive at their own solutions may stop talking.

▶ 35.8

Many parents dread the arguments of adolescence, but arguments represent engagement, and continued engagement is a key to effective monitoring. Nancy Darling and colleagues[4] have found that adolescents raised in permissive households do not disclose their thoughts or behaviors in an effort to spare their relationship with their parents. Permissive parents may assume their friendly style of parenting diminishes the barriers of communication, making it more likely their teens will disclose. In fact, they often withhold information rather than risk disappointing their parents. They don't view this as lying, just as sparing their parents. On the other hand, youth raised with the authoritative parenting style, where they received both warmth and boundaries, were most likely to disclose.[4]

The work of Darling and colleauges[4] also supports the idea that parents should be flexible around rules in order to keep their children continually engaged. This is part of the responsiveness considered key to authoritative parenting and absent from authoritarian parenting. They point out that parents should have clear rules and acknowledge those rules sometimes generate discussion, even arguments. These arguments represent engagement, a "verbal wrestling" of sorts, and are far better than silence or lying. In fact, conflict may be healthy as it can result in increased agreement over time.[23] When young people make a reasonable case for an exception to the rules or for an expanded scope of freedom, and have demonstrated responsibility, it is worthwhile for parents to demonstrate flexibility. This way, adolescents learn that reasonable negotiation pays off and will continue engaging with their parents.[4]

■ The Benefits of Group Rules and Norms

One of the fundamental questions for older children and adolescents is, *"Am I normal?"* Sometimes they will make unwise decisions to prove they are normal. If they are given clearer or stricter boundaries than their friends, they may feel as if they are being treated unfairly or even rebel. On the other hand, when parents work together to create common expectations, teens do not feel like they are being treated differently and may be more likely to comply with the rules.

■ Discipline

Discipline is a vital part of monitoring for adolescents. It is important to remind parents that the word discipline means "to teach"; it does not mean to control. In fact, effective discipline increases a young person's sense of control. This is best done when adolescents learn that the freedoms and privileges they receive are directly linked to the responsibility they demonstrate. For a deeper dive into one recommended style of discipline for adolescence, link here to an edited excerpt from *Building Resilience in Children and Teens: Giving Kids Roots and Wings,* published by the American Academy of Pediatrics in 2011.

■ Talking Points

There are several ways to discuss the importance of effective communication about rules and boundaries.

- Reinforce that **parents should trust their own reactions.** You may say, *"Anytime your gut tells you that you're dealing with a safety issue, trust that feeling and act on it to create protective boundaries."*

- You can help parents recognize that one of the best ways they can protect their teens is to **get to know the parents of their friends.** This may help parents be more comfortable calling to check in and confirming plans. You may suggest that parents develop common rules within their community—or at least between a few households—so that adolescents are less likely to feel they are unreasonable.

- Rules are so important for safety. They tell teens their parents care enough to protect them. However, as children grow older, they may begin to see the rules as parents attempt to control them, and ultimately may reject those rules. You may help parents **reframe discussions about rules so they are more clearly focused on safety:** *"It's so important you tell your children that the rules exist for their safety. Let them know how excited you are that they are growing up and that boundaries are there to make sure they stay safe while exploring new life experiences. Let them know that they will continue to get new freedoms as they show they can handle them through continued responsible choices."*

- Peers are so important to adolescents that they tend to reject parents' opinions about their friends. They think that parents do not have a right to intrude in that part of their personal lives. One good strategy to make it more likely they will have healthy friendships is to **ensure they are involved in positive activities.** When a parent thinks that a friend might be trouble, approach the conversation in a way that frames their concern about safety rather than condemning the friend.

- Parents should **clearly define rules** so there are no surprises. However, at times, a teen will ask for an exception or might ask a parent to consider rethinking a rule altogether. You might suggest, *"Never give in if safety is at stake, and always make sure that they have to show you how responsible they are. But, it's a really good strategy to let your child convince you sometimes to reconsider your rules. This will keep him talking, and that is exactly what you want. He'll also be more likely to follow your rules when he knows you are really thoughtful about them and that all he has to do to get more freedoms is to earn them through responsible behavior."*

●● Group Learning and Discussion ●●

1. A first step to being able to promote effective parenting is to consider how you were parented. It may be that you were parented quite differently by each of your parents or guardians. If so, it is important to consider how that affected your relationship with them and your own behavior. There are 2 major reasons why being aware of how you were parented is an important first step to guiding the parents you serve. First, we often assume that how we were parented was the "right" way because we turned out okay. Second, it is critical to offer parents guidance toward having a more effective style without judgment and while reinforcing the positive things they are doing. If you did not uniformly appreciate the style in which you were parented, a parent whose style resembles that of your parents may trigger in you a judgmental, or even hostile, reaction that could disempower you as a change agent.

   It may be that your group determines that the safest way to come to this self-awareness is through personal reflection. If it fits into your organizational culture, a group discussion may be mutually enriching.

2. Practice shifting parenting styles toward a balanced approach. Your goal is to promote warmth, responsiveness, and effective monitoring. Ideally, you can also offer strategies on how to monitor in such a way that young people will stay engaged and choose disclosure.

   Reinforce the existing positive aspects of a parent's style while gently guiding them toward using some of the strategies consistent with a more balanced parenting style. Work through the following cases:

Case 1: A mother brings her 16-year-old daughter to you for routine care. They are sitting next to each other and genuinely seem to enjoy each other. When you explain that part of the visit will involve some private time, the mother responds, *"No problem! We're like best friends. She'll tell me everything later anyway. I really trust her. Don't I darling?"*

Case 2: A mother and father bring in their 15-year-old son. Their son is very polite, is doing well enough in school, and is wearing a heavy metal shirt with a large marijuana leaf on his necklace. The mother says she is concerned about a new set of friends. The father chimes in and says that the mother is overprotective and that he doesn't want any "momma's boy." He goes on, *"I had a wild side myself, you know kids need to be kids so they'll be able to figure out life."*

Case 3: A father and a grandmother bring in 13-year-old twin girls. Their mother died 2 years ago. The girls are very polite and doing very well in school. The girls are relatively silent and their guardians speak. The father needs to travel for work often. The grandmother says, *"I want them to grow up to be polite young women who mind their elders. They are living in my house and my philosophy is 'my house, my rules'! They are to speak when spoken to."*

Case 4: A father brings in his 12-year-old son to discuss healthy male sexuality and puberty. He knows it is his "job" to have these conversations, but sheepishly asks for "a little help." He spends a lot of time with his son, goes to the park, takes him fishing, and talks in front of his son about how proud he is of him. They live in a neighborhood that can be a little rough, so he is pretty clear that his son needs to be home before dark and that he can't go to any friend's home unless there is adult supervision.

▪▪▪▪▪▪▪▪ Continuing Education ▪▪▪▪▪▪▪▪

If you are applying for continuing education credits, a test is available online. For more details, visit www.aap.org/reachingteens.

■ References

1. Baumrind D. The influence of parenting style on adolescent competence and substance use. *J Early Adolesc*. 1991;11(1):56–95

2. Steinberg L, Lamborn SD, Darling N, Mounts NS, Dornbusch SM. Over-time changes in adjustment and competence among adolescents from authoritative, authoritarian, indulgent, and neglectful families. *Child Dev*. 1994;65(3):754–770

3. Maccoby E, Martin J. Socialization in the context of the family: parent-child interaction. In: Hetherington EM, Mussen PH, eds. *Handbook of Child Psychology: Vol. 4. Socialization, Personality, and Social Development*. New York, NY: Wiley;1983:1–101

4. Darling N, Cumsille P, Caldwell LL, Dowdy B. Predictors of adolescents' disclosure to parents and perceived parental knowledge: between and within-person differences. *J Youth Adolesc*. 2006;35(4):659–670

5. Coplan RJ, Hastings PD, Lagace-Seguin DG, Moulton CE. Authoritative and authoritarian mothers' parenting goals, attributions and emotions across different childrearing contexts. *Parent Sci Pract*. 2002;2(1):1–26

6. DeVore ER, Ginsburg KR. The productive effects of good parenting. *Curr Opin Pediatr*. 2005;17(4):460–465

7. Blitstein JL, Murray DM, Lytle LA, Birnbaum AS, Perry CL. Predictors of violent behavior in an early adolescent cohort: similarities and differences across genders. *Health Educ Behav*. 2005;32(2):175

8. Fromme K. Parenting and other influences on the alcohol use and emotional adjustment of children, adolescents, and emerging adults. *Psychol Addict Behav*. 2006;20(2):138–139

9. Castrucci BC, Gerlach KK. Understanding the association between authoritative parenting and adolescent smoking. *Matern Child Health J*. 2006;10(2):217–224

10. Huebner AJ, Howell LW. Examining the relationship between adolescent sexual risk-taking and perceptions of monitoring, communication, and parenting styles. *J Adolesc Health*. 2003;33(2):71–78

11. Ginsburg KR, Durbin DR, García-España JF, Kalicka EA, Winston FK. Associations between parenting styles and teen driving, safety-related behaviors and attitudes. *Pediatrics*. 2009;124(4):1040–1051

12. Smith D. *Parenting and Delinquency at Ages 12 to 15*. Edinburgh, UK. The Edinburgh Study of Youth Transitions and Crime, No. 3; 2004

13. Dornbusch SM, Ritter PL, Leiderman PH, Roberts DF, Fraleigh MJ. The relation of parenting style to adolescent school performance. *Child Dev*. 1987;58(5):1244–1257

14. Rothrauff TC, Cooney TM, An JS. Remembered parenting styles and adjustment in middle and late adulthood. *J Gerontol B Psychol Sci Soc Sci*. 2009;64(1):137–146

15. Ackard DM, Neumark-Sztainer D, Story M, Perry C. Parent–child connectedness and behavioral and emotional health among adolescents. *Am J Prev Med*. 2006;30(1):59–66

16. Darling N, Cumsille P, Martínez ML. Individual differences in adolescents' beliefs about the legitimacy of parental authority and their own obligation to obey: a longitudinal investigation. *Child Dev*. 2008;79(4):1103–1118

17. McElhaney KB, Porter MR, Thompson LW, Allen JP. Apples and oranges: divergent meanings of parents' and adolescents' perceptions of parental influence. *J Early Adolesc*. 2008;28(2):206–229

18. Kerr M, Stattin H. What parents know, how they know it, and several forms of adolescent adjustment: further support for a reinterpretation of monitoring. *Dev Psychol*. 2000;36(3):366–380

19. Kerr M, Stattin H, Trost K. To know you is to trust you: parents' trust is rooted in child disclosure of information. *J Adolesc*. 1999;22(6):737–752

20. Smetana JG. "It's 10 o'clock: do you know where your children are?" Recent advances in understanding parental monitoring and adolescents' information management. *Child Dev Perspect*. 2008;2(1):19–25

21. Smetana JG, Metzger A, Gettman DC, Campione N. Disclosure and secrecy in adolescent–parent relationships. *Child Dev*. 2006;77(1):201–217

22. Aldridge B, Himmler M, Aultman-Hall L, Stamatiadis N. Impact of passengers on young driver safety. *Transp Res Rec*. 1999;1693:25–30

23. Collins WA, Luebker C. Parent and adolescent expectancies: individual and relational significance. *New Dir Child Dev*. 1994;(66):65–80

■ Related Video Content

36.0 Balanced Parenting: A Key to Adolescent Success and Healthy Behaviors. Ginsburg.

36.1 Offering Boundaries and Being Role Models: Adults' Critical Role in the Lives of Adolescents. Ginsburg.

36.2 Parental Involvement: Balancing Consistency and Flexibility. Campbell.

36.3 The Critical Role of Continued Parental Involvement During the Teen Years. Campbell.

36.4 A Focus on Parenting Teens With Chronic Diseases: Balancing Protection With the Need for Youth to Make and Recover From Mistakes. Pletcher.

36.5 Case Example: Supporting Balanced Parenting: Guiding a Teen to Navigate Through an Unhealthy Relationship. Sugerman.

36.6 Case Example: Supporting Balanced Parenting: Guiding a Teen to Navigate Through a Serious Internet Error. Sugerman.

34.2 Guiding Parents and Teens to Understand the Shifting Balance Between Parental Control and Teen Decision-Making. Sugerman.

34.5 Addressing Worrisome Behaviors and Addictions: Partnering With Parents to Create Safe and Appropriate Boundaries. McAndrews.

35.8 Listening: The Key to Guiding Your Child. Ginsburg.

■ Related Handouts/Supplementary Materials

Effective Monitoring: Make Your Rules about Safety, Not Control

Effective Monitoring: Keeping Your Child Talking to You

Effective Monitoring: Joining with other Parents to Set Common Rules

Parent Involvement: The Key to Helping Parents Make Wise Choices

Positive Discipline Strategies

■ Related Resource

To view a handout that supports parents to use a balanced style of parenting to prevent substance use, go to www.drugfree.org/wp-content/uploads/2011/07/partnership_components_tool_revised_031612.pdf.

CHAPTER 37

Delivering Upsetting News to Parents: Recognizing Their Strengths First

Kenneth R. Ginsburg, MD, MS Ed, FAAP, FSAHM

 Related Video Content

37.0 Delivering Upsetting News to Parents: Recognizing Their Strengths First

■ Why This Matters

When we work with adolescents in a confidential setting, we sometimes become aware of problems before parents do. Although we must honor confidentiality in order to maintain an environment where youth can seek responsible adults and safely disclose their concerns, we also understand that parental involvement can be pivotal in whether or not teens will successfully overcome challenges. We can usually do our best work when partnering with parents.

Parents of even well-functioning adolescents sometimes feel demoralized as their children push them away in the quest for independence. However, parents of teens who are struggling with challenges may feel particularly overwhelmed, burdened, or demoralized. When these parents become aware of bad news, they may experience a swirl of emotions, including shock, frustration, anger, and guilt. This may block them from giving the teen needed support and guidance.

You cannot take away shock, and perhaps have no right to lessen anger, but you can dissipate guilt when you recognize parents' strengths. When we work with parents while focusing on building their existing assets, we empower them to more effectively support their children.

> When parents are told bad news, they may experience a swirl of emotions, including shock, frustration, anger, and guilt. This may block them from giving the teen needed support and guidance. You cannot take away shock, and perhaps have no right to lessen anger, but you can dissipate guilt when you recognize parents' strengths.

■ How to Engage Parents While Protecting the Teen

Overview

Trustworthy professional-parent relationships play an especially important role when breaking bad news. At these times, families often turn to us for psychological support.[1]

Some strategies for delivering bad news with empathy include discussing matters in person when parents have a support person present; demonstrating a sense of caring, compassion, and connection to the teen and family; and staying attuned to parents' emotional state and pacing the discussion accordingly.[2] Other suggestions include avoiding jargon, eliciting parents' ideas, ensuring parents do not blame themselves and, finally, recommending referrals and support resources on the same visit as the news is delivered.[2]

It is also important not to "catastrophize" the news. Both the parent and teen may be experiencing shock and may be operating from a crisis mode. When this is the case, their minds may reflexively consider worst-case outcomes. Your calm demeanor serves as reassurance that the situation can be managed.

Parents Need to Remain the Strongest Voice Promoting Positive Behaviors

Perhaps the most critical reason that we should use a strength-based approach with parents is that we need them to feel empowered, rather than diminished, in times of crisis.

Many of the behaviors we fear in adolescents, ranging from drug use to eating disorders, offer quick, easy fixes and can, therefore, be quite seductive. Even when teens hope to make healthier choices, a metaphorical inner voice sometimes remains a negative influence reminding them of the benefits of the current behavior. It is imperative, therefore, that there are responsible counter-forces guiding the teen to make wise decisions. This is one of the reasons that a positive peer group is a cornerstone of efforts to reinforce alternative safe behaviors. A critical role for professionals is to be another force that promotes wise choices, hopefully by facilitating the inner wisdom of youth. But, it is parents whose role is pivotal. When they feel shamed or ineffective, we lose them as allies, and their children lose them as a strong, stable, positive voice in their lives.

Sometimes a young person who is struggling to make healthier decisions needs caring adults surrounding him or her stating, *"I can be stronger than the voice in your head that is encouraging you to _____."*

The Good News/Bad News Approach

In times of crisis, it is ideal to get parents involved as soon as possible. However, you have to first assess whether it is safe for the teen to involve his or her parent and then consider how to involve the parent in a way likely to lead to the best outcome. In some cases, disclosure to parents should not occur until the teen is well situated with other support systems, particularly when you suspect parents may not be appropriately supportive. In other cases, the teen may need a cool-down period before he can appropriately present his views and circumstances. In other cases, disclosure is inadvisable because of a real risk to the teen's well-being.

When you suggest that you would like to involve parents, don't be surprised if the first thing a teen says is, *"But they'll kill me!"* At this point, explore what she means. Likely she will say that her parents will be very disappointed. You might point out that her parents will be more disappointed if the problem escalates and they are not invited to help deal with it.

There are, of course, some problems, like sexually transmitted infections, that can be dealt with on the spot without parental involvement. Other issues, like pregnancy or drug abuse, will require long-term intervention. If the teen suggests that she will be in physical danger or kicked out of the home for sharing this "bad news," safety should remain the priority and confidentiality must be strictly maintained. However, if it seems that the teen is only afraid of disappointing her parents, you may suggest that you know how to deliver news so that parents will be supportive.

Emotional reactions parents may have to upsetting news may include anger, fear, disappointment, guilt, and shame. The combination of anger and shame is a volatile mix that may lead parents to feel the need to make you understand they are not responsible for their adolescent's behavior. They may do this by using your office as the place to verbally attack their teen: *"Didn't I tell you that I would kick you out of the house if you ever got a girl pregnant?"* or *"Didn't I tell you no drugs were allowed in this house and you would be out on your own if you ever used any?"* There are 2 reasons your office may be the place where the verbal onslaught could occur. First, parents may not be able to delay their response. Further, parents may be concerned that you, as an authority figure, think they are bad parents or are to blame for their adolescent's choices. Again, you cannot take away shock, and perhaps have no right to lessen anger, but you can dissipate guilt.

Now is the time to recognize the strengths of parents, and, in so doing, reduce their shame. The "good news" is about their presence and that their child wants them involved. Think about how many parents you wish would come to your office. It really is something worth celebrating when a teen wants his parents involved. The "bad news" is that there is a challenge you need them to address.

The Choreographed Conversation

- You might first state that you often work with teenagers, and that the law says that you have to keep their information private. As a result, you are unable to include parents even when, in your best judgment, they should be included. A likely response by a parent may be, *"Well that law is wrong. I'm the one who pays the bills and takes care of my child."*
- At this point, you may state, *"Well, the laws exist to ensure that all kids can talk to an adult, especially if for some reason they don't want to talk to their parents, sometimes just because of how much they fear disappointing them. But privacy laws don't even matter today. Your daughter said to me that, although you get angry sometimes and occasionally blow your stack, you always support her when she really needs it.* (Note: You have laid out expectations—it's okay to express your anger, just be supportive afterward.)
- Now is the time to celebrate the parent's presence: *She said to me, 'You can tell my mom anything, I really need her now.' So I have to thank you for being here. I wish all kids had parents that they wanted involved."*
- The parent is likely to say to their adolescent, *"That's right, you know you can come to me for anything."*
- Having determined beforehand whether you or the adolescent was going to make the disclosure, deliver the news. Expect that rage and anger may be released by the parents. However, more likely than not, the parents may decide to follow your precise "instructions" and be supportive of their adolescent.

Of course, this strategy does not work every time. Regardless, it may make it easier for the parents to return to you later for support after their own cool-down period, because they will recall that you do not blame them for their adolescent's predicament.

■ Never Lower Expectations

It may be that the worst outcome of a problem is not the struggle itself but the lowered expectations that follow the challenge. Central to resilience theory is that youth live up or down to the expectations that we set for them. Therefore, you have a critical role in guiding parents to not view their child only in the context of this problem. Reassure parents that normal development is full of crises large and small, and that forward movement is sometimes followed by a step or 2 backward. Help them understand that this crisis doesn't mean they have lost their child or that their teen has suddenly become a different person. After navigating the crisis, they, in fact, may have a stronger relationship, especially if their son or daughter has learned how reliable they can be. Tell them that it may be that their unwavering support is all their teen needs to get through this challenge, but reinforce that even the strongest families sometimes need professional guidance.

The best resilience-based advice you can offer to parents during crises is to never lower their expectations. Teens are fully aware when parents' disappointment and anger overwhelms them. Countless teens have told me they have nothing to lose because their parents have lost trust in them. They have used this as an excuse to use drugs, cut school, even to have a baby. Other teens noticed that their exhausted parents have given up and begun to display that dangerous "kids will be kids, what can I do?" attitude. As a result, teens learn that the only way to get attention is to engage in whatever behavior provokes a strong enough reaction to shake their parents' complacency.

Remind parents that, despite their anger and disappointment, when parents continue to hold their teens to high expectations, kids tend to strive for those standards (see Chapter 38).

●● Group Learning and Discussion ●●

Case Discussion
As a group, recall cases where parents needed to be informed of a challenge. How did they react? What were the emotions they were experiencing? Were there any situations that got out of hand? What was done to calm the situation? Can you recall a time when parental involvement further demoralized the young person?

Practice
Break into pairs and follow the suggested choreography by breaking news to parents in the following scenarios:

- A 16-year-old young woman is 9 weeks' pregnant. Her mother was a teen mother and raised her to delay pregnancy until her education was completed.
- A 15-year-old boy is in a gang. This has been his parents' biggest fear. The only way he will be able to get out of the gang is if the family figures out a way to move him out of gang territory.
- A 17-year-old young man is smoking marijuana heavily and beginning to experiment with Xanax. His grandfather is an alcoholic and his aunt died of a drug overdose at 24 years old.
- Make up other scenarios that may better fit the population you serve.

■■■■■■■ Continuing Education ■■■■■■■■

If you are applying for continuing education credits, a test is available online. For more details, visit www.aap.org/reachingteens.

■ References

1. Ha JF, Longnecker N. Doctor-patient communication: a review. *Ochsner J*. 2010;10(1):38–43
2. Levetown M; American Academy of Pediatrics Committee on Bioethics. Communication with children and families: from everyday interactions to skill in conveying distressing information. *Pediatrics*. 2008;121(5):e1441–e1460

■ Related Video Content

37.0 Delivering Upsetting News to Parents: Recognizing Their Strengths First. Ginsburg.

37.1 Parental Involvement Is Critical to Helping Teens Navigate Through Crises. Ford.

CHAPTER 38

When Parents' Resilience Reaches Its Limits

Kenneth R. Ginsburg, MD, MS Ed, FAAP, FSAHM

 Related Video Content

38.0 When Your Own Resilience Reaches Its Limits

■ Why This Matters

The best parents reach their limits at times. They might reach that point because parenting sometimes feels like a mystery; no matter what they do, they are not getting the results they want. Parents need to know how normal it can be to experience extreme frustration with their teens, especially if their teens are involved in risk behaviors. They also need to understand that even teens from the most functional families sometimes reject their parents.

It is important to support parents through the highly ambivalent, even resentful, feelings they may sometimes have toward their children. Our role can be to help them maintain or restore their relationships with their teens. At the minimum, we need to guide parents to understand that, no matter how futile their efforts might sometimes feel, their continued engagement and close monitoring remains critical in their adolescents' lives.

> **Many teens push their parents away. It really may be what they "want." Our job is to help them to understand that what they "want" is not necessarily what they "need."**

■ Assessment

We may become aware of family conflict when adolescents ask for our help communicating with their parents, or to inform their parents about a problem needing intervention (see Chapter 37). At other times, parents come to us with their worries and frustrations. In either case, the first step in determining any course of action is listening to all parties' concerns.

Adolescents engaging in risk behaviors or suffering from depression might be particularly challenging to parents. Sometimes parents will know or suspect their teen is engaging in a worrisome behavior and may share those concerns. However, many parents might notice a change in behavior or complain about conflicts at home without considering that risk behaviors, such as substance use, might be fueling the discord. Further, parents often react to their teens' volatility without knowing that irritability can be a hallmark of depression in adolescence. For these reasons, it is imperative that after a parent's concerns are aired, the professional has a private interview with the teen (see chapters 14 and 18).

It is important to consider that parental behaviors could be causing or exacerbating tension. It can be helpful to start by offering reassurance that young people drawing away from (even hating) their parents can be a normal developmental process. Ultimately, however, we want to help parents consider whether they might have something to do with the deterioration in their relationship. A nonconfrontational way to begin to explore this is to ask whether their patience might be wearing thin either because of their own stressors or because of their teen's behaviors or interactions.

■ Supporting Parents Whose Resilience Is Challenged

Our primary goals include (1) helping parents understand that tension can be a normal part of even a healthy parent-teen dynamic; (2) keeping parents engaged so they do not diminish their support or monitoring; (3) helping parents understand that they must never lower their expectations, because adolescents rise or fall to the expectations set for them; and (4) determining when family or individual counseling or another higher level of intervention is needed.

The following sections include talking points that offer possible responses to struggles parents might present. They are not meant to serve as a script. You know how best to reach each family. Rather, they are given to illustrate the key points you may wish to make.

Most importantly, none of the talking points replace listening. Sometimes all a frustrated parent needs is to be heard and to have a professional validate their emotions.

Parent-Teen Tension Can Be Normal

Family tension may represent a normal developmental process. As teens struggle to individuate and gain independence, their job is to answer the fundamental question of adolescence: *"Who am I?"* Part of that answer has to be, *"I am not my parents."* Precisely because their parents have shaped the adolescents' values, teens sometimes go through the process of rejecting their parents' views. Particularly when adolescents resemble their parents, teens become embarrassed by their presence. Many parents do not understand how common and transient a process this can be. Even parents with an understanding of adolescent development can become demoralized.

Perhaps the worst outcome of this period of tension is if parents relinquish their involvement precisely when it may be needed most. Parents may be less likely to give up if they understand that while the tension and conflict can be exhausting, it is usually temporary and can be normal. In many cases, the conflict can even be reframed in a positive light. For example, it may be the profound safety and security a child feels with a parent that allows her to take out her general frustrations on her parents while maintaining a *"what me worry?"* stance in school and with friends. Being aware of this may also help parents gain insight into the fact that there may be something troubling their child. This may activate their parenting instincts and allow them to depersonalize the conflict and set aside their own defensiveness and anger. It also can help them to understand that withdrawing would be a mistake at a time when their teen may actually need them most.

Parents may be relieved to understand that sometimes it is precisely because of how deeply they are loved that children rebel and push them away. This is a phase where they need to test their own wings. No one would want to fly from a comfortable nest; teens simply have to imagine it as nearly uninhabitable. Parents need to be reminded that teens do not really hate them; they only hate how deeply they feel connected.

Helping Parents Stay Engaged Even Through Troubled Times

Parents may believe they no longer matter. They might receive messages that reinforce this feeling from the media, popular books, or even other parents. They may be led to believe that peers have replaced them in importance. However, when parents withdraw in the face of hostility, life may feel easier but they have lost a vital role that their teens continue to need.

Parents can be counseled to understand that the rejection represents a struggle for autonomy. Although their instincts may be either to relinquish involvement or become more tightly controlling, they should honor their teens' growing need for independence by offering them freedoms in response to demonstrated responsibilities. They should maintain clear boundaries around safety, but allow a lot of leeway within those boundaries. Parents can be reassured that when they support teen autonomy in a healthy way, their children will return when they feel comfortable that they can stand on their own.

Following are a few talking points that may help parents understand the importance of their enduring engagement:

- *"Many teens push their parents away. It really may be what they 'want.' Our job is to help them to understand that what they "want" is not necessarily what they 'need.'"*
- *"Normal development is full of fits and starts, bumps and bruises. Just because you are in the midst of a crisis doesn't mean you have lost your child. On the other side of the crisis may be a deeper relationship and a son or daughter who has once more learned to turn to you."*
- *"No matter how powerless you might feel sometimes, your involvement does make a difference. Your child may pretend that she doesn't want you in her life, but she needs you to give her the clear boundaries to keep her safe. We know a lot about what kind of monitoring works to keep young people safe. Would you like to talk about that?"* (See Chapter 36.)
- *"It may be that your steady presence is all your child needs to right herself, but don't forget that the best of families sometimes need professional guidance. The health of your relationship is worth investing in; assuming that 'it will all work out in the end' might be a mistake."*

Helping Parents Understand the Power of Unconditional Love and the Need to Keep High Expectations

The literature highlights the critical importance to building resilience of at least one adult believing unconditionally in a child and holding him or her to high expectations. It may be difficult, however, for parents to maintain that idealized stance while teens are acting out or actively pushing them away. A professional can help parents understand that unconditional love does not mean blanket acquiescence to unacceptable behaviors. Further, parents who are deeply disappointed by their teens' behaviors need guidance to understand that if their disappointment translates to a lower level of expectations, their teens may determine they have nothing to lose if they continue undesired behaviors.

Following are a few talking points/narratives you may consider adapting to meet the needs of your families:

- *"The power of your influence lies in the unconditional love you maintain for your child. There is only one place in the world where a child can count on that depth of security. You must remain a stable force so your child can securely navigate a challenging world."*
- *"Unconditional love gives teens the knowledge that all will be okay in the long run. Even when we dislike or disapprove of their behaviors, they must always know we stand beside them. Unconditional love doesn't mean unconditional approval. You can reject a behavior without rejecting your child. Love is never withdrawn or withheld based on a behavior. If you approach even alarming concerns in this way, your adolescent will not go down the dangerous path of believing she has nothing to lose. Even as she may send you strong*

signals of rejection, she will eventually want to return to the greatest security she knows, your unwavering presence."

 35.5

- *"Despite our anger and disappointment, we must never lower our expectations. When parents hold children to high expectations, kids tend to strive for those standards. We expect effort and the character traits of consideration, respect, honesty, a sense of fairness, generosity, and responsibility."*

- *"Children are fully aware when parents' disappointment and anger overwhelms them. You never want your teen to believe she has nothing to lose because you have already lost trust in her. Sometimes teens ratchet up their behavior a notch to continue to get the only kind of reaction they can still get. If they notice you have given up and begun to believe 'kids will be kids, what can I do?' they may learn that the only way to get attention is to provoke a strong reaction in you."*

- *"Another way of lowering your standards is to decide to be your child's friend. We are all vulnerable to this urge when we go through rough patches with our kids. When they don't like us, it feels like a bargain to be their friend. Especially in times of crisis, your teen needs a parent with strong, predictable values more than they need a friend."*

Create Opportunities to Fall Back in Love

Too often, teens' and parents' relationships focus on issues that create tension or pressure. Parents need to develop a strategy to repair their relationship. For many, a first step to restoring their relationship may be reminding themselves of their profound and deep connection they have with their children.

- *"It's not easy to turn off the anger when confronted with a major crisis or deep disappointment. It's hard to heed the advice to maintain constant love and high expectations when you're worried out of your mind or seething with anger. You need something that will allow you to draw that deep breath to reassess how best to approach the situation. It is time to give yourself the gift of falling back in love. You fell in love the moment you looked into your child's eyes, and you were swept away when your baby grasped your finger. Well, your child might be a teen now, but can we think for a moment about some of the wonderful experiences you had raising your child? (Listen) Please tell me your favorite thing about your son. The knowledge of who your child really is can remind you of the highest expectations and greatest dreams you hold for your child. It may give you the fortitude to continue to love your teen even as you are being pushed away."*

- *"You need a reset button. You can't count on him to make the first move. You need some time together with no friction; the opportunity to enjoy each other again. Go out to dinner, to a beach, or to a theme park. Promise each other a vacation from arguments—a 'no-nag zone.' Let him see that he is not rejected. Hopefully he will learn there is something to be gained by restoring your relationship and modifying his behavior."*

Finally, we must remind all parents that precisely when worrying about their child consumes every drop of their energy, they need to remember to care for themselves. Their teens need their strength to last (see Chapter 39).

•• Group Learning and Discussion ••

Sometimes parents will be forthcoming that they are at their rope's end; other parents will feel a great deal of shame regarding their depth of anger with their adolescents or their passive acceptance that they believe their relationships have been irretrievably damaged. Because parents' ongoing care and monitoring remains so vital to the well-being of adolescents, it is important that we keep our sensors high so that we can be supportive to families—even when not directly asked—when we interact with parents whose resilience has reached its limit. Our goals include helping them realize they still matter, that conflict can be normal, that they deserve to take care of themselves and, most importantly, that relationships can be repaired. It is also important for them to understand when ongoing counseling might help their family function better.

Break into pairs (professional and parent) or trios (professional, parent, and teen) to practice your skills with the following scenarios.

Scenario 1: Mrs Scott asks for "private" time with you before you see her 16-year-old daughter. She shares that everything she does feels wrong. She dresses wrong, she talks wrong, she even feels like she breathes wrong. Her daughter is a good student, has a lot of friends, and *"even the neighbors think she is lovely,"* but *"I feel like a prisoner in my own home." "We used to be so close, people used to call her my little shadow."* She goes on to tell you that she doesn't feel angry anymore, just sad. Really sad. She has been sober for 18 years, and she doesn't want to turn back to drinking.

Scenario 2: Jackson has a purple Mohawk and is dressed in all black. He is here for a ninth-grade physical required for entrance into the high school. He is polite to you, but dismissive of his father. His father seems like a straight-laced man who runs his own small business. He seems more than quiet; he seems removed. In a private setting you learn that Jackson is using drugs pretty heavily, but refuses to allow you to share it with his father. He also looks sad when you talk about his father. He says he doesn't care about what his father thinks—*"We used to hang out when I was little, but now he works all the time."* His father comes in for a wrap-up session with both of you.

▪▪▪▪▪▪▪ Continuing Education ▪▪▪▪▪▪▪

If you are applying for continuing education credits, a test is available online. For more details, visit www.aap.org/reachingteens.

▪ Suggested Reading

Ginsburg KR, Jablow MM. *Building Resilience in Children and Teens: Giving Kids Roots and Wings.* 2nd ed. Elk Grove Village, IL: American Academy of Pediatrics; 2011

▪ Related Video Content

38.0 When Your Own Resilience Reaches Its Limits. Ginsburg.

35.5 The Power of Unconditional Parental Love to Help Teens Get Through Even the Hardest Times. Vo.

CHAPTER 39

The Importance of Self-care for Parents

Kenneth R. Ginsburg, MD, MS Ed, FAAP, FSAHM

 Related Video Content

39.0 The Greatest Gift You Can Give Your Child Is to First Care for Yourself

■ Why This Matters

Parenting an adolescent can be deeply satisfying, but it can also be challenging. In order to remain up to that challenge, parents need to maintain their own strength because parenting is a long-haul proposition; burnout is simply not an option. Nevertheless, many parents are so devoted to meeting their children's needs that they forget to care for their own. This may be particularly true for parents who have a teen with special needs, a chronic illness, or behavioral health concerns.

> **Parents need to understand that self-care is not selfish; it is a strategic act of good parenting.**

Parents need to understand that self-care is not selfish; it is a strategic act of good parenting. Parents are role models of what adults are supposed to look like. When they work hard for tomorrow but enjoy themselves today, they demonstrate that life is also about the journey, not just the destination. When they address their own problems, they make it safe for their children to admit personal limitations. When they reach out to others, they model that strong people seek support and guidance. When they live a balanced life while also caring for others, they prove it is possible. Perhaps most importantly, when they model healthy coping strategies, they demonstrate that there are positive ways to manage stress.

Professionals are well positioned to guide parents to care for themselves. Parents who are too busy caring for others to consider how they might be ignoring, or even harming, themselves may listen to a message about self-care when it is framed in the context of being able to more effectively parent.

■ Selfless Parenting

Parents under stress often conserve their limited energies for caring for their children and may even feel guilty or selfish when they consider their own needs. A wide range of stressors can lead parents to forgo their personal needs. Parents whose stressors are primarily economic, including having food or housing insecurity, may do everything they can to preserve scarce resources for their children to the detriment of meeting their own basic needs. Parents who have had to focus on their own illness or who have to navigate a divorce and single parenting may lament the time "taken" from their children. Parents who care for a child with a medical or behavioral challenge may consciously or subconsciously feel guilty and be determined to focus entirely on their child's well-being. Many parents are distraught that they are not able to both serve their careers and their families to the fullest. They feel as if they are cheating their children of time and make every available moment child-centered. At the extreme of this phenomenon is "the professionalization" of parenting, where parents try to apply the same standards of productivity to child rearing that they expect of themselves in the workplace. For these parents, their child's "success" represents their own productivity; focusing on themselves feels like a distraction.

■ Parents as Role Models of Balance and Well-being

"What you do speaks so loudly that I cannot hear what you say."
Ralph Waldo Emerson

Parents are hardwired to meet the needs of their children. Early on, it is a matter of survival. Babies require every drop of attentiveness parents can muster. Toddlers need parents to entertain them constantly, fill their brains with knowledge, and watch them closely to keep them safe. Children are like sponges as parents share their values, experiences, and wisdom.

Adolescence, however, is the time when children like to figure things out on their own. In fact, telling them too much or hovering too closely can backfire as it flies in the face of their need for developing independence. But, they are watching so closely. They notice signs of hypocrisy in adults and wonder why they are being told to behave differently than the adults they see. If we can help parents to understand that, during adolescence, their children learn the most from watching them, we may be able to help parents care better for themselves as they become the role models they hope their children will learn from. This highlights that there is a strategic reason parents should be demonstrating wise decision-making and self-care.

Beyond strategy, parents need to understand how much adolescents want their parents to be okay. They feel calmer and more confident when they see their parents are taking care of themselves. It gives them the security to navigate the world as they try to figure out their role in it. ▶39.1

■ Counseling Adolescents, but Always With Attention to Parental Modeling and Self-care

Parents may come to you as a professional to discuss the challenges they are having with their adolescents. This offers an ideal opportunity to address how important it is that they care for themselves with the same degree of commitment with which they protect and nurture their child (see Chapter 38). However, it may be appropriate to discuss parental self-care in routine visits as well. It can be approached from 2 viewpoints. First, it is reasonable to ask whether the parents' lives have been so consumed with child rearing that they may have put their own needs on a back burner. It can then be factually stated that teens thrive in environments where they can see that their parents are caring for themselves as well. Second, parents should be informed that the best teaching in adolescence comes through role modeling.

It is not unusual for adolescents with mental or behavioral health issues, such as depression, anxiety, attention-deficit/hyperactivity disorder, or substance use, to have a parent dealing with similar issues. In these cases, parents can be either a facilitator or barrier to the teen receiving needed care. They may be particularly sensitized to professionals blaming them for their teens' conditions. Parents can benefit from an "agnostic" approach where you do not assume that you can explain the source of any problem, but where you are certain that parents can be part of the solution. They are part of the solution when they make it safe to admit vulnerability and personal limitations. If they share similar challenges, they become a critical part of the solution when they model that actively addressing an issue with professional help is an act of strength that can lead to an improved state of well-being. (A note of caution: It is not our role to push a parent to seek help before they are ready or to even raise a subject they are not ready to discuss. Such attempts can backfire. On the other hand, when parents do raise their own concerns or they become evident, an empathetic approach that is concerned about both parent and child can be therapeutic.)

Young people with perfectionism can benefit dramatically from parents modeling comfort with their own unevenness. Perfectionism can be fueled from multiple sources, including parents. Again, while parents may or may not have contributed to the problem, they certainly are a critical part of the solution. It starts by them modeling a resilient mindset where mistakes are seen as opportunities for growth rather than catastrophes (see Chapter 48).

Parents can be critical to helping their child avoid risk behaviors when they teach about and model appropriate coping strategies. In childhood through early adolescence, their focus should be on teaching their children the multitude of ways in which to deal with emotional discomfort. In addition, they can work to expose their children to healthy coping strategies (eg, play, art, music, prayer, sports). However, demonstration becomes the key to helping adolescents grasp the array of positive coping strategies. Teens watch as their parents reach for a cocktail to drown out the day. They notice if instead they come home, hit the gym, and process the day with their spouse. Parents can increase the likelihood that their modeling is being noted if they add occasional "self-talk" to their actions. ▶ **39.4**

> *"This is a gigantic work assignment to finish in just a week. I'm going to break it down into smaller parts that I can handle."*

> *"I really need a few minutes to myself after the day I've had. I'm going to soak in the bathtub for a half hour."*

> *"I'm so angry I can't think straight. If I make a decision now about how to deal with you, you won't like it. Right now I need some time to cool off. I'm going for a walk to relax. Then we're going to deal with this problem."*

> *"When I paint this picture, it tells a story of how I feel. That way, I don't have to keep all my feelings inside."*

As you expose the teens in your care to stress-reduction strategies, you can magnify the effect when the parents are present. Don't be surprised if the teens occasionally lecture their parents about their need to care for themselves. Sometimes you can facilitate an agreement where the adolescent and parent take on strategies to manage stress together as a "contract" the teen will accept if they see their parent also taking positive actions (see chapters 31 and 32).

Some parents may remain resistant to self-care, perhaps because they have grown comfortable with being able to focus outside of themselves. Others may not feel the need to change their approach because their children are thriving and what they have been doing thus far seems to have paid off well. They may be right. But, if your professional instincts tell you that either the teen would benefit from increased independence or that the parent may be reaching their threshold, you may consider reminding parents that their parenting goal has to look beyond raising successful 17-year-olds—it is to raise healthy 35-year-olds poised to be happy and successful. On an individual level, help parents really focus on their own child's future for a moment. A parent may take pride in her sacrifices, but ask her if she wants her daughter to grow up and focus all of her energies on caring for her children while losing herself in the process. Remind her that she is the model for a healthy, well-balanced adult. It is a gift to her children's future happiness to show that good parents are child-centered but also maintain a rich adult existence.

•• Group Learning and Discussion ••

When parents bring their adolescents for care, their expectation is that the focus of your attention will be on the teen. However, you may do your greatest good by promoting self-care in the parent. The challenge is to do so in a way that neither puts the parent on the defensive nor makes them feel pitied. A good strategy to accomplish this is to position them as a role model. Alternatively, if their child is under the stress of living with a chronic or long-lasting medical or emotional condition the parents may be guided that they need to maintain their own strength to continue to be able to support others.

Break into groups of 3 and practice the following scenarios (or use recent cases):

Scenario 1: John is a 16-year-old with long-standing anxiety and depression. He has missed 3 months of school for abdominal pain. His mother has taken family medical leave and worries she will not be able to return to work. Lydia, his 13-year-old sister, is beginning to act out.

Scenario 2: Amber is a 15-year-old who seems to be withdrawing at home and acting out in school. In a private interview she shares that she is smoking cigarettes to "relax." Her mother has a high-stress job that leaves her almost no free time. She comes home after dinner and usually has a cocktail to relax. Her father travels most of the time and retreats into his room when he is home. Amber worries about their marriage.

■■■■■■■■ Continuing Education ■■■■■■■■■

If you are applying for continuing education credits, a test is available online. For more details, visit www.aap.org/reachingteens.

■ Suggested Reading

Ginsburg KR, Jablow MM. *Building Resilience in Children and Teens: Giving Kids Roots and Wings.* 2nd ed. Elk Grove Village, IL: American Academy of Pediatrics; 2011

■ Related Video Content

39.0 The Greatest Gift You Can Give Your Child Is to First Care for Yourself. Ginsburg.

39.1 Our Feelings Are Contagious: We Help Our Children When We Care for Ourselves. Vo.

39.2 Modeling Resilience for Your Children: Defining and Defending Your Priorities. Sugerman.

39.3 Adolescents With Chronic Disease Need Parents Who Care for Themselves. Pletcher.

39.4 Parents Model Healthy Versus Unhealthy Coping. Ginsburg.

■ Related Handout/Supplementary Material

The Greatest Gift…You Can Give Your Child is to Care for Yourself

Mental, Emotional, and Behavioral Health

Adolescents' health is tightly linked to the behavioral choices they make and their mental and emotional well-being, which, in turn, is heavily influenced by the environment they navigate.

The section begins by underscoring the importance of healthy lifestyle choices in promoting resilience to challenging situations. Subsequent chapters then address the environmental forces in adolescents' lives that could have a positive or negative effect (eg, peers and the media), as well as those that produce trauma or present serious adversities (divorce, abuse, bullying, unhealthy relationships, and violent communities). This section also includes discussions on selected behavioral morbidities (substance use, teen pregnancy, eating disorders), as well as a behavior that is both a healthy developmental milestone toward independence and the leading contributor to teen deaths (driving). Other chapters address learning differences, including attention-deficit/hyperactivity disorder. Finally, challenges to mental health and well-being, including depression, anxiety, somatization, grief, and perfectionism, are explored.

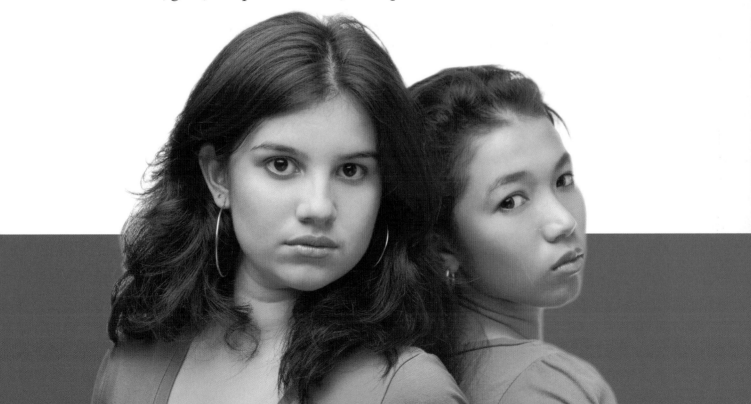

CHAPTER 40

The Role of Lifestyle in Mental Health Promotion

Nimi Singh, MD, MPH, MA

 Related Video Content

40.0 The Role of Lifestyle and Healthy Thinking in Mental Health Promotion

■ Why It Matters

Current estimates are that 1 in 5 adolescents will experience a mood disorder at some point before reaching adulthood. There is a substantial body of scientific evidence that, for many individuals, lifestyle and environment (including stress, nutrition, physical activity, and sleep) significantly affect mental functioning[1]. Further, there is growing evidence that addressing these basic issues can play a critical role in restoring mental and emotional well-being. Optimizing lifestyle may be critical to managing stress, anxiety, and depression, as well as other lifestyle-related diseases such as hypertension, dyslipidemias, insulin resistance, metabolic syndrome, and coronary artery disease.

> **A key to improving mental health is remembering "grandmother's wisdom": "Eat your veggies, get enough exercise, go out and play, get enough rest...and take time to relax."**

For all of these reasons, it is critical for us to support youth in restoring their optimal health by addressing these fundamental issues both preventively and as part of our treatment plan for mood disorders and stress in adolescents.

■ Alternative Definitions of Mental Functioning

In light of how stress is known to affect cognition and mood, what if we were to consider anxiety and depression as the temporary loss of the ability to self-right psychologically? The "stress" response keeps getting triggered, producing distorted thinking, uneven moods, and poor behavior (see Chapter 27). Mental health might then be seen as the ability to return to normal functioning after experiencing psychological stress.

■ Treating Psychological Distress

Treating psychological distress, whether anxiety or depression, then can be thought of as optimizing the body's own ability to shut off the stress response and return to optimal functioning. Critical first steps include good sleep hygiene, optimal nutrition, and adequate physical activity. Specific stress-management techniques are also extremely helpful and include self-regulatory techniques, such as progressive muscle relaxation, deep breathing, and mental imagery. Body movement therapies, such as yoga, Tai chi, Qigong, and engaging in enjoyable recreational activities, also all contribute in lowering baseline stress levels and improved coping with stress. Finally, actually learning cognitive behavioral strategies allows one to learn to disengage from and discount negative thoughts. This can be achieved through traditional cognitive behavioral approaches, such as dialectical behavioral therapy, as well as more strength-based strategies, such as health realization and mindfulness-based stress reduction (see chapters 27 and 32).

Screening: The Basics (What to Ask Youth)

Sleep

- *"What's your typical routine before you get into bed?"*
- *"What time do you get in bed?"*
- *"How long does it take for you to fall asleep?"*
- *"Do you stay awake thinking about things? What things?"*
- *"Do you wake up sooner than you want? If yes, is it hard to fall asleep again?"*

Nutrition

Whole foods versus processed foods? Phytonutrient intake (dark leafy greens, colorful fruits and vegetables)?

Multivitamin, supplements?

Exercise

How often? How much? If not, was there a time when you did?

Body movement therapies (Yoga, Tai chi, Qigong, etc)?

Recreation and Relaxation

Recreational activities (creative vs passive is better, such as art, music, journaling, hobbies, etc...)?

What do you do to relax (familiarity with breathing strategies, meditation, etc)?

Optimizing Homeostasis

Sleep

A 2003 National Survey of Children's Health revealed that 15 million US children and teens get inadequate sleep. This alone has been found to be a risk factor for anxiety and depression. Anxiety and depression, in turn, lead to poor sleep quality and quantity. Optimal hours of regenerative sleep, when cortisol ought to be at its lowest level and growth hormone at its highest, is between 10:00 pm and 2:00 am. Many adolescents miss some or part of this optimal period of sleep. The National Sleep Foundation defines sleep hours for adolescents as inadequate if they receive less than 8 hours per night, borderline if 8 hours per night, and optimal if more than 9 hours per night. Eaton et al[2] looked at the 2007 Youth Risk Behavior Survey and found that almost 70% of adolescents reported getting inadequate sleep, and only 8% reported getting optimal sleep.

What gets in the way of obtaining optimal sleep? School schedules, intellectually stimulating activities (TV, Internet, reading), and caffeine-containing foods and beverages. What helps? Limiting daytime naps, exercising during the day, and optimizing the sleep environment (the room should be quiet, dark, with minimal to no distractions). Having a regular sleep routine, where the last meal or snack is ideally no less than 2 hours before sleeping.

31.3.4

Nutrition

There is a growing recognition that, in the United States, much of the population is malnourished. We don't suffer from a macronutrient deficiency (we get enough calories from carbohydrates, proteins, and fats), but rather from a micronutrient deficiency. Micronutrients include vitamins, minerals, and the "phytonutrients" in colorful fruits and vegetables, all of which serve as critical cofactors for the enzymatic processes that allow us to convert carbohydrates, fats, and proteins into energy.

Without an adequate daily supply of these micronutrients, we run the risk of our cells functioning suboptimally, or even malfunctioning. Unfortunately, most Americans have diets high in processed foods, which are depleted in these critical micronutrients. Even foods artificially fortified with vitamins and minerals don't allow the body to absorb those nutrients nearly as efficiently as do whole foods as they occur in nature.

The beneficial, protective anti-inflammatory effects of omega-3 fatty acids are being documented for a wide variety of chronic inflammatory conditions, and are also being recognized as improving response to psychotropic medications, suggesting that, in some cases, anxiety and depression may be, in part, pro-inflammatory states. This could explain, in part, the presumed rise in mood disorders (part of the rise is likely improved help-seeking and reporting), given that other chronic inflammatory conditions are also on the rise (allergies, asthma, eczema, to name a few).

Vitamins found in dark leafy greens, such as thiamine, niacin, pyridoxine, folate, cobalamin, and co-enzyme Q10, are all understood to be critical to nervous system health. All youth with mood disorders (and any chronic inflammatory disorder, for that matter) should be screened for vitamin D deficiency and supplemented as needed. Important minerals that serve in important enzymatic processes include calcium, chromium, iodine, iron, magnesium, selenium, and zinc. For this reason, someone struggling with anxiety or depression may benefit from being started on a good multivitamin as a helpful first step toward improving nutrition, since it is difficult to change one's diet overnight. Over time, however, it's best to slowly increase one's consumption of whole fruits and vegetables as the best way to optimize cell functioning.

Finally, timing of food is also very important. A 2005 study by Mahoney and colleagues[3] demonstrated a relationship between breakfast composition and cognitive functioning in elementary school children. Breakfast should optimally include protein plus complex carbohydrate plus essential fatty acids (omega-3 fatty acids). These were found to help in maintaining focus, producing higher-quality work, and improving mood. Skipping meals such as breakfast creates the risk of developing low blood sugar, with the result of increased hunger, overeating, a spike in insulin, and subsequent low blood sugar, starting the cycle over again. Smaller, more frequent meals, alternatively, are associated with a more steady supply of glucose to brain.

31.3.3

Physical Activity

A growing number of studies have linked exercise with beneficial effects on mental health. Purported mechanisms of action include increased release of dopamine, the neuro-transmitter associated with pleasure and happy moods, increased blood flow, increasing oxygen and nutrients to the brain, reduced inflammation, altering brain wave activity, and increasing restful sleep, to name a few. Research has found positive effects for the following specific types of exercises: aerobic activity (including brisk walking), strength training, and yoga.

As Dr Kathi Kemper suggests in her 2010 book, *Mental Health Naturally*,[1] the best exercise is one the individual enjoys and will maintain over time. Ideally, it should occur 3 to 5 times a week, 20 to 30 minutes at a minimum. There is evidence to suggest that we get most benefit from exercise in the first 30 minutes, so that is a perfectly reasonable goal for most people.

▶ **31.3.1**

Recreational Activities

Finally, we often discount the value of encouraging adolescents to engage in hobbies, have some quiet unstructured time, spend time in nature, and engage in some form of creative activity or play. Passive entertainment, such as watching TV, does not engage the brain in the same beneficial way as the activities mentioned above.

•• Group Learning and Discussion ••

Mental, emotional, and behavioral health are often considered the "new morbidity," as they drive so many problems. Discuss as a group whether you tend to be more reactive to these problems or whether you have also incorporated prevention into your approach. If not, consider how to most effectively promote wellness in your setting. View the materials associated with this chapter to see some strategies on how to present the importance of sleep, exercise, nutrition, and relaxation. Then consider how to convey these points in a way that would be most helpful to the teens you serve.

■■■■■■■ Continuing Education ■■■■■■■

If you are applying for continuing education credits, a test is available online. For more details, visit www.aap.org/reachingteens.

■ References

1. Kemper KJ. *Mental Health Naturally: The Family Guide to Holistic Care for a Healthy Mind and Body.* Elk Grove Village, IL: American Academy of Pediatrics; 2010
2. Eaton DK, McKnight-Eily LR, Lowry R, Perry GS, Presley-Cantrell L, Croft JB. Prevalence of insufficient, borderline and optimal hours of sleep among high school students—United States. *J Adolesc Health.* 2010;46(4):399–401
3. Mahoney CR, Taylor HA, Kanarek RB, Samuel P. Effect of breakfast composition on cognitive processes in elementary school children. *Physiol Behav.* 2005;85(5):635–645

■ Suggested Reading

Beasley PJ, Beardslee WR. Depression in adolescent patients. *Adolesc Med.* 1998;9(2):351–362

Birmaher B, Ryan ND, Williamson DE, Brent DA, Kaufman J. Childhood and adolescent depression: a review of the past ten years. *J. Am Acad Child Adolesc Psychiatry.* 1996;35(12):1575–1583

Brown S. *Play: How it Shapes the Brain, Opens the Imagination and Invigorates the Soul.* New York, NY: Penguin; 2010

Hamrin V, Magorno M. Assessment of adolescents for depression in the pediatric primary care setting: diagnostic criteria and clinical manifestations of depression in adolescents. *Pediatr Nurs.* 2010;36(2):103–111

Hyman M. *The UltraMind Solution.* New York, NY: Scribner; 2010

Murphy JM, Pagano ME, Nachmani J, et al. The relationship of school breakfast to psychosocial and academic functioning: cross-sectional and longitudinal observations in an inner-city school sample. *Arch Pediatr Adolesc Med.* 1998;152(9):899–907

Ratey JJ, Hagerman E. *Spark: The Revolutionary New Science of Exercise and the Brain.* New York, NY: Little, Brown and Company; 2008

■ Related Video Content

40.0 The Role of Lifestyle and Healthy Thinking in Mental Health Promotion. Singh.

31.3.1 Stress Management and Coping/Section 2/Taking Care of My Body/Point 4: The Power of Exercise. Ginsburg.

31.3.2 Stress Management and Coping/Section 2/Taking Care of My Body/Point 5: Active Relaxation. Ginsburg.

31.3.3 Stress Management and Coping/Section 2/Taking Care of My Body/Point 6: Eat Well. Ginsburg.

31.3.4 Stress Management and Coping/Section 2/Taking Care of My Body/Point 7: Sleep Well. Ginsburg.

CHAPTER 41

Friendships and Peers

Sara B. Kinsman, MD, PhD

 Related Video Content

41.0 Peers and Friendships: Insights Into the Complex Positive and Negative Impact Youth Have on Each Other

■ Why This Matters?

When teens spend what can seem like an excessive amount of time talking, texting, skyping, and just simply hanging out with peers, it is important to remember that they are doing incredibly important developmental work. They are learning to manage conflict and get along with friends. To become a young adult capable of living, studying, and working with peers—independent from their parents—teens need to spend much of the second decade of their lives understanding who these people are and how to get along with them.

Parents and professionals equipped with a better understanding of peer culture and how to guide youth in navigating peer relationships will be positioned to support both safe behaviors and growing independence.

> **Peer relationships are the template for adult social, romantic, economic, and collegial relationships. In fact, peer interactions develop essential life skills connected to success, such as the ability to respond and grow from constructive criticism and develop leadership and collaborative strategies. For these reasons, it is important that we view youth separating from adults, adopting their own norms, and attending to their peers as a sign of appropriate developmental progress.**

■ Appreciating Growing Independence and the Developmental Necessity of Peer Relationships

Most teens end up not too dissimilar from their parents, but rarely does a teen or young adult want to be exactly like their parent. Instead, teens create a unique generational subculture. Nevertheless, most teen subcultures to some degree do mimic the adult social life reflected in their families. In this way, teens can say, *"I am going to grow up, be an adult, but not exactly like my parents. I am independent."* If teens never developed a sense of separateness from their parents, they would be limited in taking care of themselves and ultimately in functioning as adults.

The need to attach to peers, however, is more than a stepping-stone toward independence from parents. It is a biological necessity that represents the first step toward romantic relationships and functioning as adults. Peer relationships are the template for adult social, romantic, economic, and collegial relationships. In fact, peer interactions develop essential life skills connected to success, such as the ability to respond and grow from constructive criticism and develop leadership and collaborative strategies. For these reasons, it is important that we view youth separating from adults, adopting their own norms, and attending to their peers as a sign of appropriate developmental progress. If, on the other hand, we deride peer cultures altogether, or become overly controlling in an effort to undermine peer relationships, adolescents will reflexively reject our views and actions as impeding their drive toward independence and self-sufficiency.

■ The Peer World

There are many layers of social complexity and many directions in which teens can influence one another.

Crowds

Studies over several decades have found that many adolescents self-identify with 1 of 4 general crowds: elites/populars, athletes/jocks, academics, and deviants.[1] A fifth group comprises those who fall outside the 4 main crowds or socialize between. Teens in this crowd have referred to themselves over time as "normals," "nobodies," "hybrids," "outcasts," or "loners," to name a few. The general tenor of the 4 major crowds has stayed consistent in US non-minority schools in the last few decades though the names of some crowds have changed over time. (Deviants have self-identified as "stoners," "druggies," "burnouts," "freaks," "punks," and "hoods.") Understanding crowd affiliation helps outsiders get a quick overview of how teens see themselves and their social world. When asked, teens may tell you how they do or do not fit into a crowd. This can be helpful, because you can start to understand the school culture the teen is dealing with and the benefits and pressures of fitting in, especially if a teen explains they have 2 sets of friends, the "skaters" and the "math geeks," for example.

Self-identified crowd affiliation may also tell us something about risk exposure. Brown and other's[1] findings suggest that students who say they were part of a deviant group were more likely to smoke cigarettes, use illicit drugs, and engage in nonconforming behaviors—perhaps, a way to join nonmainstream adult roles, including musicians, artists, or tradesmen. Students who were part of a popular group were more likely to use alcohol or have sex—perhaps taking on a lifestyle that mimics their ideas about college. Crowds are a general affiliation, and we must be aware to not over-stereotype. For example, the tattooed "deviant-looking" teen may be the leader of the math team.

Cliques

Because general associations do not tell us how individual teens make decisions, it can be helpful to understand the next layer of potential peer influence.[2] Cliques or smaller peer groups create subsets of teens who are more closely affiliated than crowds. Cliques can have a negative connotation because the peer group creates cohesion, in part, by separating themselves from or excluding others. For example, a group of 6 guys who are excellent football players (in the jock crowd) start elite training to ensure future scholarships, study hard, and avoid alcohol and all party-related activities. By creating a subset with unique norms, this clique within a crowd has a different set of health-risk issues (eg, becoming overly focused on nutrition and body fat) than their general crowd affiliation (eg, drinking alcohol).

Cliques typically have a hierarchy. One young student explained,

> Bob was at the top, number 1, and Max was number 2. They were pretty much the most popular people. Then there was a jump between them and the rest of the group. Nobody was at 3, but Marcus was a 3½, and so were 3 other guys. A few people were at 3¾, then Josh was a 4 and John was a 4. Everyone else moved between 3½ and 4, including me.[2]

Top-tier students generally maintain their rank, while lower-ranked students rarely ascend to the upper ranks. A good deal of research suggests that breaking into the top tier is very hard. The top tier comprises popular clique leaders who are well liked by their friends and almost serve as role models. It is not that these teens act like adults, but they definitely know how *not* to act like a child. These higher-status teens are more likely to look physically older; act a little older; be attractive; have excellent social skills; come from a high socioeconomic background; and actually initiate, or insinuate that they are initiating, slightly more mature behaviors.[3] For example, a 15-year-old may brag that she knows how to drive so well that, if she could, she would take her test today. She is certain that she would pass, and she is sure that her dad would be so impressed that he would let her drive everyone to the beach. None of this may be realistic, but the idea that she is thinking ahead and sounding so confident can make other teens in the group admire her and be a little envious simultaneously. For minority youth, maintaining status can be a bit more complex because they need to maintain their own cultural identity within a school structure that may differ in cultural values and perspectives.[4]

The clique represents a group that does not mind conforming to one another. Tightly conforming cliques peak during early adolescence, when there is a strong desire to conform. Eleven- to 13-year-olds are more apt to conform to perceived group opinions and are more likely to question themselves, not their peers, when confronted with a discrepancy.[5] This need to conform is usually not bearing down from the group leader or the other members of the clique. Rather, it is a teen's internal desire to avoid appearing different and risk not conforming. If you think about how a school of fish swims, 1 or 2 fish do not command the others to follow, rather the leaders and followers read one another well enough to stick together. Interestingly, not only does age affect how a teen will conform, but younger teens are more apt to conform to positive or pro-social behaviors and older teens are more apt to take risks. Older teens' desire to easily conform starts to wane as their tolerance for risk increases.[6] These studies suggest that pressure to conform is multidimensional. It varies by age, gender, direction of influence (positive and negative), type of behavior (pro-social and deviant), clique, and crowd affiliation.[5-8]

One of the tricky issues when we study peer pressure is deciding what behavior is deviant. When are teens following cues from peers and moving away from adult norms? Interestingly, peers spend a great deal of time talking, gossiping, and trying to figure out how to look like and become a young adult. Most times when a teen follows their peers, they are experimenting with behaviors that they assume will make them look older. The most likely behaviors that lend themselves to peer influence are age-inappropriate (eg, drinking alcohol and having sex) and not socially deviant (eg, stealing or physically harming others).[9] This is important, because most parents do not need to veer our teens away from risky peers, rather we need to be prepared that peers with slightly higher status will role-model or suggest age-inappropriate behaviors.[10,11]

If a teen does veer away from good friends to spend time with higher-risk peers, a caring adult needs to take a step back and wonder if there is a bigger problem. Teens who abruptly and completely redirected their friendships toward crowds and cliques that are not consistent with previous affiliations are struggling. This is not an expected part of adolescent social development. Without being critical of the new affiliations, a caring adult needs to understand why this change came about rather than berating the new peers.

> Brea, a ninth grader who has always enjoyed spending time with friends from grade school and playing her flute, announces that she hates being in the band, is quitting, and finds her old friends stupid. She has started hanging out with kids who are known to skip school, smoke cigarettes, and dress provocatively. When you ask about the positives of spending time with her new friends, she explains, *"They are realistic about life. They know that almost everything in life is*

fake—just a show. They don't take any bullsh-t." After you affirm that a "take no BS attitude" might be helpful in some situations, Brea agrees. She then tells you that she saw one of her parent's e-mail accounts and learned they are having an affair. They are repeatedly lying "to everybody" about having to go on "business trips," even missing her birthday.

Taking time to understand her dilemma, which was signaled by her change in friends, allowed a caring adult to step in and help her with this painful secret.

Maturity

Markers of maturity and independence are moving targets that are continually being reinterpreted. For example, a marker of increased independence at one age—cool blue Kool-Aid dyed hair—loses its currency and seems passé quickly. How peer groups message about continuously changing norms can be subtle. With gaze, gestures, stance, touch, teasing, chitchat, gossip, storytelling, and sometimes direct instruction (eg, how to French kiss or how to put on eyeliner), teens correct one another just enough to be creative, but not too far from the agreed-on norms of their clique's roadmap toward becoming an older version of themselves. Importantly, usually peer influence is very subtle, but sometimes the peer group can be overtly directive.

In an 11th grade health class, students were asked to write down their private questions about sex and sexual health. The teacher read one card, *"Is there something wrong with you if you're a virgin at 16?"* As the question was read, the class boomed out of control. All the students, both boys and girls, were pointing and yelling to one another, *"Who is a virgin?"* Accusingly, they would point at different girls and said, *"Yeah, you're a virgin!"* The taunting continued, and the girls in question would respond, *"No, I'm no virgin!"*

This type of peer pressure dramatizes the power of peers to profoundly influence how a teen feels about her (or his) private decisions. In this school context, being a virgin was not the norm. In another school context, being a virgin could be the norm. What is interesting about moments of overt peer pressure is that we can all easily sympathize with how difficult it can feel to be the only one who is different. Of course, the teen who raised the question privately was not the only virgin, but the class response would lead each teen present to feel that they may be the only "deviant" teen in the class. These types of interactions are not typical in classrooms, but they are ever-present in more subtle dynamics. Their impact is best grasped when we understand they occur just as teens are hoping to pretty much look like everyone else, while keeping up with their peers, all while grappling with the internal desire to feel a bit more mature and a bit less like a child.

■ What Can Parents and Adults Do to Support Good, Healthy Friendships?

Professionals can play a pivotal role in supporting positive adolescent behaviors when they prepare them to manage the peer environment. However, our highest yield may be in guiding parents in how to prepare their children to navigate the world happily and safely.[12,13] Ideally, this preparation would happen early in childhood. Therefore, this section models how you might also discuss peers and friendships with parents of younger children. The talking points presented are divided among developmental ages, but should not be thought of as distinct. In fact, parents who have open communication and active involvement in the early years set the tone for ongoing deeper conversations during more advanced developmental stages.

The Early Years

- Starting from the preschool years, you can be present and available when your children are playing with others. You can provide instruction about sharing and resolving conflicts without hitting or demeaning friends. These early play times allow you to see how your child interacts with other children and highlights your child's internal social strengths and challenges. If your child is very shy, you will be able to help warm up initial interactions and, conversely, if your child is very social, you will be able to help him learn how to make room for a quieter friend.
- Even from the very start, children get very angry with friends. This gives you the opportunity to teach how to feel the emotional and physical sensation of anger and express anger without verbally or physically hurting others. It is also key to remember that anger is temporary. Your child needs to learn not to ruin a relationship out of momentary anger or frustration; the moment will pass.

The School-aged Years

- Adults often think "children need to work it out themselves." Sometimes they do. But rarely do people learn the fine art of friendship without some support or role-modeling about healthy friendships.
- Children with different social skills will require different coaching about friendships. The shy child will need to learn to not respond to peer conflict with fear, worry, and increased isolation. The child with attention-deficit/hyperactivity disorder will need to be coached to slow down or filter their thoughts so that they can give their friend "a break" before being too direct or harsh. A very physically active child will have to be sure to avoid hurting friends when filled with frustration and anger. Children who have grown up in a home where a lot of anger is expressed or children who have experienced or witnessed physical violence at home will need specific skills to slow down their physical and verbal response to a threat.
- Welcome your child's friends to your home. Be sure that they can follow the rules of your home. If speaking with respect and asking permission to have a snack is a core value in your family, be sure that your child's friends can accept and accommodate these rules. If a friend is difficult for you to manage, this will give you good information about what your child is coping with and whether you need to be involved in supporting or redirecting this friendship choice.
- If there is any chance that you can join your child's school, sport, or club event, get involved. Some preteens may ask that your involvement not "embarrass them," but still be present. In these settings, preteens may ignore you and almost forget you are there. You will get the chance to see your child in action and appreciate how they get along with their peers.
- Be sure that you, as a parent, are involved in creating social plans. There is no reason to encourage texting or phone use before a child needs it to keep in contact with you. Once she is able to remotely communicate with peers, be sure you know who she is communicating with, how much time she is in communication, and the nature of what she is communicating about. Devices should be put away when the family is hanging out (parents included).
- Though friends are important, emphasize early that so too is family time.
- Some children will identify a best friend. This can be very helpful, as the duo can take on new challenges and bounce ideas off one another. Knowing your child's best friend's family can be helpful. You can help your child decide when the friendship is supporting her to take on new developmental challenges and when one or the other child might feel burdened by being a best friend to the exclusion of others. Early best friends allow you

to start the dialogue about the lifelong challenge of balancing time with close friends, groups of friends, and family.

- Remember that peer relationships are the most important relationships, beyond the family, to teach children empathy. You can help your child identify how she feels when a friendship creates a disappointment. You can help her identify her own emotions, such as feeling rejected, angry, hurt, or sad, and then pay attention to the larger social interaction. This can allow her to empathize with her friend rather than just feel her own emotion. Guide her to learn that she should act only after her own emotions have been identified and she has considered her friend's emotions or motives.

- Friendships offer the opportunity to learn about talking and listening. Children and adults need to learn that when you talk to a friend, that friend needs to be able just to listen. This is an ideal point to role-model.

- Parents can use friendships to drive home essential points about resilience. When a child chooses to talk to a friend about a concern, issue, or anything that made them upset, it is a sign they are a good friend. Figuring out how to communicate well with other people can be a significant source of strength.

- Teach that working things through with a friend is smart—you can avoid a fight (which usually only leads to more fighting anyway), save face because you took on (for boys, "manned up" to) the problem and, most importantly preserved meaningful friendships. Teaching children to preserve friendships with all their ups and downs is a tremendous skill that will bring lifelong stability in all personal relationships, including romantic ones.

- When a good friend moves away, this is a significant loss. But it also gives your child a chance to maintain a friendship over a distance. These friendships can provide a respite from school or sport friendships that have to deal with day-to-day hassles.

The Adolescent Years

- Many risks that teens take on are proxy markers of maturity—signals that teens send to others that they are ready to be seen as a young adult. This is when you worry about negative peer influences. It is true that most of the major health risks in life are started during adolescence and in the presence of peers—cigarette smoking, alcohol use, exposure to sexually transmitted infections, and possibly even obesity. It is understandable and important for you to have concerns about the potentially negative aspects of peer influence. However, it is also important for you to remember that peer influence can also be protective and peer support can be invaluable.

- Children at different ages require more support. First it is important to know when your child is most vulnerable. Younger adolescents are most apt to conform to perceived group opinions and more likely to question their own opinion than even younger children or older peers. Your child may pass through this stage at age 11 to 13 or 13 to 15, and some late bloomers will be more vulnerable later. Knowing how your child is maturing in relation to their peers is important.

- In middle school, friends and friendships can seem to change. A friend who always loved to play with dolls will decide that such play is immature and want to be on her iPad texting others. A group of guys who could play street soccer all day now opts to stay inside and just play video games.

- Know your child's "crowd" and understand how fitting into that crowd might create a "role" for them. For example, if your child is a popular student they may be a bit more adept socially than their peers, look or act a bit older, and can be influential. This can all be quite positive. But, they sometimes are aware that they have to try to act older than their peers to keep their popularity up. This can be a risk for them.

- As teens reach high school, friends get involved in different activities and friendship groups can become more diverse, but close friends might be better matched than in the earlier years. Some friends who have a new boyfriend or girlfriend will seem to just disappear.

- Teens develop social skills by hanging out with their peers. How to meet new people, converse in a group, make small talk, be teased and gently tease back, and generally share funny stories or jokes is one of the most important parts of friendship. Later in life, good friends will meet after a long break and often say it feels as comfortable to talk as when they first met in their teen or young adult years. In part, that is because they quickly get to the core of who the other person is, have a shared past, and often laugh at the same type of humor. Learning how to share your sense of humor with friends is critically important for social development because it can offset conflicts, mitigate criticism, and make life in general more fun.

- Encourage your teen to talk about all kinds of things with their peers. In conversations with peers, teens can have a back-and-forth discussion that feels more mutual than with adults who may have "already made up their mind" and inadvertently do not allow the teen to explore a range of ideas. Peers can be protective of your teen.

- Having a caring adult who is adept and "friended" without limits on your teen's social network page is important. It ensures that you "know" to some degree the feel, humor, and different types of people that your child connects with.

- Rather than blaming a teen who is vulnerable to peer pressure for "not being able to stand up" to others, it can be helpful to know that you will need to rely on "face-saving" strategies to help your child stay safe. This will better allow your child to be different from peers. Parents deciding that a preteen cannot go on a sleepover to a home with poor adult supervision makes the parent look like "a huge pain," but the preteen is spared potentially difficult decisions at the sleepover that he was not ready to face.

- One of the best things you can do to support good behaviors is to connect with the parents of your teen's friends. Remember that one of the fundamental questions for adolescents is, *Am I normal?* and sometimes they will make unwise decisions to prove they are normal. If they are given clearer or stricter boundaries than their friends, they may feel as if they are being treated unfairly and rebel as a result. On the other hand, when parents work together to create common expectations, your teens do not feel like they are being treated differently and will more comfortably comply with the rules.

■ Teaching a Young Person Peer Navigation Skills[14]

A young person can be well informed, highly motivated to do the right thing, and poised to take action and still find herself unable to follow through on her intentions if she is not equipped with the skills that will enable her to implement her plans successfully.[15] The importance of possessing skills is a vital part of any behavioral change strategy. Without skills, any action is unlikely to meet with success, and the subsequent failure may generate frustration that will increase stress and may prevent a person from trying again.[16] Skills are essential to creating the genuine sense of competence that gives a person well-earned confidence. The skills needed to promote safe behaviors range from properly using a bike helmet or seat belt to correctly using a condom. The discussion here, however, will focus on the skills youth need to successfully navigate the pressures and influences of their peers.[17] These skills can be broken into 3 categories. ▶ 41.1

1. Learning to say no
2. Recognizing manipulation and successfully navigating around it
3. Shifting the blame to save face

These skills may be ideally taught in the presence of parents because they can reinforce the lessons and are actually integral parts of the plan for adolescents. You can directly teach the skills in an office visit or raise the subject and distribute the supplemental materials.

Learning to Say "No!"

When the word "no" is used equivocally, it leads to conflicting double messages, particularly in sexual circumstances. When "no" is said with a smile or giggle, it is interpreted as "keep asking." These mixed signals can lead to continual pressure or even date rape. Too often, adolescents explain that they don't like to say no because "it sounds mean." You are not asking them to be mean, just to be clear. In fact, suggest that, when they mean yes, they should also just say "yes" and then take steps to ensure they are safe.

Teens need to learn to say no in a clear, firm tone and make it nonnegotiable. Even consider practicing this vital skill with youth in your office. Be prepared that this may be somewhat embarrassing, and they may do so with a smile. This gives you an opportunity to point out how a smile coupled with the word "no" conveys a confusing message.

In preparing parents for adolescence, we can guide parents of younger children to use the word "no" rarely, and to reserve it for only when they mean it. Many children learn early in life that, if they continue to ask, they can turn their parents' initial denial into a "well, maybe," and finally a "yes." Learning that "no means no" in their early years can make it easier for preteens and teens to understand that message clearly when they have to say no themselves. Parents should feel comfortable saying "maybe" or "I'll have to consider it," instead of a reflexive "no" when they may just be tired or don't really mean no.

Recognizing Manipulation and Successfully Navigating Around It

Peer pressure is usually subtle. Often, words are not even exchanged. Rather, it is internally driven: *"If I do this, I'll fit in."* or *"If I do it just once, I'll earn my way into the popular crowd."* or *"He really will love me if I just let him."* Although most peer pressure is internally driven, young people still do receive pressure-filled, manipulative messages from peers.

A commonly taught way to prepare young people to deal with manipulation is to teach them to recognize a line and then to respond by reversing the pressure. For example, *"Let's get drunk. I'll bet you'll be a funny drunk. You're my best friend and everybody else is already doing it every weekend,"* would elicit a response like, *"Well, I'm not like everybody else, and I don't need to drink with you to be your friend."* This strategy ignores how much teens are driven to be accepted. While they may understand how to implement this technique, they may not actually use it if it puts them in conflict with their friends.

A slightly modified way to handle this kind of pressure allows adolescents not to have to challenge their friends while still controlling their own actions. The technique has 3 stages.

1. They need to be able to recognize a line. Parents can reinforce this skill using commercial manipulation as a teaching tool or while watching television. You can also suggest they do it while driving around and witnessing teen behaviors. The key to minimizing resistance is to keep the discussion away from situations that are personal to the teen.
2. They need to be taught how to firmly state their positions with no ambivalence without being argumentative, accusatory, or condescending. *"I'm not getting drunk." "I'm not ready for sex." "I'm not cheating."*
3. They offer an alternative that allows them to continue the relationship on their terms but doesn't challenge the friendship. *"I won't get drunk, but if you can still stand up, I'll shoot hoops with you later." "I love you, too, but I'm not ready for sex. I still want to be with you and we can have fun, even feel good, in other ways." "I'm not bad at biology, so if you want, I'll get you caught up."*

Shifting the Blame to Save Face

Adolescents are better equipped to deal with peer pressure and other negative influences if they can get out of difficult situations without losing face or compromising standing with peers. Teens may know the rational decision to make, but if that choice doesn't play well in peer culture, they may choose not to follow their own common sense.[18] The following 2 techniques are designed to offer adolescents a way out while still fitting in, essentially by shifting blame to their parents.

The Check-in Rule

The check-in rule is a logical extension of parental monitoring. It is a bedtime routine not unlike the one families may have with younger children. While it is unusual for a younger child to get to bed without some parental involvement—a story, a bath, prayer, or help with homework—adolescents often go to bed without such a routine. They are sometimes allowed to arrive home after parents have themselves gone to sleep.

The check-in rule has to be used every time, no exceptions. No matter what time the adolescent arrives home, she must say goodnight to her parent(s), even if it means awakening them. This creates opportunities for some very important discussions. Having a nightly "check-in rule" also helps adolescents shift blame to parents. Teens have a face-saving reason to avoid drinking or staying out too late: *Are you kidding? My mom smells me!* This strategy of parental monitoring allows a teen to better maintain self-control. The teen also may be more likely to do the right thing just because he knows his parents care enough to be paying attention.

Code Words

With this technique, the parent and adolescent choose a code word or phrase not to be shared with friends and to be used only in an emergency. "Emergency" is defined as any situation in which the adolescent needs to leave a risky social situation and feels uncomfortable or at risk for not being able to get out safely on his own. He calls or texts home in front of his friends, ideally so they can clearly hear or view his end of the conversation. He informs his parents that he will be out late or tells them where he will be going, presumably to ask permission. He casually inserts the code, perhaps *"Yeah, I won't be home so I can't walk Sparky."* Sparky is their agreed-on code word. When the father hears it, he knows his son is in a difficult situation, so he raises his voice loud enough for the friends to overhear and demands his son comes home. If the son can get home safely, he leaves, all the while complaining about his overbearing father. If he can't get home on his own, he rejects his father's instructions to return home, prompting his father to demand he meet him outside in 5 minutes. The code word works best when it comes with an agreement that teens will not be punished for reaching out for help, even if they were involved in something parents would not approve of.

A code word is an ideal addition to the "Contract for Life" promoted by Students Against Destructive Decisions.[19] In that contract, the teen promises to call home for a ride if there is any reason to believe driving may not be safe, particularly if the driver has been using substances. In turn, the parent(s) agrees to provide a safe ride without an accompanying punishment. The contract assumes the teen will have the ability to call parents from within a social, peer-charged context. If a code word is added to the contract, it may make it easier for the teen to place that call or text home.

●● Group Learning and Discussion ●●

Break into pairs. First, practice having a conversation with parents about their important role in supporting healthy friendships. Then, practice guiding teens on how to navigate peer culture safely by discussing the key communication skills and negotiation skills discussed in this chapter. Finally, hold a discussion with parents on the check-in rule and implementing a code word as firm family safety rules.

▪▪▪▪▪▪▪▪ Continuing Education ▪▪▪▪▪▪▪▪

If you are applying for continuing education credits, a test is available online. For more details, visit www.aap.org/reachingteens.

■ References

1. Sussman S, Pokhrel P, Ashmore RD, Brown BB. Adolescent peer group identification and characteristics: a review of the literature. *Addict Behav.* 2007;32(8):1602–1627

2. Adler PA, Adler P. *Peer Power: Preadolescent Culture and Identity.* Piscataway, NJ: Rutgers University Press; 1998

3. Coleman JS. *The Adolescent Society: The Social Life of the Teenager and Its Impact on Education.* Oxford, England: Free Press of Glencoe; 1961

4. Fordham S, Ogbu J. Black students' school success: coping with the "burden of acting white." *Urban Rev.* 1986;18(3):176–206

5. Costanzo PR, Shaw ME. Conformity as a function of age level. *Child Dev.* 1966;37(4):967–975

6. Berndt T. Developmental changes in conformity to peers and parents. *Dev Psychol.* 1979;15(6):608–616

7. Brown BB, Lohr MJ, McClenahan E. Early adolescents' perceptions of peer pressure. *J Early Adolesc.* 1986;6(2):139–154

8. Clasen DR, Brown BB. The multidimensionality of peer pressure in adolescence. *J Youth Adolesc.* 1985;14(6):451–468

9. Kinsman SB, Romer D, Furstenberg FF, Schwarz DF. Early sexual initiation: the role of peer norms. *Pediatrics.* 1998;102(5):1185–1192

10. Snyder J, Dishion TJ, Patterson GR. Determinants and consequences of associating with deviant peers during preadolescence and adolescence. *J Early Adolesc.* 1986;6(1):29–43

11. Dolcini MM, Adler NE. Perceived competencies, peer group affiliation, and risk behavior among early adolescents. *Health Psychol.* 1994;13(6):496–506

12. Romer D, Black M, Ricardo I, Feigelman S. Social influences on the sexual behavior of youth at risk for HIV exposure. *Am J Public Health.* 1994;84(6):977–985

13. Fletcher AC, Darling, NE, Steinberg L. The company they keep: relation of adolescents' adjustment and behavior to their friends' perceptions of authoritative parenting in the social network. *Dev Psychol.* 1995;31(2):300–310

14. Ginsburg KR, Jablow MM. *Building Resilience in Children and Teens: Giving Kids Roots and Wings.* 2nd ed. Elk Grove Village, IL: American Academy of Pediatrics; 2011

15. Prochaska JO, DiClemente CC. Stages of change in the modification of problem behaviors. *Prog Behav Modif.* 1992;28:183–218

16. Bandura A. *Social Learning Theory.* Englewood Cliffs, NJ: Prentice Hall; 1977

17. Velicer WF, Prochaska JO, Fava JL, et al. Smoking cessation and stress management: applications of the transtheoretical model of behavior change. *Homeostasis.* 1998;38:216–233

18. Gardner M, Steinberg L. Peer influence on risk taking, risk preference, and risky decision making in adolescence and adulthood: an experimental study. *Dev Psychol.* 2005;41(4):625–635

19. SADD Contract for Life. SADD, Inc., 2005. http://www.sadd.org/contract.htm. Accessed June 25, 2013

■ Related Video Content ▶

41.0 Peers and Friendships: Insights Into the Complex Positive and Negative Impact Youth Have on Each Other. Kinsman.

41.1 Peer Negotiation Strategies: Empowering Teens AND Parents. Ginsburg.

41.2 Media as a Super-peer. Rich.

41.3 Peer Relationships Can Tell Us so Much if We Don't Interrupt Disclosure With Judgment. Pletcher.

41.4 Peers, Partners, Friends, and Even Partners of Friends: Widening Circles of Influence. Diaz.

41.5 Peers and Friendships: The Voice of Youth. Youth.

34.6 Case Example: Guiding a Parent and Teen to Work Together to Address Substance Use. Sugerman.

59.5 Helping Youth With Chronic Illness Navigate Peer Relationships. Pletcher.

■ Related Handouts/Supplementary Materials

Doing the Right Thing…and Still Keeping Your Friends

Saying "NO!"…When You Really Mean It

Effective Monitoring: Joining with other Parents to Set Common Rules

■ Related Web Sites

Friends Are Important: Tips for Parents

www.healthychildren.org/FriendsAreImportant

This brochure ties in with the *Connected Kids* theme of the benefits of positive communication with your child about the benefits of friendships.

Connected Kids

www.aap.org/connectedkids

This is one practical approach for pediatricians to provide anticipatory guidance protocols such as Bright Futures and Guidelines for Health Supervision. The approach focuses positive friendships, anger management as a way of emphasizing the important of violence prevention.

KidsHealth: Helping Kids Cope With Cliques

http://kidshealth.org/parent/positive/talk/cliques.html

CHAPTER 42

Depression

Sara B. Kinsman, MD, PhD

 Related Video Content

42.0 Supporting Youth Through Depression

■ Why This Matters

At some point in time, almost 9% of teens will suffer with clinical depression. For many teens, depression goes unnoticed or undiagnosed and can lead to serious outcomes, including poor school performance, difficulty in peer and family relationships, and withdrawal from important developmental growth experiences. Withdrawing from participation in normal social experiences (ie, clubs or sports teams) or self-medication with substances (ie, use of alcohol or drugs to avoid feelings) worsen social isolation, increase the risk of self-harm in the short term, and may lead to lasting maladaption to stress. Identifying adolescents with depressive symptoms and providing them appropriate care can reduce short- and long-term risks, promote normal adolescent development, and possibly protect from recurrent depressive episodes in adulthood.

> **Remember that asking questions about suicide openly and with interest can decrease isolation for teens who may feel stuck in negative thinking about a behavior that they find intolerable, even crazy. Asking questions about suicide does NOT stimulate a new interest in suicide among teens.**

■ What to Listen for When Talking to Teens

In order to be able to screen for depressive symptoms in adolescents, it is essential to first understand what depression looks like in teenagers. Depression can look quite differently in adolescents than in adults. Many people expect to see the classic "vegetative" symptoms of depression in adolescents, such as fatigue, disinterest, listlessness, poor grooming, and over- or under-eating. Those symptoms can exist in some teens, but others are irritable or act out with rage. Further, adolescents are less able to articulate specific emotions and fears compared to adults. They are more likely to exhibit changes in behavior, raise concerns about how their body feels, and express those feelings that have been well developed since early childhood, such as anger or frustration.

Once the language of a teen's depression is understood, it can be much easier to step into her world and further explore other risks or feelings without immediately labeling her set of feelings into a "diagnostic category." If a clinician too early attaches a label to an adolescent's experience, the teen may feel judged, uncomfortable, and further isolated from the adult trying to serve her. For example,

> Lily is a 16-year-old who explains how she started to feel dizzy during band practice in the summer, had moments when she could not concentrate on the music, and forgot what she was doing during the routines. Initially, she thought

this may be related to being dehydrated or a viral infection, but, as a seasoned band member, she knew these symptoms felt different. She asked her parents to stop band and take time to rest, which they found concerning but trusted that she would soon feel better and would easily catch up. After 2 weeks, she felt more fatigued and increasingly nauseous, her acne worsened, and she stopped even trying to spend time with her close band friends. As school started, she found that she couldn't concentrate well enough to read and spent most of her time playing one video game. She denied any major stressors. She acknowledged that her parents had changed their living arrangements, but she was sure this was for the best. When asked about sleep, she stated she was having trouble sleeping—mostly when she visited her dad and slept on the air mattress in the living room. This was her only complaint regarding the departure of her father from the family home. She didn't like sleeping on the air mattress and it was even weirder when her father and his new girlfriend offered Lily and her sister their bedroom. It took several weeks before Lily could put into words her sadness about her family's breakup and her deep sense of loss. She missed each parent when she spent time with the other. She was confused about whether her family had ever really been happy or whether her parents had been faking it all along. She also expressed confusion about how she should act toward her father's new girlfriend, who is really nice.

Though Lily expressed many of the symptoms of depression (other diagnostic labels could be grief reaction or adjustment disorder), by helping Lily to put the pieces together, she came to understand that it was reasonable that she might be deeply sad and that this sadness could affect her body and social behaviors. She was able to put her feelings into words and begin to see the need to participate in doing uncomfortable but necessary things to improve her physical symptoms and functioning. To the many adults in her life, it was obvious that something was wrong. Though Lily's parents were strongly making the case to their daughters that this was a new but not unexpected step toward increased happiness in their family's life, they did not seem to notice the degree of her distress. As parents, they were too vulnerable and filled with guilt to accept that their child's suffering could be triggered by their own necessary but difficult choices. Other adults noted that this teen gave up the activity that she loved most in life, developed worsening somatic symptoms, and became increasingly unable to function at a developmentally appropriate level at school or with peers. With calm, steady support Lily was able to articulate the depth of her feelings, her fear of those feelings when she painfully thought, "it doesn't matter if I am here," and her anger and confusion toward her father, his girlfriend, and her mother ("who let it happen").

■ Interviewing Teens When Concerned for Depressive Symptoms

Early awareness that a teen is at risk or suffering from depressive feelings can be lifesaving. Assessment tools can help with detection and assessment of mood severity (see depression resources at the end of this chapter), but optimal screening also relies on a direct interview by a clinician who can engage teens in understanding their emotional feelings and, with time, be able to actively participate in emotional wellness.

The SSHADESS screen is a strength-based comprehensive screening tool that is meant to be a set of questions that teens are comfortable answering when the interviewer has appropriately set the stage for a trustworthy interaction (see chapters 14 and 18). Questions start with a point of strength and then ask about meaningful issues that most teens hope some adult in their life will be comfortable enough to "put it out there," to open the door for a nonjudgmental discussion. When interviewing a teen who is suffering from depression, the provider might notice the following:

- **Strengths:** When asked about strengths, the teen may have difficulty explaining what he enjoys doing or what he is good at. You might hear: *"I used to be a good soccer goalie,"* or *"Strengths, things I'm good at, I'm not sure right now."*
- **School:** The teen who used to like school may now be struggling academically or report *"feeling confused."* She may want to avoid school because, *"I don't like being around so many people."* She may admit to missing many days or half days. When asked about the future, she may say, *"I don't know any more,"* or *"I used to want to be an artist."*
- **Home:** Teens may describe recent changes in home life, but not be able to fully explain why there was a change.

> Teen: *"Last year, I lived with my mom and now I moved in with my grandma."*
> Provider: *"Why did you move?"*
> Teen: *"She* [teen's Mom] *was getting on my nerves."*

It is really important to ask about functioning and health of family members.
— *"Is anyone at home having trouble with work in this economy?"*
— *"Is anyone sick at home?"*
— *"Has anyone recently passed away in your family?"*
— *"When was the anniversary of your brother's death?"*
— *"Is anyone deployed overseas?"*

Teens are not "in charge" when a family member is not able to function or is ill. For example, if a beloved family member has passed away, adults may think it is best to not "bring up something sad," leaving the teen to cope with an anniversary or memories on his own without the support and love of the adults in his life (see Chapter 45).

- **Activities:** Teens who are feeling down may have difficulty spending time with friends or may seek out friends who participate in behaviors that provide an escape. Some teens will start online relationships with other youth who are feeling down and can provide support and understanding without facing the day-to-day interactions or the stigma that can go along with face-to-face expressions of depression (including crying in front of peers or adults). Understanding the extent of these online relationships and how beneficial they may be, or, conversely, how they may negatively reinforce a down mood, will be very important as treatment options are considered.
- **Drugs/Substance Use:** Teens may be able to explain how a substance helps them to cope. For example, a teen might explain, *"I started smoking weed because it made me less angry and I could deal with my dad now that he's back from Afghanistan,"* or *"My head stops spinning when I'm high."* In addition to asking about how it makes the teen feel, understanding how much the teen is using and whether she is using alone can assess the degree to which the teen is using substances to cope with her mood and independently developing a substance issue (see Chapter 50).
- **Emotions/Eating/Depression:** One of the hallmarks of mood changes is a feeling of irritability (*"Everyone is on my nerves"*) or frustration (*"No one gets what I am saying"*) or anger out of proportion to the situation (*"I don't f…ing care what my teacher says, I am not redoing my f…ing quiz. I just don't care."*). Some teens will be able to describe themselves as stressed, but often they will explain that other people in their lives are stressing them. Not only is that developmentally normal, but, given that this may be the first time a teen is feeling sad from the inside, he is understandably looking to external factors to explain his mood. Another hint that a teen might be depressed is that he expresses boredom. A teen who was very engaged in school last year may say all his classes are boring. He doesn't want to see that movie because it is boring. This poses a challenge

because it can be hard to get adolescents with very low energy or low engagement in life to participate in positive coping strategies.

Ask directly, *"Have you been feeling down, sad, or depressed?" "Have you ever tried to hurt yourself?"* Because the SSHADESS conversation has already covered a lot of ground, most teens are pretty sure by this point that you are nonjudgmental and aware that life isn't going smoothly, and that you are there to help. Teens often answer these questions directly and can feel great relief sharing their deeper concerns about their own well-being and safety. (See more about suicide screening in the following text.)

Be aware, however, that some youth may not be self-aware (or comfortable) enough to respond to the words "down," "sad," or "depressed." The words might denote stigma. These same teens may be more comfortable responding to questions about stress or anger.

- **Sexuality:** Lesbian, gay, bisexual, transgender, and questioning youth are at increased risk for isolation from family and peers. It is critical, therefore, to be open-minded when asking about sexual feelings and health. Remember to ask about relationships: *"Are you attracted to anyone?"* (either in a gender-neutral way or through offering options ["either guys, girls, or both"] to indicate that you are comfortable discussing all sexual preferences). Remember to ask about self-identity: *"Are you comfortable with who you are? Are you comfortable with your body? Do you wish things were different?"* Another group of teens that are at high risk are those who use sex to provide quick, intense moments of physical comfort and emotional release (casual and frequent sex). Finally, ask the teen, *"Are you worried at all that you are pregnant or have an STI?"* This allows a teen to open a door regarding a fear that may seem insurmountable yet can easily be addressed with the help of a caring adult.

- **Safety:** Some teens with depression will have experienced unsafe situations or traumatic experiences when they were younger. Be sure to ask, *"How do people get along at home?" "Has anyone in your home been physically or emotionally hurtful to you or to others?"* This may open the door to discussions about what happens in the home now as well as when they were younger. It can be useful to link these discussions to safety in current romantic friendship. A teen may put up with an unsafe romantic partner if that person provides relatively more safety than they have experienced at home. It is important to know if a teen is being bullied in person or online. Bullying creates a deep sense of fear in young people and can lead to depression and feelings of hopelessness, especially because the adults in the teen's life are not providing adequate protection (see Chapter 55). Asking about sexual trauma is critical and can easily flow into this line of questions (see Chapter 57). Finally, it is important to know if an adolescent has thoughts of harming others or has a weapon. Though not common, depression can lead to confused thoughts and paranoia that put the young person and those around him in a high-risk situation.

■ Medical Evaluation Is Essential

Depressive symptoms can result from a number of medical conditions. A full medical workup can ensure that medical conditions, such as malnutrition with or without vitamin deficiency, endocrine disorders, anemias, cardiac issues, autoimmune disorders, neurologic issues, or acute infections, are ruled out. A full family history should ask about depression, mood disorders, substance use, and health history of siblings, parents, aunts and uncles, and grandparents. The health professional will want to know if there has been a suicide or attempts in family members.

■ Stigma and Shame Associated With Depression

Once it is clear that an adolescent is suffering from depressive symptoms, it is important to find ways to explain this experience to the teen and her caregivers. We usually explain that depressive symptoms arise from the interplay of genetic susceptibility and an environmental trigger (or set of sequential triggers). Many people have negative feelings about the diagnosis of depression or other mental health issues. Teens may hear, *"Why do you choose to be depressed?" "Your life isn't that bad. Why are you acting sorry for yourself?" "Why can't you just be happy for what you have?" "Only weak people get depressed; stop worrying!"* Then youth have the dual problem of sharing some of these negative social views and feeling incompetent. Depression takes away the ability to cope normally, making depressed teens feel increasingly bad about themselves. That's why it is so important for caring adults to be able to explain the various causes of mood changes, remove stigma, and energize a teen and her family with hope and a pathway to healing. For example, you might say, *"For a number of reasons, the neurotransmitters in your brain are making you feel sad, making it hard for you to stay active in life, and making it really hard for you to see how special you really are. This type of sadness sometimes happens during the teenage years and, luckily, we know a lot of ways to help you feel more like your old self. It is important for you and your family to know that you are not choosing to feel this way and it is not your fault. We wouldn't blame you if you had asthma, so, likewise, we are not going to blame you for having depression. We are going to start today to try to help you feel stronger."*

■ Supportive Treatment

Recommendations about how to provide support for the teen with depression are based on (1) how serious the depression is, (2) how many other treatments have been tried, (3) family involvement and support, and (4) concern regarding lethality of suicidal thoughts.

Adolescents with mild depressive symptoms who are eager to talk often feel very relieved to be given psychoeducation and support by the caring adults in their life. Close monitoring of a mildly depressed teen for several weeks can help the teen feel empowered to take steps toward minimizing symptoms and improving function. If this approach is not sufficient, teens can be transitioned to more intensive therapy. It is important to let families know that each child responds to treatment in a unique way. There is not one therapy that will work for everyone: *"With strep throat, we usually know the exact treatment to get someone to feel better and treat the infection. With mood changes, we need to remember that not everyone will benefit from every type of therapy. So we will try some approaches that may help a lot of people and see if these will help you. These approaches include moving your body, feeding your body what it needs, getting sleep, and reenergizing all the great ways that you might have coped in the past. In addition, there are some treatments that involve counseling or trying medications if you want to talk more about these."*

Most teens with mood disturbance heal best with a combination of healing strategies.

1. Regular daily routine and exercise. Exercise has proven to be an effective approach to treating depressive symptoms in adults. Finding ways for teens to become physically active can change their neuroendocrine milieu and enhance a sense of well-being.
2. Eating foods that promote a positive mood can be helpful. Adolescents with a low vitamin D level will benefit from vitamin D supplementation. Adolescents with no obvious vitamin insufficiencies will know that they are taking care of themselves, especially if they cannot eat a perfect diet, by taking a vitamin supplement. Some families will be interested in taking a supplement such as Omega-3. As long as the adolescent is interested in trying holistic modalities, families may choose these options.

3. For some teens, focusing on sleep hygiene will be one of the most important ways to help a teen feel stronger and less vulnerable to their own feelings. Empowering a teen to revisit successful coping strategies can significantly enhance well-being (see chapters 31 and 40).

Explaining potentially effective counseling therapies to teens and their families is one of the best ways to jump-start success. There are a number of counseling therapies that may help young people with depression, and explaining the differences can inform therapy decisions. You might say, *"There is one type of counseling called CBT—this stands for cognitive behavioral therapy. This type of counseling can refocus how you think about things so that you can feel more positive emotions and physically stronger. It helps you to recognize and then stop uncomfortable thoughts that can worsen your mood."* Families who are worried about having to "dredge up" painful issues sometimes are agreeable to this form of counseling because, while it acknowledges challenges, the counseling style is directive and solution focused. Other families will be more interested in interpersonal therapies that focus on the individual adolescent's needs and rely on empathy, affirmation, and providing general support. Finally, families that have experienced significant disruption, such as illness, divorce, or a recent move, may benefit from family therapy that explores and addresses the environmental triggers that have contributed to the depressive feelings.

Teens with a significant family history of depression or suicide, whose depression symptoms started before puberty, whose scores on standardized tools are high, or who are functioning very poorly may benefit from psychopharmacological interventions. It is critical for all teens and their families to know that psychopharmacological interventions usually are reserved for major or chronic depression and need to be started along with counseling. Medications are not a substitute for counseling for adolescents with depression. Comprehensive approaches should involve close primary provider monitoring, patient self-monitoring, family support, and support from key adults in an adolescent's life, including teachers, school counselors, coaches, and extracurricular advisors or teachers. This enhances the likelihood of success because the depressed teen will have active social links to many caring adults. These connections are one of the best ways to keep adolescents safe as we treat their depression.

■ Suicide

Suicide is the third leading cause of death in the United States, and the second killer of adolescents. Approximately 4,600 adolescents die each year by suicide.

- Males are more likely to die; females are more likely to attempt suicide.
- Some ethnic or cultural groups are at extremely high risk, including Native American youth.
- Sexual minority youth are at higher risk of suicide. This is further reason to break down any isolation that these youth may experience and to be supportive of their needs to gain acceptance.
- Youth who feel bullied or isolated may be at increased risk.
- Adolescents who have made an attempt to die in the past are the highest risk group for suicide.

The above points on suicide risk are useful, but, every time you read a statement on proportionate risk, remember you have only one teen in front of you. Every teen needs to be screened for depression whether or not they are in a risk group. This can be done easily at each visit. All depressed youth should be screened for suicidal thoughts and behaviors. In fact, all teens should be asked if they ever entertain these thoughts, because some youth who attempt or complete suicide do so impulsively without a clear history of depression.

Remember to include suicidality as a limitation of confidentiality when you are explaining the nature of your relationship and limits of privacy.

Adolescents who express thoughts of serious self-harm need to have a careful assessment, increased support from those around them, and possibly an increased level of care to ensure physical safety. Although most providers know that asking questions about suicide does not stimulate a new interest in suicide among teens, many providers still find this a tough set of questions to address with a young person. Remember that asking these questions about suicide openly and with interest is one of the best ways to decrease isolation for teens who may feel stuck in negative thinking about a behavior that they find intolerable, even crazy. The Guidelines for Adolescent Depression in Primary Care (GLAD-PC) suggests the following questions to assess safety:

- *"Have you ever felt badly enough that you wished you were dead?"*
- *"Have you had any thoughts about wanting to kill yourself?"*
- *"Have you ever tried to hurt or kill yourself or come close to hurting or killing yourself?"*
- *"Do you have a plan?"*
- *"Do you have a way to carry out your plan?"*

The more detailed the plan and lethal the means (*"I would shoot myself with my dad's gun."*), the more quickly to intervene with a psychiatric evaluation to see if a teen would benefit from a stay in a monitored unit. Once the clinician has completed the screen and feels that the teen does not need an acute psychiatric assessment, planning for safety with teens and their care providers can be very reassuring. As potential risks are removed from the environment, teens begin to feel safer. (See www.healthychildren.org/ChildDepression.) Caring adults are usually able to secure access to firearms; decrease exposure to prescription and, importantly, nonprescription medications; lock all sources of alcohol; and monitor teens' comings and goings to limit access to alcohol or other drugs at this high-risk time. Some families resist these safety measures: *"I don't want Alex to think I don't trust him."* When reassured, the adolescent and even reluctant families are more willing to work on limiting access to lethal means of suicide attempts. Most importantly, caregivers and families find it supportive when they are guided to understand that their mere presence is critical in letting their child know that they are not alone with their suicidal thoughts. Their child will know that they can count on the caretaker or parent to understand that this is happening, be available to talk, and be responsive if a teen has worsening thoughts and needs an increased level of care or evaluation.

•• Group Learning and Discussion ••

Break into pairs and consider the following scenario.

Dylan is a 17-year-old young man. He is generally popular, friendly, and a good student. His parents are concerned because he has begun withdrawing at home. He seems fatigued, is eating less, and has become gaunt. He is going to school, but has been late 4 days in the last 2 weeks because he is having trouble waking up. His grades are about the same, but he finds school "lame and boring." He is still going out with friends, but his friends have become annoying. When he gets home, he goes right to his room. He used to run track, but he quit the team last season. His parents have tried to share with him how concerned they are about him, but he often stares straight ahead and seems distant.

Their concern became heightened when they told him they were worried about him, loved him, and wanted to help and he responded, *"What for? It just doesn't matter."* They asked him to come and see you and he responded *"whatever,"* but he got in the car. Now he is sitting in your office, unkempt and with a downward gaze.

1. Perform a SSHADESS screen with particular attention to assessment for mood. Go into greater depth by assessing for depression. Practice the GLAD-PC recommended screening questions for suicide.

2. Dylan is able to offer insight into the fact that he is *"not myself."* He tells you that things just feel *"dark."* He tells you that he has thought about being dead, but does not want to kill himself now, has not tried in the past, and does not have a plan. He adds, *"That would really hurt my mom. I don't want to do that."*

3. First, help him to understand the following key points:
   a. Seeking help is an act of strength.
   b. He is not alone, *"both his parents and you will give him the support to become himself again."*
   c. Then, discuss with him wellness strategies (exercise, nutrition, and sleep) as well as the role of counseling and the potential role of medication.

(You may want to review Chapter 33, Chapter 40, and the sections on exercise, nutrition, relaxation, and sleep in Chapter 31.)

▪▪▪▪▪▪▪▪ Continuing Education ▪▪▪▪▪▪▪▪

If you are applying for continuing education credits, a test is available online. For more details, visit www.aap.org/reachingteens.

▪ Related Video Content

42.0 Supporting Youth Through Depression. Kinsman, Feit, Chaffee.

42.1 Depression Case: Assessment and Referral to Counseling. Feit.

42.2 Teen Testimonial: Survival, Resilience, and Overcoming Depression. Youth, Ginsburg.

42.3 Case: Working With a Young Man Self-medicating Depression With Drugs. Sugerman.

18.18 Case: 11-Year-Old Girl With Chronic Disease and Depression. Peter.

39.2 Modeling Resilience for Your Children: Defining and Defending Your Priorities. Sugerman.

45.0 Supporting Youth Through the Grieving Process. Kinsman.

■ Related Resources

DEPRESSION

American Academy of Pediatrics. *Addressing Mental Health Concerns in Primary Care: A Clinician's Toolkit.* http://tinyurl.aap.org/pub112382
> This toolkit, in the form of a CD-ROM, can be updated through the Web to provide current management advice, care plans, documentation and coding advice, parent handouts, and community resources to help address a variety of mental health concerns, including depression, anxiety, attention issues, substance use, learning differences, and other mental health concerns.

Cheung A, Zuckerbrot RA, Jensen PS, et al. Guidelines for Adolescent Depression in Primary Care (GLAD-PC): II. Treatment and ongoing management. *Pediatrics.* 2007;120(5). http://pediatrics.aappublications.org/content/120/5/e1313
> Part 2 of the guidelines that explain the rationale of the recommendations for the management of adolescent depression in primary care. Suggestions are provided for the monitoring of mildly depressed youth, evidence-based medication and psychotherapeutic approaches in cases of moderate-to-severe depression, approaches to monitoring side effects of medications, ways to coordinate care with mental health specialists, how to follow response to treatment, and actions if the adolescent is not improving as expected.

Foy JM, Perrin J; American Academy of Pediatrics Task Force on Mental Health. Enhancing pediatric mental health care: strategies for preparing a community. *Pediatrics.* 2010;125(suppl 3):S75–S86. http://pediatrics.aappublications.org/content/125/Supplement_3/S109.full
> This article helps providers identify logical approaches to the evaluation and treatment common mental health concerns in children and adolescents.

HealthyChildren.org. Childhood Depression: What Parents Can Do To Help www.healthychildren.org\ChildDepression
> This online resource provides a brief overview of what parents can do to take protective action at home when their adolescent is depressed, including increasing social support and reducing exposure to suicide risks such as drugs, alcohol, and guns.

National Institute of Mental Health
> Depression and High School Students. http://www.nimh.nih.gov/health/publications/depression-and-high-school-students/depression-high-school-students.pdf
> > This handout provides answers to frequently asked questions that teens or their parents may have about depression.
> Depression in Children and Adolescents Fact Sheet
> http://www.nimh.nih.gov/health/publications/depression-in-children-and-adolescents/index.shtml
> > This handout provides a brief overview about child and adolescent depression treatments.
>
> Questions and Answers about the NIMH Treatment for Adolescents with Depression Study (TADS)
> http://www.nimh.nih.gov/trials/practical/tads/questions-and-answers-about-the-nimh-treatment-for-adolescents-with-depression-study-tads.shtml.
> > Provides clinicians with a brief overview of this multisite clinical research study examining the short- and long-term effectiveness of an antidepressant medication and psychotherapy in combination and alone for the treatment of depression in adolescents ages 12 to 17.

Ratey JJ with Hagerman E. *Spark: The Revolutionary New Science of Exercise and the Brain:* New York, NY: Little, Brown and Company; 2008
> This book explains how exercise affects mental health and well-being, and specifically how it helps depression and anxiety.

Williams SB, O'Connor E, Eder M, Whitlock E. Screening for child and adolescent depression in primary care settings: a systematic evidence review for the US Preventive Services Task Force. *Pediatrics.* 2009;123(4):e716. http://pediatrics.aappublications.org/content/123/4/e716.full
> The USPSTF suggests screening adolescents (12 to 18 years of age) for major depressive disorder.

Zuckerbrot RA, Cheung AH, Jensen PS, Stein REK, Laraque D; GLAD PC Steering Group. Guidelines for Adolescent Depression in Primary Care (GLAD-PC): I. Identification, assessment, and initial management. *Pediatrics.* 2007;120(5). http://pediatrics.aappublications.org/cgi/content/full/120/5/e1299

> Part 1 of the guidelines explains the rationale of the recommendations for the management of adolescent depression in primary care. Suggestions are provided for the monitoring of mildly depressed youth, evidence-based medication and psychotherapeutic approaches in cases of moderate-to-severe depression, approaches to monitoring side effects of medications, ways to coordinate care with mental health specialists, how to follow response to treatment, and actions if the adolescent is not improving as expected.

SUICIDE

If you are concerned about yourself or someone you care about, call the National Suicide Prevention Lifeline 24/7 for free, confidential help (800/273-8255).

American Academy of Pediatrics Committee on Adolescence. Suicide and suicide attempts in adolescents. *Pediatrics.* 2000;105:871–874. http://pediatrics.aappublications.org/content/105/4/871.full.pdf+html

> Supports clinicians' efforts to screen for depression and suicidal behavior and improve care in the office, patient's home, school settings, and community.

Centers for Disease Control and Prevention. Promoting Individual, Family, and Community Connectedness to Prevent Suicidal Behavior. http://stacks.cdc.gov/view/cdc/5275

> Published in 2008, this document describes the Centers for Disease Control and Prevention's work to prevent suicidal behavior by strengthening connectedness among individuals, families, and communities.

Recommendations for Reporting on Suicide
www.reportingonsuicide.org

> Developed in collaboration with a multidisciplinary set of journalism and public health organizations, these recommendations provide reporting guidelines to the media that help reporting on suicide minimize risk or contagion to vulnerable groups.

Suicide Prevention Resource Center (SPRC)
www.sprc.org

> This organization conducts a broad range of activities intended to improve the development, implementation, and evaluation of suicide prevention programs and practices.

US Department of Health and Human Services Substance Abuse and Mental Health Services Administration Center for Mental Health Services. Preventing Suicide: A Toolkit for High Schools. http://store.samhsa.gov/product/Preventing-Suicide-A-Toolkit-for-High-Schools/SMA10-4515

> Recommends how schools can work to prevent suicide including implementing policies to prevent abuse, bullying, violence, social exclusion and strongly promoting social connectedness. Also, suggests that school staff can be trained to recognize students at potential risk of suicide and refer to appropriate services.

US Surgeon General. The 2012 National Strategy for Suicide Prevention. http://www.surgeongeneral.gov/library/reports/national-strategy-suicide-prevention/full-report.pdf

> The US Surgeon General and the National Strategy for Suicide Prevention Task Force presents a national agenda for suicide prevention based on the principles that "suicide is preventable, suicidal behaviors are treatable, and the support of families, friends, and colleagues are critical protective factors."

CHAPTER 43

Anxiety

Sara B. Kinsman, MD, PhD

 Related Video Content

43.0 Anxiety

■ Why This Matters?

Anxiety is an emotional and physical state of prepared-
ness that anticipates a potential stress or threat. Anxious
feelings and behaviors include mild fear, anticipation,
preparation for an upcoming event, and drawing up
contingency plans for the unexpected. Anxiety can be
beneficial, even lifesaving, and, in moderation, allows
individuals to prepare for upcoming stressors and
function well. However, when anxiety gets too high, or
is misdirected, it can limit functioning and lead to significant emotional or physical discomfort. When anxiety
gets in the way of healthy adaptive functioning, we call this
an anxiety disorder. Practitioners caring for adolescents can
help teens and their parents understand the positive aspects of
anxiety while also knowing how to get help when it becomes dysfunctional.

> **Practitioners car-
> ing for adolescents can
> help teens and parents
> understand the positive
> aspects of anxiety while
> also knowing how to get
> help when it becomes
> dysfunctional.**

■ How to Destigmatize Anxiety

While some adolescents will come seeking help for anxiety, most will give more subtle cues
that they are struggling. Frequent somatic concerns, missed school, inability to complete
school work, avoidance of previously enjoyed activities, and irritability are all cues that
an adolescent may have an anxiety disorder. While it is important to diagnose the specific
disorder and hone in on treatment, the first step is to whittle away at the stigma many
people associate with feelings of anxiety; the next step is to develop a richer understanding of how the anxiety is affecting the adolescent and family. Once an adolescent and her
family share your belief that anxiety is not shameful, she may be more willing to share
her internal experience. For example, if I suspect that a teen or her parent is embarrassed
about symptoms of anxiety, I sometimes find it helpful to explain that anxiety is one of
the most important and powerful human emotions.

> *"We don't know exactly why so many people have this emotion, but we believe
> that, as humans evolved, those individuals who were a little more 'on alert' had a
> crucial survival trait that benefitted the entire community. Imagine a family troop
> crossing a savanna; each troop member would have his or her own job. Some
> members would navigate the way, others would search for food, and others would
> have the critical role of being on constant lookout—they were keeping the entire
> troop safe. Those 'on alert' troop members would NOT ignore an unusual pattern
> in the grass, they would notice it, pay careful attention, and assess quickly if the*

pattern was a snake, a lion, or simply wind blowing the grass. This ability to look at the normal environment and pick up on potential dangers is one of the most protective traits we have. Individuals who have this trait are uniquely skilled to stay on alert, repeatedly check and recheck, not miss a risk, and warn others. Sure, it also meant that they sometimes over-called a snake in the grass when it was really a rabbit, but better for some people to be highly sensitive than to miss the snake altogether. In other words, some degree of anxiety is a highly valued skill."

By flipping our understanding of anxiety around from a frailty to a strength, we open a door to destigmatize this emotion and gain the teen's and family's trust. This positions us to more easily listen as the teen begins to share her sometimes distressing anxiety symptoms.

■ Anxiety Disorders

Anxiety disorders affect approximately 10% of adolescents, making them the most common mental health concerns for youth. The causes of these disorders are not fully understood. Genetics and parenting style may both increase risk. Experiencing a stressful event or maltreatment can also predispose a child to anxiety. We do know, however, that professional support can guide a young person to a lifelong positive approach that effectively manages anxiety and increases general well-being.

The spectrum of anxiety disorders includes generalized anxiety disorder (GAD), separation anxiety disorder, social anxiety disorder, panic disorder, specific phobias, obsessive-compulsive disorder (OCD), acute stress disorder, and post-traumatic stress disorder (PTSD). The specific criteria to diagnose each can be found in the *Diagnostic and Statistical Manual of Mental Disorders, Fifth Edition (DSM-5)*. For most caring adults working with teens, it is not critical to know specific diagnostic criteria, but it can be helpful to understand the various ways that anxiety affects adolescents so that we can spot when a teen's emotions, attitudes, or behaviors signal that he is anxious and needs our help. The more quickly a young person knows that he can get nonjudgmental and effective help, the more positive he can begin to feel about himself and life in general.

The following sections describe different types of anxiety and what we might see in an anxious teen.

Generalized Anxiety Disorder

Adolescents with GAD may worry about potential problems to a degree that seems out of proportion and unrealistic to those around them. Most adolescents will know that they are worrying too much. Some may experience painful teasing from peers (*"Can't you just chill?"*) or family members (*"She's always been my worrywart!"*). Even when teens know that they are overly worried, they may not be able to calm down or turn off their worries. Some teens may feel irritable and, conversely, others may feel exhausted. Most teens with GAD will report difficulty concentrating or sleeping and somatic complaints. Occasionally, GAD will initially present with substance abuse as the adolescent "self-medicates" to manage the discomfort.

Monica came to visit for a recheck of her hearing test. She looks a bit strained. You ask if she is at all worried, and she tells you that she is a tiny bit worried about her class trip. Then her mom jumps in and laughs, *"You call that a tiny bit worried?"* Monica's mother goes on to tell you that Monica is playing the "what if game?" *"What if the bus gets lost?"* *"What if we start the tour late?"* *"What if we get separated from our tour guide?"* *"What if we get locked in the museum overnight?"* *"What if Mom calls the police to report a missing teen?"* *"What if the police suspect Mom?" "What if Mom has to go to jail?"* Monica looks very embarrassed that her mother shared this story. As a practitioner, you ask Monica if you can ask her a few questions privately.

Practitioner: *"Do you find that you worry a lot?"*

Monica: *"All the time."*

Practitioner: *"Do you wish you could worry less?"*

Monica: *"Yes, but I can't get myself to stop."*

Practitioner: *"I can see that your family thinks you worry too much. Do they also think that you exaggerate your fears?"*

Monica: *"Yeah, and this one girl at school says that I'm a 'drama queen' and I'm trying to get attention, but really I get so worried and I start talking."*

Practitioner: *"It is really hard that your friends are reacting that way. Do you ever feel so worried or nervous that you can't do things you really want to do?"*

Monica: *"I really don't want to go on this trip. I have a feeling something is going to go wrong."*

At this point, the practitioner can see Monica is really suffering from anxiety and is not sure how to help herself. In addition, her family and friends are reacting, but in a way that alienates Monica and makes her feel less supported. One positive note is that Monica can express her thoughts, so providing pycho-education and referring for cognitive behavioral therapy (CBT) training may be a first step.

Separation Anxiety Disorder

For young children, separation anxiety is a normal stage in development. But, for adolescents, separation anxiety results in significant impairment. This disorder occurs when a teen cannot bear to be apart from the object he is attached to (eg, his parent or home). The teen will fear losing the object and, more generally, may fear being alone. It is not uncommon for the teen to ask to sleep with siblings or parents, experience repeated nightmares, or express strong somatic complaints.

> Josh is a 14-year-old whose parents report that he has been having trouble going to school for the last 2 months, especially on Monday mornings. He had gotten into the habit of hanging out at home over the weekend and not visiting friends. He "camped out" in the family room to watch TV and play video games. When his parents tell him that he must stay with his best friend for the weekend so they can go out of town, Josh "freaks out." He throws things, curses at his parents, and screams over and over, *"I'm not going."* This is very unusual behavior for Josh and reminds Josh's parents of his anxiety episodes when he was younger and tried to refuse to visit relatives for the holiday. Josh's parents let him know that they could see how upset the idea of staying away from home is making him feel. While they understand this, they also know that he loved being at his best friend's house this past summer for a full week. They want to understand what has changed. When given a calm space and understanding, Josh was able to share how much calmer he feels at home. When he is out, even at his best friend's house, he doesn't feel comfortable and is constantly thinking about getting back home to the family room. With this insight, the family can begin to explore how Josh's anxiety is manifesting and consider ways of coping that can help him leave home and do things he enjoys.

Social Anxiety Disorder

The hallmark of a social anxiety disorder is the intense, persistent fear of being judged by others. The teen fears that she will do something that will embarrass or humiliate herself. Most people know that these fears do not make complete sense, but still will avoid situations that might evoke anxiety symptoms such as blushing, sweating, trembling, and difficulty talking. Some people will have more limited worries, such as fear of public speaking. This is a common disorder and can present in children as excessive shyness or in adults who maintain few social connections. Social anxiety disorder can start in mid-adolescence and can initially be confused with the self-consciousness associated with the teen years.

Ty is a 15-year-old who was a talented soccer player in middle school. In ninth grade, his coach noticed that he kept more to himself and started checking himself—almost second-guessing himself—on the field. Now he is in 10th grade and seems less connected with his teammates, and is even stepping away from the ball. He seems nervous and stutters short answers when his coach tries to see how he's doing. One day, when he missed the ball, his coach yelled, *"Ty that was your ball. You should have had it."* Ty stopped what he was doing and walked off the field. The next day, Ty left his soccer jersey in his coach's office. His coach checks in with other teachers and guidance counselors and learns that Ty is having a hard time participating in class. He doesn't go to the lunch room. His English teacher says that he startles every time she calls on him and gets sweaty and flushed when he has to read out loud in class—she is avoiding calling on him and hoping he will "calm down." Another teacher wonders if he is anxious about something. The coach offers to check in.

Coach: *Thanks for coming to see me Ty. I'm sorry if I was too hard on you last week.*

Ty: *No, that's not it.*

Coach: *I know how good you are at lots of things, and I am wondering if you are ok.*

Ty: *I'm not good at stuff. I try and I just look weird out there. I make myself look like a doof.*

Coach: *Are you saying that you don't feel comfortable on the field?*

Ty: *Actually, I don't feel comfortable anywhere. I make myself look so stupid over and over.*

Coach: *Do you think other people think you look stupid?*

Ty: *Well, yeah. I hate being here, being around everyone, having everyone judging me. It's too hard.*

Coach: *You feel like giving up soccer?*

Ty: *Yeah, soccer, school, life.*

Coach: *I got it. You're feeling pretty awful about yourself. You know, you are an amazing kid even if you don't feel that way right now. Can we talk to Ms Marshall (guidance counselor)? I don't want you to feel this bad. I really want to support you, and I'm pretty sure she can help us get you feeling better with a little more support.* (Either the coach or the guidance counselor, if the visit is immediate, needs to explore what Ty meant when he included "life" as one of the things he feels like giving up.) *Thanks for talking to me.*

Obsessive Compulsive Disorder

Obsessive compulsive disorder (OCD) commonly presents in childhood at about 10 years of age and in young adulthood at about 21 years of age. Young people with OCD have persistent, recurring, intrusive thoughts (obsessions) and repetitive behaviors or rituals (compulsions) that are done in order to alleviate the worries that are stirred up by the obsessions. Adolescents can feel extremely ashamed and embarrassed by their OCD symptoms. This places adolescents with OCD at increased risk for self-harm. In addition, the symptoms are often quite time-consuming and can significantly impact daily functioning, especially since many thoughts or behaviors are kept hidden from others.

> Anna is a 12th-grade straight-A student, who found that she was having difficulty for the first time in her life completing her homework assignments before 2:00 am and was becoming increasingly physically ill with abdominal pain and exhaustion. She identified her strengths as doing well in school and being able to help others in her home be organized (both she and her mother laughed). Anna enjoyed school and did not feel the work was too hard, got along well with her parents and sister, played second violin in the school orchestra, did not endorse using any drugs or having sex, denied depression or suicidality, and reported feeling safe in all aspects of her life. But as she spoke about not being able to finish her schoolwork, she became flushed, sweaty, and almost tearful. As we spoke about her after-school routine, it was clear that there are a few hours that appeared to be missing. When asked about this, she looked more upset. When it was reflected back that she looked anxious and we were talking together to try to help her, Anna explained that she felt anxious in specific situations. Slowly, Anna was able to describe how she kept the anxiety away when she completed her homework. First, she needed to reorganize everything on her desk, then count her pens and pencils and place them in a specific order. She repetitively sharpens her pencils. She would start from scratch and redo an assignment if it did not appear "to look right." Anna noted that, as long as she did these behaviors, she really didn't feel anxious, but now the only problem was that it took too much time to get her schoolwork done. We were able to see that she was spending approximately 4 hours nightly trying to manage what appeared to be significant anxiety and OCD.

By removing the stigma, relieving Anna of the burden of secrecy, and addressing her question, *"Am I crazy?"* we then were able to start talking about her underlying fear of not getting into the college of her choice. We were able to brainstorm ways to manage stress that did not trigger the significantly time-consuming ritualized coping strategies. Her mother shared how Anna's father developed and learned to manage a significant bout of obsessive compulsive behavior when he studied business in graduate school. With support and counseling, he has learned to manage his anxiety and has always been a positive role model for Anna.

Panic Disorder

Panic attacks can occur outside a panic disorder. Both are likely to present during late adolescence, with a higher prevalence among young women. Panic attacks and panic disorder often occur together with other anxiety disorders or depression. A typical panic attack might include excessive sweating, increased heart rate or palpitations, trembling or shaking, chills or hot flashes, the sensation of shortness of breath or choking, chest pain, nausea, dizziness, numbness or tingling, feeling detached, and fear of going crazy or dying. Adolescents with the disorder will have recurrent attacks, worry about future attacks, and change behavior to avoid potential triggers.

Specific Phobias

Adolescents do not usually make others aware of specific phobias unless they find that they can't function normally. With a phobia, the young person may have a persistent fear out of proportion to the actual danger and experience intense anxiety when exposed to the object or situation. Adolescents with a phobia usually know it is irrational but will still avoid the feared object. For some adolescents, the thought of facing their feared object or situation can bring on a panic attack.

> Zoe, a civic-minded college student, has the chance to travel abroad with her church to do a much needed service project in a developing country. She desperately wants to go, but feels that she has to say no. You ask her why and she explains, *"You are going to think I'm crazy, really crazy, but I can't go there because everyone, everyone, tells me there are these snakes—they are really hard to see and they can come into your hut at night. It happened to my friend when she went over, and I can't do it. I would die. I'm dying even talking about this. I know you think I am crazy, but I just can't do it. I can't do it. No way."* You reflect back to her that you can appreciate from her tone and message that she feels that she cannot go. You also add that phobias like this are treatable. If she is willing, there are a couple of approaches that can really address this fear and allow her to take advantage of this great opportunity to serve others.

Acute Stress Disorder

Acute stress disorder can follow a traumatic event and result in a feeling of numbness, feeling that one is watching oneself go through the motions, or having a sense that the world is not real. Young people may re-experience the trauma or sensations related to the trauma and avoid anything that reminds them of the trauma. Acute stress disorder can last up to 4 weeks after a traumatic experience. This reaction occurs commonly after an assault, motor vehicle crash, or witnessing of a shooting.

> "JC" was on his way home from the convenience store and was walking in a dark section of his block when he thought he heard something behind him. Before he could look around, he felt a cold metal object pointed at his back and the man said, "Slowly hand me your money or I'll shoot you." "JC" took his wallet out of his jeans; the man grabbed it and pushed him really fast and hard to the pavement. "JC" remembers just lying still and feeling scared to death. He got up, realized that no one was around or noticed, and started to walk home, but he felt like he was watching his feet move. In the next few days, he was so angry. He kept thinking that he should not have walked down the darker side of the street. He kept saying to himself that he knew something was going to happen and he kept checking to see if something was behind him. He was having trouble sleeping and had nightmares that he was shot. He stopped drinking the orange soda that he had gone to the store to buy. But after about 2 and half weeks, "JC" stopped talking about being held up all the time, he started sleeping better, and resumed drinking his favorite drink. He still modifies how he comes home from the convenience store.

Post-Traumatic Stress Disorder

Post-traumatic stress disorder (PTSD) may develop after experiencing, witnessing, or being involved in a life-threatening event or serious injury. Responses include fear, helplessness, disorganization, or agitation. The event is re-experienced with intrusive thoughts, upsetting dreams, the feeling that an event is recurring, and intense psychological or physical reactions to cues that are reminders of the event. Hypervigilance and arousal, including irritability or outbursts of anger, can occur. Not every traumatized person develops full-blown or even minor PTSD. Symptoms usually begin within 3 months of the incident, but occasionally emerge years afterward. They must last more than a month to be considered PTSD.

> Mark is a 16-year-old who came to the pediatrician's office to have numbing sensation in his legs checked out, which has been recurring on and off for the past 2 months. Initially, he focuses on this sensation and casually mentions that it is really a problem because he has to help his mom after her most recent surgery. In bits and pieces, he tells you about her multiple surgeries after a severe crash, and then you ask about the event. He becomes uninterruptable as he tells you about the SUV landing on their car, the moment when he thought he would die, and the pain in his leg after the impact. He describes looking at his mom in the driver's seat and thinking she looked dead, then getting his 2 little sisters out of the car and not being allowed to go back and get his mom out. He remembers telling his little sister she was all right. Then he says that what is so weird is that he was doing so well after the crash and helping to take care of his little sisters while his mom was in the hospital. Then he started to get nightmares. He refuses to go to driver education at school, is afraid to ride in the passenger's seat, and when in the car yells out directions to look out for other drivers. He can't concentrate, and he now has this pain in his leg.
>
> Practitioner: *"Do you think about the car crash often?"*
>
> Mark: *"Pretty much every day. Well whenever I need to get in a car."*
>
> Practitioner: *"What do you think about when you think about the crash?"*
>
> Mark: *"I still can't believe that we all didn't die. I still can't believe it."*
>
> Practitioner: *Do you feel like you are actually going through it again?*
>
> Mark: *"Just when I get those nightmares. This leg pain is weird too."*
>
> Practitioner: *"Do you avoid being around things that remind you of that time?"*
>
> Mark: *"Not really, but I don't care what people say, I really don't care. I don't need to drive and I don't want to drive."*
>
> Practitioner: *"Mark, I am not surprised that you are affected by such a bad crash and are making decisions to keep you and others safe. I'm wondering, though, if you might want to work on some strategies to put the pain of the crash behind you and in the past. Mind you, I'm not saying to forget it. I'm just saying to place it where it belongs, in the past, so you can have more room in your mind for what is going on around you now and what you want to do going forward."*

■ Psychosocial Screening and Structured Screening

In addition to carefully listening to presenting concerns, the SSHADESS Screen can help identify triggers or explanations for anxiety, including early childhood trauma, witnessing trauma, abuse (physical or emotional), neglect (now or in the past), fear of abandonment, feelings of depression, and fear of specific social situations. It can also reveal a substance use history (including use of substances that may be used to cope with anxiety or substances that may mimic anxiety, such as highly caffeinated beverages). A more focused history can help better identify different types of anxiety, including phobias, panic disorder, or PTSD. In addition to an in-depth interview, screening questionnaires can help practitioners identify anxiety disorders and can be accessed through the resources listed at the end of the chapter.

■ Medical Evaluation Is Essential

Anxiety is a general symptom that can result from a number of medical conditions. A medical evaluation with attention to possible etiologies can be helpful, including endocrine disorders such as hyperthyroidism or Cushing's syndrome, cardiac arrhythmias, overuse of prescription drugs for asthma or attention-deficit/hyperactivity disorder, misuse of amphetamine-like drugs, or withdrawal from benzodiazepines or alcohol. A thorough family history is helpful, because other people in the family that may have dealt with anxiety can be identified, and because treatment strategies that have been used by other family members, such as counseling and/or appropriate medication, can be discussed. In addition, negative coping strategies, such as detrimental alcohol use or benzodiazepine addiction, can be identified. For adolescents with new onset OCD, consider the possibility of pediatric acute-onset neuropsychiatric disorders.

■ Tips for Health Professionals (and Those Who Refer to Them)

- Teens who present with symptoms of anxiety deserve a medical evaluation to rule out a physiological cause of the symptoms of anxiety. (See above.)
- Adolescents with anxiety may be more likely to have physical manifestations of their emotions. This is not faking; the physical symptoms are real (see Chapter 44).
- It is common for clinicians to become anxious about their inability to more effectively relieve physical symptoms or diagnose their cause. In parallel, parents or teens may have increasing anxiety as the symptoms persist. When you experience this anxiety yourself or are absorbing it from others, allow yourself a pause to gain insight into the possibility you may be caring for a teen or parent whose primary issue is anxiety.
- However, do not assume that just because there is anxiety there is not also a physical problem. Remember that people who feel poorly worry about their own health and become anxious that we might miss something. The anxiety you may be witnessing may be a reaction to the illness rather than a cause of the symptoms. It is important to be both aware of the possibility that stress/anxiety is the driver of some or all of the physical symptoms *and* that there may be an underlying physical cause.
- The teen or parent who presents with significant worries related to a physical complaint may be exquisitely wary of exploring emotional concerns. Help families bridge the gap between physical and mental symptoms and come to awareness, without shame, that the body and mind are integrally related. A key to early and effective treatment is to help families lose their fear of mental health diagnoses and gain an understanding of the emotional and physical sequelae of anxiety (see Chapter 44).
- Sometimes, parents are resistant to accepting a psychological cause because they are worried that if their teen's diagnosis is anxiety, you will not be able to help and their child will have to live with this challenging disorder. Other times, they are concerned they will be "passed along" to mental health services and lose the relationship with you or that you will be less thoughtful in considering physical concerns. Finally, parents may have experienced less-than-compassionate care themselves and want to spare their child. Reassurance that you will remain both thoughtful and involved can help families more easily accept mental health diagnoses.

Supportive Treatment

For mild anxiety that is minimally affecting function, creating a space where a young person or family member can talk through her experience while a professional listens without judgment is an invaluable first step. Talking openly about worries and subsequent behaviors can be cathartic and healing. Young people gain a sense of control with self-discovered insights, and control can diminish anxiety. Many of these adolescents will do quite well with close follow-up alone.

Adding a set of positive stress-management and coping strategies will enhance adolescents' ability to mitigate their anxiety (see Chapter 31). In addition, healthy lifestyle choices, including appropriate sleep, good nutrition, and exercise, can help young people manage mild anxiety (see Chapter 40). Exercise, in particular, can help adolescents manage both baseline stress or discomfort and acute bouts of anxiety. You might say, *"Stress or really bad anxiety makes you feel as if a tiger is chasing you. So the answer is to run!!! Really you can do any kind of exercise that moves your legs—running, swimming, dancing, jumping rope, biking, or any kind of sports that have you move. When you don't run, your body thinks there is still a tiger lurking ready to attack you. Of course you can't concentrate or think of anything else if there might be a tiger hanging out. When you exercise, you communicate to your body that you have escaped."* Young people with school-related anxiety may tell you that they don't have time to exercise. Your response should be, *"You don't have time not to exercise. You will be far more focused and efficient if you just take 20 minutes for a hard sweat. You are not supposed to be doing schoolwork when a tiger is chasing you. Trust me, one of the few things I can guarantee is that you will focus better if you exercise first."* ▶ 31.3.1

For anxiety that significantly impacts function in the social or functional realms, consider adding therapy to address and reshape fears and worries. Cognitive behavioral therapy has been shown to be effective in treating some adolescents with anxiety disorders. Cognitive behavioral therapy focuses on identifying worries or negative thoughts, boosting positive thoughts, challenging the possibility or evidence for a fear or worry, testing adaptive thoughts against maladaptive beliefs, and creating a coping plan for anticipated fearful situations. The main goal of treatment is to rearrange and prioritize thinking. By actively quieting anxiety pathways and building calmer problem-solving pathways, adolescents can learn to approach stressful situations with a healthy amount of anxiety and healthy degree of positive coping.

Treatment with medication can sometimes be helpful for children and adolescents with severe anxiety in combination with CBT or other therapies. Serotonin reuptake inhibitors may be an effective approach to treating an adolescent with anxiety, and some trials have shown that, for significant anxiety, combined treatment with medication and CBT counseling can be more effective than just monotherapy.

Summary

Practitioners caring for adolescents can be very effective in helping teens modulate anxiety. Learning to use anxiety when it is helpful and finding effective coping strategies when it is not is one of the most important skills a young person can develop to ensure lifelong steadiness and well-being.

●● Group Learning and Discussion ●●

Break into groups of 3 and work through a case that has presented in your setting or choose one of the scenarios given in this chapter. One of you should play the part of an anxious parent who has his or her own history of an anxiety disorder and who is very worried about his or her child.

1. Perform a SSHADESS screen in private with the teen while paying particular attention to the assessment for anxiety.

2. Help the teen to understand the following key points:

   a. Anxiety can be a protective emotion. There is no shame or stigma in having anxious feelings. Practice giving the explanation offered in this chapter, or develop one that feels comfortable to you.

   b. Seeking help is an act of strength.

   c. You are not alone, *"Both your parent(s) and I will give you the support to become yourself again."*

   d. Then, discuss wellness strategies (exercise, nutrition, and sleep) as well as the role of CBT and the potential role of medication.

(You may want to review Chapter 33, Chapter 40, and the sections on exercise, nutrition, relaxation, and sleep in Chapter 31.)

■■■■■■■■ Continuing Education ■■■■■■■■

If you are applying for continuing education credits, a test is available online. For more details, visit www.aap.org/reachingteens.

■ Related Video Content

43.0 Anxiety. Kinsman.

43.1 Managing School-Related Anxiety. Ginsburg.

31.3.1 Stress Management and Coping/Section 2/Taking Care of My Body/Point 4: The Power of Exercise. Ginsburg.

31.3.2 Stress Management and Coping/Section 2/Taking Care of My Body/Point 5: Active Relaxation. Ginsburg.

■ Related Resources

GENERAL

Ratey JJ with Hagerman E. *Spark: The Revolutionary New Science of Exercise and the Brain.* New York, NY: Little, Brown and Company; 2008

This book explains how exercise affects mental health and well-being, and specifically how it helps depression and anxiety.

FOR ADOLESCENTS

Substance Use and Mental Health Service Administration. In the Wake of Trauma: Tips for College Students.
http://store.samhsa.gov/shin/content//KEN01-0092R/KEN01-0092R.pdf

> Developed by Substance Use and Mental Health Service Administration in 2007 to help college students cope with the mental health effects in the aftermath of trauma. Explains normal reactions, emphasizes the importance of talking about feelings, and offers tips for coping. Includes resources for more information.

TeensHealth. What Is Anxiety?
http://kidshealth.org/teen/your_mind/mental_health/anxiety.html

> TeensHealth is a Web site designed for teens (with parallel sites for parents and younger children) that provide clear, developmentally appropriate health information. This topic explains what anxiety is, different options to help cope with anxiety, and what to do if it becomes a problem.

FOR PARENTS AND CARETAKERS

American Academy of Child and Adolescent Psychiatry (AACAP)
The Anxious Child Facts for Families. http://www.aacap.org/App_Themes/AACAP/docs/facts_for_families/47_the_anxious_child.pdf

> From the AACAP, this fact sheet highlights that anxiety in children can be treated and that early treatment can prevent future difficulties, such as loss of friendships, failure to reach social and academic potential, and feelings of low self-esteem.

Obsessive-Compulsive Disorder in Children and Adolescents. http://www.aacap.org/App_Themes/AACAP/docs/facts_for_families/60_obsessive_compulsive_disorder_in_children_and_adolescents.pdf.
December 2011

> From the AACAP, this fact sheet explains the onset of OCD and how it can interfere with day-to-day functioning.

National Institute of Mental Health

> Anxiety Disorders in Children and Adolescents. http://www.nimh.nih.gov/health/publications/anxiety-disorders-in-children-and-adolescents/anxiety-disorders-in-children-and-adolescents.pdf
>
> > This fact sheet explains how anxiety disorders affect children and adolescents and the direction of future research.

> Substance Use and Mental Health Service Administration
> Tips for Talking With and Helping Children and Youth Cope After a Disaster or Traumatic Event: A Guide for Parents, Caregivers, and Teachers. http://store.samhsa.gov/Tips-for-Talking-With-and-Helping-Children-and-Youth-Cope-After-a-Disaster-or-Traumatic-Event/SMA12-4732
>
> > Developed by Substance Use and Mental Health Service Administration in 2012 to help parents and teachers recognize common reactions children of different age groups (preschool and early childhood to adolescence) experience after a disaster or traumatic event. Offers tips for how to respond in a helpful way and when to seek support.

FOR PROVIDERS

American Academy of Pediatrics. *Addressing Mental Health Concerns in Primary Care: A Clinician's Toolkit.*
http://tinyurl.aap.org/pub112382

> This toolkit, in the form of a CD-ROM, can be updated through the Web to provide current management advice, care plans, documentation and coding advice, parent handouts, and community resources to help address a variety of mental health concerns, including depression, anxiety, attention issues, substance use, learning differences, and other mental health concerns.

Beesdo K, Knappe S, Pine DS. Anxiety and anxiety disorders in children and adolescents: developmental issues and implications for DSM-V. *Psychiatr Clin N Am.* 2009;32:483–524

> A summary of the complex epidemiological risk factors and long-term outcomes related to anxiety disorders in childhood.

Brewer S, Sarvet B. Management of anxiety disorders in the pediatric primary care setting. *Pediatr Ann.* 2011;40:541–547

    A follow-up article that lays out treatment options with a clear explanation of cognitive behavioral therapy that can easily be explained to patients and families.

Sarvet B, Brewer S. Anxiety disorders in pediatric primary care. *Pediatr Ann.* 2011;40:499–505

    An excellent summary of how anxiety disorders present in primary pediatric care and considerations for diagnosis.

Walkup JT, Albano AM, Piacentini J, et al. Cognitive behavioral therapy, sertraline, or a combination in childhood anxiety. *N Engl J Med.* 2008;359:2753–2766

    Describes the benefits of CBT alone and sertraline alone over placebo and the combined benefit of CBT and sertraline over either single modality therapy.

CHAPTER 44

Somatic Symptoms

Sara B. Kinsman, MD, PhD

 Related Video Content

44.0 Managing Somatic Symptoms

■ Why This Matters?

We all commonly experience somatic physical sensations or pain. Some people have "butterflies" before a big test, others experience headaches when stressed out, and still others get sweaty palms when they are attracted to someone. Adolescents experiencing these feeling for the first time may feel confused or concerned. They may wonder, "What is happening to my body? Am I sick?" It can be helpful to explain that these sensations are common and are sometimes a signal that one needs to be aware of a stressor or environmental challenge.

> **Adolescents experiencing somatic feelings for the first time may feel confused or concerned. They may wonder, "What is happening to my body? Am I sick?" It can be helpful to explain that these sensations are sometimes a signal that one needs to be aware of a stressor or environmental challenge.**

■ Common Somatic Concerns in Adolescence

All people have somatic symptoms as our bodies react to our environment. Fleeting moments of anxiousness tense our muscles or cause a sinking feeling in our bellies. In most cases, we barely notice these changes because they pass quickly. In times of higher or prolonged stress, these changes sometimes generate fear or anxiety as we develop concerns over our well-being.

Adolescents frequently complain of body aches and pains. It is estimated that 10% to 30% of school-aged children complain of recurrent somatic concerns. The most common concerns are headaches (approximately 10%–30%), stomachaches (approximately 10%–25%), and limb pain (approximately 5%–20%). Adolescents with recurrent symptoms do not typically meet diagnostic criteria for somatoform disorders. Teens tend to have 1 or 2 somatic concerns; they can reoccur, but are often self-limited and resolve as the adolescent gets more experience and support in coping with life's challenges. Problems develop when somatic conditions are incredibly uncomfortable, interfere with function, or help a teen cope with or avoid a challenge. Then physical symptoms can become increasingly severe or unremitting.

Young adolescents can be intensely concerned about normal developmental changes in their body, and their increased attention can make them hyperaware of otherwise mild to moderate sensations. For example, some girls experience pain with breast budding. Although this is common, it can be frightening if unexpected. For an adolescent or her mother who has also witnessed breast cancer, normal breast budding can be alarming.

In this situation, you can ask questions that explore fears and provide reassurance that mildly painful breast budding is normal and unrelated to cancer.

■ Other Somatic Conditions

Conversion disorder occurs when teens feel they have involuntary loss of control over their ability to regulate movement or their sensory experience. A psychological stressor may precede the symptom and can be associated with the symptom or deficit, but the teen may not recognize this association, especially if the stressor occurred during the preverbal years (before age 3 years). Common conversion disorders include pseudoseizures, which are movements that look like seizures but are not accompanied by electrical brain wave activity. Other teens will present with extremity weakness or difficulty coordinating their legs, which can interrupt participation in school or sports. The key to taking care of common conversion disorder is engaging physical therapy early.

It is less common for adolescents to have *hypochondriasis,* which is a belief or fear of having a specific serious disease. When a teen shares repeated worries about having an illness, these concerns may be related to other behaviors or traumas too difficult to talk about. For example, the young man who repeatedly wants HIV testing may be trying to share information about current or past sexual risks.

Many practitioners become frustrated when they believe that a teen may be manipulative, malingering, or feigning illness. For example,

> One young man came into the emergency department with severe neck pain and a vague history of having fallen. He was placed in a neck collar, but refused to let anyone examine him or take x-rays. The medical team felt he might be malingering. One provider said, *"Robert, I'm not sure you know this, but the nurse noticed that you start crying out before they have touched your head or neck. One person worried that your pain seems out of proportion to what happened or you might be overdoing it a bit."* Robert responded, *"I can't leave here. I can't go to school."* The provider said, *"I got it. You need to stay here. Okay. Are you hungry?"* Robert said he was mostly thirsty. After he had a drink, the provider asked about his strengths. Robert explained that he takes care of his family, especially since his dad died. He explained it is hard to get money when people won't give you a job. He feels bad for his mom and younger siblings and wants to help. Then he says, *"I didn't really mean to get into it. I thought I would just get a little money around Christmas. It would make things easier for my mom. But she found out when CJ got shot and now everything's a mess. I don't know what to do."* With some more gentle questions, the provider learns that Robert has been running drugs. His mom found out when CJ was shot and has insisted that he promise to quit. He thought it would be cool with the guys, because he wasn't "too deep," he was only a runner. But they told him that if he tried to pull out, they would shoot him next.

This case demonstrates that malingering, exaggerating, or "faking it" is a tool a teen might use to seek help. If we strive to understand this, rather than becoming angry about being manipulated, we can position ourselves to make a difference.

Munchausen syndrome or *Munchausen syndrome by proxy* are especially concerning because the teen or parent will create a problem to prompt the medical team to do sometimes invasive studies or treat with unnecessary medications. For example,

> One young woman presented with blood in her urine and no symptoms of pain. Even though the symptoms did not make sense to the medical team, the team did a careful workup. Everything looked normal and the symptoms would come

and go. One team member did a thorough examination and noticed that the teen was biting the inside of their lip. The patient adamantly denied putting blood in her urine, but the team was able to take a step back and wonder if there were any factors in her life that would make the teen feel safer being in the hospital and suffering through medical studies than being at home. Some team members were concerned about her relationship with her older brother. When asked, the teen shared that she really loves her older brother, but she feels uncomfortable when he insists on coming into her bathroom to watch her shower.

Though this syndrome can be frustrating to treat and place the teen at risk, a team with the right mindset can explore the teen's cry for help and attention.

■ Why Are Adolescents at Increased Risk for Somatic Symptoms?

Adolescence is a time of significant brain maturation when teens can begin to appreciate a wider breadth of emotions, including those that are contradictory and ambivalent. Children and younger teens are often more accustomed to expressing their anxiety or worries in physical terms because they may not recognize their feelings or have the vocabulary to express them. A sixth-grade boy who is being teased for being overweight may not be able to verbalize the need for a "mental health" day to take a break from the repeated jabs at school, but his morning nausea may provide a good reason to stay home. As children mature, they can learn that morning queasiness may mean they are getting stressed at school and can either start to manage their stresses by mobilizing adult support or employing effective coping strategies.

Teens are struggling to understand their rich array of new emotions. Younger children are pretty clear when they are happy, mad, sad, or jealous. But when an eighth-grader feels happy that her best friend got the winning goal in the soccer game, jealous that she herself didn't get that goal, and sad that the team seems to celebrate only the best friend's final goal and not earlier contributions made by all the players, the young teen can feel confused. Sometimes they are embarrassed that they have negative feelings. If they can overcome that embarrassment and talk to an adult, the adult may shut down discussion of the natural muddle of feelings. *"You shouldn't be jealous. That's not nice. She did a great job and you should feel happy for her."* So as teens develop the ability to simultaneously experience several emotions, it is important that they have adults who appreciate their emerging emotional capacity and can support discussion. The adult may say, *"It makes total sense that you have a mix of feelings. Excitement for your friend, frustration, and maybe even jealousy, because it wasn't you. We all feel a mix of emotions when something like that happens. It's really good to talk about it."*

Somatic concerns may be linked to an emotion or event, but the teen and even her parents may not appreciate that connection. The stressor may have happened when she was much younger, but she is only equipped to begin to understand the meaning of the event now.

Sonya is a 13-year-old with new symptoms of occasional confused speech. The practitioner noticed that Sonya was fine until they started talking about her acting classes. When asked what this made her think about, Sonya launched into a complex story about how her mother decided that they would drive to Hollywood to audition for a movie when she was 4 years old. When she didn't get the part, her mom was barely able to function. After that trip, Sonya moved in with her dad and barely saw her mom. She cannot remember any feelings from that time, but her father remembers her fear and how sad it was to take visitation away from Sonya's mother when she would not take her schizophrenia medications. Sonya interrupts and asks, *"What is schizophrenia? Mom liked to act and she was sick, maybe that's happening to me. Do I have what Mom has?"*

For this young woman, having a somatic symptom opened the door to communicating about her confusion about the past and fears about her future. Both she and her father were relieved to learn that she did not have a life-threatening illness and they could begin talking about the challenges they overcame and others they are still working through.

Adolescents have not had the experiences of coping with new challenges alone. When they were younger, parents and teachers helped navigate new experiences. Now teens are flying a bit more solo. Performing with the jazz band in front of the whole middle school, juggling several class projects at the same time, missing a critical field goal for your football game that means your team will not make it to the state championship, trying to be noticed (but not too noticed) by a person who you really want to have as your boyfriend are all examples of first-time challenges, and the teen has to call the shots and deal with the consequences. The problem is that teens are learning coping skills as they go along, so they might not have the right skills to meet each new challenge. The body absorbs stress when the mind is struggling to make sense out of complex emotions.

While their capacity to gain these insights emerges, teens start to try to make sense of things that happened to them when they were younger. The teen who wonders about why his parents divorced may reexperience the "tummy aches" he had whenever he missed the parent he was away from. The teen whose mother died when she was a toddler may "remember" her mom's death in the same way she experienced it at age 2—a general physical discomfort because no one else in the family knew how to hold and comfort her like her mother did. Children exposed to difficulties when they are younger may need to take a little time in adolescence to ask questions and think through things that they were not capable of doing earlier.

Teens who survived traumas such as neglect, abuse, or witnessing of abuse may have lifelong alterations in baseline cortisol levels and exaggerations in cortisol responses to stress. Their brain may be rewired to be reactive. This "neurologic vigilance" can result in significant physical responses to environmental cues and stressors, such as an exaggerated startle reflex and sensitivity to their environment. Fortunately, the brain neuroplasticity that accompanies the teen years allows young people exposed to traumas to remap their brain and develop healthier and physically calmer ways of reacting to their environment.

■ Who Sees Teens With Somatic Symptoms?

Adolescents frequently see their primary care provider with concerns related to physical function and pain. Sometimes they will seek a specialist, such as a gastroenterologist, to help with abdominal discomfort. But, much more often, somatic symptoms are noticed first by parents, teachers, school nurses, counselors, and coaches. These adults have a vital role in teaching teens about somatic symptoms. When suggesting the teen visit a doctor, it might be helpful to say, *"When you get your jaw pain checked out, it might be good to mention that you've been studying really hard for your SATs. They may be able to figure out if your body is getting a bit tired out or if you are clenching your jaw as you study."* Caring adults can help teens learn that bodily discomfort is both real and commonly linked to stress.

■ The Medical Visit

Most clinicians will be told the reason for the visit is a physical concern. To schedule an appointment, most parents or teens provide a "legitimate medical complaint" to the office personnel. It will be a wonderful advance in our understanding of stress and the body when teens can schedule a visit because they are feeling stressed and having daily afternoon headaches.

When assessing a problem, it can be helpful to add this observation, *"Sometimes when people are dealing with a lot of stuff going on at school or at home, the extra energy or effort it takes to deal with everything can take a toll on the body. I was just wondering how things are going for you."* With this brief comment, the teen knows you are interested not just in the physical complaint, but also in the teen's general well-being. You have opened the conversation to include potential stressors.

Understanding the Teen's Symptoms

When sensing a teen may have a somatic concern, you may want to try the following approach:

- Listen to the patient's whole story. Ask the teen to start at the beginning: *"Tell me when you last felt well."* Be sure to pay attention to events that occurred the day or week prior to the start of the symptoms. Remember to ask about any anniversaries or birthdays.
- Retell the story you heard to the teen and family. Ask if you fully understood all of the symptoms. The patient or parent may say, *"Yes, except…."* In this case, retell the story with the additional information. Remember that listening to the teen, understanding his physical symptoms and empathizing with his discomfort can in and of itself be healing.
- Be sure to get a broad understanding of the teen's life. You will learn about emotional stresses and what strategies may help to strengthen effective coping strategies. For example, if you learn that a parent just returned home from deployment with significant physical disabilities and post-traumatic stress disorder, you may focus on ensuring proper mental health support for the entire family.
- Spend time alone with the teen to understand what he sees as his strengths and what is on his mind. Use SSHADESS to guide your discussion.
  - **S**trengths: Assess a teen's strengths and positive coping strategies before asking about more sensitive questions.
  - **S**chool: Understanding the complex cycle of school stress is important for healing teens with somatic concerns. Peer relationships and school functioning are a critical part of a child and adolescent's development. Be attuned to changes in (a) friendships, (b) being harshly judged or bullied at school, (c) physical or social differences that set the adolescent apart from their main peer group, (d) changes in the school or school environment, (e) academic disabilities, or (f) the need for academic perfection. Both academic and social challenges at school can cause overwhelming stress. As somatic symptoms worsen, these symptoms increase challenges at school, but also create a temporary escape from the stress of school. Adults thinking the teen is making excuses to get out of school may worsen a teen's esteem and further inhibit his ability to manage school stress.
  - **H**ome: Explore both positive family relationships and stress related to changes in family functioning, such as (a) divorce; (b) loss of a parent; (c) parental physical or mental illness; (d) parental job loss; or (e) deployment, reentry, and reintegration of a military parent.
  - **A**ctivities: It is important to know if the symptoms are impacting any activities *and* how upset the teen is (especially compared to his parents) about not participating. Sometimes a teen can't tell his parent that he is ready to give up an activity or sport (especially if the parents are counting on the teen earning a scholarship for college),

but, by having a somatic concern, the teen may gain the dual benefit of not having to participate and not having to confront his parents with the decision to stop participating.

— **D**rug use/substances: Ask about substances that can exacerbate symptoms (eg, tremors can be related to stimulant use or cigarette smoking). Adolescents will also self-medicate somatic symptoms with drugs or alcohol. For example, a college student might tell you, *"I don't get that stomach stuff before an exam anymore, because I take just one shot of Jack Daniels—just one shot—and I am ready to go."*

— **E**motion/eating/depression: Since somatic concerns are frequently the presenting sign of a mood disorder, such as depression, anxiety, obsessive-compulsive disorder, panic disorder, and substance-related disorders, it is important to consider psychiatric comorbidities as an essential part of the evaluation (see chapters 42 and 43). **S**exuality: Sometimes the trigger for a somatic concern may be hard to bring up spontaneously. Check in on how teens are faring with their sexual preferences, sexual orientation, romantic relationships, and gender identity.

— **S**afety: It can also be hard for adolescents to bring up some safety issues. A somatic complaint may be one way a teen can gain attention and compassionate listening. Sometime teens are just hoping that the caring adult will not be afraid to ask about their safety at home, on the way to and from school, in school, in relationships, and on campus. For some teens witnessing domestic violence and verbal abuse is incredibly painful. They are old enough to feel they should help, but still are too young to effectively intervene (see Chapter 18).

After a thorough psychosocial evaluation, a careful and gently executed physical examination is necessary. Start by gaining the patient's trust by asking his permission to examine areas that are reported to be painful. Be sure to not exacerbate discomfort or inadvertently demean the patient by pointing out inconsistencies.

The Differential Diagnosis and Evaluation

Illness in adolescents does not always follow the same course as in a younger child or an adult. Adolescents may minimize or amplify symptoms. They do not know how to effectively communicate how they feel. Therefore, it is our responsibility to give extra thought to the teen's symptoms. All potentially serious or progressive debilitating diagnoses need to be excluded. Rather than share your full differential diagnosis with the patient and family, discuss the teen's specific medical concerns, including a somatic diagnosis, and explain that you are thoroughly considering all the possible sources of the symptoms.

Some practitioners worry that if they entertain the thought that a teen has a somatic symptom at the time of initial presentation, they may start to subtly judge the teen and inadvertently overlook a "real" disease process. If we can appreciate that somatic symptoms are as "real" as other diagnoses—based on neurotransmitter dysregulation—and commit to completing a full differential diagnosis, we will not have to worry about including a somatic explanation from the start. In fact, by including somatic concerns in the initial differential diagnosis, we ensure that unnecessary testing and treatments are avoided and that mind-body symptoms are routinely discussed at each visit. If we wait until the "medical workup" is completed and then mention a somatic explanation, teens and their families will think we don't know and are "pointing the finger" at the patient's inability to manage stress. Some families will feel that you have given up. Others may worry you did not look deeply enough for the true diagnosis. In these situations, families may request further testing or seek second or third opinions. When we integrate somatic concerns into our initial discussions, we place this diagnostic possibility on par with others, and do not inadvertently perpetuate the pervasive societal stigma associated with physical symptoms related to stress. Leaving it as "unspeakable" only reinforces and perpetuates shame and stigma.

If symptoms do not warrant further evaluation, tests should not be ordered. Avoid ordering tests to "prove" to the patient and family that they are not ill. When tests are indicated, explain your expectations regarding the results.

> *"I think those extra movements you are having may be your body's way of letting us know that Algebra II is feeling like it is "too much" for your brain right now. We knew that this class would be a real challenge with your math disability, and I think these headaches are a sign that your brain is working overtime and is frustrated with this class. As you know, my job is to do the extra worrying. So I am going to order some tests, but I expect that these will all be normal. Luckily, we can start helping you feel better today."*

If a family really wants a confirmatory diagnosis, the practitioner might say,

> *"We do not have a specific test to explain why you are not moving your right foot, but we know your nerves are working, your brain is safe, and your symptoms are completely consistent with what we call a conversion disorder. Some research tells us that these symptoms are caused by changes in the blood flow to different parts of your brain. We do not do functional MRIs routinely, but this is so common and we are so good at getting young people better, that we can start treatment right away."*

After assuring the family that somatic symptoms are not life-threatening or progressively debilitating, you can explain the mind-body connection.

Explaining Somatic Symptoms and the Mind-Body Connection 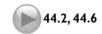 44.2, 44.6

- Some teens will easily grasp the mind-body connection and how stress affects emotional and physical feelings. Other teens and families will benefit from a more medical, neurobiological explanation, especially in the beginning of care.
- Sometimes the mind-body connection can be most easily explained by using physiological or animal models that make both practical and intuitive sense.
  — Example 1: Tension headaches rooted in shoulder, neck, and cranial muscular tension: *"Can you think of an animal that tenses its back muscles when it is stressed or upset? Exactly, a cat! Where do you also have cat muscles? When you are tense, those muscles at the back of your neck will become tense and can trigger one muscle after another to squeeze too tight, including those that connect to the base of your neck* (touch the occiput or nape of the neck) *and those that circle your head."* (touch the temples where they likely have experienced a squeezing or pulsing sensation)
  — Example 2: *"Belly pain can be caused because much of your blood is going to the wrong place. When you are relaxed, 40% of your blood is hanging out in your gut to calmly digest food. When you are stressed you feel like you should be running, so the blood is shifted to your leg muscles; that leaves your belly feeling very uncomfortable and functioning poorly."*
  — Example 3: *"Many people have to run to the bathroom when they get stressed. In fact, it makes a lot of sense. If you watch a film of a gazelle running from a leopard, you will see them jumping, swerving, running in herds, all while emptying their bowels. It is a matter of survival. They can run faster and jump higher without the weight. Some people just have really strong gazelle bellies."*

- For some families, trying to get the teen or parent to understand and "buy into" the mind-body connection will not feel therapeutic. Families may have strong preconceived notions that "weak" people experience stress. Others may suffer from an inability to identify and talk about internal emotions (alexithymia). In these cases, providing a symptom-based diagnosis consistent with the teen's concerns (eg, abdominal pain) can be reassuring and makes more sense to those unable to appreciate emotions.

- A primer on how neurotransmitters operate can break down old notions about the mind being separate from the body. You might say, *"The body has messengers called neurotransmitters that connect the brain, heart, stomach, and all the muscles. For example, if you burn your hand, the damaged skin sends your brain a message. Your brain then signals your hand to move and speeds up your heart rate. You might yell 'ouch' and you might feel angry. We don't think about these actions; the brain and the body are so well connected, it happens automatically. Sometimes this system gets worked up for other reasons. For example, when someone gets ready to go to college, the brain might get worried in advance about the upcoming change. A young person may not get restful sleep, and, therefore, may become tired or achy. This can be confusing when the summer is such fun. There are a lot of things we can do to help people whose neurotransmitters are 'gearing up for a change.'"*

■ Judgments, Stigma, and Terminology Impact How We Help Teens With Somatic Concerns

A patient with somatic symptoms may receive messages from peers or adults that she might be "faking it" and acting like a "drama queen," or that the physical discomfort or symptoms are "all in your head." This can be demoralizing. It can also undermine the therapeutic alliance you are trying to form because the teen or family may become invested in searching for a "real problem" or "medical diagnosis." You might let the teen and family know that they may hear this from people who just don't understand that pain can be related to all kinds of things—past events, current events, anniversaries, working really hard, or looking forward to a big event. Sometimes we don't know what the specific trigger might be; still, we can always help people feel better and figure out ways to communicate with uninformed people in their lives. A teen might explain to their soccer team, *"Hey guys, can you stop hassling me—look, I'm not exaggerating the pain, my doctor explained that it is common to get neck cramps every now and then and he really doesn't want me to head any balls while I'm trying to deal with it, but I can still play when I feel well."*

Other ways of taking away shame and stigma include reinforcing that somatic symptoms are universal.

- You may turn to your own experience to teach about somatic symptoms, while being careful not to cross boundaries. Tension headaches that develop when studying for a test, stomach discomfort on test days, and sweating when nervous are all examples of somatic concerns we have overcome or learned to deal with. Often, with this firsthand appreciation for the somatic symptoms, you can normalize the experience.

- It can also be helpful to share how other adults have overcome these symptoms. A parent may share how a beloved aunt or uncle's body responds to stress. *"Not sure if you know this, but, when Uncle Jimmy works too much, he gets really bad back pain and that's why he stretches and exercises every day when we vacation together."*

- You can also encourage the parent to share how they feel when they are stressed: *"When I'm stressed, I get these terrible headaches."* Sometimes a parent will use this opportunity to share the level of stress in their own lives and, in turn, the teen can let the parent know if this is added to her own stress or even the main stress. When this occurs, the practitioner is given an opportunity to talk about self-care as a first step to supporting the child.

Preparing the Teen to Use the Right Terminology

When returning home, teens are inevitably asked, *"So what did the doctor/nurse say?"* Though some will be comfortable explaining the mind-body connection, others may worry about disapproval or negative judgments. It is important to spend a few moments discussing how to explain the symptoms and treatment plan to others. Often, teens prefer to use a label that simply describes the symptoms and general approach to the care plan. The adolescent may benefit from a brief role-play before leaving the office.

> A 14-year-old had worsening of her recurrent abdominal pain (RAP). She practiced what she would tell her worried grandmother and officious school nurse: *"My doctor says I have RAP, which means recurrent abdominal pain. My mom, my doctor, and I are doing a bunch of different things to deal with the really bad stomach pain. Sometimes my gut might get a little tensed up, so we are going to work on ways to calm it down, including relaxation exercises and deep breathing. We also think it will help to stay active in school and sports."*

■ Initial Approach to Alleviating Concerns

Using a Diary

- Some teens will find it helpful to keep a diary or log of their symptoms. The diary should include activities, foods, and social activities that might exacerbate or relieve symptoms. For example, in the case of chest pain, it could include the pain's relationship to exercise, food, the amount of homework a teen might have, and if there were any issues at school, online, or at home. The diary can help identify both things that make symptoms worse and what alleviates discomfort. For example, a teen might see that he never gets nausea at his aunt's home and come to realize that his parents' constant fighting is actually getting to him. In addition, the diary can list things he enjoys doing or that help him cope.

Care Versus Cure Approach

- Adopt a "care versus cure" rehabilitative approach, which encourages return to usual activities and responsibilities even if symptoms persist. A detailed, realistic, graded plan that addresses all aspects of a teen's life will help the teen to learn to manage symptoms and regain function. The goal is to develop a collaborative process that empowers the patient to function to the fullest.

Treatment Team

- It is most helpful to establish and work with a treatment team. Typically, the team will include the adolescent, the family, the health clinician, the school nurse, the guidance counselor, an individual or family therapist or child psychiatrist who is knowledgeable of somatic symptoms, and other complimentary providers. These may include a physical therapist, chiropractor, massage therapist, acupuncturist, homeopathic therapist, or yoga teacher.

Resuming a Routine

- Ask which activities can be resumed immediately and work together to reintroduce them. Ideally, the adolescent can quickly return to some routines, such as waking at school time, showering, getting dressed, joining the family for breakfast and dinner, completing some household chores, and starting to catch up in 1 or 2 subjects.

- Returning to school can be overwhelming for adolescents with many absences who have not kept up with schoolwork. Coordinate a catch-up plan with the school guidance counselor and teachers. Many adolescents do not have sophisticated executive functioning skills that would enable them to multitask and "catch up" in several subjects simultaneously. Parents might ask the school to permit part-time attendance and a plan to complete makeup work. In-school accommodations and tutoring programs may be helpful. For example, adolescents with severe irritable bowel symptoms may benefit from access to a private bathroom. Adolescents may feel reassured that they can "rest" in the nurse's office or other calm space if necessary. School nurses are always core members of the treatment team.

Physical Reconditioning

- Physical reconditioning is often the first step in recovery. Conditioning goals should be achievable. If the adolescent has been "couch-bound," suggest walking out to get the mail every day and circling the dining-room table twice every 2 hours. What may seem like minimal progress will enable the adolescent to propose a healing regimen and take things at a pace that ensures success, advancing every few days. Some adolescents will ask if they might attend their teams' practices, but not participate; this can be a great motivator and will facilitate valuable peer contact. Others will make great strides by working with a physical therapist to stretch painful muscles, release trigger spots, and use deep breathing. Programs that support intense aerobic reconditioning have reported very successful short- and long-term wellness.

Individual and Family Therapy

- Most patients and families will benefit from working with an individual or family therapist experienced with somatic complaints. In making a referral, it is crucial to ensure that the selected therapist is skilled in this area. He or she should be able to help the adolescent interpret physical sensations and discomfort, identify strengths and coping skills that can be used to manage symptoms, and address the inevitable disappointments, such as changes in peer relationships, that may accompany disruption in normal school activities. The therapist should also be able to help family members learn to respond appropriately as improvements occur and should encourage positive parenting skills. If there is resistance to therapy, remind the teen that her pain is traveling through her nerves. The coordinator of all of their nerves is the brain. Counseling can help use the brain to learn to calm the signals the nerves are sending.

Pain Management

- Almost two-thirds of somatic complaints include an element of pain or discomfort. Pain management may be needed while the adolescent works to increase overall functioning, and even after full function has returned. A number of non-pharmacological and pharmacological approaches may be effective.
- Massage, tender-point release, acupuncture, and stretching exercises included in yoga, tai chi, or Pilates may alleviate musculoskeletal pain. Hypnotherapy and visualization or meditation techniques have also proven helpful. These approaches may also help teens deal with stress, which in turn affects their symptom experience and overall well-being.
- Intermittent use of non-steroidal anti-inflammatory medications can ease discomfort as physical therapy is initiated, but the most important message for adolescents with somatic concerns is that there is no "magic pill," and that many different non-medication modalities should be explored as you work together to increase function and manage symptoms.

- If a practitioner is concerned that the teen has a concurrent mood disorder, evaluation by a psychiatrist who can carefully consider the risks and benefits of treating concomitant mood disorders with medications such as tricyclic antidepressants, serotonin reuptake inhibitors, and mood stabilizers. (When choosing a medicine, always consider suicidality, since medications have varied lethality in an overdose.) When a well-functioning multidisciplinary team is working in harmony, the teen's complex need can be addressed on multiple levels.

■ Ongoing Treatment Plan

- Once a plan and healing team are in place, schedule frequent visits to assess symptoms, monitor progress, and minimize setbacks that can occur with the stress of getting back into a regular routine. You can also coordinate communication with members of the medical team and the adolescent's high school, college, or workplace.
- Some adolescents will regain function and see their symptoms resolve very quickly. For these patients, continuing to provide support and remaining accessible is essential. When the teen is feeling better, plan to talk about the somatic symptoms and consider what elements of the treatment plan worked so that if new stressors cause symptoms, the teen has a plan that may quickly be put into place to minimize future impairments in function.
- Frequent contact with other team members is essential to ensure that everyone is giving the teen the same message and working together to address the evolving needs and concerns.
- When the adolescent's symptoms take time to resolve, stay vigilant for potential diagnoses that were not initially obvious. Also remember that teens with somatic disorders also get other diagnoses. Youth with chronic abdominal pain still get appendicitis; adolescents with reflex sympathetic dystrophy can still get Lupus.

■ Summary—Putting It All Together

Educating adolescents about the mind-body connection is one of the most important preventive health messages we can offer. We achieve this by expressing empathy for the adolescent's symptoms and the caretaker's concerns. With this understanding, we can then guide youth to discover the connection between their emotions and physical experiences. When we encourage effective coping strategies for different emotions, we promote lifelong wellness.

•• Group Learning and Discussion ••

Discuss how youth with somatic symptoms have presented in your setting. If you work in a non-health setting, what might your institution be doing to support young people to reengage as fully as they can, or, conversely, might your setting be inadvertently stigmatizing their experience?

Case for Health Professionals

Break into groups of 3, splitting roles of youth, parent, and health professional.

Taylor is a 13-year-old with belly pain for about 3 weeks. It is mostly around her navel. She also has diarrhea almost every night and vomits most mornings when she brushes her teeth. Her pain is worse around lunchtime. She is really upset about this because Marita, her best friend, sits with her at lunch. She really needs time with her because they had a fight a month ago and she needs to make up. She can't even go to school about twice a week and is really anxious because she already didn't "get" algebra.

Case for Community-Based Programs

Discuss as a group how to come up with a plan to welcome Chase back to your program.

Chase is a 15-year-old who has not been coming to your program for 5 weeks. Even when he was coming in the last couple of months, he was on the sidelines a lot with headaches, or a "weak" ankle. You know how much he needs your program as a place to connect with adults and vent his frustrations. It has been especially important since his big brother was shot and has had severe difficulty communicating and drags his leg while walking. Chase has been in the hospital for the last week; you are not sure if it was an acute care or mental facility. You are aware that, about 6 weeks ago, one of the youth workers said to him, *"You're just going to have to stop moping around, there is nothing you can do for your brother."* Another said, in attempted good humor, *"Man don't pull that weak ankle line on me, you've just lost your jump shot!"*

Case for Educational Settings

Discuss as a group how to help Marcos reintegrate into school.

Sixteen-year-old Marcos is an outstanding student who has been out of school for 6 weeks. Prior to this stretch he had mono for 2 weeks and missed school. His doctor thought he was better, but, after a couple of days back at school, he became even more tired and had terrible headaches. He was very frustrated that he was so behind and that he got a D on a make-up physics exam. He turned in an English paper 3 days late and it was much lower quality than his norm; he received a C-. After a week of being back in school, he stayed out for the last 6 weeks nursing his pains and sleeping much of the day. His nurse practitioner says he is ready to return now, but needs you to help plan his reentry. Prepare for a meeting with Marcos and his parents.

▪▪▪▪▪▪▪ Continuing Education ▪▪▪▪▪▪▪

If you are applying for continuing education credits, a test is available online. For more details, visit www.aap.org/reachingteens.

■ Suggested Reading

American Psychiatric Association. *Diagnostic and Statistical Manual of Mental Disorders.* 5th ed. Arlington, VA: American Psychiatric Association; 2013

Campo JV, Fritz G. A management model for pediatric somatization. *Psychosomatics.* 2001;42(6):467–479

Dell ML, Campo JV. Somatoform disorders in children and adolescents. *Psychiatr Clin North Am.* 2011;34(3):643–660

Kinsman SB. Caring for adolescents with somatic concerns. *Adolesc Health Update.* 2004;16:1–9

Shapiro B. Building bridges between body and mind: the analysis of an adolescent with paralyzing chronic pain. *Int J Psychoanal.* 2003;84(3):547–561

■ Related Video Content

44.0 Managing Somatic Symptoms. Kinsman.

44.1 Why Stress Affects Our Body, and First Steps Toward Healing. Singh.

44.2 Helping Adolescents Understand (Without Shame!) How Stress Affects the Body. Ginsburg.

44.3 Helping Your Child Whose Physical Symptoms Might Be Related to Stress. Kinsman.

44.4 Mindfulness as a Tool That Allows Us to Better Be Present With Others' Pain. Vo.

44.5 The Use of Skillful Self-disclosure to Reinforce That ALL People's Bodies React to Stress. Vo.

44.6 Using Insight Into How the Body and Mind Are Integrated to Reduce Somatic Symptoms. Ginsburg.

32.1 The Body Scan. Vo.

■ Related Resources

There are a limited number of academic resources that are free of language that may feel judgmental for some patients or families. We suggest using handouts associated with coping (see Chapter 31). Some patients or families with conversion disorders may benefit from this Mayo Clinic resource, which may help families understand that conversion symptoms are well recognized and can improve.

Mayo Clinic Health Information for Patients Conversion Disorder: www.mayoclinic.com/health/conversion-disorder/DS00877

CHAPTER 45

Grief

Alison Culyba, MD, MPH
Sara B. Kinsman, MD, PhD

 Related Video Content

45.0 Supporting Youth Through the Grieving Process

■ Why This Matters

Grief is a universal experience. Approximately 2 million children and adolescents in the United States have experienced a parental death. Half of all marriages end with divorce, creating family conflict for countless teens. Neighborhoods are gripped by violence, with teens losing family and friends unexpectedly. Caregivers suffer from chronic physical and mental illnesses that render them unable to fully participate in family life. Loved ones are deployed for extended periods to serve our nation. All of the youth we care for will experience grief at some point. Helping adolescents effectively cope with loss builds resilience and allows them to develop a coping skill set that they can carry forth into adulthood.

> Grieving adolescents learn an essential life skill—how to survive loss. As they grieve, they develop a deeper understanding of their emotions. They come to understand their profound capacity for love. And they ultimately find that, despite the depth of sadness, they are able to heal and again find joy.

■ Grappling With Loss

Grief can emerge for adolescents through the loss of a parent, a sibling, a grandparent, or a very good friend, or loss of an animal that is considered part of the family. Grief can also occur due to serious medical or mental illness in the family that renders someone unable to connect in a meaningful way. When families are separated by divorce or military deployment, adolescents can also experience grief at the change in family structure. Some losses, such as those experienced when family members suffer from terminal illness, are prolonged. Others are sudden and unexpected, such as the loss of a friend to gun violence. Violent deaths can cause severe stress responses as well as a strong desire to seek revenge. Both foreseeable and unexpected losses can bring with them profound grief. Understanding the depth of the loss requires insight into the individual relationship between the adolescent and their deceased family member or friend.

Adolescence is a particularly challenging time to grapple with grief and loss. Teens attempt to seek out meaningful and lasting relationships with both adults and peers. They begin to form unique relationships, with each relationship providing them with a special kind of connection. When one of these relationships ends abruptly, it can be particularly jarring. Further, in contrast to younger children, adolescents have a more complete understanding of the permanence of death.

Losing a loved one is a physically painful process. It can be all-consuming and over-whelming. For many, the adolescent years will be the first time they experience these intense emotions. They may be surprised by the depth and intensity of emotions they feel in response to the loss. They often feel as though their world has come to a stop. Yet they see the busy world around them continuing to carry on while they struggle with intense sadness. You may hear adolescents say things like, *"How can these people be out getting coffee when my grandmother just died?"* or *"How are they laughing?"* They grapple with how to fill the void left by the person who passed on.

■ Loss Affects Family Functioning

Loss becomes more complicated because it affects the way an entire family functions. When the loss involves a member of the nuclear family, it usually causes the family to function poorly. Suddenly, family roles can change. An adolescent who thought of her mom as the family foundation becomes confused when she sees that her mom cannot cope with her father's death. As parents deal with their own grief, they may become less available to their children and cease to function as leaders of the family. People around them may say things like, *"You just lost your grandmother, but your mom is here."* or *"You are so lucky to have such a great dad to help you through this."* However, in reality, the mom or dad may not be functioning well in their parenting role following a loss. Teens are very perceptive regarding these role changes. They may feel abandoned. The sense of, *"Oh no, who is taking care of me?"* can be very real.

■ Making Sense of a Loss

Teens can react in many ways to loss. Teens (and adults suffering a loss of someone they are very connected to) may continue to experience a loved one's presence. Sometimes you will learn that the teen continues to sense the presence of the person they lost and will even feel comforted talking with that presence. Adolescents may say, *"My mom is always with me. I feel she is always there."* or *"My grandmother talks to me while I am sleeping."*

Other teens will experience comfort in the smell or feel of their loved one. Younger adolescents often seek out physical items such as clothing and accessories that belonged to the lost loved one in order to further solidify this bond. These are helpful ways for adolescents to cope with the loss and transition from having their loved one close by.

■ Common Adolescent Behavior Changes

Adolescence is a developmentally complicated period in which individuals are exploring their own self-identity and defining their relationships. They are seeking more independence. They are also moving from very concrete to more abstract thought processes. These developmental changes can be challenging under the best of circumstances. However, in times of stress, these processes become even more challenging.

It is important to keep these developmental changes in mind when thinking about normal adolescent responses to grief. In some ways, adolescents deal with grief similarly to adults. The adult classic model of the stages of grief first described by Dr Elisabeth Kubler-Ross in 1969 (denial, anger, bargaining, depression, and acceptance) applies to some degree to adolescents. However, it is essential to explore adolescents' grief responses within a developmental framework in order to understand the deeper driving forces. While adolescent development occurs on a continuum, it is helpful to explore the distinct responses of early and late adolescents.

Early adolescence (about ages 12–14) is a particularly challenging time to experience loss. During this time, adolescents are working to withdraw emotionally from parents in order to gain more independence and gain peer acceptance. There is often tremendous internal conflict between wanting to be dependent versus independent. Early adolescents' grief frequently manifests as anger as they struggle with these 2 forces. They may wish to avoid all emotional expression, especially any public display of emotion. They can become angry or dismissive if an adult begins to cry in front of others. They may allow their emotions to come out in private, often crying alone in their rooms. This can create tension within a family because older adults feel the teen pulling away just in a moment when most adults seek closeness. And while early adolescents want to spend more time with friends, they are extremely apprehensive about confiding in friends for fear of being rejected by their peer group.

Some younger adolescents tend to become busy with their school and extracurricular activities following the loss of a loved one. Boys in particular respond to grieving this way. They may immediately want to go back to school. They fill their days with schoolwork, games, and activities. This offers a distraction from the all-encompassing grieving that is typically going on at home. Some youth may be talkative and pepper family with questions. Others will be less cooperative and more demanding of attention than usual. This can be challenging for families because teens can become difficult as they seek out attention through acting out. However, undesired behavior can serve an important role. It forces engagement, which causes grieving families to regroup.

> Henry is a 12-year-old who just learned that his dad's cancer returned. Henry had been a constant source of support and humor during his father's first and second treatment regimens. When his mom and dad told him that his dad would have to restart medicines and travel to another city for treatment, he responded with irritation: *"OK, fine. So who is going to take me to baseball practice?"* His parents understood that Henry had enough understanding to know that this was very bad news, but at that moment he couldn't take it all in, process yet another loss of his father to cancer, and know that he would have to bear another loss of "normal life." Mostly, he felt deeply scared, and his parents knew that when he was ready, at random times, he would ask the questions that were difficult to speak out loud: *"Is Dad really ever going to get better?"* or *"Is Dad going to die?"* But for now, it made sense that Henry wanted to know how to keep going on with his life and manage this difficult news in small increments.

Older adolescents (about ages 15–17) tend to experience grief in ways more similar to adults. They often have intense emotions, such as sadness and despair, that interfere with normal functioning. Because they are able to think more abstractly, they have a better sense of the permanence of death and also understand the implications that the loss will continue to have on their own life. They mourn specific aspects of their relationship with the deceased, but also mourn the loss of how that relationship would have evolved over time. For instance, teens may say things like, *"Who is going to help me move into my dorm room?"* or *"Who is going to be there when my first child is born?"* Older adolescents also worry about their own mortality in light of the current death. They become intensely focused on things such as the heritability of medical conditions from which their loved ones suffered. In contrast to younger adolescents who tend to focus almost exclusively on themselves, older adolescents have a greater ability to empathize with others suffering around them. They tend to be more willing to spend time with family following a loss. However, they still struggle to find balance between their own needs and caring for other family members. They turn to friends and intimate partners for support, but are still keenly aware of the possibility of rejection from their peer group.

Many teens will also experience sleep disruption. For some, this will manifest as difficulty falling asleep. Teens may lie awake trying to process their loss; others will have nightmares. Nightmares can be related to the actual death or may bring forth other unrelated fears. Sleep difficulties make it hard for teens to get the rest needed to cope with stress.

Adolescents will often test parental boundaries following a loss. They may talk back or refuse to do chores. They may stay out late with friends or experiment with alcohol or drugs. These behaviors serve as an escape from their emotional reality. They also challenge caregivers to set limits. Adolescents are seeking out adults that can reinforce family structures that may have been disrupted by the loss.

Some adolescents will regress. Rather than participating in peer activities, they may wish to spend all of their time with family. For instance, a 16-year-old who used to enjoy going on school trips, playing soccer with a community team, and sleeping overnight at friends' houses may instead now want to stay home. Or a younger adolescent may refuse to go to school. Teens may act younger in a hope that adults around them will focus more on taking care of them. While their behavior can seem childlike, it is a mechanism for coping with emotional intensity; they shut out feelings to attempt to return to a simpler emotional state. They may also be so distraught that they cannot fully participate in activities in which they typically excel.

Sometimes withdrawal from activities may stem from a heightened sense of responsibility to take care of family members, especially if caregivers are so fraught with grief that they are unable to perform their traditional family roles: *"Are they going to be okay? Are they too depressed? Do they need help? Who will take care of my younger siblings if I go out?"*

■ Guilt Is a Normal Part of Grieving

Some adolescents, especially younger teens, grapple with guilt. Younger children may worry they caused a parent's death because they had wished their parent was dead once when they were arguing. Adolescents have a more nuanced sense of guilt. They may think things such as, *"Even though this does not fully make sense, is there a part of me that caused this to happen? If I hadn't been such a pain at home, then maybe she would have gone to the doctor sooner."* Guilt helps explain the loss they have experienced; by giving themselves a role, they find a way to take charge of the situation.

■ Grieving Takes Time

Losing a loved one is life-altering and it takes time to rebuild a network of meaningful relationships. During their initial stages of coping, many adolescents busy themselves with activities, fully immersing themselves in their former lives. This can create confusion for adults, who assume they must not be grieving because they are able to carry on. Adults may say, *"Look how great she is doing. She is still getting straight 'As' and playing varsity soccer."* But, grieving can be extremely unpredictable. Emotions come forth at unexpected moments for months or even years. For instance, a teen may be excited about prom for weeks and beam with joy as she steps out in a new dress. However, when the band plays a song that her ill mother would not allow her to listen to, she may burst into tears and race home. Teens can become incapacitated by grief without notice. Eventually, the unpredictable nature of their grief lessens as adolescents come to terms with the loss.

> Emily is a 15-year-old who comes to see you because she can't stop crying. She learned that she has to go on a gluten-free diet and says, *"This is too, too much, I can't do it."* You know Emily to be a practical young person who rarely gets shaken by challenges. So you ask what else is going on. Her mother and best friend, who have both come to the visit, mention Jamie. Emily sits with tears

streaming down her face. Jamie, her boyfriend for the last year, broke up with her through a text and told her that he was seeing another girl. Emily couldn't talk. She just teared. When you spend time alone with her, you learn that she can't believe this is happening. She doesn't know what she will do. You ask if she has thoughts of not wanting to be here or wanting to hurt herself or be dead. She clearly says no: *"Who would take care of my younger brothers and my mom?"* You can see that she really doesn't have words to describe how much pain she is in, and you ask her if she remembers being in this much pain before and she responds, *"Only when Daddy died."* and she begins to cry harder. You ask her if she might be having "pain on top of pain" or "piggyback pain." That is, when one loss brings up the memories and deep sadness of an earlier loss. She cries and says all she is dreaming about is her dad. She explains that she was only 10 when he died. Her mom was so sad that Emily started helping around the house and getting the boys off to school. Her mom cried most of that time and struggled to find a job to support the 3 kids. I asked Emily if there was any chance that she could take some time to be sad for the loss of Jamie, but also mourn, more like an adult, the loss of her dad. She looked so relieved. Finally, the "over the top" feelings about breaking up with Jamie (she adds at this point in the conversation that he was really not the best boyfriend*)* make sense, and Emily starts to share with you (with tears and a little laughter) some funny stories about her dad, whom she hadn't talked about with anyone in a long time.

■ Grief Builds Life Skills

While dealing with loss is one of life's greatest challenges, it also creates opportunity. It is important to remember that grieving adolescents are learning an essential life skill: how to survive loss. As they grieve, they develop a deeper understanding of their emotions. They come to understand their profound capacity for love. And they ultimately find that despite the depth of sadness, they are able to heal and again find joy. These are profound life lessons that carry forth into adulthood. Adolescents must have the room and the support to move through this process so they can become stronger, compassionate adults.

■ Assessment of the Grieving Adolescent

Caring for adolescents who are grieving is an extremely important part of participating in someone's life and helping them move forward. Being able to explore their unique experiences while also helping them understand what is normative is one of the gifts you can give to youth as they heal. Caring adults can support young people by asking questions, listening deeply to their experience, and providing guidance.

- When speaking with grieving youth, it is essential to acknowledge the loss. Acknowledge that grief is an individual experience. Let the adolescent know that you are here to support him or her through the process.
- Take time to explore the adolescent's relationship to the person. Ask about what they enjoyed doing together, a favorite memory, a special personality trait. While some teens may shut down or act angry, others will open up and reveal incredible stories that provide you with a glimpse into their loss. By creating the space for storytelling you allow the adolescent permission to speak openly. By actively listening, you can start to forge a trusting bond that is essential for the healing process.

- It can be very helpful to discuss common symptoms of grief. Let them know that it is normal to feel angry, devastated, guilty, lonely, numb, or indifferent. It is acceptable to not want to deal with it now. Prepare them to feel many different ways over the coming weeks; it is common to have feelings of sadness emerge unexpectedly.

- Understand how the loss has impacted their functioning. Are they going to school? Are they still participating in sports? Have they changed peer groups? Are they able to do things they still enjoy? Are they spending more time alone? Have they been using substances to help cope? Have they made any decisions about relationships or their bodies that they regret? Do they have someone they can talk to about their loss?

- Talk about physical complaints. The mind and body are inherently linked. As adolescents grieve, they often suffer with headaches, abdominal pain, fatigue, chest pain, and insomnia (with or without upsetting dreams) and literally feel that they have a "broken heart." These symptoms can be disabling, especially if they are similar to symptoms experienced by the deceased. Adolescents may worry that they, too, are suffering from a serious affliction (like the lupus that just took their aunt's life). Taking their symptoms seriously and providing reassurance empowers adolescents to understand their body's physical response to grief. Offer advice about the importance of sleep, exercise, a well-balanced diet, and social interaction to help guide them through the healing process (see Chapter 44).

- Ask about how the loss has changed family functioning. *"Losing someone puts tremendous stress on the whole family. How have things changed in your family since your dad moved out?"* This allows you to assess the degree of dysfunction within the grieving family as well as identify caregivers who may be coping well.

- Ask adolescents if they have suffered previous losses. Listening to discussions about coping with previous loss provides invaluable information about an individual's understanding of grief and the skills he or she developed through the process.

- Identify supportive adults. Ask, *"Who in your life can help you through this?"* Explore whom the teen has reached out to already and brainstorm other potential sources of strength within their network. Ask if it would be helpful for you to speak to these family members, or for you all to meet together, to discuss the healing process.

- Next, it is essential to understand the depth of their loss. Adolescents grappling with acute grief are all struggling to manage their emotions. Care providers must determine which adolescents require immediate professional support due to the severity of their grief experience. Becoming familiar with normal grieving responses as well as signs of more serious disorders is essential (Table 45.1). Are they feeling so sad and confused that they cannot participate in life? Are they wishing they were with the person who is gone? Are they wishing to be dead themselves? These are adolescents who need immediate professional help to ensure they remain safe.

■ Guiding the Youth Toward Help

Many adolescents in the throes of grief will be reluctant to seek help. Care providers should emphasize that seeking help is a sign of personal strength.

> *"Sometimes when you are grieving, you might feel that life will never get better, or even is not worth living. That is the time to get help. Help is a way to go through a path of grieving, to map it out, to accept all of the difficulties, and to move forward in a way that is helpful for you and those around you. It is hard work. It takes incredible strength. Those who do it are brave."* Provide adolescents with support to know that their strength will serve themselves and others. *"You need to do it for yourself, you need to do it for the person who passed away, and you need to do it for the rest of your family."*

Table 45.1
Range of Common Grief Manifestations in Children and Adolescents[a]

Normal or Variant Behavior	Sign of Problem or Disorder[b]
Shock or numbness	Long-term denial and avoidance of feelings
Crying	Repeated crying spells
Sadness	Disabling depression and suicidal ideation
Anger	Persistent anger
Feeling guilty	Believing guilty
Transient unhappiness	Persistent unhappiness
Keeping concerns inside	Social withdrawal
Increased clinging	Separation anxiety
Disobedience	Oppositional or conduct disorder
Lack of interest in school	Decline in school performance
Transient sleep disturbance	Persistent sleep problems
Physical complaints	Physical symptoms of deceased
Decreased appetite	Eating disorder
Temporary regression	Disabling or persistent regression
Being good or bad	Being much too good or bad
Believing deceased is still alive	Persistent belief that deceased is still alive
Adolescent relating better to friends than to family	Promiscuity or delinquent behavior
Behavior lasts days to weeks	Behavior lasts weeks to months

[a]Reprinted with permission from American Academy of Pediatrics Committee on Psychosocial Aspects of Child and Family Health. The pediatrician and childhood bereavement. *Pediatrics*. 2000;105(2):445–447.
[b]Should prompt investigation; mental health referral is recommended.

Adolescents in crisis may have difficulty identifying supportive people. Find out who has helped them through previous stressful times. *"When you are looking for someone to help you get through grief, it is really important you find someone you are comfortable speaking to. You need somebody who has been through it and who you trust, someone who is older and can give you their wisdom."* Help adolescents explore their relationships with parents, grandparents, adult siblings, aunts and uncles, family friends, teachers, school counselors, coaches, and health care professionals. *"Who do you think will be the most helpful for you? When will you have a chance to talk?"* For adolescents you identified as high risk, formulate a plan to ensure prompt follow-up with a mental health professional to ensure their safety.

■ Helping Families Support Grieving Adolescents

Surviving loss puts tremendous stress on families. Parents attempt to support their children while simultaneously grappling with their own grief. It is important for parents to maintain expected family roles to the best of their abilities. Parents should maintain routines and discipline. They should be prepared to de-escalate conflicts that often arise between grieving family members. Teens often feel abandoned and alone following the death of a loved one. Being surrounded by others who are working to maintain a supportive family environment can be extremely healing. It is helpful for parents to identify other adults who can step up to handle family responsibilities if the parent is too overwhelmed by grief.

Honesty is essential to help families move forward. Encourage parents to openly discuss the circumstances surrounding the loss. Parents often want to shield their children from death, hoping to lessen the grief they experience. However, adolescents understand death and feel betrayed when adults are being secretive. Allow teens to ask questions and answer them as openly as possible.

Help parents understand that adolescent grief looks different from adult grief. Anger is often very pronounced and can be directed at surviving family members. Regressive behavior is common. Teens often have erratic emotions in the weeks to months following a death, with emotions emerging at unexpected moments. It is important that parents create a safe space for teens to express their emotions. Younger adolescents, who are often embarrassed by public displays of emotion, may benefit from more structured times to reminisce. Bringing the family together to do an activity that was meaningful to the deceased provides a wonderful opportunity to share memories.

Parents need to be mindful that just because their teen has resumed activity as usual and seems to be coping well, they are still working through profound suffering. Older adolescents often feel that they must "keep it together" for the sake of the family; they worry that, if they take time to grieve, their family will fall apart. Parents need to be alert to this tendency and make sure that teens know it is all right for them to work through their own grief. This may mean that teens miss several days of school, do not keep up their grades, or decline trying out for the soccer team. Grieving teens are participating in an incredible project. That project is learning about loss and about surviving loss. When we expect adolescents to bypass normal emotions so they can keep getting As in school, we will have foregone immeasurably important life lessons. We will have set up unrealistic expectations and will not have helped them develop into strong, resilient adults.

Participating in bereavement rituals can be very healing. Offer adolescents the opportunity to participate in memorial services. Find out what portions of the services they wish to attend, but do not force them to join if they do not want to. Many teens will want to pay tribute to their loved one by speaking, reading a poem, or creating a photo montage. Other teens will find more solace through personal journal writing. Reflecting on treasured memories is an important part of the healing process. Parents should be sure to honor their child's individual approach to grieving while providing opportunities to mourn with others in their community.

Help parents identify supportive peers. By late adolescence, peers are a strong source of emotional support. Parents can help identify trusted friends to be present through the grief process. This allows grieving adolescents to continue on their developmental trajectories. Having emotional outlets outside of the family can also help reduce conflict within the family.

Inform family members of the warning signs of severe grief. Parents know their children best, so they are well poised to seek help for their struggling teen. Discuss that it is very common for adolescents to struggle following a loss. Assess parental willingness to seek help from a health professional and provide resources so that parents feel empowered to help their teen. Discuss referral for professional counseling for teens exhibiting severe symptoms. Research suggests that participation in structured psycho-educational support groups can improve outcomes for both adolescents and parents.

Encourage parents to care for themselves. Parents may be so focused on protecting others that they do not meet their own basic needs, let alone process their own loss. Reassure parents that it is not selfish to care for themselves; indeed it is a strategic act of good parenting (see Chapter 39). Explain that children respond to adversity best when their parents remain stable and serve as models for healthy coping.

A Path Forward

There are many different ways to work through grief. Some of it is time. Some of it is talking with family, trusted adults, and health care professionals. Some of it is getting back to usual activities and busying oneself. Sometimes it is a feeling that you are fulfilling a mission of the person who passed away by doing something in their honor.

Care providers play a fundamental role in helping youth move forward. By creating a safe environment to explore grief and listening to adolescents' stories, they can begin the healing process. Youth often describe a feeling of emptiness following a loss. They seek various strategies to fill this void. Some of these strategies, such as alcohol and drug use and sexual promiscuity, put vulnerable teens in high-risk situations that can jeopardize their futures. Steering teens toward positive strategies, in contrast, strengthens their repertoire of coping mechanisms.

> Justin is a 17-year-old who came into the office for a routine physical. He wore a baseball cap that cast a long shadow over his forehead as he sat slumped in an examination room chair. His eyes fixed on the floor as he answered questions about his medical history with short sentences. We eventually moved on to discuss his social history. I asked, *"Whom do you live with?"* The question, which for most adolescents serves as a harmless introduction to discuss more sensitive topics, hung heavy in the air. *"It's complicated,"* he shrugged. I asked, *"What does complicated look like?"* He discussed how he had been bouncing around between foster families for the past 2 years. *"I move around a lot because I keep getting in fights."* When I asked him what made him angry enough to fight, he said, *"People are always messing with me, talking s**t about me."* He revealed that he was suspended from school for fighting and on the verge of being kicked out of his district. I asked him who he used to live with before entering foster care. He described how his father left when Justin was very young and his mother has been in and out of rehab for alcohol and heroin use. *"Was there anyone in your family you used to be close to?"* I inquired. *"My grandmother was always there for me. She took me in and raised me while my mom was away. She took good care of me, made sure I had a good home-cooked dinner, was always nagging me to do my homework, made sure I pressed my shirt for church on Sunday morning…."* His voice trailed off and then he said, *"But she is dead now. Died of cancer a few years ago. And my mom, she didn't even come to the funeral. Only thing she gives a d**n about is getting high. And so I had nowhere to go."* After a pause I said, *"I can tell you loved your grandmother deeply. What do you think it was about her that made her so special?"* As he told stories of his grandmother teaching Sunday school, bringing neighborhood kids into her home who were in search of a warm meal, picking up trash that littered the sidewalk, and gathering old winter coats to donate to a local shelter, Justin's eyes lit up. For the first time during our visit, he cracked a small smile. *"And it's just not right that she is gone while all these other losers are still hanging around in the neighborhood,"* he said. *"Your grandmother sounds like she was an amazing person, and I can tell that her death was tremendously hard. What do you think she would say if she were here now?"* He sat silently for a while, and then said softly, *"She'd tell me I gotta keep going and I can't give up."* I reflected to him that he had already shown a tremendous amount of strength to move forward. I asked him what he wanted to do with his life and he said, *"I want to be a counselor to help kids when they hit rough spots."* I looked him right in the eye and said, *"Your grandmother would be so proud."* He allowed himself to cry.

From there, we talked about how fighting could get in the way of his desire to honor his grandmother's memory. We came up with strategies he could use to get out of fights. And we figured out that he could volunteer at a local library helping neighborhood kids with their homework. By listening to the story of his loss and helping him figure out how to pay tribute to his grandmother through his actions, Justin was able to move forward.

Assisting adolescents in honoring the legacy of lost loved ones can be healing. It allows them to take charge. It allows them to channel their feelings in a positive direction. Creative expression is another powerful tool to promote healing following a loss. Journal writing, poetry writing, and drawing give adolescents a safe space to express their emotions. They may choose to share portions of their work with family, friends, or caring professionals, or they may choose to keep their expressions private. Youth are often surprised by the power of their own words. They are able to explore the depths of their sadness and relive bittersweet memories. Creative outlets allow them to begin to move forward to become compassionate and resilient adults.

45.1

●● Group Learning and Discussion ●●

1. Prior to this session, assign one member of the group to find local resources for grieving youth.
2. Discuss the wide range of ways youth in grief have presented in your practice setting.
3. Break into pairs and choose a case in which a youth "acted out" to deal with her grief, sought revenge, or even her own death as a means to handle her emotions. If you do not have a case, use one of the 2 below. Guide these youth toward channeling their grief by honoring the legacy of those they have lost.
    a. Cicely is a 14-year-old who has recently lost her grandmother. She has argued incessantly with her mother recently. She implores, *"I am nothing like her!"* She palpably misses her grandmother, whom she visited weekly at the elder community. Her grandmother always showed her off to all of her friends, and she used to even play cards with them. She tearfully says that she wishes she could be with her grandmother.
    b. Shane comes into the community center and things just seem different. He is irritable and seems to intentionally foul the other men on the court. The youth worker takes him aside and comments that something seems to be on his mind. He fumes, *"D**n straight I'm angry. My cousin was shot and he has a little girl. Just a baby. He wanted to be a cop. Showed off her picture all the time, had big dreams for her. She's never gonna know him. It's alright though, I'll find out who did it."*

▪▪▪▪▪▪▪ Continuing Education ▪▪▪▪▪▪▪

If you are applying for continuing education credits, a test is available online. For more details, visit www.aap.org/reachingteens.

▪ Related Video Content

45.0 Supporting Youth Through the Grieving Process. Kinsman.

45.1 Dealing With Grief by Living Life More Purposefully. Ginsburg.

■ Related Resources

American Academy of Child and Adolescent Psychiatry
Facts for Families: Children and Grief. http://www.aacap.org/cs/root/facts_for_families/children_and_grief
> This information sheet reviews common grief symptoms and behavioral manifestations. It highlights concerning symptoms for which parents should seek help from mental health professionals.

American Academy of Pediatrics
Addressing Mental Health Concerns in Primary Care: A Clinician's Toolkit
http://tinyurl.aap.org/pub112382
> This toolkit provides up-to-date management advice, care plans, documentation and coding advice, parent handouts, and community resources to help address a variety of mental health concerns including grief, depression, anxiety, attention issues, substance use, learning differences, and other mental health concerns.

American Academy of Pediatrics Committee on Psychosocial Aspects of Child and Family Health. The pediatrician and childhood bereavement. *Pediatrics*. 2000;105(2):445–447
> This article reviews children and adolescents' response to grief and provides guidance for pediatricians to use when caring for patients and families following a loss.

HealthyChildren.org
www.healthychildren.org/EmotionalWellness
> This site focuses on helping parents promote emotional wellness across all ages.

Christ GH, Siegel K, Christ AE. Adolescent grief. "It never really hit me…until it finally happened." *JAMA*. 2002;288(10):1269–1278
> This article uses a teen's narrative to explore developmental models of grief, with a specific focus on coping with loss in relation to a terminally ill parent. It provides age-specific helpful strategies for engaging youth throughout the illness, death, and mourning periods.

Christ GH. Impact of development on children's mourning. *Cancer Pract*. 2000;8(2):72–81
> The author uses a qualitative approach to analyze interviews with grieving children and then highlights features of the grief response across the age spectrum. The article specifically discusses what grief looks like, what parental attributes are mourned, key developmental characteristics, and parental tasks to facilitate coping in 5 different age groups.

Dehlin L, Martensson L. Adolescents' experiences of a parent's serious illness and death. *Palliat Support Care*. 2009;7:13–25
> This qualitative study uses interviews with grieving teens to describe the threat of parental death, how adolescents manage this threat, and how they cope with loneliness following death. It includes multiple interview excerpts that allow teens to describe the grieving process in their own words.

Kubler-Ross E, Kessler D. *On Grief and Grieving: Finding the Meaning of Grief Through the Five Stages of Loss*. New York, NY: Scribner; 2007
> This book builds on the author's classic *On Death and Dying*, which changed the way we talk about death. It added understanding on the grieving process.

Kirwin KM, Hamrin V. Decreasing the risk of complicated bereavement and future psychiatric disorders in children. *J Child Adolesc Psychiatr Nurs*. 2005;18(2):62–78
> This article synthesizes various theoretical models of grieving and explores psychological factors that affect the grieving process. It outlines the importance of support from families and care providers to improve long-term mental health outcomes for grieving youth.

Lancaster J. Developmental stages, grief, and a child's response to death. *Pediatr Ann*. 2011;40(5):277–281
> This article examines the stages of grief through a developmental lens. It also discusses myths surrounding childhood grief and risk/protective factors that impact bereavement.

Moreno M, Furtner F, Rivara F. Advice for patients: when a loved one dies. *Arch Pediatr Adolesc Med*. 2012;166(3):296
> This patient handout explains children's and adolescents' response to grief and provides concrete tips parents can use to help their families after a loss.

Riely M. Facilitating children's grief. *J Sch Nurs*. 2003;19(4):212–218

This article focuses on the role of school health professionals in guiding children through the grieving process. It provides suggestions for school-based therapeutic interventions and outlines guidelines and resources for implementing grief support programs for children and families.

Substance Abuse and Mental Health Services Administration

www.samhsa.gov/MentalHealth/Anxiety_Grief.pdf

This informational handout for patients provides basic information about grief as well as online resources.

CHAPTER 46

ADHD in Adolescents

Susan T. Sugerman, MD, MPH, FAAP

 Related Video Content

46.0 ADHD: From "Disorder" to Manageable Difference

■ Why This Matters

Attention-deficit/hyperactivity disorder (ADHD) is one of the most common neurobehavioral disorders of childhood, affecting 9.5% of children in the United States.[1] Often persisting into adulthood,[2] ADHD is characterized by developmentally inappropriate levels of inattention and hyperactivity resulting in functional impairment in academic, family, and social settings.[3]

> To begin to understand what it might feel like to receive the diagnosis ADHD, it is important to point out that the label has 2 words in it: "deficit" and "disorder." Our job is to help the young person understand this condition in a way that reduces shame and stigma.

Without adequate recognition and management, children and teens with ADHD often develop long-term impairments in self-esteem, academic performance, difficulties in family and social relationships, and problems with self-protective decision-making. They are also more likely to have other mental health and neurodevelopmental conditions (including learning disabilities, problems with conduct, substance use, anxiety, and depression) and to experience activity restrictions, school problems, grade repetition, and poor parent-child communication.[4] Compared with teens without ADHD, young drivers with ADHD are 2 to 4 times more likely to be involved in motor vehicle crashes, 3 times more likely to sustain injuries in crashes, 4 times more likely to be at fault, and 6 to 8 times more likely to have their license suspended.[5,6] The multidimensional effect of ADHD on daily life functioning can culminate in significant costs attributable to greater health care needs, more frequent unintentional injury, co-occurring psychiatric conditions, and work loss.[7] The reassuring news is that many of these problems, including substance use and poor driving performance, are significantly reduced with appropriate ADHD management.[8,9]

It is important to recognize that people with ADHD also tend to have abundant strengths. Many adolescents who have ADHD may feel demoralized, having received a lifetime of negative messages about the condition, their interaction styles, or their school performance. Therefore, it is especially important when working with these youth to use a strength-based approach that reinforces those assets that may position them to better be able to overcome their challenges and build on their potential.

■ Criteria to Make the Diagnosis of ADHD

The key behaviors of ADHD are inattention, hyperactivity, and impulsivity. These are symptoms of underlying differences in brain function, not causes of the disorder itself. Therefore, it is imperative to always consider other diagnoses when evaluating for challenges to focus and attention as well as impulsivity. For example, anxiety, depression, and learning differences often interfere with one's ability to focus; similarly, the irritability that is often associated with depression in children and teens can appear very much like the impulsivity characteristic of ADHD. Given the high degree to which other mental health conditions coexist in youth with ADHD, clinicians must be vigilant in ensuring their diagnostic assessment includes contributing conditions that may confound, mask, or accentuate typical symptoms of ADHD and related impairments.

The American Psychiatric Association's *Diagnostic and Statistical Manual of Mental Disorders, Fifth Edition (DSM-5)* is used by mental health professionals to help diagnose ADHD.[3] This diagnostic standard helps ensure that people are appropriately diagnosed and treated for ADHD.

DSM-5 Diagnostic Criteria for ADHD

The following diagnostic criteria are reproduced with permission from the American Psychiatric Association. Diagnostic and Statistical Manual of Mental Disorders. *5th ed. Arlington, VA: American Psychiatric Association: 2013;59–66.*

A. A persistent pattern of inattention and/or hyperactivity-impulsivity that interferes with functioning or development, as characterized by (1) and/or (2):

1. **Inattention:** Six (or more) of the following symptoms have persisted for at least 6 months to a degree that is inconsistent with developmental level and that negatively impacts directly on social and academic/occupational activities:

   Note: The symptoms are not solely a manifestation of oppositional behavior, defiance, hostility, or failure to understand tasks or instructions. For older adolescents and adults (age 17 and older), at least five symptoms are required.

   a. Often fails to give close attention to details or makes careless mistakes in schoolwork, at work, or during other activities (eg, overlooks or misses details, work is inaccurate).

   b. Often has difficulty sustaining attention in tasks or play activities (eg, has difficulty remaining focused during lectures, conversations, or lengthy reading).

   c. Often does not seem to listen when spoken to directly (eg, mind seems elsewhere, even in the absence of any obvious distraction).

   d. Often does not follow through on instructions and fails to finish schoolwork, chores, or duties in the workplace (eg, starts tasks but quickly loses focus and is easily sidetracked).

   e. Often has difficulty organizing tasks and activities (eg, difficulty managing sequential tasks; difficulty keeping materials and belongings in order; messy, disorganized work; has poor time management; fails to meet deadlines).

   f. Often avoids, dislikes, or is reluctant to engage in tasks that require sustained mental effort (eg, schoolwork or homework; for older adolescents and adults, preparing reports, completing forms, reviewing lengthy papers).

   g. Often loses things necessary for tasks or activities (eg, school materials, pencils, books, tools, wallets, keys, paperwork, eyeglasses, mobile telephones).

   h. Is often easily distracted by extraneous stimuli (for older adolescents and adults, may include unrelated thoughts).

   i. Is often forgetful in daily activities (eg, doing chores, running errands; for older adolescents and adults, returning calls, paying bills, keeping appointments).

2. **Hyperactivity and impulsivity:** Six (or more) of the following symptoms have persisted for at least 6 months to a degree that is inconsistent with developmental level and that negatively impacts directly on social and academic/occupational activities:

Note: The symptoms are not solely a manifestation of oppositional behavior, defiance, hostility, or failure to understand tasks or instructions. For older adolescents and adults (age 17 and older), at least five symptoms are required.

   a. Often fidgets with or taps hands or feet or squirms in seat.
   b. Often leaves seat in situations when remaining seated is expected (eg, leaves his or her place in the classroom, in the office or other workplace, or in other situations that require remaining in place.)
   c. Often runs about or climbs in situations where it is inappropriate. (**Note:** In adolescents or adults, may be limited to feeling restless.)
   d. Often unable to play or engage in leisure activities quietly.
   e. Is often "on the go," acting as if "driven by a motor" (eg, is unable to be or uncomfortable being still for extended time, as in restaurants, meetings; may be experienced by others as being restless or difficult to keep up with).
   f. Often talks excessively.
   g. Often blurts out an answer before a question has been completed (e.g., completes people's sentences; cannot wait for turn in conversation).
   h. Often has difficulty waiting his or her turn (eg, while waiting in line).
   i. Often interrupts or intrudes on others (eg, butts into conversations, games, or activities; may start using other people's things without asking or receiving permission; for adolescents and adults, may intrude into or take over what others are doing).

B. Several inattentive or hyperactive-impulsive symptoms were present prior to age 12 years.

C. Several inattentive or hyperactive-impulsive symptoms are present in two or more settings (eg, at home, school, or work; with friends or relatives; in other activities).

D. There is clear evidence that the symptoms interfere with, or reduce the quality of, social, academic, or occupational functioning.

E. The symptoms do not occur exclusively during the course of schizophrenia or another psychotic disorder and are not better explained by another mental disorder, personality disorder, substance intoxication or withdrawal).

Specify whether:

Combined presentation: If both Criterion A1 (inattention) and Criterion A2 (hyperactivity-impulsivity) are met for the past 6 months.

Predominately inattentive presentation: If Criterion A1 (inattention) is met but Criterion A2 (hyperactivity-impulsivity) is not met for the past 6 months.

Predominately hyperactive/impulsive presentation: If Criterion A2 (hyperactivity-impulsivity) is met and Criterion A1 (inattention) is not met for the past 6 months.

■ Assessment/Screening/Tools

Attention-deficit/hyperactivity disorder is a clinical diagnosis based on symptoms and findings noted above and cannot always be determined by a single diagnostic test. Several screening tests may help identify and differentiate subtypes of ADHD in the context of possible confounding factors, such as depression, anxiety, and other behavior disorders. They help clinicians obtain and interpret information from parents, teachers, and others about symptoms and functioning across various settings for assessment and can be helpful for monitoring the effects of treatment.

Validated Screening Tools

- NICHQ Vanderbilt Assessment Scale and Follow Up (for Parent and Teacher)
- Parent-completed Child Behavior Checklist
- Teacher Report Form (TRF) of the Child Behavior Checklist
- Conners Parent and Teacher Rating Scales
- ADD-H: Comprehensive Teacher Rating Scale (ACTeRS)

When basic screening and a clinical interview fail to adequately identify the primary cause of symptoms or dysfunction, comprehensive neuropsychological or psychoeducational testing can be helpful. These evaluations can function like an "MRI of the mind," providing a "picture" or explanation of how the brain thinks, rather than what it looks like. Licensed psychologists choose from a battery of well-studied, validated testing instruments to assess issues related to attention, distractibility, learning styles, multiple components of intelligence (several types of IQ testing), thought patterns, mood concerns, personality profiles, family/sibling conflict, etc.

Good testing helps children to understand themselves and assists parents in directing efforts at support and intervention. Results can help teens understand why certain situations are hard for them and others are not. They can help with choices of schools or colleges, learning environments, and even career choices. A comprehensive testing report can guide a clinician in choosing medication (if necessary) and help a counselor select the best form of therapy.

■ Helping Teens Understand ADHD

To begin to understand what it might feel like to receive the diagnosis or label "ADHD," it is important to hear clearly 2 words imbedded in the name—"deficit" and "disorder"—that can create shame and generate stigma. This highlights the importance of teens understanding what this condition means for them, including both the challenges they need to work around as well as the likely strengths they also possess. **46.0**

As you sit down to discuss this with the young person and family, consider trading chairs. Give the young person your chair that spins, adjusts up and down, and has wheels. Give him permission to go for a ride and spin if he would like. At some point deep into the conversation, while he is looking pretty preoccupied with the spinning, ask him to repeat what you said. His parents may just be amazed to find that he was actually listening better when allowed to move.

First Things First: What Does It Mean?

The first thing a young person needs to understand is that ADHD may be a bit different in every person and that the label does not predict how you will think, act, or feel. Generally, however, ADHD is about having trouble blocking out interrupting or distracting thoughts. Dr Edward (Ned) Hallowell,[10] coauthor of *Driven to Distraction: Recognizing and Coping with Attention Deficit Disorder*, describes the ADHD brain as a "turbo brain" in overdrive. Sometimes this charged up brain gets kids in trouble and other times it produces the best and most creative ideas.

Young people need to understand that thinking is not their problem; organizing all of the thoughts they do have, however, may be troublesome. For this reason, having organizational strategies and reminders to help put on the brakes can be key to managing ADHD successfully.

ADHD is not necessarily a deficit of attention. People with ADHD pay attention just fine—to the pencil dropped across the room, the clicking of heels in the hallway, the starting and stopping of the air conditioner system, the conversation on the other side of the library carrel, etc. People with ADHD are very easily distractible and often hypervigilant to changes in their environment. This makes focusing on one task more difficult than average for peers of comparable age and developmental stage, especially if the task is boring or mundane. In contrast, when the task is something compelling or extremely interesting, those with ADHD can often hyper-focus to the exclusion of all other stimuli. This explains why some youth can't make it from the kitchen to carpool without losing their lunch and their homework, but have no problem losing themselves for hours in a novel or video game.

ADHD is not necessarily a disorder. Imagine we are a society of cave people who decide to go out hunting for deer. How must we behave to catch a deer? Imagine that everyone in the hunting party stays totally focused, still, and silent during the deer hunt, looking only for the deer. What is likely to happen? We won't see the tigers sneaking up on us from the back! (Or the signs that the warring tribe is ready to ambush us, let alone the storm clouds and flash floods that could risk everyone's lives.) Our society needs both the focused, task-oriented performers at the core of the group (the deer hunters) as well as the "lookouts" on the fringes who can see the big picture and challenge us to see things a little differently. However, don't write off the "lookouts" as potentially good hunters themselves. They are the ones who may have noticed the brush moving and who can then hyper-focus on the prey.

We live in a society of deer hunters. Our education system in particular rewards those who can put their blinders on and stay focused on the regimented, prescribed tasks at hand. We are expected to sit still, pay attention, mind our own business, and not look away from our own desks or cubicles. These are not the strengths of students with ADHD. In a highly structured (ie, boring, dull, or repetitive) learning environment, individuals with ADHD are more likely to daydream, doodle, talk to a neighbor, or even fall asleep. They may read ahead or do different work altogether. The student with ADHD may be fidgety or just plain hyperactive, sometimes to the point of having to get out of his or her seat. These are not traits that please teachers trying to train future deer hunters.

The problem with being a lookout. When appropriately motivated, individuals with ADHD will keep trying to pay better attention, to keep track of assignments, or to remember to bring their lunch or instrument to school. They promise to talk less in class or to stop barging in their sister's room without permission. Though well-intentioned, their success rate is not always high. They do not wish to disappoint or anger their teachers and parents. Yet they face daily reminders of how they can't seem to "behave" or "perform" as well as their peers or siblings. Most importantly, they are accused of "not living up to their potential." When adolescents don't understand why learning is hard for them, and when they cannot "fix it" themselves, they may begin to internalize the feeling that they are "stupid" or "lazy." It can be easier for a child to "check out" or claim not to care than to keep banging his or her head against the wall trying to improve at something that never seems to get any better. Especially in families where parents or siblings are seen as successful, a child may feel it is easier to be seen as "bad" rather than "dumb."

Back on the farm... Students who are easily distracted may struggle to stay on task in traditional academic settings, but learn the same concepts and life skills through artistic activities such as theater or art. In contrast to deer hunting, if we raised children on farms, they would learn science by studying crop cycles, develop math skills while cooking for 50 farm hands, practice critical thinking skills by assessing and responding to inventory needs in relationship to demand for agricultural products, and engineering through repairing farm equipment. Students with ADHD often respond quite well to active experiential learning environments that encourage creativity and independent task completion with visible, tangible results. They enjoy frequent breaks and changes of venue. A day that starts in the milking parlor and ends in the corn field by way of the chicken coop, "mess hall," general store, and stables can leave you feeling exhausted but productive. Especially for someone with ADHD, it can be hard to get that same level of satisfaction sitting still in a deer blind for 8 hours. "Finding their farms"—learning and work environments that keep them engaged but also productively stimulated—can help those with ADHD achieve necessary educational and vocational goals. Programs offering more "hands-on" and holistic ways of teaching and reaching students may better serve this talented and creative group of young people who may otherwise be failed by our mainstream educational systems.

Apples don't fall far from trees. Quite often a child with ADHD has a parent with similar characteristics, whether or not they carry the diagnosis. In a "best-case scenario," a fairly disorganized, impulsive, creative parent has thrived in spite of—and often because of—those tendencies. The family may benefit from considering how that parent has learned to compensate and accommodate for those symptoms over a lifetime. More concerning examples include parents with ADHD traits who found significant life difficulties leading to personal or professional failures or even problems self-medicating with drugs or alcohol. Even in this case, it can be useful to help a young person understand how ADHD can affect one's life and begin to develop strategies to work toward better outcomes.

Highlighting the Positives and Taking Away Shame

Rather than a weakness or disability, ADHD can be a strength when channeled in productive directions. Of course, people with ADHD have a wide variety of personalities, and we shouldn't assume positive traits any more than we assume negative ones, but there are some general assets common to people with ADHD. The characteristics common to individuals with ADHD—distractibility, impulsivity, and hyperactivity—are often seen in those with creative energy and problem-solving skills. They see what others do not see, connecting dots out of order as their ideas bounce around in unexpected ways, and come up with solutions more linear thinkers could not have envisioned. They are visionaries, big thinkers, and risk-takers; many are our artists, writers, poets, inventors, and entrepreneurs. All social entities, from small businesses to large governments, need the dreamer who is willing to challenge norms and think outside the box in addition to the realist who can keep the process organized and accountable and who can get things done. People with ADHD can be quite successful professionally when they keep their eye on the big picture and delegate the details.

When working with a young person with ADHD, it is important to understand both his strengths and limitations. Certainly he needs to know how to exist in a deer hunter society, particularly because most of his education will be delivered in a style that assumes one can stay focused for great lengths of time. However, he also needs to know the great benefits that having a different way of thinking, when well-managed, can be for his future success. The deer hunter/lookout metaphor can be useful both in helping youth describe what it feels like to have ADHD (being always aware of their environment, including things large and small, easily evident and hidden) and to minimize their shame in having it. Young people need to understand that although a revved up brain can definitely find it difficult to stay focused on one subject at a time or to live in a body that is told it must sit still, there are some real advantages to being so charged up.

The best way of reinforcing a young person's strengths is to ask her to elicit a list of positive things she believes a person with ADHD might have. The list of positives includes being energetic, passionate, funny, driven, sensitive, and creative. Consider sitting down at a computer with a young person and using the search phrase "the good things about having ADHD." Your favorite search engine will populate with scores of sites. Look through a few together with the youth and parent(s), then invite them to do the same at home as a family.

■ ADHD Is Both Over- and Underdiagnosed

It can be all too easy to diagnose and treat based on the key features of ADHD—distractibility, impulsivity, and hyperactivity—without recognition of alternative or contributing causes or comorbidities. On the other hand, the personal and family frustration resulting from long-term consequences of unrecognized and untreated ADHD can lead to cycles of blame, shame, and significant life dysfunction, which could be dramatically improved by appropriate diagnosis and treatment. It is the responsibility of the diagnosing professional to evaluate for other causes of these symptoms, including learning differences/disabilities, stress, and mental health disorders.

- **"Plain" ADHD:** Native difficulty maintaining vigilance while attending to relevant stimuli (or filtering out irrelevant stimuli) describes ADHD in the classical sense. Youth with this type of difference in brain function respond well to psychostimulant and other approved ADHD medications.
- **Learning differences/disabilities:** Students with significant learning disabilities will have difficulty sustaining attention when being taught in ways inconsistent with their optimal learning styles. When unable to compensate, frustration or disappointment in their performance may lead them to secondary problem behaviors, which can easily be seen as disrespectful or sometimes impulsive. For example, a child with an auditory processing disorder may do well enough in elementary and middle school doing worksheets and group projects but begin to show signs of distractibility and trouble focusing when teachers start lecturing in high school. While ADHD medication may, in part, improve attention, it will do nothing to address the underlying learning disability.
- **Mental health concerns:** A teen with significant depression or anxiety will have a hard time staying focused on learning. Even youth who are stressed will have difficulty focusing on tasks. For example, we cannot expect youth whose parents are constantly fighting to keep from being distracted by worries about what is happening at home. ADHD medication has the potential to exacerbate rather than alleviate problems for these individuals. In some cases, failure to recognize the underlying causes of their symptoms can have serious implications.

Be particularly attentive for young people who carry other "labels" or have been presumed to be behavioral problems during childhood. Some of these adolescents have ADHD and will be far better served with the appropriate label rather than one that implies delinquency. Similarly, always look for youth with school failure, or who have been described as "lazy" or not living up to their potential. Many of the adolescents have ADHD or another learning difference and may have given up on their ability to learn. Further, routinely consider whether the substance-using teen is self-medicating ADHD or another behavioral health disorder.

■ Management Strategies

A comprehensive treatment strategy should include organizational strategies and basic wellness principles regarding exercise, sleep, and nutrition, and may include medication.

ADHD Medication

Medications can be an important part of an overall strategy to manage ADHD, particularly in fostering school success or increasing driving safety.[11] However, they must not be seen as the sole mode of ADHD treatment. It is beyond the scope of this chapter to describe different medication regimens. If a medical professional determines medication may be useful, it is important that adolescents, parents, and teachers all offer feedback on its effectiveness.

Teens deserve an honest discussion where you can help them consider all of the benefits and potential side effects of medication. Most importantly, they should understand that side effects should only be tolerated as a last resort and that they should work with their health professionals until they can settle on a regimen with minimal or no undesired effects.

Some young people may be concerned that medications will flatten their personality. The fact that you have approached ADHD from a strength-based perspective may make youth more comfortable sharing this fear. In fact, some people do experience a change in personality while on medication. The good news is that these are not permanent changes, and many medications wear off on a daily basis. The teen deserves reassurance that she will be the same person on or off medications. For example, her love of animals or passion for soccer will not change. Further, some of the ways the medication may affect her may actually make her more likeable. For example, she may find that she is able to be a better listener. Finally, help the adolescent understand that the goal of medication should always be to achieve the benefit (in this case increased focus) on the smallest dosage possible. In the case of ADHD, the lowest dosage can be achieved when it is also "treated" by learning effective organizational strategies and incorporating wellness strategies into a healthy lifestyle.

Organizational Strategies

Youth with ADHD tend to be disorganized, partly because they pay too much attention to what others would call extraneous stimuli. Also, they may be working on one task, but will become distracted by another they find more interesting or immediate. In effect, they lack an internal file cabinet that neatly organizes and prioritizes the items they need to work on. A critical part of ADHD management, therefore, is to help youth understand that precisely because they may have more trouble organizing or prioritizing, they need to figure out how to be even more organized and to have better prioritization tools than someone without ADHD. They have to learn to create an external file cabinet. At its simplest level, this includes making lists that prioritize tasks. They also benefit from reminders, repetition, structure, and clear limit setting. While electronic devices sometimes provide temptation for distraction, many functionalities of common applications included in mobile phones and online calendars can be set to send reminders of upcoming tasks, appointments, and deadlines. Further strategies can be developed with an educational specialist equipped to help youth build organizational skill sets.

Wellness Strategies

The standard of evidence has not yet produced the "ideal" ADHD diet, exercise plan, or sleep regimen. It is beyond the scope of this chapter to cover the range of thinking on these matters. Suffice it to say that general wellness strategies on exercise, sleep, and nutrition will benefit everyone's ability to focus and may hold particular significance for people who already have difficulty with distractibility and task management (see Chapter 40).

Exercise

Exercise has been found to significantly reduce ADHD symptoms.[12,13] It uses up some of the excess energy associated with ADHD. The importance of exercise can be described to young people using the deer hunter/lookout model. Their "job" is to be a scout or lookout, to go up hills and down hills, and to make sure others will be safe from predators or attacking villagers. When a young person who is a "lookout" exercises, he satisfies his biologic need to be running while scanning the environment. When possible, encourage morning exercise to start the day. **31.3.1**

Nutrition

The optimal ADHD diet would help the brain function better and decrease restlessness and distractibility. Current research on ADHD diets is limited, and results are mixed.[14,15] Many experts do believe that diet likely plays a role in mitigating some ADHD symptoms. We can start by assuming that whatever is good for the brain is likely to be good for ADHD. Therefore, it is reasonable to suggest that eating a balanced diet of high-quality protein; complex carbohydrates like whole grains, fruits, and vegetables; and limited healthy fats (as well as fewer simple or highly processed carbohydrates) may ensure optimum brain metabolism. This, in combination with limiting simple sugars or highly processed carbohydrates, will also decrease brain blood sugar fluctuations, and, therefore, may improve concentration. **31.3.3**

Sleep

Most teenagers do not meet the recommended standards of 8 to 9 hours of sleep per night.[16] This limits their ability to learn, listen, and concentrate. Therefore, while sleep is important for all youth, it is even more critical for youth with ADHD who already have baseline challenges in these areas. In fact, sleep restriction has been found to critically influence the formation of long-term memory in youth with ADHD.[17,18] **31.3.4**

•• Group Learning and Discussion ••

It is beyond the scope of this chapter to focus on ADHD diagnosis; rather, we want to focus here on management. The first step of management is removing shame from the diagnosis. You might consider using the deer hunter/lookout metaphor to do so. In fact, you might find that metaphor will offer a clue that someone may have ADHD when the adolescent says, *"That's me, I'm a lookout."* (However, that statement of self-recognition is not enough to make a diagnosis.) Another strategy to remove shame and stigma from the diagnosis is to make the list of "the good things about having ADHD," perhaps using the Internet to help prime the list. After you have helped the young person develop a sense of pride in her difference, she will be more likely to join with you in developing a comprehensive strategy to manage ADHD. Such a strategy may include medication and should include organizational strategies, good nutrition, enough sleep, and appropriate exercise. If it includes medication, help the youth to understand how the "changes" the medication might produce can be beneficial.

Break into pairs and use the following scenarios to practice this strength-based approach to ADHD. Alternatively, use your own cases.

Case 1: Samantha is an 8th grade girl brought into your office by her parents. They say that she is falling behind in school. She responds, *"Who cares, school is stupid anyway."* Her parents explain that the school psychologist tested her as having ADHD, predominately inattentive subtype. She recommended that Samantha consider medication. Samantha states, *"I'm fine just the way I am, I already told you school is stupid, and besides those pills made my friend a zombie."*

Case 2: Charles is a 10th grade student who was diagnosed with ADHD in first grade. His mother says, *"He never could sit still."* He has been on medications since then and his mother says they do help, and that he is still "a terror" on weekends when he is off his medications. He has never tried anything but pills. When you ask if they help, he says, "Whatever." You are not even sure he was listening because he was squirming. His mother says, *"Charles, be respectful and listen. Now sit still and pay attention!"*

■■■■■■■ Continuing Education ■■■■■■■

If you are applying for continuing education credits, a test is available online. For more details, visit www.aap.org/reachingteens.

■ References

1. Centers for Disease Control and Prevention. Increasing prevalence of parent-reported attention-deficit/hyperactivity disorder among children—United States, 2003 and 2007. *MMWR Morb Mortal Wkly Rep.* 2010;59(44):1439–1443

2. Kessler RC, Chiu WT, Demler O, Merikangas KR, Walters EE. Prevalence, severity, and comorbidity of 12-month DSM-IV disorders in the National Comorbidity Survey Replication. *Arch Gen Psychiatry.* 2005;62(6):617–627

3. American Psychiatric Association. *Diagnostic and Statistical Manual of Mental Disorders.* 5th ed. Alexandria, VA: American Psychiatric Association; 2013

4. Larson K, Russ SA, Kahn RS, Halfon N. Patterns of comorbidity, functioning, and service use for US children with ADHD, 2007. *Pediatrics.* 2011;127(3):462–470

5. Barkley RA, Guevremont DC, Anastopoulos AD, DuPaul GJ, Shelton TL. Driving-related risks and outcomes of attention deficit hyperactivity disorder in adolescents and young adults: a 3- to 5-year follow-up survey. *Pediatrics.* 1993;92(2):212–218

6. Barkley RA, Murphy KR, Kwasnik D. Motor vehicle driving competencies and risks in teens and young adults with attention deficit hyperactivity disorder. *Pediatrics*. 1996;98(6 pt 1):1089–1095

7. Matza LS, Paramore C, Prasad M. A review of the economic burden of ADHD. *Cost Eff Resour Alloc*. 2005;9(3):5

8. Wilens TE, Biederman J. Alcohol, drugs, and attention-deficit/hyperactivity disorder: a model for the study of addictions in youth. *J Psychopharmacol*. 2006;20:580–588

9. Cox, DG, Merkel RL, Moore M, Thorndike F, Muller C, Kovatchev B. Relative benefits of stimulant therapy with OROS methylphenidate versus mixed amphetamine salts extended-release in improving the driving performance of adolescent drivers with attention-deficit/hyperactivity disorder. *Pediatrics*. 2006;118(3):e704–e710

10. Hallowell EM, Ratey JJ. *Driven to Distraction: Recognizing and Coping with Attention Deficit Disorder*. New York, NY: Anchor Books, Random House; 2011

11. American Academy of Pediatrics Subcommittee on Attention-Deficit/Hyperactivity Disorder, Steering Committee on Quality Improvement and Management. ADHD: clinical practice guideline for the diagnosis, evaluation, and treatment of attention-deficit/hyperactivity disorder in children and adolescents. *Pediatrics*. 2011;128(5);1007–1022

12. Ratey JJ, Hagerman E. *Spark: The Revolutionary New Science of Exercise and the Brain*. New York, NY: Little, Brown and Company; 2008

13. Halperin JM, Healey DM. The influences of environmental enrichment, cognitive enhancement, and physical exercise on brain development: can we alter the developmental trajectory of ADHD? *Neurosci Biobehav Rev*. 2011;35(3):621–634

14. Millichap JG, Yee MM. The diet factor in attention-deficit/hyperactivity disorder. *Pediatrics*. 2012;129;330; DOI: 10.1542/peds.2011–2199

15. Newmark SC. Nutritional intervention in ADHD. *Explore*. 2009;5(3):171–174

16. National Sleep Foundation. Teens and Sleep. http://www.sleepfoundation.org/article/sleep-topics/teens-and-sleep. Accessed July 22, 2013

17. National Sleep Foundation. ADHD and Sleep. http://www.sleepfoundation.org/article/sleep-topics/adhd-and-sleep. Accessed July 22, 2013

18. Prehn-Kristensen A, Molzow I, Munz M, et al. Sleep restores daytime deficits in procedural memory in children with attention-deficit/hyperactivity disorder. *Res Dev Disabil*. 2011;32(6):2480–2488

■ Related Video Content

46.0 ADHD: From "Disorder" to Manageable Difference. Ginsburg.

31.3.1 Stress Management and Coping/Section 2/Taking Care of My Body/Point 4: The Power of Exercise. Ginsburg.

31.3.3 Stress Management and Coping/Section 2/Taking Care of My Body/Point 6: Eat Well. Ginsburg.

31.3.4 Stress Management and Coping/Section 2/Taking Care of My Body/Point 7: Sleep Well. Ginsburg.

40.0 The Role of Lifestyle and Healthy Thinking in Mental Health Promotion. Singh.

■ Related Web Sites

Children and Adults with Attention Deficit/Hyperactivity Disorder (CHADD)

www.chadd.org

An organization that provides education, advocacy and support for individuals with ADHD.

Centers for Disease Control and Prevention. Attention-Deficit/Hyperactivity Disorder (ADHD)

www.cdc.gov/ncbddd/adhd/index.html

National Institute of Mental Health. Attention Deficit Hyperactivity Disorder (ADHD)

www.nimh.nih.gov/health/topics/attention-deficit-hyperactivity-disorder-adhd/index.shtml

The National Resource Center on ADHD (A program of CHADD)

www.help4adhd.org/index.cfm

■ Related Resources

American Academy of Pediatrics Subcommittee on Attention-Deficit/Hyperactivity Disorder, Steering Committee on Quality Improvement and Management. ADHD: clinical practice guideline for the diagnosis, evaluation, and treatment of attention-deficit/ hyperactivity disorder in children and adolescents. *Pediatrics.* 2011;128(5):1007–1022. http://pediatrics.aappublications.org/content/early/2011/10/14/peds.2011-2654. Accessed June 26, 2013

American Academy of Pediatrics Task Force on Mental Health. *Addressing Mental Health Concerns in Primary Care: A Clinician's Toolkit* [CD-ROM]. Elk Grove Village, IL: American Academy of Pediatrics; 2010. http://tinyurl.aap.org/pub112382. Accessed June 26, 2013

American Academy of Pediatrics. *Caring for Children With ADHD: A Resource Toolkit for Clinicians,* 2nd ed. [CD-ROM]. Elk Grove Village, IL: American Academy of Pediatrics; 2011. http://tinyurl.aap.org/pub169531. Accessed June 26, 2013

Ratey JJ, Hagerman E. *Spark: The Revolutionary New Science of Exercise and the Brain.* New York, NY: Little, Brown and Company; 2008

American Academy of Pediatrics. Reiff MI, ed. *ADHD: What Every Parent Needs to Know.* 2nd ed. Elk Grove Village, IL: American Academy of Pediatrics; 2011

CHAPTER 47

Learning Differences

Marina Catallozzi, MD, MSCE
Susan T. Sugerman, MD, MPH, FAAP

 Related Video Content

47.0 Learning Differences in Adolescents

■ Why This Matters

Many young people with learning differences have been diagnosed well before adolescence; however, some come to us during adolescence with presentations far subtler than "I think I learn differently." They may be demoralized, falling behind, or "not living up to their potential." They may feign laziness or be exploring an alternative lifestyle rather than face the discomfort school engenders within them.

Our sensors need to be high if we are to catch these youth and point them in the direction of the assessment and intervention that can restore their confidence in their ability to learn. Further, we can help these youth who have sometimes lost confidence to find within themselves the strengths they possess so that they can grasp how their learning difference may bring with it an untapped gift in another area.

> **When young people don't understand why learning is hard for them, and when they cannot "fix it" themselves, they may begin to internalize the feeling that they are "stupid" or "lazy." It can be easier to claim not to care than to keep banging your head against the wall trying to do something difficult that never gets any better. Especially in families where parents or siblings are seen as successful, it may feel easier to be seen as "bad" rather than "dumb."**

■ What Are Learning Differences?

Learning differences refer to different ways that the brain processes information. Everyone learns differently. While some people learn best by seeing something written down (visual learners), others learn better by hearing (auditory learners), and still others by doing things hands-on (experiential learners).

All adolescents vary in their preferred learning styles. Delays or inconsistencies achieving specific skills may be normal within an individual adolescent. Differences become concerning only when they interfere with how a young person functions, particularly with regard to their ability to learn basic academic or life skills.

Our role is to celebrate differences in style while being sensitive to uncovering concerning learning differences that are persistent (recur over time) and pervasive (begin to affect multiple areas of their lives).

When someone has a learning difference, it means that they can have problems with how information is received, how information is processed or interpreted, and/or how information is communicated back to the outside world. These learning differences are present at birth, can have many different causes, and sometimes run in families. They have nothing to do with intelligence, but affect how someone performs specific skills or tasks. Learning differences can affect how someone listens or speaks (spoken language); how they read, write, and spell (written language); how they calculate or conceptualize things (arithmetic); and how they organize and integrate their thoughts and ideas (reasoning).

It should be noted that those young people who are not diagnosed with learning differences until adolescence likely have strengths that have compensated for their challenges throughout childhood. Therefore, when thinking about adolescents with learning differences, it is vital to think about their strengths in the face of these specific weaknesses and to build interventions on existing competencies.

■ Why Do Learning Differences Matter?

Many young people with learning differences have higher intelligence than their academic performance would indicate; however, their specific cognitive difficulties impact their ability to achieve academically. Their learning difference means that, when they are taught, they cannot learn because of the way the information gets to them or is processed. This is different than a young person with attention-deficit/hyperactivity disorder (ADHD) who is impulsive, distractible, or cannot filter information. It is also different from a young person with mental health or environmental issues, such as anxiety, depression, trauma, or malnourishment. Sometimes, it can take time to sort out these issues.

Learning disabilities are diagnosed when these differences in the ability to process information interfere significantly with school performance and the capacity to do important tasks in life. Learning disabilities are common, affecting an estimated 8% to 12% of American youth younger than 18, with most having challenges with reading and language skills.[1] The National Joint Committee on Learning Disabilities has operationalized the general term "learning disabilities" to include a group of varied disorders that interfere with the ability to acquire and use listening, speaking, reading, writing, reasoning, or math skills.[2] While the disorders do run in families, they are thought to be specific to the young person, indicate some dysfunction of the brain's ability to process, and will likely persist through life. While these learning disorders can be associated with other disabilities (ADHD, mental retardation, serious mental health issues) or outside factors (English as a second language, inadequate school exposure for whatever reason), the disabilities don't result from these issues or conditions.[1,2]

Learning disabilities can be diagnosed and qualify as disabilities protected by the Individuals with Disabilities Education Act.[3] Children and adults with learning disabilities are entitled to services such as Individualized Education Plans (often referred to as IEPs) that allow them to receive accommodations and modifications that will help to maximize their ability to learn and function in both school and work environments.

■ What Are the Specific Learning Disabilities?

Listed briefly below are some specific learning disabilities and the ways they might present.[4]

Dyslexia (or difficulty reading) is a general problem with language or reading. The young person may mix up letters or words, have difficulty spelling words correctly, or have problems distinguishing right and left. In later grades, different reading issues arise when reading is more connected to comprehension.

Dysgraphia (or difficulty writing) is a problem with forming letters or producing legible handwriting. In later grades, this can show itself in problems with spelling and grammar and with expressing ideas in writing.

Dyscalculia (or difficulty with mathematics) are problems with math concepts and symbols. In later grades, problems go beyond numbers and are more connected to issues with reasoning, so students have difficulty approaching the math problem or checking that the solution is correct.

Dyspraxia is a problem when language comprehension does not match language production (may mix up words while talking).

Visual and Auditory Processing Disorders are difficulties processing and remembering language-related tasks even though vision and hearing are normal.

Nonverbal learning disorder is when there is trouble with nonverbal cues, motor coordination, visual-spatial organization, and social skills.

Please note that ADHD is covered elsewhere (see Chapter 46). While its association with distractibility, impulsivity, and hyperactivity can impede academic success, young people with ADHD may or may not have associated learning disabilities.

■ What Are the Signs of a Learning Disability?

While learning disabilities should be diagnosed as early as possible, they are sometimes missed. Remember, a young person may compensate for the disability because of high intelligence or other strengths. The diagnosis of a learning disability should be considered if a young person in middle or high school is still spelling incorrectly, avoiding assignments that involve reading and writing, cannot answer open-ended questions, has a poor memory, has difficulty with transitions, cannot work quickly, has difficulty with abstract concepts, ignores or focuses on details, and/or does not read directions appropriately.[4]

■ What Adults (Both Parents and Professionals) Can Do to Support Adolescents

Most students in most schools should be able to do well enough to pass (C or higher) most classes most of the time. When a child cannot meet passing standards, attention issues, mental health problems, social stressors, or learning differences may be the cause. A child who processes visually may do well through elementary school but have difficulty when teachers begin to lecture in middle and high school. A tactile learner can succeed easily with hands-on projects but fall behind when more reading is required. Students with dyslexia tend to perform well in dynamic, interactive learning environments but then fail when asked to complete independent study outside the classroom.

We need to be aware of "red flags" that indicate that there may be a learning difference. These can include

- Change in motivation to do well in school
- Problems with organization and task management
- Excessive time required to complete homework
- Failure to turn in assignments (even if they are completed)
- Extreme frustration in certain subjects
- Significant drop in grades
- Self-labeling as "stupid"
- No longer trying at all

When young people don't understand why learning is hard for them, and when they cannot "fix it" themselves, they may begin to internalize the feeling that they are "stupid" or "lazy." If these young people could have fixed the problem, they would have. It can be easier to claim not to care than to keep banging your head against the wall trying to do something difficult that never gets any better. Especially in families where parents or siblings are seen as successful, it may feel easier to be seen as "bad" rather than "dumb."

This partly explains why learning differences can be associated with depression and behavioral problems.

Unless the reasons for school performance problems (and related mood issues) are obvious, students in these situations benefit from a comprehensive assessment that provides a full evaluation of possible causes of the behavior or learning problems. Simple screening tests may help point out possible learning differences or signs of ADHD. Other tests can evaluate signs or symptoms of depression, anxiety, or obsessive compulsive disorder. Professional evaluation through comprehensive neuropsychological or psycho-educational testing can be extremely helpful. These evaluations can function like an "MRI of the mind," providing a "picture" or explanation of how the brain thinks, rather than what it looks like. Licensed psychologists choose from a battery of well-studied, validated testing instruments to assess issues related to attention, distractibility, learning styles, multiple components of intelligence (several types of IQ testing), thought patterns, mood concerns, personality profiles, family/sibling conflict, etc.

Good testing helps young people to understand themselves and helps parents to support them. Results can help an adolescent understand why certain situations are hard for them and others are not. They can help with choices of schools or colleges, learning environments, and even careers. A comprehensive testing report can guide a clinician in choosing medication (if necessary) and help a counselor select the best form of therapy. It also can re-instill hope in parents and young people. Parents who know that things can get better can become more effective advocates.

Pointers for Parents 47.2

- **Try not to focus on grades.** Adolescents understand that how you do in school matters, but try not to make their value as a person be based on how they do in school.
- **Advocate for the right environment for your child's learning style.** A school where sitting still and being quiet is the rule, with no hands-on learning, may not be right for your adolescent.
- **Make sure to focus on what your adolescent is good at** because if they are not doing well in school (where they spend most of their time), they are likely feeling bad about themselves. Even though it may seem that they don't, adolescents thrive on adult approval and need to feel that they are valued.
- **Words like "lazy" and "stupid" should not be part of your or your adolescent's vocabulary.** Poor performance and a bad attitude are symptoms of a learning difference, not its cause. When adolescents understand why they are having trouble in school and how they can get help in the areas they need support, they can believe again in their potential for success.
- **Know when to strengthen and when to avoid a weakness.** If an adolescent has dysgraphia (poor handwriting) and his school requires written exams, then it may help to get him occupational therapy to improve his hand-eye coordination. If his school allows him to take notes on a laptop and he types well, encourage him to do so. Sometimes a combination of approaches is the way to go.
- **Praise the process instead of the outcome.** Praising a young person for his effort *("I can tell you really thought that through.")* rather than the outcome *("You are good at math!")* can lead to more confidence.
- **Help kids use their strengths to find confidence and to help compensate for their weaknesses.** Figuring out an adolescent's talent can help to drive her sense of self-worth.

- **Understand the dangers of perfectionism.** Expecting perfection can only lead to eventual disappointment. Learning to put up with mistakes and even failure helps adolescents deal with the realities of the world, where things don't always turn out as planned, even if we try really hard.
- **Use the right interventions for the right reasons.** The goal of interventions should not be to change grades, but to support healthy growth and development.

Pointers for Professionals

Professionals are responsible for helping in the diagnosis and management of learning differences and disabilities, and for ensuring adolescents and families have appropriate resources.[5] Particularly when learning disabilities are diagnosed at the later stage of adolescence, young people and their families need to know their legal rights and the agencies available to help them get appropriate supports and interventions. Garnering appropriate resources sometimes requires significant advocacy.

Professionals need to be attentive to parents' concerns and have a low index of suspicion for learning differences or other factors that may interfere with learning (adolescents with a family history of learning differences, history of developmental delay, psychosocial and environmental stressors, mental health concerns). A comprehensive medical evaluation is an essential first step since there is significant overlap of learning differences with behavioral, neurologic, and genetic issues. This should include a history and physical, specific testing for hearing and vision, and other medical testing when indicated by history and examination. A focus on the adolescents learning history (compiled from the adolescent, parent, and teachers if possible) and a developmental history are crucial.

A special effort should be made to identify the adolescent's strengths, as this is vital for creating a plan for future success and combating the demoralization that often accompanies learning disabilities. While adolescence is considered a late diagnosis for learning differences and disabilities, knowledge is power that can help adolescents and their families access the help they need to succeed in current academic and future work environments.

●● Group Learning and Discussion ●●

Prior to the group learning session, gather a list of local professionals who do neuropsychological or psychoeducational testing. Then discuss a series of cases in which learning differences presented in your setting. Finally, discuss the cases below and next steps you might take to diagnose and address the disability. In each case, discuss the accompanying compensatory strengths and consider how you might leverage them as you initiate the intervention.

Scenario 1: Zeke is a really musical kid (he taught himself piano and guitar) who did okay in school until he started high school. He is in a big school and he doesn't get to take music until his junior year. His new school uses a lot of textbooks and he cannot keep up with the readings. His backpack is filled with incomplete homework assignments that he has not handed in to his teachers. He is spending a lot of time in his room listening to music with the lights off.

Scenario 2: Veronica's mother is really frustrated with her. Veronica takes down messages when people call and her mother cannot read them. When she asks Veronica what it says, she says she doesn't know and cannot remember. Veronica loved social studies in middle school, but her mother just found out that she failed a US history exam. When she looks in Veronica's notebook, she doesn't see any notes—just doodles. Her teacher says that she doesn't use a textbook and asks the students to rely on class notes. While Veronica seems interested in class, she doesn't take any notes.

▪▪▪▪▪▪▪ Continuing Education ▪▪▪▪▪▪▪▪

If you are applying for continuing education credits, a test is available online. For more details, visit www.aap.org/reachingteens.

■ References

1. National Institute of Neurologic Disorders and Stroke. NINDS Learning Disabilities Information Page. http://www.ninds.nih.gov/disorders/learningdisabilities/learningdisabilities.htm. Accessed June 26, 2013

2. National Joint Committee on Learning Disabilities (NJCLD). *Operationalizing the NJCLD Definition of Learning Disabilities for Ongoing Assessment in Schools. American Speech-Language Hearing Association, 1997.* www.asha.org/docs/html/RP1998-00130.html. Accessed June 26, 2013

3. LD Online. *IDEA 2004.* http://www.ldonline.org/features/idea2004 Accessed June 26, 2013

4. LD Online. *LD Basics: What is a Learning Disability?* http://www.ldonline.org/ldbasics/whatisld. Accessed June 26, 2013

5. Bravender T. School performance: the pediatrician's role. *Clin Pediatr (Phila).* 2008;47:535–545

■ Related Video Content

47.0 Learning Differences in Adolescents. Catallozzi.

47.1 Case: Learning Differences Can Present in Adolescence With Mood Disorders or Substance Use. Sugerman.

47.2 Your Role in Supporting Your Child With Learning Differences. Catallozzi.

47.3 Clues That Offer Insight Into the Possibility of a Learning Disability. Feit.

46.0 ADHD: From "Disorder" to Manageable Difference. Ginsburg.

CHAPTER 48

Perfectionism

Kenneth R. Ginsburg, MD, MS Ed, FAAP, FSAHM
Susan T. Sugerman, MD, MPH, FAAP

 Related Video Content

48.0 Perfectionism: A Barrier to Authentic Success

■ Why This Matters?

We prepare youth to be successful when they are poised to be high achievers rather than perfectionists. Perfectionists feel unacceptable unless they produce a flawless product or performance.[1] Perfectionism is associated with a host of problems in adolescents, including eating disorders,[2-4] obsessive compulsive disorder (OCD),[5,6] depression and anxiety,[7,8] somatic symptoms,[7] and suicidality.[9]

The literature discusses adaptive and maladaptive perfectionism with the understanding that some degree of the drive toward being perfect may actually be good.[10] Here, a person with adaptive perfectionism will be termed a "healthy high achiever" and the maladaptive perfectionist will be referred to as a "perfectionist."

> **Teach parents how to support "healthy achievement" while minimizing the drive to maladaptive perfectionism, which may prevent outside-of-the box thinking and limit creative and innovative potential. Help parents teach their children to use mistakes and failures as learning opportunities for growth that generate long-term character and values and more genuine lifelong success.**

Perfectionists don't enjoy the creative process because their fear of failure is greater than the joy of experiencing success. They see mistakes as proof that they're unworthy. They are suspicious of others' praise because they view themselves as "imposters" whose faults remain undiscovered. They may experience constructive criticism as reinforcement of their inadequacy. Perhaps most limiting to future success, the thought of not doing something well may prevent them from thinking outside of the box, limiting their creative and innovative potential.

In contrast, healthy high achievers aren't satisfied until they've done their best and prove resilient when they fall short of perfection. Healthy high achievers enjoy the process and excitement as they work their hardest. They see mistakes as opportunities for growth and failures as temporary setbacks. They value constructive criticism as informative. They look for creative solutions and are willing to take healthy risks.

Not all perfectionists are high performers. Fear of failure may cause them to avoid a task entirely. Sometimes they project an image to make the pressure stop. Being perceived as "lazy" or even as a drug user can be viewed positively by some teens, whereas being anxious is not. The pressure of being perfect makes them go out of their way to build a strong case for indifference. This possibility should be considered when young people have a sudden drop in performance. These youth often receive negative feedback from home and may need professional guidance to be able to say, *"I act like I don't care because I care too much."*

What Factors Create Perfectionism?

There may be a biological component to perfectionism as evidenced by its link to eating disorders[2-4] and OCD.[5,6] Here we will focus on those environmental factors that may contribute to or exacerbate perfectionism.

Inappropriate Praise

Carol Dweck and colleagues[11] study the effect that praise and criticism have on performance and write about a "growth mindset" compared to a "fixed mindset." Young people with a growth mindset believe their intelligence can be developed with effort. When they do not produce desired results, they don't see themselves as failures, but as learners. People with a growth mindset want feedback because they understand they need others' assessments to learn to do things better. Dweck writes, *"The passion for stretching yourself and sticking to it, even (or especially) when it's not going well, is the hallmark of the growth mindset."*

In contrast, people with a fixed mindset (including maladaptive perfectionists and others) believe people are either smart or not and failure proves you're not. In fact, hard work suggests one doesn't have natural intelligence. Their goal becomes to avoid failure at all costs since they need consistent feedback to affirm they're smart. Dweck explains that people with a fixed mindset view situations from the prism of, *"Will I succeed or fail?" "Will I look smart or dumb?" "Will I win or lose?"* People with a growth mindset feel successful when they can do something they couldn't do before, whereas those with fixed mindsets feel smart when they avoid errors.

Dweck's research reveals that how a child is praised contributes heavily to whether she develops a growth versus fixed mindset. In brief, those praised for being smart are more likely to grow to fear being seen as anything else, and those noticed for effort develop a passion for growth.

Academic Pressures and a Competitive College Admissions Process

Parents and children alike see getting a college degree as important for long-term success and financial security. This often translates into external and internal pressure not simply to attain high grades and test scores, but also to build extensive resumes filled with impressive extra-curricular achievements. The competition is not limited to those applying to elite universities. Increases in the perceived importance of secondary education across society as well as the rising costs of tuition lead to anxiety among all students about competition for admission and scholarship dollars, especially in the context of difficult economic times.

Sensationalism of Success and Failure (ie, Who Are Our Heroes?)

Our culture reveres success and ridicules failure. The heroes in our society tend to epitomize a perfect performance in their fields and are rewarded with the greatest external trappings of success. Whether the highest-scoring athlete, the top-grossing recording artist, or the most beautiful movie actress, our sports stars and entertainment figures receive enormous attention, especially when at the "top of their game." When they have a transgression, the media quickly focuses on their problems. Youth receive the message that, to gain recognition, you must be at the top, and, once there, you had better not make a mistake.

Increase in a Permissive Style of Parenting

Permissive parents are very warm and supportive to their children but offer few boundaries or rules, often taking on a tone of "friendship" more than mentorship in their approach to parenting (see Chapter 36). The result is that teens' behavioral control is achieved largely through their desire to please parents. Achieving perfection can ensure the child pleases his parents, especially if the definition of what counts as "acceptable" is not clear.

Fear of Disappointment

Many perfectionists have a strong desire to avoid disappointing their parents, especially when raised in a permissive parenting style as noted above. Others are driven by the fear of disappointing themselves. Children who see themselves as valuable only when achieving success may experience significant cognitive dissonance when trying to accept a failure or limitation in performance or abilities. As a result, they pursue perfectionism as a means to avoid disappointment at all costs.

Applying Professional Standards to Personal Parenting

Some parents highly prepared for the work world apply the same standards of efficiency, productivity, and performance to family life. When this happens, their children's perceived successes or setbacks become markers of the parents' own success. This may intensify stress on children either directly through parental pressure or through their own drive to please adults.

Desire to Spare Stressed Parents

Teens sometimes have an intense need to spare a parent whom they perceive as stressed. Children whose parents suffer from trauma, illness, or divorce may try to be perfect children. They may keep their own anxieties and struggles as tightly held secrets, always showing parents their best face. Parents who explicitly verbalize feelings of being overwhelmed to their children or who excessively rely on their children as confidants about adult problems could exacerbate this.

■ Solutions

The professional can have 3 major roles in serving the adolescent with perfectionist tendencies: (1) assess for comorbid conditions (eg, anxiety, OCD) that may benefit from appropriate referral and treatment, (2) offer parents guidance on how to prevent or minimize perfectionism, (3) help youth who "have gotten off the playing field" and are perceived as being "lazy" to address their fear of failure. This can be healing for families because anger and disappointment can transform to more appropriate support.

Parents may or may not be one of the sources of perfectionism, but they certainly can be part of the solution. The above points present the areas you can use as topics of discussion. It is important in these discussions to remember that even parents who put a lot of pressure on their children do so with their children's best interest in mind. They should be gently guided to understand perfectionism not only feels uncomfortable but also interferes with success; the fear of failure associated with the need to be perfect can stifle creative and innovative thought and generate discomfort with constructive criticism. Following are a few topics you may want to draw from in your discussion with parents.

Effective Praise and Criticism

It is important that parents learn to praise effort rather than product. The statement, *"Just try your best,"* may be misunderstood by people with a high degree of internalized pressure. Those who have been capable of high performance or perfect scores in the past may take this to mean they should meet that standard on every task in the future. Instead, keep feedback and encouragement targeted. Explain that someone can try really hard yet perform quite differently in different subjects due to uneven strengths. **48.2**

- For example, instead of parents saying, *"Don't worry, I just expect you to do your best,"* say something like, *"All I expect is for you to put in a good effort. I care less about your grades and more about the fact that you are learning. Some things come easily to me, and with even a little effort I will always do well—for you, that's math. In other subjects, I might work really hard and still not do as well as I wish I could. But, all I want from you is to stretch yourself and learn; it's not the grades that matter. I know writing is hard for you, I'm proud when I see you keep working on it."*
- Teach parents to guide teens through self-evaluation based on the process rather than the outcome. They can ask, *"Do you think you spent a reasonable amount of time working on the project (or studying for the test)?" "Do you feel you learned what you needed to?" "Is there something you wish you did differently that you can change the next time?"* When youth learn from their own "imperfect" experiences without internalizing negativity, they can make real and meaningful changes to improve the process (and possibly outcome) in the future.
- Provide perspective about the costs of perfectionism (ie, just because you can doesn't always mean you should).

Most parents intuitively recognize the need for balance in managing the tasks of daily life. They can help their children work toward the same goal by teaching that perfectionism comes with costs to emotional and physical health. Time and energy are limited resources; one cannot sleep and study simultaneously. Extra time spent on a project may mean less time connecting with friends or doing a rewarding extracurricular activity. Parents may have to advocate for their children's need to get enough sleep, even when homework is not finished. Parents seeing their children suffer symptoms of exhaustion, isolation, anxiety, or depression may need to set limits on numbers of advanced classes taken or the degree of participation in outside activities.

Model Self-acceptance

Help parents present a "human" face to their children. Explain that children learn to internalize humility and self-respect when they see a parent admit and correct a mistake or failing, while witnessing parental self-deprecation for less than perfect achievement or talent sets children up to accept nothing less from themselves. Encourage parents to acknowledge their own limitations while celebrating their strengths, and hopefully their children will do the same.

Making Realistic Heroes

Talk to parents about the importance of discussing the real heroes all around us—those who choose to teach and to heal, those who choose to protect us and to serve our communities and nation. Encourage parents to talk about the acts of kindness they witness among neighbors. When children see realistic heroes and hear positive messages about the actions of real, accessible people, they learn a broader definition of success within which they, too, can feel valued.

Parents Need to Communicate That They Are Not Spared When Adolescents Keep Their Feelings Inside

You might consider discussing with parents whether their children notice their level of stress. As always, encourage parents that one of the best things they can do for their children's emotional well-being is to take care of themselves—to "put on their own oxygen mask first." (See Chapter 39.)

- Consider encouraging them to explain that, although they might be burdened, their greatest pleasure and most important job remains to parent them. You may consider encouraging them to say something like, *"I know you want to protect me from more worries, and I appreciate how much you care about me. But, the one thing I want to do right now more than anything is to be your mom/dad. Please let me to do that; I want to always be there for you."*

Encourage Parents to Be Clear About Their Definition of Success

Children absorb the definition of success from the media and broader culture. Some of those messages do not sit well with parents. Encourage parents to clarify and communicate their own views of success. You can't tell parents what those should be, but you might suggest some worthy contenders.

- Happiness, contentment
- Commitment to hard work, tenacity
- Resilience
- Generosity
- Compassion and empathy
- Desire to contribute
- Capacity to build and maintain meaningful relationships
- Collaborative skills
- Creativity and innovative potential
- Capacity to accept and learn from constructive criticism

Encourage Parents to Give Kids Opportunities for Self-discovery

Many parents assume that more is better—extra activities will build their resume. Enrichment activities are good, but we need to also encourage child-driven play and some down time.[12] To parents who would never let their kid be a "quitter," reframe it as "pruning." When kids feel overwhelmed, they can't focus on anything or learn where they excel. When they can prune away what no longer interests them, their strongest interests and greatest talents will flourish.

Unconditional Acceptance

If perfectionism is a state of discomfort driven by a fear of being unacceptable, the greatest antidote is unconditional acceptance. Parents need to consistently reinforce that their teens are acceptable just as they are.

You can reinforce that the most essential ingredient in raising resilient children is the connection parents form when they love or accept their children unconditionally and hold them to high but reasonable expectations. "High expectations" does not refer to grades or performance. It refers to their expectations for effort and of integrity, generosity, empathy, and other core values. Remind parents not to compare their adolescents to siblings or neighbors, because such comparisons impede feeling fully acceptable. Finally, although parents don't intend to imply conditional acceptance when they overfocus on grades and scores, children can misinterpret this attention as, *"If I bring home better grades, you'll love me more."*

Seeking Professional Help

Perfectionists may be so anxious and uncomfortable that they deserve professional help. First, the school should know how anxious the student is so that parents and the school together can convey supportive messages that reduce external pressures. However, sometimes a teen's perfectionism is internally driven by unhealthy thought patterns that reinforce what they "must" or "should" do lest their actions lead to catastrophic outcomes (eg, *"If I don't get an A, I will never get into college, I will never be able to become a doctor, and I will lose the love of my parents."*) In these cases, consider referral to a mental health specialist who includes cognitive behavioral therapy in treatment plans.

●● Group Learning and Discussion ●●

There are several key challenges in discussing perfectionism with adolescents and their families. The first is to do so without making the parent feel guilty or responsible; the key here is to emphasize that perfectionism comes from multiple sources and they may or may not be part of the problem, but they are certainly part of the solution. Second, it is important to help anxious parents understand that your goal is not to help their child achieve mediocrity; to the contrast it is to position him for authentic success. The third is to help parents understand that their "lazy" child may in fact care too much and may be masking his discomfort. In parallel, you hope to help the young person to be able to express that he is not lazy, it is just that he cares too much. Finally, it is your role to assess whether a higher level of care is needed, such as cognitive behavioral therapy, or even medication, in the case of anxiety or OCD.

Discuss in a group how perfectionism manifests among the teens you serve. Then break into pairs and work through the following cases.

Case 1: A 15-year-old girl is the daughter of immigrant parents. They have told her that the only way to make it in America is through an education. She has been told that there are no A minuses in their family. She studies until 1:00 to 2:00 every morning, taking breaks only for her violin lessons. She has daily abdominal pain, but has been told she is constipated. She loves her parents very much. They work 16- to 18-hour days so that she and her 2 siblings can go to the very best college. She doesn't want to disappoint them.

Case 2: A college professor brings in her 17-year-old son. His father is on international travel closing a business deal. He used to do quite well in school until he began changing. Now he has long blue hair and acts like he doesn't care at all about school. He is getting Cs and Ds except for in English class, where he loves talking about the innuendos hidden throughout the works of Shakespeare and Chaucer. He says his English teacher is cool, but the rest of school is lame.

Case 3: A distraught couple brings in their 13-year-old daughter. She studies all the time, sleeps little, and does not seem to be social. She worries incessantly that she is going to fail out of school, but what she means is that she might not get a 100 on her tests. Her parents insist that they just want her to be happy. They feel terrible that they used to tell her to study harder last year when she spent so much time at the mall with her friends. In a private interview, the girl tells you that she just knows her teachers will hate her if she fails out. She also knows that she'll never get to be a doctor if she fails now. To make sure that she does well, she spends a lot of time staying organized. All of her schoolwork and books are color-coded and in alphabetical order. She also worries about getting sick because she can't afford to miss school. To stay healthy, she keeps her room spotless and washes her hands repeatedly to make sure they are germ-free.

▦▦▦▦▦▦▦ Continuing Education ▦▦▦▦▦▦▦▦

If you are applying for continuing education credits, a test is available online. For more details, visit www.aap.org/reachingteens.

■ References

1. Greenspon TS. *Freeing Our Families From Perfectionism*. Minneapolis, MN: Free Spirit Publishing; 2002

2. Kirsh G, McVey G, Tweed S, Katzman DK. Psychosocial profiles of young adolescent females seeking treatment for an eating disorder. *J Adolesc Health*. 2007;40(4):351–356

3. Castro J, Gila A, Gual P, et al. Perfectionism dimensions in children and adolescents with anorexia nervosa. *J Adolesc Health*. 2004;35(5):392–398

4. Soenens B, Vansteenkiste M, Vandereycken W, Luyten P, Sierens E, Goossens L. Perceived parental psychological control and eating-disordered symptoms: maladaptive perfectionism as a possible intervening variable. *J Nerv Ment Dis*. 2008;196(2):144–152

5. Libby S, Reynolds S, Derisley J, Clark S. Cognitive appraisals in young people with obsessive-compulsive disorder. *J Child Psychol Psychiatry*. 2004;45(6):1076–1084

6. Ye HJ, Rice KG, Storch EA. Perfectionism and peer relations among children with obsessive-compulsive disorder. *Child Psychiatry Hum Dev*. 2008;39:415–426

7. Stoeber J, Rambow A. Perfectionism in adolescent school students: relations with motivation, achievement, and well-being. *Pers Individ Dif*. 2007;42(7):1379–1389

8. Hewitt PL, Carmen F, Caelian CF, et al. Perfectionism in children: associations with depression, anxiety, and anger. *Pers Individ Dif*. 2002;32(6):1049–1061

9. O'Connor RC. The relations between perfectionism and suicidality: a systematic review. *Suicide Life Threat Behav*. 2007;37(6):698–714

10. Enns MW, Cox BJ. The nature and assessment of perfectionism: a critical analysis. In: Flett GL, Hewitt PL, eds. *Perfectionism: Theory, Research and Treatment*. Washington, DC: American Psychological Association; 2002: 33–63

11. Dweck C. *Mindset: The New Psychology of Success*. New York, NY: Ballantine Books; 2006

12. Ginsburg KR; American Academy of Pediatrics Committee on Communications, Committee on Psychosocial Aspects of Child and Family Health. The importance of play in promoting healthy child development and maintaining strong parent-child bonds. *Pediatrics*. 2007;119(1);182–191

■ Related Video Content

48.0 Perfectionism: A Barrier to Authentic Success. Ginsburg.

48.1 Raising Children Prepared for Authentic Success. Ginsburg.

48.2 Using Praise Appropriately: The Key to Raising Children With a Growth Mind-set. Ginsburg.

48.3 We Must Not Assume "Perfect" Youth Are Problem-Free: They Need Us to Hear Their Struggles and Assess Their Behaviors. Campbell.

48.4 Because We Need to Learn How to Recover From Failure, Adolescence Needs to Be a Safe Time to Make Mistakes. Ginsburg.

48.5 Teen-Produced Song: Paper Tigers. Youth, Toro.

43.1 Managing School-Related Anxiety. Ginsburg.

54.2 Children of Divorce Can Become Perfectionists to Spare Their Parents. Sonis, Ginsburg.

63.1 Addressing Perfectionism in Military Youth. Youth, Lemmon, Ginsburg.

■ Related Handouts/Supplementary Materials

Don't Spare Me! Help Your Child Understand that You Want to Be There When They Need You, Even if You are Busy or Stressed

Helping Your Child...be a High Achiever instead of a Perfectionist

CHAPTER 49

Eating Disorders

Rebecka Peebles, MD, FAAP
Laura Collins Lyster-Mensh, MS
Richard E. Kreipe, MD, FAAP, FSAHM, FAED

 Related Video Content

49.0 A Comprehensive Approach to Serving Youth With Eating Disorders

■ Why This Matters

Eating disorders are common and dangerous conditions that present challenges to patients, families, and professionals. It is hard to talk to a family who has watched their adolescent struggle with eating for months, and sometimes years. Parents often feel disempowered by the illness and worry that they did something wrong that resulted in their child developing an eating disorder. Patients are often interested in recovery, but can also feel "stuck" in their illness, and this ambivalence can make a therapeutic rapport difficult. These diseases are life-threatening in more ways than one—they have inherent and significant mortality risks, but they also greatly impair quality of life. The professional's role in early identification and treatment is critical to successful recovery.

> **Eating disorders are not anyone's "fault," including parents. Indeed, parents are a critical part of the solution. We know that by achieving weight restoration effectively and quickly through evidence-based treatment, patients and families can reverse many of the symptoms and complications of these serious illnesses.**

■ Background

Eating disorders have been reported to be quite prevalent, with conservative estimates demonstrating anorexia nervosa (AN) in 0.5% of adolescents, bulimia nervosa (BN) in 2%, and the combination of other specified feeding and eating disorders (OSFED) and unspecified feeding and eating disorders (UFED) in an estimated 5%. Note: The diagnostic categories have been updated in the *Diagnostic and Statistical Manual of Mental Disorders (DSM-5),* with anorexia and bulimia broadened and avoidant restrictive food intake disorder and binge eating disorder added. Other specified feeding and eating disorders and UFED have replaced the category formerly termed eating disorders not otherwise specified. See *DSM-5* for diagnostic criteria (www.dsm5.org/Documents/Eating%20 Disorders%20Fact%20Sheet.pdf). In addition, disordered eating behaviors are very common, with 80% of early teens reporting dieting to lose weight, 25% of high school girls and 11% of boys reporting disordered eating severe enough to need evaluation, and 9% of high school girls and 4% of boys vomiting daily to control their weight. While these diseases used to be thought of as only affecting a small subset of society (largely affluent females), they are now recognized to impact millions of Americans, cross all racial and socioeconomic lines, and occur in both males and females.

Eating disorders used to be conceptualized as chronic diseases that often resulted from control struggles and sometimes trauma. We did not have effective interventions to ensure long-term recovery, and, as a result, we often hesitated to diagnose them in pediatric patients, as the diagnosis itself often felt hopeless. Diagnosis was also made more difficult because diagnostic criteria were originally developed for adult females. These criteria were then translated to pediatric patients even though they frequently did not "fit" classic molds. For example, all diagnostic criteria for AN may not apply in a pediatric population—patients may not be cognitively able to verbalize abstract concepts such as fear of weight gain or body distortions, they may not have lost dramatic weight, but may simply not be growing well over time, and they may be early in puberty or male, so amenorrhea may not be relevant. Therefore, many adolescents with eating disorders best meet criteria for OSFED or UFED. This can be problematic, as these eating disorders are often misinterpreted as less severe than AN or BN, although they are not.

We now know that eating disorders are not anyone's "fault," including parents. Indeed, parents are a critical part of the solution. We also know that, by achieving weight restoration effectively and quickly, patients and families can reverse many of the symptoms and complications of disordered eating: hunger and fullness cues can normalize, eating-disordered cognitions can reduce, pubertal and growth milestones can resume, and other organ systems can start to heal.

Health professionals can also be very useful to youth and families who struggle with these disorders. We can work to recognize changes in growth patterns early, before severe weight loss or other disordered behavior has occurred, thus improving prognosis by initiating early intervention.

■ Common Mistakes

Younger patients are often "atypical" in their presentation. Their weight may appear normal because they may not have grown or gained weight appropriately over the past year. Their linear growth may be stunted, and this is easy to miss. Adolescents are often unable to express classic disordered eating cognitions as noted above. If we look only for "classic" eating disorders, we will miss many opportunities for early identification and intervention.

■ Screening

One validated screening measure developed in England for primary care is called the SCOFF questionnaire. Answering "yes" to 2 or more of the following questions (with American equivalents in parentheses) has been shown to be 100% sensitive and 88% specific for the presence of an eating disorder:

S Have you ever made yourself sick (thrown up) to lose weight?

C Have you ever eaten a lot of food at once, in a way that you felt out of control and couldn't stop?

O Have you recently lost more than one stone (14 lb) in 3 months?

F Do you think you're fat when others don't?

F Do you feel that food has taken over your life?

In addition, asking about the quality and feelings behind exercise, rather than just the amount, may be helpful. Adolescents who exercise compulsively often feel that they cannot go a day without exercise, so this is a useful question to ask during an interview. Finally, because they lead to different health risks than restricting or purging behaviors can, asking about laxative or diet pill use may be helpful.

Some early eating problems that begin in childhood, but have been linked to the development of eating disorders, are selective eating (also sometimes called "picky" eating, or eating only a very selective and narrow number of foods), food hoarding (eating in secret, often leaving wrappers that parents later find), and swallowing or vomiting phobias. These behaviors also often require early intervention if reported.

■ Special Considerations

Males and Eating Disorders

Males get eating disorders as well, with increasing prevalence now than in years past. They are actually more likely than females to get binge-eating disorder, and, by the latest estimates, they account for about 15% of cases of AN. It is important to keep a heightened sense of suspicion for these illnesses when adolescent males present with weight loss, vomiting, or other related concerns. Otherwise, these illnesses can go undetected and unchecked longer in males because they are not recognized as quickly and referred for good care. It is also very important to reassure males that eating disorders are not "female" illnesses and to reinforce that there is no shame in acknowledging that they struggle with eating issues.

Obesity and Eating Disorders

We are constantly reminded about the epidemic of obesity. This is certainly a problem facing adolescents and deserves thought. However, some obese youth suffer from disordered eating, and a subset will be vulnerable to AN, BN, and other eating disorders. While we screen routinely for signs of insulin resistance and dyslipidemia, we are not as practiced at screening for disordered eating behaviors, even though they are equally common conditions. We can also be biased toward only looking for eating disorders in thin patients, which can be dangerous. If we miss emerging AN in an obese patient who is embarking on weight loss in an unsafe manner, we miss an opportunity to intervene early and instead run the risk of only "catching" the eating disorder when it has become far too entrenched, often actually congratulating the patient on weight loss in the meantime. It is important to remember that weight loss from an obese state is difficult to accomplish, and that, when we see consistent and rapid weight loss over time, we should always screen for eating disorders and make sure that there are no extreme weight control behaviors emerging. Research has shown that patients who are normal weight and overweight but have a clinical eating disorder can still experience life-threatening complications.

Young Adults

Young adulthood is a critical phase of development and typically a time of increased autonomy. The additional difficulty with an eating disorder during this time is that a young person may be legally allowed to make medical and other decisions, but the eating disorder may be impairing their ability to make decisions about food and activity in a safe manner. Clearly, we need to promote care that respects legal boundaries; however, we need to also remember that just because someone has turned 18 does not mean they should be expected to fight a life-threatening illness all on his or her own. Family members can still be an incredibly helpful part of the treatment team. It is important to have a frank discussion early in care about how the young person may allow their involvement.

■ Interview

While it is always helpful to spend some time alone with the adolescent when obtaining a history of disordered eating, parental or caregiver histories are often just as valuable. As a result, it is important to spend time alone with both the youth and parent(s). Studies have shown that many patients with eating disorders underreport their symptoms compared to their parents at presentation. It is important to hear parent concerns because they are on the "front lines" with this illness, often long before bringing their child to the health professional. It is equally important that we not pathologize their concerns as overbearing or overinvolved, as parents can seem highly anxious at presentation. Remember that this is not their natural state; rather, it results from the anxiety that builds from watching their child eat less and less over time.

In addition to this natural worry, parents often feel guilty and even defensive in this first interview, as they may have already heard or read incorrect and dated presumptions that parents in some way cause eating disorders. As a result, the simple act of letting parents know that their child's illness is not their fault, and that you view them as part of the solution, can be very powerful and healing. Be careful to be truly nonjudgmental, ▶**49.1** and view these parents as you would any other caregivers.

Patients also benefit from this same nonjudgmental approach, as they can also feel guilty for causing their loved ones so much worry. Reassuring patients that this disease is not their fault either, and that you wish to hear what they have to say and how they are feeling is helpful. Professionals and parents alike can sometimes become impatient or lack empathy for adolescents with eating disorders, as eating more does not seem on the surface as though it should be a complicated task. However, it is important to remember that the adolescent's brain is captive to the illness itself. These disorders are not volitional; therefore, eating is not a simple or rational process. Eating-disordered cognitions do not tend to respond to long discussions of why food is important and why weight gain is helpful; therefore, a concise explanation of any new recommendation is a good idea, but engaging in circular discussions regarding your reasoning is not. It is often necessary to remind patients and parents that sometimes "listening" and "agreeing" are different, and you will always be honest about what treatment entails, even if that feels uncomfortable or makes the eating disorder angry.

With eating disorders, it is important to remember that we should not be afraid of a tough discussion, and we cannot be afraid of addressing what the young person with an eating disorder might find most uncomfortable. For example, if a teen wishes to run cross-country, but you do not think this is safe, it is important to just present that in a straight-forward manner, rather than avoiding the discussion out of concern that she might become upset. This sends a message that you are stronger than the illness, which will be an important message throughout treatment.

■ Medical Assessment

Assessing for strengths through the interview is important in both the parent and the adolescent. If a broad medical diagnosis is being considered, which happens frequently with weight loss, vomiting, or lack of appetite, it is still important to bring up the possibility of an eating disorder early in your evaluation. Be straightforward that this is one of the most common causes of such symptoms and may be present here. If families don't hear that an eating disorder is a possibility until an extensive medical workup has been completed, they often lose trust in the process.

Discussing the details of medical complications and differential diagnoses is outside the scope of this chapter. However, it is important to remember that, if an eating disorder is suspected, medical urgency is warranted. These are life- and quality-of-life–threatening illnesses, yet they are illnesses in which the patient often feels well and is functioning well in numerous arenas, such as academics and athletics. Anosognosia, a state wherein a patient with a disability or illness is unable to recognize that they have the disability or illness, is a common feature of AN and other eating disorders. This is what makes the treatment of eating disorders so different from other life-threatening illnesses, in which patients know that they are ill and wish to get better.

Because of anosognosia, using the physical examination and vital signs to point out how their current state reflects malnutrition is often helpful to both patients and families. For example, explain findings of acrocyanosis by tying it to poor eating by stating, *"Your hands and feet look purple to me. This can happen when your heart is tired from not receiving enough energy through nutrition, and has to, therefore, make tough decisions about where to send blood. It decides that the hands and the feet aren't that important, so they become more purple."* It can help families to understand why it is urgent that they mobilize as a team to fight this illness now, even if the adolescent is not yet fully accepting of the need for treatment. Letting families know that the body is tired, and that you see signs of malnutrition on examination, is a good way of starting to help adolescent patients "connect the dots" and understand that, while they may think they feel well, their bodies may disagree.

■ Healthy Weight, Healthy State

Eating disorders can affect all body systems, causing multiple serious complications, such as low bone density, cardiac arrhythmias, and liver damage. Many or most of the complications are reversible, although they become less so with increased duration and severity of illness. In order to achieve complete healing, full weight restoration is crucial. A healthy weight would be a healthy "state," where eating patterns have normalized, pubertal progression or prior milestones like menses have resumed, linear growth has resumed if it is expected, vital signs and labs are normal, and thoughts have normalized as well.

A healthy weight is different from person to person. Factors like mid-parental height, as well as birth weight and birth history, may be useful in assessing if the young person was growing well before the eating disorder started. Examining prior body mass index (BMI) growth curves can be very helpful, as typically we aim for patients to return to their pre-illness growth patterns. The exceptions to this are when patients were either very underweight or overweight prior to their eating disorder; in that case, we may aim for them to be at a slightly higher (if previously underweight) or lower (if previously overweight) BMI percentile than they were before. Another exception is the patient who has arrested linear growth prior to presentation—often then you have to aim for a weight that would match the height that he should have achieved rather than one appropriate for his current height in order to catch up linear growth. If no prior growth curves are available, as a starting point, you can use a median body weight that is based on the 50th percentile BMI for age, as long as you follow the body's signs of recovery, understanding that some patients will be most healthy above the median and some below. The important thing to remember is that there is no one-size-fits-all number that will work for everyone, and that all weight goals are really just an educated guess as to when someone might reach a healthy "state." We will still really need to see how he is doing as he gets closer to his goal. We recommend emphasizing to parents and adolescents that goal weights are also "moving targets" throughout adolescence, as normal teens are growing throughout that time, so a healthy weight at 15 years old should be higher than a healthy weight at 14 and a half.

Because of all of the above factors, an educated guess as to goal weight is necessary and helpful when treating adolescents with eating disorders, but patients may be well before reaching that weight, and they may need to keep going and gain a few more pounds than estimated. Framing the goal weight as a moving target, and subject to change based on a patient's "state" as they approach it, is very helpful.

Should patients know their weight? This question is often asked by parents, team members, and patients. The anxiety around weight is strong, and it can be tempting to do "blind" weights as a result. In general, this is not recommended, as the exposure to normal weight and growth, and working through the resultant anxiety that may arise, are important parts of recovery. Again, this is individualized. There may be some patients, especially those who are very young, for whom it makes more sense to keep the focus away from weight as a specific number and instead to focus on weight change and growth at visits. In addition, professionals themselves can sometimes become overly focused on numbers, and understanding that weights can be fluid and vary physiologically is important for providers to keep in mind as well. The important goal to keep at the forefront of treatment is restoring normal growth patterns, and consistent weight trends will be more important than one single data point.

■ Nutritional Needs

The calorie needs of patients recovering from eating disorders, particularly those involving weight loss and restriction, can often be quite surprising. It is not unusual for patients to need 3,000 to 5,000 calories/day to achieve effective weight gain; serious athletes often need even more. Patients also continue to be hypermetabolic, meaning that their bodies burn and require more energy to function, for up to 2 years after they achieve weight restoration, so it is important to remind parents and patients that these calorie goals may not be temporary. Young people may expect only to need these large amounts of food for weight gain, but they may also end up requiring them to maintain weight as they get back to normal activity.

Do not be surprised when the amount of food it takes to supply the necessary calories is shocking to young people with disordered eating and to their parents. It is often helpful to remind parents that adolescent caloric needs are typically far greater than adult needs even in a healthy state, let alone in a state in which weight gain is required and metabolic needs may be further increased. It is important, therefore, to always keep the focus on restoring health when talking to young people with eating disorders: *"Our goal is for you to be healthy and safe, and this is the amount of nutrition your body and mind need to be healthy. We will not feed you any more or less than what you need."*

■ Treatment

There are many types of treatment available to patients with eating disorders, including individual supportive therapy, cognitive and dialectical behavioral therapies, group therapy, intensive outpatient and partial hospitalization programs, and longer-term residential care. The most evidence-based treatment at this time for the treatment of restrictive eating disorders and bulimia nervosa in adolescents is family-based treatment, (FBT). In studies of FBT, about 70% to 80% of patients are doing much better after 6 months, and, while this therapy doesn't work for everyone, it is becoming the gold standard for newly diagnosed pediatric patients, as 50% are completely in remission at 1 year, with a significant proportion of the rest doing quite well. It also seems to be better at preventing relapse.

Family-based treatment with regard to AN and other eating disorders means something very specific and does not refer to traditional family therapy. It rests on the idea that insight-oriented therapy is not particularly useful when the adolescent brain is malnourished and aims to reverse complications of malnutrition early so that more insight can develop in time. While it supports adolescent maturation and autonomy, FBT also recognizes that the eating disorder has arrested the normal developmental process, and that parents are usually the people best equipped to restore their child's normal adolescent functioning. It has many key features in its philosophy.

1. It is *agnostic* as to cause, meaning that exploring any possible triggers or causes of the eating disorder is not central to treatment and can in fact be a distraction; if causative factors emerge, that is fine, but the focus is on finding ways to move forward. Treatment focuses on eliminating both blame and guilt while still finding practical roles and responsibilities for each member of the family.

2. It is *parent-empowered*. Parents become equal parts of the treatment team, and their strengths are assessed and used. They are not pathologized or made to feel that they should back off; instead, work is focused on how to empower them to help and support their child to eat in whatever healthy ways work for their family.

3. The focus is on *restoring healthy eating*. Parents are reminded that they always fed their children well in the past, and now they are encouraged to serve foods that used to be enjoyed in their household, before the eating disorder.

4. Patients and parents are reminded that the illness is a *separate* force, causing the adolescent to make decisions that he or she would not normally make. Separating the illness from the child is also helpful in reminding parents that we are not fighting their child, we are fighting the disease. It can also help parents and caregivers enhance empathy and reduce criticism when faced with extremely challenging behaviors, as they can sympathize with the difficulties the illness has created for their child.

5. Therapists and pediatricians act as *consultants* to the parents, who are reminded that they have their own expertise in their child. We avoid being overly directive; nutrition and activity decisions are often made in therapy by parents in this type of treatment. All professionals are responsible for reminding parents of their skills and reinvigorating them when they feel fatigued or discouraged.

Typically, the therapist coaches families through 3 phases of treatment.

Phase 1: This phase focuses on early and complete weight restoration. To best achieve this, parents and/or caregivers are asked to take charge of all meals, including meal preparation and serving. The child's only job is to eat; it is not recommended the patient have any other involvement related to food (no reading labels, helping cook, choosing menus, etc). This phase typically continues until the adolescent is fully weight restored, not just partially so. Activities are minimized during this time—usually the child attends school, but often other activities are modified or paused during this phase.

Phase 2: Age-appropriate autonomy is slowly transitioned back to the child/adolescent; this will look different for a 12-year-old than for a 19-year-old.

Phase 3: Any remaining developmental issues identified by the family that may impact the adolescent's ability to achieve and maintain recovery from his or her eating disorder are addressed during this phase.

It is important to remember that FBT does not work for all patients and families. In addition, there may be rare cases of abuse and neglect that make involving families inappropriate, as well as some parents who may refuse or be unable to participate in treatment. However, many of the above principles can be helpful regardless of the type of therapy used.

In brief, the following principles, while seemingly basic, have pushed the field of eating disorders forward and allowed us to work in a much more collaborative, positive way with families:

1. Separate the patient from the disease. Help parents see that their "little boy" or "little girl" still exists. The disease might try to push them away, but their child needs their love and support.

2. Avoid pathologizing parents and instead look for their strengths. This is a much more positive, empowering way of treating these illnesses regardless of the type of treatment chosen by the family.

3. Treat parents as a part of the treatment team, and respect their thoughts and opinions. Focus on their strengths and how these can best be used to help their child.

■ Talking Points: How You as a Professional Can Help

1. Pay attention to any disruptions in growth curves for your patients—early. Malnutrition and eating disorders are much easier to treat the earlier they are diagnosed. These illnesses are not a "phase," and patients do not "grow out" of them. Noting if patients are losing weight or arresting their pubertal growth or linear height is key to early intervention.

2. Ensure a thorough medical assessment is completed for possible non–eating disorder etiologies as well as for possible complications that need attention.

3. Be clear that you know that parents do not cause eating disorders. Just that simple statement can be very powerful and healing to the entire family, as they may have felt implicit or explicit blame from others.

4. Take care to emphasize that eating disorders are life-threatening and require urgent intervention, but that they are also quite responsive to early and evidence-based intervention and carry a favorable prognosis in most cases.

5. Involve families in care, and maintain a nonjudgmental stance. Appointments should involve both parents and patient, as the parents need to be informed about treatment in order to help their adolescent succeed in recovery. Parental histories are also often critical to understanding how patients are progressing in their home environment.

6. Role-model calm limit-setting in the office. Do not be afraid of what the eating disorder is afraid of, and do not be afraid to deliver difficult news. Do not escalate if the adolescent starts to escalate.

7. Frame difficult decisions (activity restriction, goal weights, hospitalization, calorie goals) as being about safety—because they are. Punishment and reward systems are typically not relevant or helpful, but letting patients and parents know that these decisions are really just about what is safe usually helps to keep everyone focused.

8. Avoid triangulation of different team members by the illness. It is common for adolescents to be very angry and uncomfortable early in treatment. While it is fine to empathize with the difficulty of changing behaviors and how irritating treatment and refeeding may be, it is critical to remember that the therapist and other team members are very likely to be unpopular early in treatment, and this doesn't necessarily mean that any team members, including parents, are doing anything wrong—it may mean that they are doing everything right!

9. Expect parents to feel weary and discouraged at times. This is an exhausting illness, treatment is labor-intensive, and feeling tired does not mean the treatment is not working. Reminding parents of all of their strengths and how they are helping their child is key to helping them persevere.

10. Be clear that the goal is true health—age-appropriate activities, weight, cognitions, puberty, and autonomy.

●● Group Learning and Discussion ●●

It may be helpful to have a case in mind as you reflect on the questions below. If you do not have an adolescent in your practice to consider, you may wish to use one of those presented in Chapter 4.

1. Working with the adolescent while simultaneously working with parents is an important factor in treatment success. Striking a good balance in this can be challenging, especially given that your recommendations will likely focus on getting parents to take charge of nutrition early on, which may anger the patient and make them feel that you haven't "heard" them. Practice shifting your focus during an interview from the teen to the parents. Your goal is to listen to and communicate with all parties while maintaining a nonjudgmental stance. What are some ways you might achieve this? Do you have any worries about this? What pitfalls should you watch out for, and how might you overcome them?

2. Throughout all discussions the provider must keep a calm but persistent focus on the task at hand, which is how to best refeed the adolescent, and set limits around the eating disorder behaviors. This can be difficult to do when patients become angry during the discussion, and parents often seek to calm them down. What are some ways you might do this? How can you be honest and empathetic while being firm and limit-setting at the same time?

■■■■■■■■ Continuing Education ■■■■■■■■

If you are applying for continuing education credits, a test is available online. For more details, visit www.aap.org/reachingteens.

■ Suggested Reading

American Psychiatric Association. *Diagnostic and Statistical Manual of Mental Disorders.* 5th ed. Arlington, VA: American Psychiatric Association; 2013

Austin SB, Ziyadeh NJ, Forman S, Prokop LA, Keliher A, Jacobs D. *Screening high school students for eating disorders: results of a national initiative. Prev Chronic Dis.* 2008;5(4):A114

Bravender T, Bryant-Waugh R, Herzog D, et al. *Classification of eating disturbance in children and adolescents: proposed changes for the DSM-V. Eur Eat Disord Rev.* 2010;18(2):79–89

Bryant-Waugh R, Markham L, Kreipe RE, Walsh BT. *Feeding and eating disorders in childhood. Int J Eat Disord.* 2010;43(2):98–111

Hudson JI, Hiripi E, Pope HG Jr, Kessler RC. *The prevalence and correlates of eating disorders in the National Comorbidity Survey Replication. Biol Psychiatry.* 20071;61(3):348–358

Kenney L, Walsh BT. Avoidant/restrictive food intake disorder (ARFID). *Eating Dis Rev.* 2013;24(3). http://www.eatingdisordersreview.com/nl/nl_edr_24_3_1_html. Accessed June 26, 2013

Le Grange D, Swanson SA, Crow SJ, Merikangas KR. *Eating disorder not otherwise specified presentation in the US population. Int J Eat Disord.* 2012;45(5):711–718

Lock J, Le Grange D, Agras WS, Moye A, Bryson SW, Jo B. *Randomized clinical trial comparing family-based treatment with adolescent-focused individual therapy for adolescents with anorexia nervosa. Arch Gen Psychiatry.* 2010;67(10):1025–1032

Lock J, Fitzpatrick KK. *Advances in psychotherapy for children and adolescents with eating disorders. Am J Psychother.* 2009;63(4):287–303

Morgan JF, Reid F, Lacey JH. *The SCOFF questionnaire: assessment of a new screening tool for eating disorders. BMJ.* 1999;319(7223):1467–1468

Nicholls DE, Lynn R, Viner RM. *Childhood eating disorders: British national surveillance study. Br J Psychiatry.* 2011;198(4):295–301. Erratum in: *Br J Psychiatry.* 2011;198(5):410

Neumark-Sztainer D, Hannan PJ. *Weight-related behaviors among adolescent girls and boys: results from a national survey. Arch Pediatr Adolesc Med.* 2000;154(6):569–577

O'Toole J. Determining Ideal Body Weight [blogpost]. 2008. http://www.kartiniclinic.com/blog/post/determining-ideal-body-weight/

Rosen DS; American Academy of Pediatrics Committee on Adolescence. *Identification and management of eating disorders in children and adolescents. Pediatrics.* 2010;126(6):1240–1253

Stiles-Shields C, Hoste RR, Doyle PM, Le Grange D. *A review of family-based treatment for adolescents with eating disorders. Rev Recent Clin Trials.* 2012;7(2):133–140

Weltzin TE, Fernstrom MH, Hansen D, McConaha C, Kaye WH. *Abnormal caloric requirements for weight maintenance in patients with anorexia and bulimia nervosa. Am J Psychiatry.* 1991;148(12):1675–1682

■ Related Video Content

49.0 A Comprehensive Approach to Serving Youth With Eating Disorders. Kreipe, Peebles.

49.1 Working With Families of Adolescents With Eating Disorders. Peebles.

49.2 A Story of Hope: A Young Patient With an Eating Disorder. Auerswald.

49.3 Model Eating Disorder Interview. Peebles.

49.4 Insights Into Approaching Adolescents With Eating Disorders and Their Families. Kreipe.

49.5 Dr Peebles Offers Personal Reflections. Peebles.

49.6 Dr Kreipe Offers Personal Reflections. Kreipe.

49.7 Promoting Health Rather Than Focusing on Weight or Shape. Peebles, Kreipe.

26.1 Motivational Interviewing With a Young Woman With an Eating Disorder. Kreipe.

34.5 Addressing Worrisome Behaviors and Addictions: Partnering With Parents to Create Safe and Appropriate Boundaries. McAndrews.

■ Related Handout/Supplementary Material

Parents' Guide to Eating Disorders

■ Related Web Sites

F.E.A.S.T. (Families Empowered And Supporting Treatment of Eating Disorders)
www.feast-ed.org

Maudsley Parents—a site for parents of children with disordered eating
www.maudsleyparents.org

Academy for Eating Disorders
www.aedweb.org

National Eating Disorders Association
www.nationaleatingdisorders.org

■ Related Resources

BOOKS

Alexander J, LeGrange D. *My Kid is Back: Empowering Parents to Beat Anorexia Nervosa.* New York, NY: Routledge; 2010

Arnold C. *Decoding Anorexia: How Breakthroughs in Science Offer Hope for Eating Disorders.* New York, NY: Routledge; 2012

Brown H. *Brave Girl Eating: A Family's Struggle with Anorexia.* New York NY: William Morrow; 2010

Collins L. *Eating With Your Anorexic: How My Child Recovered Through Family-Based Treatment and Yours Can Too.* New York, NY: McGraw-Hill; 2005

Lock J, LeGrange D. *Help Your Teenager Beat an Eating Disorder.* New York, NY: The Guilford Press; 2005

Norton CP. *Feeding Your Anorexic Adolescent.* Nutripress; 2009

O'Toole J. *Give Food a Chance.* Portland, OR: Perfectly Scientific, Inc; 2010

VIDEOS FOR FAMILIES AND PROVIDERS

www.youtube.com/watch?v=JhA_CShr7tU&lr=1

http://vimeo.com/50460378

www.youtube.com/watch?v=pPSLdUUlTWE&list=PLmy40N4PX61Yb46HMETtFC5Vc8vZ3V69u&index=34&feature=plpp_video

www.youtube.com/watch?v=wE3fyQV_chI&feature=share&list=PLmy40N4PX61Yb46HMETtFC5Vc8vZ3V69u

CHAPTER 50

Talking to Teens Who Are Using or Abusing Substances

Jonathan R. Pletcher, MD, FAAP

 Related Video Content

50.0 Working With Youth Who Use Substances

■ Why This Matters

Motor vehicle crashes, homicide, and suicide account for more than 70% of all deaths among adolescents and young adults. Substance use and abuse are associated to some degree with each of these mortalities and contribute substantially to morbidity as well. Use of alcohol and illegal substances will have direct and indirect effects on the life of virtually every adolescent, through personal use, parental use, peer use, and/or family and community impact. According to the 2009 Youth Risk Behavior Survey of the Centers for Disease Control and Prevention,[1] 1 in 5 high school students has used marijuana within the prior 30 days. Double that number reported for ever using marijuana. More than 2 in 5 had at least one alcoholic drink in the prior 30 days, and half of these teens had more than 5 drinks in a row on a given day. Twenty percent of teens reported using a prescription drug, such as a stimulant or benzodiazepine, without a doctor's prescription. Rates are lower, but significant, for inhalants, amphetamines, cocaine, and heroin.

> There is rapidly growing evidence that substance abuse can be a sequela of trauma. Traditional service delivery approaches can exacerbate or trigger counterproductive reactions in trauma survivors. For example, strict adherence to policies that refuse care for minor infractions of office policies or expecting a teen to wait or be interviewed unclothed in an examination room will undermine trust and rapport.

The good news is that the inverse of these often-referenced statistics informs us that most teens are not engaging in regular patterns of use. Substance use, in fact, is not a normative experience. Nonetheless, teens who are choosing not to use substances benefit from screening and discussion as they face regular opportunities to initiate use, and will need to navigate social situations where substances are being used.

Although every professional who sees teenagers has the opportunity to intervene, this topic is often viewed as too complex and time-consuming to make a routine part of visits. This attitude contributes to a loss of human potential and significant cost to society.

Through regular screening, many youth can be identified who are at risk of developing more serious problems, or who may be at risk of suffering an associated health problem. Brief interventions are relatively easy to learn and work into everyday practice. When we are aware of community resources and use effective communication strategies to assess for problems and motivate for change, we are positioned to make referrals that can lead to treatment and recovery.

Basic Principles

The golden rule of communication with teenagers is that the professional should enjoy seeing them. We must also have the capacity to involve family members while maintaining developmentally appropriate confidentiality for sensitive subjects (see Chapter 14). It is equally important that the strengths of teens are recognized, and that they do not get the impression that we see them only as walking risk-takers. While our knowledge of the profound impact of substance use through epidemiologic statistics informs our practice, we cannot project these statistics on every teen we encounter.

It is important that we not feel intimidated in addressing the sensitive matter of substance use. Many professionals feel they neither have the time nor skill to address substance use in the office. Research demonstrates that the following basic principles set the foundation for honest discussion and brief office-based interventions.[2,3]

1. Greet and shake hands with the adolescent first, then parents.
2. Focus on the reason for the visit and initial history. Particularly when there is a hidden agenda of discussing substance use, reflecting and reframing based on the initial history can be very effective.
3. Maintain a positive attitude toward the teenager. Discovering that a teen is using substances should not diminish any of their accomplishments or affect your rapport.
4. Avoid giving lectures. Preaching can easily be perceived as passing judgment and disempowers the patient. Always try to stay neutral regarding moral judgments about substance use, and avoid discussing your personal attitudes, beliefs, and experiences regarding drugs and alcohol.
5. Always try to maintain your focus on what the teen is saying, stay genuine, and avoid jargon. This usually means putting down the pen or turning away from the electronic record.
6. Provide empathy toward the teen and the situations with which they are coping. Identify potentially dangerous activities without blaming. Attempt to highlight the positive aspects of how they are coping.
7. Let the teen know when you are closing the conversation. Be sure to allow the opportunity to share any final thoughts or concerns. Outline the next steps clearly, including the need to disclose sensitive information and how that can be done collaboratively.

Moving From Screening to Brief Intervention

Screening for substance use or abuse should be a standard part of annual visits and integrated into interim and problem visits related to injuries, change in school performance, problems with familial or peer relationships, and sports or driving preparticipation examinations. Several validated brief office-based questionnaires have been developed, such as the AUDIT, CRAFFT, and POSIT. Related resources are easily found through an Internet search or by contacting local adolescent health or substance disorder treatment experts.[4] For a downloadable pocket guide for alcohol screening and brief intervention, go to www.niaaa.nih.gov/youthguide. An online screening tool for alcohol and substance use can be found at www.drugabuse.gov/nmassist.

Before moving to intervention, it is important to recognize protective and risk factors related to development and progression of a substance use disorder. First and foremost is family attachment. Teens that feel connected to parents and siblings have a much lower risk of developing a substance use disorder, although they are not immune. Overly permissive parent or older sibling attitudes regarding substance use might increase risk in spite of strong connections. Other protective relationships include positive relationships at school and in the community. These relate to possessing social skills that lead to positive and mutually productive friendships. Having a sense of spirituality also may maintain a sense of purpose and interconnectedness.

Warning signs or factors that may place a teen at higher risk include low self-esteem and self-worth. Drug use by friends and family members increases exposure and leads to normalization. While teens rarely admit to feeling peer pressure, the need to fit in and anxiety about exclusion is nearly universal. Family conflict, particularly when it is between parents and involves physical violence, is a major risk factor for poor mental health outcomes. Poor grades at school can be both a cause and a consequence of substance use. Social isolation is a leading risk factor for drug use.

■ Recognizing and Building Strengths

There can be shame and stigma associated with substance use. It is likely the youth you care for have felt judged by their substance use and expect the same from you. In fact, they may be hiding their use to avoid the demoralization that follows judgment. It may be that, in order to forge an alliance, they need first to know you see their worrisome behaviors in the context of their strengths and challenges.

Substance users often possess great sensitivity. There are so many ways to manage pain; youth who use drugs are choosing to become numb because of their capacity to feel. Knowing this positions you to frame a conversation about both the short-term challenges *and* long-term strengths of feeling deeply, rather than using scare tactics or focusing only on the young person's concerning choices (see Chapter 25). **50.2**

■ Motivational Interviewing

Perhaps the most well-studied technique for talking with teens about alcohol and drug use is Motivational Interviewing (MI).[5,6] Because one of the key tenets of MI is to "roll with resistance," it becomes easier to resist the urge to correct the adolescent. Rather, listening to the teen and understanding her personal motivations and challenges for change allows you to empower them and facilitate her progress (see Chapter 26).

A useful mnemonic for practicing MI is OARS:

- *O*pen-ended questions that ask for descriptions of experience and understanding include, *"Describe for me what happens when you use marijuana." "What is your understanding of the effects of alcohol on your body?" "How does it help you to take 'Xanies'?"*
- *A*ffirmations are statements that express appreciation and recognize the teen's strengths. *"Thank you for sharing that important information with me. It is clear to me that you have survived some very scary experiences. You have amazing strength."*
- *R*eflective statements are a way of checking if you understood the meaning or emotion behind what was said. *"You must have been very anxious about your exam to take your friend's Adderall." "What a terrible experience you had growing up, that must have really affected how you deal with relationships."*
- *S*ummary statements restate key things the teen told you and shows you heard and understood. *"You know a lot about marijuana and how it affects your ability to concentrate. Do you want to learn more about the long-term effects of using it every day?"*

Another useful technique is Ask-Tell-Ask:

> Professional: *"I can see that you're ready to start making changes with the assistance of other people. Would you be interested in learning about some resources for teens who want to cut back on substance use?"*
>
> Teen: *"Okay."*
>
> Professional: *"Well, there are 2 programs that come to mind. One involves working with adult mentors in a community garden project. The other is called an intensive outpatient program that helps young people learn more about how to manage emotions comfortably and strengthen coping skills that don't involve using. Would you like to hear more about either of these ideas?"*
>
> Teen: *"Yeah. The community garden project sounds interesting. I don't want to go to a mental place. I would rather be outside and do things with my hands."*

Motivational interviewing is based on meeting teens where they are along the continuum of readiness for change and helping them consider the benefits of moving to the next stage. Many practitioners use the mnemonic DARN-C to assess desire, ability, reason, need, and commitment for change. Use of a 1 to 10 scale can be helpful. The professional can draw the scale and ask the teen to point how close they are to either extreme.

- "On a scale of 1 to 10, how much do you want to stop drinking alcohol on the weekends?"
- "On a scale of 1 to 10, do you think you are able to stop weekend drinking?"
- "What reasons can you see for changing?"
- "On a scale of 1 to 10, how important is it to you to stop drinking?"
- "On a scale of 1 to 10, how committed are you to changing?"

This can provide useful information for reflective statements and identify what the teen perceives as barriers to change.

> Professional: *"So you seem to a have a lot of reasons to change. You see it as important for your future and you want to stop drinking. Why do you think you gave a low number for your ability and commitment to changing? How can you make that number a 7 or 8?"*
>
> Teen: *"I don't have anyone who will help me. Every time I go out with friends I want to drink. They start drinking, what am I supposed to do? It's not like they're forcing me, I just feel like I can't hang out with them if I'm not drinking too. Maybe I won't be funny or they won't want me to be there."*

Reflective statements can help to identify meaning or emotion. They can also help diffuse potential conflict and reinforce that change must come from within the individual.

> Teen: *"Smoking pot lets me chill and forget about my worries. I really don't want to quit. Why do you keep asking about it?"*
>
> Professional: *"Now may not feel like the right time to talk about this. It is up to you to decide when you want to talk about it."*

The professional will not address substance cessation now and instead will first build alternative coping strategies (see Chapter 31). **26.4, 26.5**

■ Trauma-Informed Approach

There is a rapidly growing evidence base that substance abuse can be a sequela of trauma. A trauma-informed approach involves every part of the organization, including administrators, support staff, and clinicians, first gaining a basic understanding of how trauma affects lives and then assessing their practices and modifying them when necessary.[7] Traditional service delivery approaches can exacerbate or trigger counterproductive reactions in trauma survivors. For example, strict adherence to policies that refuse care for minor infractions of office policies, or expecting a teen to wait or be interviewed unclothed in an examination room can undermine trust and rapport. The goal of trauma-informed care is to understand the vulnerabilities and needs of trauma survivors so services can be supportive and avoid re-traumatization. Trauma-informed care recognizes that these experiences are extremely prevalent, and nearly universal in persons in need of medical and mental health care. This approach extends to every aspect of the practice, from receptionist to professional, from office manager to billing agent, and from hospital administrator to trainees.

Some examples of the neurobiological and behavioral consequences of trauma in school-aged children include

- Difficulty paying attention
- Variably quiet and withdrawn and upset
- Easily tearful and sad when talking about negative feelings and ideas
- Frequent verbal and physical fights with peers or adults
- Changes in school performance
- Eating more or less than usual
- Getting into trouble at school or home

Examples regarding teens include
- Talking about the event all the time or denying that it happened entirely
- Refusal to follow rules or talking back with great frequency
- Fatigue with frequent sleeping or insomnia
- Engaging in high-risk behaviors such as substance use or sexual promiscuity
- Increase in aggressive behaviors
- Social withdrawal, including from friends
- Multiple somatic complaints in the absence of underlying physiologic explanation
- Running away and delinquency

The trauma-informed approach recognizes these vulnerabilities and anticipates the consequences of trauma. Disclosure, processing, and acceptance of the past trauma are not necessary. Once the neurobiological and behavioral patterns are recognized, the focus is on empowerment, collaboration, and connectedness (see Chapter 22).

■ Connecting to Community Resources Through SBIRT

Screening and brief interventions can result in effective referrals to treatment when the professional has knowledge of, and ideally a collaborative relationship with, local community resources that focus on treatment and recovery. The Substance Abuse and Mental Health Services Administration (SAMHSA) has partnered with states and local communities across the country to facilitate this process, termed SBIRT (screening, brief intervention, and referral to treatment).[4] This includes access and training to use screening tools, technical assistance toward quality improvement regarding screening and brief intervention, and facilitation of connections with community resources for treatment. Many online training modules exist, and many more opportunities exist for professionals to connect with treatment programs.

The overarching agenda of SBIRT is "to improve linkages between general community health care and specialized substance abuse providers to facilitate access to care when needed." The framework is designed for practitioners who are not drug/alcohol specialists and based on the view that substance use exists on a continuum. A dichotomous view that an individual is either "addicted" or "not addicted" and, therefore, deserving or needing treatment can undermine recovery. In fact, SBIRT is suggested as universal screening to identify the appropriate level of services, if any, based on the identified risk level. For this reason, SBIRT can be used in any visit, whether or not you, the teen, or the family perceive a problem. Low-risk screens result in no further intervention, moderate risk in brief interventions, moderate to high risk in suggested brief treatment, and severe risk or dependency on referral to specialty treatment.

There is also an acknowledgment that substance use is often intertwined with other behavioral health problems, and referral for these services is also important. The responsibility for change is on the teen and family, and they can choose the pathway to change, including reducing use, tailoring use to minimize high-risk situations, and moving toward abstinence.

In a 2011 policy statement, "Substance Use Screening, Brief Intervention, and Referral to Treatment for Pediatricians," the American Academy of Pediatrics (AAP) offers a strategy to address substance use in adolescents that can be useful for all professionals.[8] It first asks brief screening questions to assess any substance use experience, then if there has been any exposure the CRAFFT screen is given. CRAFFT is a brief, validated screen shown to have good discriminative properties for determining level of risk in adolescents.[9] The policy statement also offers an algorithm to follow based on responses to the CRAFFT (Figure 50.1). We suggest that when exploring "Trouble," you also ask the teen if he or she is more likely to engage in a sexual behavior, that he or she would not otherwise choose, while under the influence of substances. ▶50.4

■ Guiding Principles of Recovery

The SAMHSA has a consensus definition for recovery from substance abuse and addiction, including guiding principles.[2] Reviewing this can be very useful for professionals who may feel overwhelmed by the task of "fixing" their patients. According to SAMHSA, "Recovery from alcohol and drug problems is a process of change through which an individual achieves abstinence and improved health, wellness, and quality of life."

- There are many pathways to recovery.
- Recovery is self-directed and empowering.
- Recovery involves a personal recognition of the need for change and transformation.
- Recovery is holistic.
- Recovery has cultural dimensions.
- Recovery exists on a continuum of improved health and wellness.
- Recovery is supported by peers and allies.
- Recovery emerges from hope and gratitude.
- Recovery involves a process of healing and self-redefinition.
- Recovery involves addressing discrimination and transcending shame and stigma.
- Recovery involves (re)joining and (re)building a life in the community.
- Recovery is a reality. It can, will, and does happen."

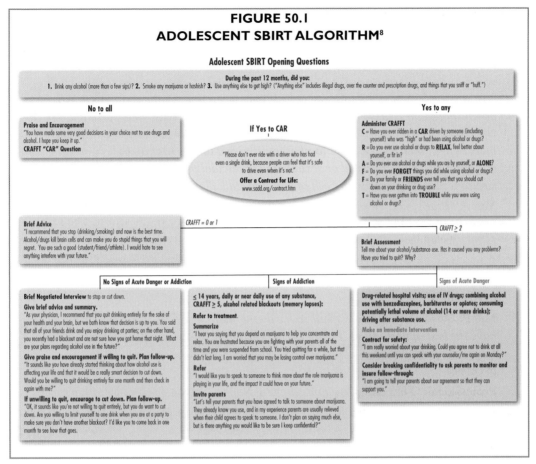

FIGURE 50.1
ADOLESCENT SBIRT ALGORITHM[8]

■ Case Study

You are about to see a 15-year-old female you have known for some time. You are aware she attends an alternative program after being expelled from her school. Her mother brings her in after discovering she has been purging after meals. She has raised her daughter alone and with minimal family support. Naomi had to learn how to be semi-independent at a relatively young age.

> Professional: *"Hello Naomi, thanks for coming in. Hello Mrs P. It's a pleasure to see you both. What would you like to talk about?"*

> Mrs P: *"I found Naomi vomiting in a closet last weekend and she tried to deny it. I have seen her change her friends and I did not say anything about it. Now I can't deal with her having an eating disorder too. I want to take her out of school because she is refusing to get help for this. She just can't made good choices on her own."*

> Professional: *"Naomi?"*

> Naomi: *"My mom is making a big deal out of nothing. Puking after I eat is the least of my worries. She just doesn't get it."*

> Professional: *"What do you feel she doesn't understand, Naomi?"*

> Naomi: *"I don't know, it's hard to explain. I mean there's all this pressure to be a certain way, or do a certain thing. I just want to be. Things just don't seem fun anymore, and…it sounds weird…but I feel better after I puke."*

Professional: *"Hmmm. I think we should take a few minutes to talk more about this so that I can give you both helpful advice. It's important that we review what confidentiality means, since I can provide the best service after we talk alone Naomi. Remember that I will not go behind your back with any information that you may not be ready to share with the adults who love and care about you. I will give you the best advice that I can, which may mean that we make a plan to talk about important issues with your mother, but that will be with your participation. Of course, if there is anything that I learn about that could put your life in immediate danger, then we will have to plan to discuss it today. That includes reporting any concerns about physical or sexual abuse, suicidal plans, or plans to hurt someone else. Is it okay with both of you if we talk alone?"*

Mrs P: *"That is exactly what I am most afraid of. When she sees a therapist, or after she talks with you, I am not allowed to know about it. How can I help her if I don't even know what is going on?"*

Professional: *"Let me ask you this. You said she is not making good choices. Do you think there is a way that she can learn to make better choices and be independent?"*

Mrs P: *"Absolutely. I have worked so hard and made sacrifices so that she can have the best opportunities. I want her to learn how to manage her stress. Maybe I messed up by working so hard so she could go to good schools and be able to go to college."*

Professional: *"I hear your fear and concern. Naomi, do you agree we're talking about how your behavior might impact the goal of your being independent?"*

Naomi: *"Absolutely. I wish she would understand that."*

Professional: *"I think we are all on the same page. Ultimately, Naomi, you are the only person who will be able to fix these things…of course with all the support and care that your mother and other caring adults in your life can offer. Mrs P, do you agree that Naomi and I should talk alone?"*

Mrs P: *"OK. I will wait in the waiting room. Will we all get to talk after you are finished?"*

Professional: *"Yes. Do you agree, Naomi?"*

Naomi: *"OK. I just want to get this over with."*

Mrs P leaves the room.

Professional: *"Naomi, do you have any questions about what we just discussed?"*

Naomi: *"Not really. She just tries to fix everything, and she used to be able to. Now everything she does just makes it worse. I don't know if it's me or her."*

Professional: *"I hear you. That is a very common experience we all have as we grow into adults and need to find our own way. Do you agree with her that your vomiting is a problem?"*

Naomi: *"Yes. It's not like I want to do it. I mean it's gross. But I have to do something to feel better. Do you think I am depressed?"*

Professional: *"Well, that is a possibility. Would you like to talk more about that?"*

Naomi: *"OK."*

Professional: *"There can be many symptoms of depression, including losing interest in things that used to be enjoyable. You mentioned that before. Sometimes people will lose interest in friends and spending time with other people. Sometimes depression contributes to feelings of guilt and worry. And sometimes depression can lead to thoughts about death. Do you have any of those symptoms?"*

Naomi: *"Well, I always worry and I don't like being with the same friends any more. I really only like being with my boyfriend, but my mom doesn't like him. I feel guilty that I am not the person she wants me to be."*

Professional: *"Thank you for sharing that. What about thoughts of death or hurting yourself?"*

Naomi: *"Not really. I mean sometimes I wish everyone else would go away, but I don't think I would ever try to kill myself or anything. I love my mom too much to do that to her."*

Professional: *"You are showing some signs of strength and resilience. It does sound like you may be depressed, but you have many positive things going for you. Do you still want to have a career in music?"*

Naomi: *"Yes! Playing music still makes me happy. That's how I met my boyfriend. He plays the guitar."*

Professional: *"Maybe we can talk about him later. That also sounds like a very positive thing in your life. Right now we need to figure out how you can get some relief and learn to cope with the mood symptoms you are having. Would it be okay if I asked you about some other common problems that young adults with depression can develop?"*

Naomi: *"Okay. You're going to ask me about drugs, aren't you?"*

Professional: *"You are so smart. Yes, that is something we should discuss. Is that okay?"*

Naomi: *"My mom knows I drink alcohol sometimes. Not every day, only once in a blue moon. I did get in trouble for drinking at a school football game. Will you tell her if I am doing other things?"*

Professional: *"I think you are showing a lot of interest in yourself by talking about this. We can make a plan today depending on what you tell me. Like I said, I will only go against your wishes if you are in life-threatening situations. Other than that, we'll discuss what might be best for you. What are some of the other things you want to talk about today?"*

Naomi: *"Well, I know you'll tell me it's not good for me, but marijuana really helps me relax. To tell the truth, I only vomit on days that I don't smoke. It should be legal because it works. I think I would be way worse off if I couldn't smoke."*

Professional: *"Have you tried other drugs, like pills or anything else?"*

Naomi: *"I don't know why I am telling you this, but I also have sniffed heroin. I know I'm not an addict because I don't want to shoot up. I've only done this with my boyfriend, so I know I'm safe."*

Professional: *"Naomi, it sounds like you feel like you have a lot of control over the drugs and alcohol you are using. Do you see any problems with continuing to use them?"*

Naomi: *"Kind of. I know I could get into trouble. Sometimes I forget so much that it worries me."*

Professional: *"Do you think you were ever drugged and raped, or that your physical safety was in danger?"*

Naomi: *"No, nothing like that. Like I said, I can trust my boyfriend; he would never allow anything to happen to me."*

Professional: *"How does your mother feel about your boyfriend?"*

Naomi: *"She doesn't like that I am involved with him. She liked him at first, but now she worries we're too into each other. She doesn't realize how fast I had to grow up."*

Professional: *"Naomi, it sounds like you are safe with him, but we should talk more about this at a future visit. For now it seems like the most pressing problem is your mood—like you said—that you might be depressed. I am worried that even though marijuana and other drugs help you cope, they might have a more negative long-term impact. What do you think about what I just said?"*

Naomi: *"Well, I'm glad you're not going to tell my Mom that I should stop seeing my boyfriend. I probably wouldn't come back if you did. I have been worrying about how I could get in trouble and other things I have heard about drugs. I know I could quit anytime, but then I might do other things. I don't know what to do, this is so frustrating!"*

Professional: *"Naomi, I think the first step is that you get an assessment and maybe counseling for depression. There is a person I know who can help connect you to really good programs that will help you develop better ways to cope and move away from drug use. I also think that we should discuss this with your mom so she understands the importance of helping you take advantage of this program. Okay?"*

Naomi: *"Oh no! Please don't tell her about the heroin. I think she knows that I smoke, but she hasn't said anything. Can we just talk about that?"*

Professional: *"I think that as long as you are moving forward with treatment for depression and that you are committed to cutting back on drug use, that is okay. I have to emphasize how dangerous snorting heroin can be. I know that it is addicting no matter how it gets into your body. Will you commit to not using that drug?"*

Naomi: *"Yes, I understand. You can drug test me if you want."*

Professional: *"That's a good idea. I will keep the test in mind, but let's wait until later. Is it okay if we bring your mother back?"*

Naomi: *"Okay. But you talk."*

(Mrs P re-enters)

Mrs P: *"Well that didn't take as long as I thought. What can I know?"*

Professional: *"Mrs P, your daughter has given me permission to discuss my opinion and recommendations with you. I know that you are having problems communicating sometimes, but I want to tell you how pleased I am that she really wanted to include you. That speaks to the core strength of your relationship."* (See Chapter 37.) *"She is certainly suffering from a depressed mood, and there may be more, such as anxiety or past trauma, that is making it hard for her to cope right now. The vomiting is not the only behavior she is relying on for relief. More concerning is that alcohol and marijuana have also become coping mechanisms. Is it okay if I go on?"*

Mrs P: *"I knew he was a bad influence. Naomi, you are not allowed out of the house."*

Naomi: *"I knew you would overreact. Can't you see he is the only good thing in my life? Please don't do this!"*

Professional: *"Can I say something? You both care about each other, and, Naomi, your mother only has your best interest at heart. Mrs P, I want to suggest that right now the most important thing you can do is to call this number and talk with Suzanne the intake coordinator for the Adolescent Behavioral Health Center. They will be able to see Naomi this week. If Naomi participates, hopefully she will develop the strength and ability to make these choices on her own. I am not disagreeing with you that he is a bad influence—I don't even know who he is. I am just saying that Naomi has to make these decisions. The goal that we discussed at the beginning was helping her to be healthy and independent. What do you think?"*

Mrs P: *"Ahh. I know what you are saying is true. She has been through so much and I was always worried that how her father treated me would continue to haunt her. My deepest fear was that she would repeat the same mistakes I made."*

Naomi: (Crying) *"Mom I love you and I want to feel better. Thank you for not trying to control everything. It's not your fault."*

Professional: *"Wow, you guys are an amazing team in spite of all that you have been through together. Please let me know if there is anything I can do to help you get the support you deserve. I think it would be good to see you back, Naomi, in 2 weeks so we can talk about some of the other things that we did not have time for today. Mrs P, will you schedule an appointment for her?"*

■ Parents as Critical Partners

Families in which substance use deeply affects teenagers are likely to be under enormous stress. That stress may be as a result of the substance use or may have contributed to it. The parents may be free of substances or have their own history of past or current use. Regardless, with some exceptions for families with extreme dysfunction or abuse, parents can remain critical to the recovery effort. They may be drained or demoralized themselves, may have been pushed away and feel angry and powerless, but they need to remain involved as strong "counter voices" to the pull of addiction. Youth need consistent and loving forces in their lives that can speak loudly and firmly to counter the easy answer that drugs offer.

We as professionals need to reinforce to parents how important they can be in helping their children overcome substance use. The greatest challenge is helping them strike the balance between consistent support and enabling. Professionals experienced in substance use management can work with families to create healthful environments that include emotional support, close monitoring, and appropriate limits.

•• Group Learning and Discussion ••

This chapter encapsulates many of the strength-based strategies for communication raised elsewhere (setting the stage to gain trust, eliciting and reflecting to overcome youth's sense of demoralization, MI, trauma-informed practice, and the importance of the parent-professional-teen partnership). It, therefore, serves as an opportunity to review many skills.

This chapter also introduces you to the concept of universal screening for substance use using SBIRT recommended by SAMHSA. Prior to this group session, review the AAP policy statement, "Substance Use Screening, Brief Intervention, and Referral to Treatment for Pediatricians."[8] It focuses on using brief opening questions followed by the CRAFFT screen and then offers an algorithm to follow based on risk. Any professional who serves teens can use this approach. You may also want to consider other screens and review the SBIRT Web site or search for how other organizations are implementing SBIRT. In the beginning of your session, discuss as a group how these screening strategies can best be implemented into your practice settings. In the second half, break into pairs and practice routine screening in several brief scenarios. The participant acting out the teen role should decide before each scenario to act out a different level of risk. Finally, ensure that your practice has appropriate referral strategies in place for youth who need higher levels of intervention.

▪▪▪▪▪▪▪▪ Continuing Education ▪▪▪▪▪▪▪▪

If you are applying for continuing education credits, a test is available online. For more details, visit www.aap.org/reachingteens.

■ References

1. Eaton DK, Kann L, Kinchen S, et al. Youth risk behavior surveillance—United States, 2009. *MMWR Surveill Summ.* 2010;59(5):1–142. http://www.cdc.gov/mmwr/pdf/ss/ss5905.pdf

2. United States Department of Health and Human Services. Substance Abuse and Mental Health Services Administration, Center for Substance Abuse Treatment. *Principles of Recovery.* http://www.samhsa.gov/samhsanewsletter/Volume_17_Number_5/SeptemberOctober2009.pdf. Accessed June 26, 2013

3. Halvorson A, Skinner J, Whitter M. *Provider Approaches to Recovery-Oriented Systems of Care: Four Case Studies. HHS Publication No. (SMA) 09-4437.* Rockville, MD: Center for Substance Abuse Treatment, Substance Abuse and Mental Health Services Administration; 2009

4. Substance Abuse Mental Health Services Administration. *Screening Brief Intervention, and Referral to Treatment.* http://www.samhsa.gov/samhsanewsletter/Volume_17_Number_6/NovemberDecember2009.pdf. Accessed June 26, 2013

5. Motivationalinterview.org. *MI Bibliography Filter—Substance Abuse Disorders, Alcohol, Marijuana, and other Drugs of Abuse.* http://motivationalinterview.org/Documents/bib/sads.pdf. Accessed June 26, 2013

6. Motivationalinterview.org. Manuals. http://www.motivationalinterview.org/quick_links/manuals.html. Accessed June 26, 2013

7. Elliott DE, Bjelajac P, Fallot RD, Markoff LS, Reed BG. Trauma-informed or trauma-denied: principles and implementation of trauma-informed services for women. *J Community Psychol.* 2005;33:461–477 doi: 10.1002/jcop.20063

8. American Academy of Pediatrics Committee on Substance Abuse. Substance use screening, brief intervention, and referral to treatment for pediatricians. 2011;128(5):e1330–e1340. http://pediatrics.aappublications.org/content/128/5/e1330.full

9. Knight JR, Sherritt L, Shrier LA, Harris SK, Chang G. Validity of the CRAFFT substance abuse screening test among adolescent clinic patients. *Arch Pediatr Adolesc Med.* 2002;156(6):607–614

■ Related Video Content ▶

50.0 Working With Youth Who Use Substances. Pletcher.

50.1 Guiding Parents Whose Teens Are Using Substances. Pletcher.

50.2 Sensitivity: A Common Trait of Youth Who Use Substances—A Blessing and a Curse. McAndrews.

50.3 Building a Positive Peer Network: An Essential Strategy for Moving Teens Away From Substance Use. McAndrews.

50.4 Using the CRAFFT Screen to Assess Level of Concern for Substance Use. Kinsman.

50.5 Quitting Substances: Leveraging Existing Skills. Ginsburg.

50.6 The Presentation of Substance Use in a School Setting. McAndrews.

50.7 Drugs Are Not the Only Way to Escape. Ginsburg.

50.8 Homeless Shelter Staff Speak of What Drives Drug Use and Healing the User. Covenant House PA staff.

50.9 Drugs as Self-medication. Kinsman.

50.10 Tailoring Guidance on Smoking to Developmental Stage. Diaz.

50.11 How Talking About Stress Can Lead Into a Discussion on Substances. Pletcher.

50.12 Preventing Substance Use Has Lifelong Implications. Ford.

50.13 Understanding Family Context as Part of the Assessment of the Substance-Using Teen. McAndrews.

50.14 Eliminating Parental Guilt: The First Step of Building a Team to Address Substance Use. McAndrews.

50.15 Dual Diagnoses: Substance Use With Other Mental Health Problem. McAndrews.

50.16 The Role of 12-Step Programs for Teens Who Use Substances. McAndrews.

50.17 When Teens Make Mistakes: The Long-lasting Lesson of Unconditional Love. McAndrews.

50.18 Why Substance Users (and Even Parents) Withhold the Truth. McAndrews.

50.19 Recognizing and Leveraging the Strengths of Youth Who Use Substances. Adolescent Advocates staff.

50.20 Warning Signs for Substance Use. Adolescent Advocates staff.

50.21 Screening for Substance Use. Adolescent Advocates staff.

50.22 When Substance Use Is a "Problem." Adolescent Advocates staff.

50.23 Guiding Parents Whose Children Use Substances. Adolescent Advocates staff.

50.24 Change Has to Come From Within the Substance-Using Youth, But It Takes Time and Support. McAndrews.

18.12 SSHADESS Screen: Pearls on Asking About Drugs and Substances. Diaz, Adolescent Advocates staff.

18.16 Case: SSHADESS Screen Reveals Substance Use—CRAFFT Screen Follow-up. Kinsman.

26.4 Using Motivational Interviewing to Help Substance-Using Youth Consider Change. Pletcher.

26.5 Case: Motivational Interviewing in Substance-Using Youth. Singh.

34.3 Preparing Youth to Disclose Difficult Personal Information to Parents. Reirden, Hawkins.

34.5 Addressing Worrisome Behaviors and Addictions: Partnering With Parents to Create Safe and Appropriate Boundaries. McAndrews.

34.6 Case Example: Guiding a Parent and Teen to Work Together to Address Substance Use. Sugerman.

42.3 Case: Working With a Young Man Self-medicating Depression With Drugs. Sugerman.

66.18 Testimony From Youth With a History of Unstable Housing: Don't Assume We Are Drug Addicted…But Do Understand Why We Might Use Drugs. Youth.

■ Related Resources

To view a handout that supports parents to use a balanced style of parenting to prevent substance use, go to www.drugfree.org/wp-content/uploads/2011/07/partnership_components_tool_revised_031612.pdf.

National Institute on Alcohol Abuse and Alcoholism
Alcohol Screening and Brief Intervention for Youth: A Practitioner's Guide
www.niaaa.nih.gov/youthguide

National Institute on Drug Abuse
Clinician's Screening Tool for Drug Use in General Medical Settings
www.drugabuse.gov/nmassist

CHAPTER 51

Teen Pregnancy and Parenting

Charles G. Rogers, MD

Kenneth R. Ginsburg, MD, MS Ed, FAAP, FSAHM

 Related Video Content

51.0 A Strength-Based Approach to Teen Pregnancy: Changing the Conversation From "Prevention" to "Delayed Parenting"

■ Why This Matters

Adolescent pregnancy and parenting are associated with significant social, psychological, health, and economic challenges for the mother, father, and child. Our goal must be to ensure that appropriate programs and strategies are in place to address this entirely preventable problem. However, as we approach the issue, we must not inadvertently transform the perception of pregnancy and parenting into a disease state needing to be prevented. Rather, we need to celebrate it as something that deserves planning and preparation and make a compelling case for why it should be delayed for the sake of the teens' future and their children.

> If you ask, *"What are you doing to prevent pregnancy?"* you will never learn about a teen's desire to have a baby. Start instead with, *"What are your thoughts about the right timing for pregnancy?"*

■ Background

Few issues capture the public consciousness like teen pregnancy. From articles in *Slate* to multiple reality television shows, images of pregnant and parenting adolescents, young babies on their hips, saturate our society. And this is not a new issue. In the 1980s, the Pulitzer Prize–winning reporter Leon Dash wrote a startling and brilliant work on impoverished teen mothers called *When Children Want Children*.[1] That title captures much of the popular fascination and societal challenge of adolescent pregnancy—"children" raising children. While we know that adolescents are not just big children, we also know their bodies, minds, and personalities are undergoing massive changes throughout this period of development.

A large body of literature has developed around adolescent pregnancy and parenting, and you can read several good reviews if you are interested in diving more in-depth into this literature.[2-4] A few highlights, though, are appropriate. To begin, the good news: Adolescent pregnancy and parenting rates are down. The Centers for Disease Control and Prevention reports that in the year 2009 there were approximately 38 live births per 1,000 young people between the ages of 15 and 19, compared to 48 live births per 1,000 young people in 2000.[5] In further good news, this decline appears to be related to both improvement in contraceptive use and availability and in delaying sexual activity. Improved contraceptive use accounts for 77% of the decline in adolescent pregnancies between 1995 and 2002.[6]

Despite these improvements, adolescent pregnancy appears to be associated with multiple medical challenges, ranging from anemia to preterm labor to more complicated labor and delivery.[2,3] Following the birth of the child, multiple issues continue to exist, particularly in the arena of mental health, with adolescent mothers demonstrating higher levels of depression than adult mothers.[7] Some research has found these health difficulties are no different between adult and adolescent mothers when corrected for socioeconomic status.[2,3,8] The relationship between poverty and adolescent health continues to be an important and provocative area of research, with a recent article stating that poverty is a primary cause of adolescent pregnancy and parenting in the United States.[9]

In looking toward the future lives of young mothers, the statistics continue to show long-lasting deficits and social implications. Furstenberg,[10] in the 1960s and 1970s, demonstrated that adolescent mothers had long-term difficulties with achieving life goals, finishing schooling, having stable relationships, achieving financial stability, and effectively controlling future childbearing. Many of these negative outcomes are reduced, but not eliminated, by correcting for family and socioeconomic background.[2,11]

Multiple long-term negative physical, mental, and social outcomes are found in children of adolescent mothers. Increased rates of physical and emotional abuse are perpetrated by both adolescent mothers and fathers.[2] The increased rates of abuse are particularly exacerbated in the context of dysfunctional relationships between the parents, and in the setting of limited social and economic capital.[12,13] Developmental delays, particularly in the area of behavioral control, are also seen in the children of adolescent parents.[14-16] In looking toward the future, the children of adolescent parents are more likely than their peers to become adolescent parents themselves.[8,17]

Fathers are often overlooked in research on adolescent parenthood. However, understanding adolescent fatherhood is critical to understanding and addressing the challenges of adolescent parenting. Sons of adolescent fathers are more likely to enter fatherhood themselves as adolescents.[17] Delinquent behavior, lower maternal education, living in an environment with high levels of physical danger, and dating at an early age are examples of other factors associated with increased rates of adolescent fatherhood.[17]

Social, developmental, and health outcomes for adolescent fathers are much less understood.[2] It is suspected that many of the social outcomes are similar to adolescent mothers, but this is unproven.[2] Education is one area where poor outcomes have been documented, with adolescent fathers being significantly less likely to complete high school or obtain a GED than their peers.[18] One study suggested that mothers were gatekeepers who determined fathers' involvement, and the key to the gate was their ability to contribute financially.[19]

While these challenges are real, and seem overwhelming, these young people are entering our lives and centers every day. The challenges they face in making decisions around pregnancy, parenting, and their futures are immense. We are positioned to come alongside and partner with them for a brighter future for themselves and their children.

Pregnancy Prevention Programs That Work

While the statistics on pregnant and parenting teens remain concerning, programs to reduce adolescent pregnancy are contributing to recent positive trends. However, it is beyond the scope of this chapter to review or summarize parenting prevention efforts and programs. Visit the resources below for greater details into evidence-based programs.

Healthy Teen Network. Consider viewing HTN Evidence-Based Resource Center. http://www.healthyteennetwork.org/

The National Campaign to Prevent Teen and Unplanned Pregnancy. http://www.thenationalcampaign.org

Centers for Disease Control and Prevention. Teen Pregnancy. http://www.cdc.gov/TeenPregnancy/index.htm

Using a Strength-Based Approach to Communicate About Teen Parenting

The overriding purpose of *Reaching Teens* is to help youth-serving professionals consider how our guidance might support or reinforce young people's wise decision-making. In this chapter, we hope to prepare professionals to guide youth toward becoming outstanding parents by delaying parenthood until they are fully prepared to meet their potential. We will focus on the conversations we have in our offices. It is critical to underscore that these conversations are additive to participation in evidence-informed interventions and are not meant to substitute for them. Hopefully, they may be useful in helping a young person choose participation in a program or in accessing comprehensive sexual health education services.

Although teen pregnancy can be an "accident," it is often actively or passively *("If it happens, well, it happens")* planned. Accidental pregnancies are prevented through effective education that delays sexual initiation, reduces or eliminates unprotected sexual activity, and combats prevailing myths that suggest pregnancy will not happen under certain conditions. It is further prevented by accessible birth control and barrier protections. Here, we wish to address those pregnancies that are planned.

Parental Involvement

When considering strength-based care, it is always helpful to start with the greatest potential source of positive and effective messaging—the young person's parents. Parents are ideally positioned to have clear conversations about expectations and values. They are also well situated to ensure that their children get appropriate health care, including access to comprehensive sexuality education and services.

Sometimes parents benefit from our reminding them how much they matter in shaping their adolescents' values and behaviors. They may need further education to reinforce that having open conversations about healthy sexuality and connecting their children with sexual education services does not give "permission" to have sex. Rather, it conveys that this is a serious topic worthy of full discussion.

Starting the Conversation

During your psychosocial assessment (see Chapter 18), explore the question of healthy sexuality and parenting in an open-ended way. If you ask, *"What are you doing to prevent pregnancy?"* you will never learn about the teen's desire to have a baby. Start instead with something like, *"What are your thoughts about the right timing for pregnancy?"* Ask this question even to teens that have not yet initiated sexual intercourse, because there may be some who are ready to have a baby who have not yet had sex. This may be the ideal moment in time to delay sexual initiation altogether, especially if the desire for a baby is driving the intention to have sex. The answer will allow you to distinguish between those teens who want to avoid pregnancy, those who are passive but would start contraceptive use if access barriers were minimized, those who passively desire pregnancy, and those who eagerly anticipate having a baby in the near future.

Are Teens Who Want to Become Pregnant Thoughtless and Irresponsible?

Their actions and desires may not be optimal for their well-being, but they may have admirable reasons for desiring a pregnancy. Ask them. Often you will find that they have a strong desire to be loving and nurturing. Perhaps their greatest role models are parents, and more than anything they wish to emulate them. Their pull in this direction might be stronger if there are not enough community role models who have benefitted from higher education or who are participating in the work force, furthering the effects of living in areas of concentrated poverty. Don't assume, however, that only youth who live amidst financial deprivation will find pregnancy appealing; sometimes youth with abundant resources may get every material item they want but not the attention they need. Other youth may not have had good parental models and want to give love and care that they did not receive from caregivers.

Regardless of their motivation, starting our conversations by condemning their aspirations is nearly certain to fail. We should instead congratulate them for their desire to be an involved, loving parent, and then invite them to consider that their love will still be present in a few years when the rest of their life will feel more settled.

Using Strength-Based Messaging While Simultaneously Challenging False Assumptions 51.0

Sexuality (and Pregnancy and Parenting) Is Positive—Really

In an effort to delay sexual initiation or decrease sexual activity, adults can often make sex feel dirty, or dangerous at best. This is not a very positive way to approach something so fundamentally human. Similarly, in our efforts to prevent teen pregnancy we can make it seem like a disease. Pregnancy is not gonorrhea. Parenting is not herpes. Pregnancy and parenting may be among the most wonderful phases of human existence. We need to transform the conversation into a fully honest one: Parenting is both amazing and challenging. The challenges are reduced when an individual has the rest of his or her life in order. Children benefit greatly from having parents who have completed their education, are financially secure, and have charted their life directions. *"Congratulations on your determination to be a wonderful parent! Have you given thought into how long you might delay it so that your baby will enter this world with you ready to give it absolutely everything you can offer?"* That is a conversation starter, not the last line of a lecture.

Reinforcing the Positive

Ask youth what kind of parents they hope to be. Explore why they think they will be that kind of parent. Assume that they are committed to creating the best life for their children, including love, excellent nutrition, and total security and stability. Invite them to consider whether they can provide all of that now. What might get in the way? Will they be able to do all of those wonderful things later? Might there be fewer barriers? What kind of pleasurable teen activities are they looking forward to? Will it be easier to enjoy them now if they delay pregnancy? (For all questions, expect well thought out challenges that explain how everything will work out nicely, just as it did for their friend or mother.)

Having Young People Arrive at Their Own Decision to Delay Parenting

The decision about when to parent (even if chosen through passive neglect) is a big one and cannot be dictated. This is especially true when young people see it as a genuinely positive action. They may need to weigh the benefits and downsides of delaying pregnancy. It is only when they conclude that the downsides of waiting are counterbalanced or surpassed by the benefits of being more prepared to parent that they will make the decision to delay pregnancy. Motivational interviewing may therefore be a useful technique to facilitate youth through this thought process, with one study showing that motivational interviewing was effective at reducing rapid-repeat pregnancies in adolescents.[20] (See Chapter 26.)

Having Young People Own Their Solutions

It is so clear to us that there are numerous downsides to teen pregnancy. It is natural to want to launch into a lecture enumerating all of the immediate downsides and long-term sequelae. The problem is that this abstract presentation could be humiliating and ultimately disempowering. Instead, we need to guide youth to arrive at their own conclusions through facilitated discussions. In addition to motivational interviewing, you might consider a decision tree that would allow a young person to visualize where different choices might lead (see Chapter 28).

Addressing Misconceptions

As you facilitate youth to consider rethinking their plans to have a baby in the near term, it may be helpful to help them think through 2 prevailing misperceptions. First, many youth see a baby as something that gives unconditional love. Instead, they need to understand that it needs and demands love and constant attention. Second, babies don't salvage or guarantee relationships. In fact, they stress relationships. Rather, their goal should be to find someone with whom they can partner as they navigate life through both good and challenging times. When a relationship is thoroughly tested and a commitment is firmly in place, then a secure home exists to welcome a baby. Similarly, for those who are already parents, their goal should be to find supports in their families and communities. A baby does not create a secure home; a baby requires it.

■ A Word on Teen Fathers 51.3

Many young men wish to be fully engaged parents. In some cases, they need to overcome a major financial barrier. The mother may insist on significant financial participation in order to allow visitation. This can engender shame and demoralization and force fathers away.[19] Both young men and women need to understand that male involvement can be a critical factor in the long-term well-being of the child. The price for that involvement should be time, love, and attention—and all of those things are free. Fathers who can't buy disposable diapers should be encouraged to learn to change them. They can offer the young mother their time in babysitting and child care—that is an invaluable gift of time and support. They should be encouraged to focus on their education because that remains the best guarantee of long-term stability.

■ Teens Who Are Already Parenting

Teen parents who come for services likely have extensive experience with judgment. Therefore, your ability to be a positive force in their life starts by withholding negative judgment and assuming that they desire nothing but the best for their baby or child. Teens also likely come with a dose of reality injected into their vision of what being a parent entails. This may make them very receptive to considering delaying a second pregnancy, perhaps motivated by a desire to offer their existing child the very best.

Key points you may consider

- Reinforce that their own happiness and security is critical to the long-term well-being of their babies. Inquire about what they are doing to take care of themselves. Explore their educational plans and encourage them to pursue their dreams. Remind them that it is not selfish to take time for their education, or to put resources into that education. In fact, it is the best investment they can make for their child's future. Even if they buy fewer things for their baby now, as long as she or he has essentials (shelter, nutritious food, adequate clothing, and love) the child will benefit greatly in the future by the parents' investment in their own education now.
- Talk about the importance of having both parents in the child's life (assuming a safe, healthy relationship between parents). Reinforce that time and love are the tickets for involvement, not money.
- Some young parents take a great deal of pride in the wonderful toys they buy for their child or how they dress him or her. While congratulating them for their loving attention, remember to focus on the intangibles you also notice they offer their child. Love. Attention. Nurturance. Attention to their feelings. Then make some of the following points:
  — The best toys are the simple ones that require imagination (dolls, blocks, art supplies). They build creativity and intelligence; they are also the least expensive.[21,22]
  — The very best plaything to a baby is a parent. Nothing is more fascinating than a face. Nothing is more satisfying than full attention.
  — The best way to build intelligence is to read books with your child.
- Help young parents understand that discipline is not about control. It is about teaching and keeping children safe while they have opportunities to explore the world. Reinforce that you can't spoil a child with love.
- Development is a miracle. Sometimes when we are busy or burdened we miss the opportunity to celebrate the giant successes babies, toddlers, and children accomplish every day. It is so easy to ignore milestones because they just happen; everyone does it. But, for a child, those milestones are great sources of pride and accomplishment. Ask the teen what accomplishment gives them the greatest pride. (Expect most to say, *"Having my baby."*) Ask them how it would have felt if no one was there for them or no one even noticed it was a big deal. Explain that some of the things we take for granted are that big a deal for a child. A perfect example is a first step. Every toddler takes one. But, for that child, the world changes in an instant. Then, the very next moment, the toddler falls down. In a matter of minutes, toddlers learn whether people will notice their accomplishment, cheer them on, and encourage them to get right back up when they fail, or learn that they will be ignored altogether. Every developmental milestone offers parents opportunities to build self-confident, secure children. The best parents, teen or otherwise, celebrate successes and encourage continued effort during those fleeting, but ever-present, moments of failure.

•• Group Learning and Discussion ••

Prior to this group activity, review the chapters on

- "Addressing Demoralization: Eliciting and Reflecting Strengths"
- "Delivering Upsetting News to Parents: Recognizing Their Strengths First"
- "Helping Adolescents Own Their Solutions"
- "Motivational Interviewing"

Then proceed with the following 3 cases.

Case 1: A 15-year-old is in your office. She has had the same boyfriend for more than 9 months. She is thinking about having a baby, or at least wouldn't complain if it happened. She says, *"Well, I know that if I did get pregnant, I'd keep it…and be a really good mom. Ty would be a great dad too…he's so funny and is awesome with his nephews."* She would like to be a nurse when she gets older. Her aunt is a nurse and really loves her career. She is really close with her mom, who is in the waiting area, and thinks she could talk about just about anything with her. Her mother had her when she was 16. She states, *"My mom had a rocky start, but has a good job now."*

Case 2: A 16-year-old young man comes to you for a routine visit. He is a good student and plans on going to college. He has his daughter's name tattooed on his arm. You ask about his daughter and he beams with pride as he shows you her pictures on his phone. You ask how often he gets to see her, and his mood shifts. *"Not too much, her mom and I don't get along all of the time. She says I don't care about my little girl. She says if I did, I'd be buying her more stuff. I'm planning on it too. I'm going to get a job and quit school for a little while. I'll get my GED at night."*

Case 3: A 16-year-old girl looks sullen as you speak to her, offering monosyllabic answers in the beginning of your interview, but then she begins to open up. She lives in a group home after being put into foster care when she was 13. She doesn't want to give details, but does tell you, *"Me and my mom didn't get along."* Her dad is in prison, but that doesn't really bother her: *"I never knew him anyway."* She uses marijuana regularly, *"To chill."* She has 3 siblings: 14, 12, and 5. She does everything she can to make their lives better than her own. She gives them a lot of advice and teaches them not to listen to their mom *"when she's drunk and stuff"* because she doesn't even mean what she says. *"I tell them, 'She really, really loves you.'"* She wants to be a teacher or a counselor when she gets older. Ms Vaughn, her English teacher, is the only person who ever really noticed how smart she is. Her foster care social worker, Mr Delgado, *"has stuck with me through all types of stuff."* She really wants to help kids when she gets older.

She is ready to have a baby. She's learned a lot about what children need and knows she can give the love a baby needs. She doesn't know who the father should be yet, but she's been talking to one guy for about 3 months, and he treats her really well.

▪▪▪▪▪▪▪▪ Continuing Education ▪▪▪▪▪▪▪▪

If you are applying for continuing education credits, a test is available online. For more details, visit www.aap.org/reachingteens.

■ References

1. Dash L. *When Children Want Children: The Urban Crisis of Teenage Childbearing.* New York, NY: William Morrow; 1989:270

2. Beers LAS, Hollo RE. Approaching the adolescent-headed family: a review of teen parenting. *Curr Probl Pediatr Adolesc Health Care.* 2009;39(9):216–233

3. Creatsas G, Elsheikh A. Adolescent pregnancy and its consequences. *Eur J Contracept Reprod Health Care.* 2002;7(3):167–172

4. Elfenbein DS, Felice ME. Adolescent pregnancy. *Pediatr Clin North Am.* 2003;50:781–800

5. Martin JA, Hamilton BE, Ventura SJ, et al. Births: final data for 2009. *Natl Vital Stat Rep.* 2011;60(1):1–70

6. Santelli JS, Lindberg LD, Finer LB, Singh S. Explaining recent declines in adolescent pregnancy in the United States: the contribution of abstinence and improved contraceptive use. *Am J Public Health.* 2007;97(1):150–156

7. Lanzi RG, Bert SC, Jacobs BK. Depression among a sample of first-time adolescent and adult mothers. *J Child Adolesc Psychiatr Nurs.* 2009;22(4):194–202

8. Brooks-Gunn J, Furstenberg FF. The children of adolescent mothers: physical, academic, and psychological outcomes. *Dev Rev.* 1986;6(3):224–251

9. Kearney MS, Levine PB. Why is the teen birth rate in the United States so high and why does it matter? *J Econ Perspect.* 2012;26(2):141–166

10. Furstenberg FF Jr. The social consequences of teenage parenthood. *Fam Plann Perspect.* 1976;8(4):148–164

11. Hoffman S, Foster E, Furstenberg F. Reevaluating the costs of teenage childbearing. *Demography.* 1993;30(1):1–13

12. Yookyong L. Early motherhood and harsh parenting: the role of human, social, and cultural capital. *Child Abuse Negl.* 2009;33(9):625–637

13. Moore DR, Florsheim P. Interpartner conflict and child abuse risk among African American and Latino adolescent parenting couples. *Child Abuse Negl.* 2008;32(4):463–475

14. Black MM, Papas MA, Hussey JM, et al. Behavior and development of preschool children born to adolescent mothers: risk and 3-generation households. *Pediatrics.* 2002;109(4):573–580

15. Ryan-Krause P, Meadows-Oliver M, Sadler L, Swartz MK. Developmental status of children of teen mothers: contrasting objective assessments with maternal reports. *J Pediatr Health Care.* 2009;23(5):303–309

16. Chiu SH, DiMarco MA. A pilot study comparing two developmental screening tools for use with homeless children. *J Pediatr Health Care.* 2010;24(2):73–80

17. Sipsma H, Biello KB, Cole-Lewis H, Kershaw T. Like father, like son: the intergenerational cycle of adolescent fatherhood. *Am J Public Health.* 2010;100(3):517-524

18. Marsiglio W. Adolescent fathers in the United States: their initial living arrangements, marital experience and educational outcomes. *Fam Plann Perspect.* 1987;19(6):240–251

19. Rhein LM, Ginsburg KR, Schwarz DF, et al. Teen father participation in child rearing: family perspectives. *J Adolesc Health.* 1997;21(4):244–252

20. Barnet B, Liu J, DeVoe M, Duggan AK, Gold MA, Pecukonis E. Motivational intervention to reduce rapid subsequent births to adolescent mothers: a community-based randomized trial. *Ann Fam Med.* 2009;7(5):436–445

21. Milteer RM, Ginsburg KR, Mulligan DA, et al. The importance of play in promoting healthy child development and maintaining strong parent-child bond: focus on children in poverty. *Pediatrics.* 2012;129(1):e204–e213

22. Ginsburg KR. The importance of play in promoting healthy child development and maintaining strong parent-child bonds. *Pediatrics.* 2007;119(1):182–191

■ Related Video Content

51.0 A Strength-Based Approach to Teen Pregnancy: Changing the Conversation From "Prevention" to "Delayed Parenting." Ginsburg.

51.1 Delaying Parenting for Teenagers: A Cost-effective Intervention. Jenkins.

51.2 Appropriate Access to Care Can Lower Teen Pregnancy Rates. Diaz.

51.3 Teen Fathers Need to Be Encouraged to Offer What They Can Give Now While Keeping Their Focus on How to Give More Later. Ginsburg.

26.2 Motivational Interviewing: Making Sure to Uncover the Teen's Perspective. Singh.

34.3 Preparing Youth to Disclose Difficult Personal Information to Parents. Reirden, Hawkins.

37.0 Delivering Upsetting News to Parents: Recognizing Their Strengths First. Ginsburg.

37.1 Parental Involvement Is Critical to Helping Teens Navigate Through Crises. Ford.

■ Related Web Sites

Centers for Disease Control and Prevention
www.cdc.gov/TeenPregnancy/index.htm

Healthy Teen Network
www.healthyteennetwork.org
Consider viewing HTN Evidence-Based Resource Center

The National Campaign to Prevent Teen and Unplanned Pregnancy
www.thenationalcampaign.org

CHAPTER 52

Teen Driving

Kenneth R. Ginsburg, MD, MS Ed, FAAP, FSAHM

 Related Video Content

52.0 Teen Driving

■ Why This Matters

Driving is the greatest risk to teens' safety. Teen drivers aged 16 to 19 are 4 times more likely to get in a fatal crash than drivers aged 25 to 69, and crashes are the leading cause of teen death. About 4,700 teens aged 16 to 19 die in crashes each year and another 350,000 need to be treated in an emergency department.[1,2]

A first step is to reframe how we think and speak about motor vehicle accidents by understanding that true "accidents" are rare, while crashes are preventable. As long as we think of the problem as accidental, we will be complacent and hope for the best. When we understand the problem is preventable, we will feel empowered to take action to save lives.

It may be that professionals' primary role in preventing crashes is in supporting effective parenting regarding driving.

> **If we think of crashes as "accidents," we will be complacent and hope for the best. When we understand the problem is preventable, we will feel empowered to take action to save lives.**

■ Background

The greatest lifetime chance of crashing occurs in the first 6 months after licensure,[3,4] not during the learning to drive period. This raises 2 critical points. First, the period of supervised driving allows young people time to build skills while relatively protected. Second, it is essential that safety measures, including monitoring, continue even after licensure.

Nearly three-fourths of serious teen driver crashes are due to "critical errors," with 3 common errors accounting for nearly half of these crashes.[3,5]
- Inadequate scanning. In other words, not being fully aware of the environment that surrounds the car in order to allow adequate reaction time.
- Driving too fast for road conditions (eg, driving too fast to respond to other drivers, for weather conditions, or to successfully handle a curve).
- Distractions.

There are a number of proven strategies to significantly reduce the chances teens will get in crashes. Driving is too often seen simply in terms of acquiring a set of skills, which then leads to passing a licensing test. Having the basic driving skills needed to get a license is only a first step; driving maturity only comes with experience. Further, we know seat belts are often the determining factor in whether or not a crash leads to serious injury or even death.

■ GDL: A Proven Solution to Save Lives

Graduated driver licensing (GDL) laws have been proven to prevent teen driver crashes. Research shows that most teen crashes involve "rookie" mistakes. Graduated driver licensing involves a 3-phase strategy to introduce driving privileges to new drivers while they gain experience.[3]

- The first phase (learner) allows teens the opportunity to gain experience while being closely supervised by an adult.
- The second phase (probationary/intermediate) gives a new driver the opportunity to drive alone but with certain restrictions designed to limit exposure to high-risk conditions.
- The third phase (full licensure) allows teens to drive alone without restrictions.

Graduated driver licensing has 4 key objectives.[3]

1. To expand the learning process. It provides new drivers with varied and supervised practice to gain experience. It has a holding period between the time a teen gets a permit and can take a licensing exam.
2. Minimize crash risk exposure by requiring new drivers to gain experience in lower-risk conditions (daytime driving, without peer passengers, etc) before driving in higher-risk conditions.
3. Improve driving skills by encouraging new drivers to practice while being supervised by a competent adult.
4. Increase motivation for safe-driving behaviors by acknowledging safe behaviors and reducing privileges for reckless or unsafe behaviors.

Graduated driver licensing laws vary by state. Parents must first be reminded that states set minimum requirements, and they can hold their teens at least to the highest recommended standards. These include the following:

- Unless it is necessary for your rural community and farming, do not get a learner's permit until 16 at the earliest.
- Offer at least 50 hours of adult-supervised driving practice with a minimum of 10 hours of nighttime driving (more is better).
- Allow at least 6 months of practice time from the time your teen gets a learner's permit to the time he can go for a license.
- No cell phone use (or texting!!) in the car unless it is parked.
- No teen passengers for at least the first 6 months of driving after the license. No more than one teen passenger for at least the second 6 months of driving.
- No unsupervised driving between 10:00 pm and 5:00 am.
- Continue with supervision and exposing your teen to new and varied driving conditions of increasing complexity even after licensure.[3,6]

 52.2

■ Parents: The Intervention to Save Teens' Lives

Although GDL laws are legislated by the states, it is parents who practically implement them. Parents model seat belt use and can set the rules around substance use, peer passengers, and cell phone use. They are in a pivotal position to make a difference by taking deliberate steps to ensure teens gradually and systematically gain needed experience both before and after licensing. We know that being an involved parent who sets reasonable rules and provides appropriate supervision works. In fact, teens who said their parents provided them with a mix of warmth, support, and monitoring around driving—that desirable balanced (authoritative) style of parenting—were less than half as likely to be in crashes than teens whose parents were less involved. They were also far more likely to wear seat belts, not drive while intoxicated, and forego use of cell phones while driving.[7]

A first step to prepare parents to fill their role is to guide them to be the kind of authoritative parents who can effectively monitor their children. The key here is to notice and be responsive to their teen's increasing skill level and displays of responsibility, while setting firm rules around safety. In order for teens to adhere to parents' monitoring and boundaries, it is critical that teens understand that the rules are in place for safety, not as a means to control them (see Chapter 36). ▶ **36.0, 52.1**

■ Talking Points for Teens

Professionals can reinforce all of the points listed below for parents in the presence of teens. However, it is particularly important to directly teach about why distractions are so dangerous. Many teens cannot imagine why a casual conversation with a peer, changing a radio station, biting a sandwich, or even texting *("It's not like I'm old, I can text much more easily than you can.")* would get in the way of paying attention.

Teens need to understand they have 3 seconds to avoid a crash—that is 3 seconds to notice something is wrong, to think about what to do, and then to do it. Sharing this fact can lead to conversations about scanning and following distance. It also allows you to demonstrate (while looking at a clock or snapping your fingers) how long 3 seconds last. Now take that bite of a sandwich, change a radio station, look at a friend in the passenger seat, or answer a call and demonstrate how each takes longer than 3 seconds. Tell the teen, *"If there was no child chasing a ball into the street, older lady crossing the street, or truck trying to beat a turn signal, it would be no problem. So, most times, you'll get away with it. Don't let that make you think it is okay. If your eyes are not on the road always scanning, you won't always be lucky."* ▶ **52.3**

■ Talking Points for Parents

- Teens begin learning about driving safety long before they get their learning permit. They watch you put on seat belts, slow down when the light turns yellow, come to a stop at stop signs, and sit patiently in traffic versus become full of rage. They watch you put away the phone or pull off the road to make a call.
- Setting reasonable rules and monitoring, the gradual granting of more freedom when competency is demonstrated, and discipline that ties consequences directly to the behavior at hand will help keep your teen safe and reduce the parent-child conflicts that frequently arise around driving.
- By positioning your conversations about driving around safety issues, your teen is less likely to feel as though you're trying to control him just as he's becoming independent.
- The car has long represented independence in American culture. You don't want the car to become the place where your teen rebels against you or acts out freedom fantasies. Instead, you want the car to be the place your teen demonstrates responsibility and earns the trust to gain more privileges.
- As you consider whether your teen is ready to drive, remember state laws offer a minimum age of licensure. Your teen might be allowed under state law to get a learner's permit at age 16 and a license 6 months later, but you need to be the ultimate judge of whether your teen is ready to take on this responsibility.
- The pre-permit phase is a good time to float the idea of a parent-child driving contract, which will lay out ground rules for safe driving. You don't have to nail down the details quite yet, but, by introducing the concept of a contract early, your teen won't interpret it as you being controlling just as he is celebrating passing his driver's test. Use the contract to spell out the nonnegotiable aspects of driving behavior—no speeding, no cell phones, no drinking—and clarify the ways that you will monitor your teen's performance. Consequences for breaking the rules should also be included in the contract,

including what will happen in the case of speeding or parking tickets. You should include a plan for increasing your teen's use of the car as he proves himself to be a responsible driver, because that's a good motivator.[8,9]

- Remember, your state sets minimum requirements for the length of time a teen needs to hold a learner's permit as well as the number of hours a teen has to log behind the wheel before getting licensed. Let your teen know that you will gradually introduce him to varying driving conditions—traffic volume, time of day, weather, highway versus back roads and city streets—as you see him gain skill and confidence.

- It's recommended that teens get at least 50 hours of on-the-road experience before they get their license. More is better! Professional lessons can also be helpful because the instructor is trained to deal with new drivers and is a neutral person your teen is likely to listen to.

- You should become familiar with your state's graduated driving laws. These laws slow down the licensing process and are designed to gradually expose teens to increasing complexity on the road. But, you should institute your own restrictions because your state may not have all of the restrictions in place that are known to protect teens and prevent crashes.

- Make sure other parents in your community are aware of all of the protections so your teen won't feel alone in having these measures enforced.

- Let your teen know that, in your household, rules around driving and monitoring will continue even after she gets her license. Also tell her that teaching in new driving conditions will continue.

- Talk about substance use and driving. Institute the Students Against Destructive Decisions Contract for Life (www.sadd.org/contract.htm). Add a "code word" to the contract to make it easier for your teen to call you if he is in trouble (see Chapter 41, page 335).

- Consider getting professional on-the-road driver's education instruction. But, even if your state says you can loosen any of the above restrictions because your teen has had driver's education, do not take them away.

- You should control the keys at least for the first 6 months to get your teen in the habit of saying where he's driving to and when he'll be back. Have him put the keys on a communal hook when he gets home.[10]

- Remind your teen that experience only comes with time, and that he'll need to demonstrate that he's good at the basic driving challenges before you trust him to handle even more. Even after your teen gets his license, continue to be a passenger whenever possible, and especially as he takes on more challenging conditions.

- Even with your focus on safety, be prepared for your teen to say, *"You don't trust me,"* or *"I always knew you hated my friends."* Your responses should avoid defensiveness and reiterate your commitment to safety, *"More crashes happen after dark, and until you have more experience, I just can't let you take that safety risk,"* or *"I really love your friends and care about your safety, so please let me drive all of you to the concert."*

- New tracking devices allow parents to keep tabs on where their teen driver goes, how fast she drives, and how long she stays at stopping points. In a matter of time, it may be able to check for signs of drinking and to check seat belt use. Some GPS systems will even send an alert if the driver strays from a preprogrammed route. You can decide whether to use these technologies to support your monitoring, but **they should never replace open communication.** Kids need to understand your monitoring of their driving is an act of love and concern about safety, not an effort to control them.

•• Group Learning and Discussion ••

Practice homework: Post state GDL laws and determine whether they are optimal or whether you should recommend parents enforce stricter rules.

Discuss

Many practice settings that serve youth address dangerous teen issues such as sex, drugs, and violence. Do we also discuss driving safety? Even though it is not something that attracts popular media attention, why would driving safety be a critical discussion topic?

Practice

Practice a discussion with a teen on why distractions are dangerous (cell phones, peer passengers, texting, changing the radio stations). Come up with a technique to demonstrate how it takes only 3 seconds to recognize a danger, decide what to do, and then do it.

▪▪▪▪▪▪▪▪ Continuing Education ▪▪▪▪▪▪▪▪

If you are applying for continuing education credits, a test is available online. For more details, visit www.aap.org/reachingteens.

▪ References

1. Centers for Disease Control and Prevention. Web-based Injury Statistics Query and Reporting System (WISQARS) [Online]. National Center for Injury Prevention and Control, Centers for Disease Control and Prevention; 2010

2. NHTSA. Fatality Analysis Reporting System (FARS), 2009. Washington, DC: US Department of Transportation, National Highway Traffic Safety Administration, National Center for Statistics and Analysis; 2009

3. The Children's Hospital of Philadelphia's Center for Injury Research and Prevention. Teendriversource. http://teendriversource.org. Accessed June 26, 2013

4. Mayhew DR, Simpson HM, Pak A. Changes in collision rates among novice drivers during the first months of driving. *Accid Anal Prev.* 2003;35(5):683–691

5. Curry AE, Hafetz J, Kallan MJ, Winston FK, Durbin DR. Prevalence of teen driver errors leading to serious motor vehicle crashes. *Accid Anal Prev.* 2011;43(4):1285–1290

6. Ginsburg KR, Fitzgerald S. Get a driver's license and car. In: Letting Go With Love and Confidence: Raising Responsible, Resilient, Self-Sufficient Teens. New York, NY: Avery Press, Penguin Books; 2011

7. Ginsburg KR, Durbin DR, García-España JF, Kalicka EA, Winston FK. Associations between parenting styles and teen driving, safety-related behaviors and attitudes. *Pediatrics.* 2009;124(4):1040–1051

8. American Academy of Pediatrics Committee on Injury, Violence, and Poison Prevention, Committee on Adolescence. The teen driver. *Pediatrics.* 2006;118;2570–2581

9. Simons-Morton B, Ouimet MC. Parent involvement in novice teen driving: a review of the literature. *Inj Prev.* 2006;12(suppl 1):i30–i37

10. García-España F, Ginsburg KR, Durbin D, Elliott MR, Winston FK. Primary access to vehicles increases risky teen driving behaviors and crashes: national perspective. *Pediatrics.* 2009;124(4):1069–1075

■ Related Video Content

52.0 Teen Driving. Ginsburg.

52.1 Parents' Essential Role: It's Much More Than Just Teaching Driving Skills. Ginsburg.

52.2 Graduated Driver Licensing (GDL) Laws. Ginsburg.

52.3 Help Teens Understand Why a Distraction-Free Environment Is Key to Crash Avoidance. Ginsburg.

36.0 Balanced Parenting: A Key to Adolescent Success and Healthy Behaviors. Ginsburg.

41.1 Peer Negotiation Strategies: Empowering Teens AND Parents. Ginsburg.

■ Related Web Sites

National Highway Traffic Safety Administration
www.nhtsa.gov/Teen-Drivers
Offers a comprehensive approach to teen driver safety

The Children's Hospital of Philadelphia's Center for Injury Research and Prevention
www.teendriversource.org
Offers information and intervention strategies for teens, parents, professionals, and researchers

Students Against Destructive Decisions Contract for Life
www.sadd.org/contract.htm

CHAPTER 53

Managing Electronic Media Use in the Lives of Adolescents

Michael O. Rich, MD, MPH, FAAP, FSAHM
Victor C. Strasburger, MD, FAAP, FSAHM

 Related Video Content

53.0.1 How Does Media Figure Into the Lives of Kids?
53.0.2 Media's Effect on Our Youth

■ Why This Matters

Adolescents spend more time using media than they spend in school, with parents, or in any other learning or role-modeling experience. On average, American youth between 8 and 18 years old actively use electronic media for more than 7 hours every day, they text or talk on mobile phones for an additional 2 hours or more, and they multitask with several media at a time, resulting in nearly 11 hours of exposure to media content daily.

> Just as adolescents need teaching and supervision while they learn to drive an automobile safely and responsibly, they need to be mentored in the healthy ways to use the powerful interactive media tools at their fingertips.

Some types of media use expose youth to behavioral risks and negative health outcomes, including obesity, social isolation, and poorer sleep. Other types of media use have been linked to improved visual attention, better academic performance, improved social connectedness, and increased participation in the democratic process. Providers, educators, and parents have a meaningful role in helping adolescents achieve positive outcomes and minimize risks from their electronic media use.

■ Reducing Potential Risks of Electronic Media Use

Much of the original research on the adverse affects of media exposure for children and adolescents focused on television use. Commercial television gives a picture of the broader world that may shape young people's norms. According to "super-peer" theory, which proposes that media are an ever-present and influential force in youths' lives, media can portray certain behaviors, such as having unprotected sex or violence, as expected, even attractive. Advertising that highlights the pleasure of drinking beer and eating calorically dense foods without references to moderation or potential risks is designed to encourage their consumption. ▶ 41.2

- On commercial primetime television, 75% of shows contain sexual references or content, but only 10% mention the need for contraception or sexually transmitted infection protection. Television shows and commercials that mention or advocate condom use or birth control are rarely seen on commercial networks.

- Television aimed at young audiences can contain more violence than adult television, with one-fourth of violent interactions featuring guns. Violence on children's shows is frequently portrayed as humorous or as an acceptable solution to a complex problem. The notion of justified violence may reinforce aggressive behavior and desensitize children and adolescents to violence and its consequences.

- American children and adolescents view 2,000 beer commercials per year. Most of the commercials suggest that drinking alcohol is normative and that people who do so are successful, happy, and sexy. For every antidrug public service announcement (PSA) on television, there are an estimated 25 to 50 beer commercials. Most PSAs focus on marijuana, cocaine, inhalants, or heroin use, not alcohol use—the leading substance used by American teenagers today, and a key factor in many adolescent deaths.

- Numerous studies demonstrate a link between the amount of television viewed and the prevalence of being overweight among children. The mechanisms remain unclear. Television viewing may displace more active activities, expose children and adolescents to unhealthy food choices, alter eating habits, or interfere with sleep. The average child or adolescent sees between 4,400 and 7,600 food advertisements per year on television, most of which are for snacks, fast food, and sugared cereals.

- Risks associated with television viewing increase with unsupervised screen time (eg, when a child or adolescent is permitted to have a television or Internet connection in his or her bedroom). On the other hand, parents of teenagers can improve communication with their children and adolescents by watching television together, discussing content, and substituting ongoing "little" discussions about sex, violence, and alcohol for "the big talk" about such matters. Not only can viewing challenging material together provide "teachable moments" that are less awkward, but some studies have shown that, as with other family activities, families who watch TV or play video games together have greater connectedness.

- Recommendations to reduce unsupervised screen time will become increasingly difficult as more adolescents view television on mobile devices. The Pew Charitable Fund 2009 Survey found that 79% of adolescents nationally owned an iPod or MP3 player, 75% owned a cell phone, and 69% owned a desktop or laptop computer. The changing trends in usage and ease of mobility of many of these devices challenges researchers, educators, and parents to explore how to best help adolescents benefit from increased access to media while minimizing its associated risks.

■ Maximizing the Potential Benefits of Electronic Media Use

Contemporary electronic media provide an important environment for exploring the key tasks of adolescent development. Adolescents are becoming abstract thinkers and can consider the intricacies of the larger world and express their concerns via the Internet.

- Media provide a safe way for adolescents to explore identity development and peer connections. Adolescents strive for independence—from parents, teachers, and other authority figures—and they experiment with freedom through social media, texting, and their mobile phones. Establishing their individual identities, adolescents seek out role models in their own lives and in larger-than-life figures from sports, music, movies, and television. Adolescents may "try on" a variety of identities, choosing elements that feel comfortable until they have a unique mosaic of appearance, traits, and behaviors that are their own.

- Adolescents need to learn how to connect to and get along with peers—media tools such as texting and social media provide greater perceived safety to reach out to others at a time when many youth feel self-conscious or insecure. For marginalized adolescents or adolescents with chronic illness, social media can provide an incredibly important connection to their community of peers.
- Moving beyond their nuclear families, adolescents seek experience and sensation (some adolescents are more sensation-seeking than others). They can fulfill these needs in relative safety, with everything from playing basketball to racing cars to engaging in graphically realistic warfare in the virtual worlds of electronic games.

■ Parents Need to Provide Guidance

Adolescents are digital natives, having grown up with interactive screen media, but their parents sometimes feel uncomfortable and inept with electronic devices, especially in comparison to their children. Even very young children, who may need initial instruction in the mechanics of keyboarding, mousing, or texting, are quickly at ease and adept in electronic environments. Unfortunately, what may result is parents' inability to offer oversight and guidance with media at the level they routinely exercise in other realms of their adolescent's life. As a result, many adolescents have assumed that their cell phones, social media sites, and digital communications are their private space in which ▶ **53.4** their parents have no business.

Parents of adolescents often use a great deal of media themselves, watching TV, communicating via mobile devices, etc. It is important for parents to model the same healthy media behaviors they want for their children. Remember, kids hear 1% of what you say but see 100% of what you do.

Despite their technical facility, adolescents still need guidance to develop the ability to use media mindfully and with a focused purpose, and especially to become healthy and safe digital citizens. Adolescent brains are still maturing, with uneven impulse control and ability to appreciate future consequences. Just as adolescents need teaching and supervision while they learn to drive an automobile safely and responsibly, they need to be mentored in the healthy ways to use the powerful and pervasive media tools at their fingertips. To do this, we must use the evidence of how media affect youth to encourage healthy, responsible, and effective media use. Rather than discourage media use, we need to guide youth to maximize potential benefits and minimize risks.

For example, while media offer potential for positive social connections, they also present the danger of linking with online predators, and too easily allow teasing or "teen drama" to spiral into cyberbullying. As another example, in response to justified concerns about sexting, communities are criminalizing and punishing involved youth. Instead, we can recognize that this behavior results from a combination of developmentally appropriate sexual curiosity, unmonitored media use, underdeveloped impulse control, and a limited appreciation of future consequences. Ideally, we can use this phenomenon to teach youth about normative sexual interactions and the potential risks of sexting. In this way, we can help adolescents make better online decisions going forward, and can engage parents to increase monitoring of their children's' online behaviors while ▶ **53.1, 53.3** modeling healthy media use themselves (see Chapter 36).

■ How to Provide Guidance

If we are to guide youth toward physical, mental, and social health in the digital age, parents, teachers, providers, and other adult figures in adolescents' lives not only have the right, but the responsibility to monitor and guide adolescent electronic media use.

- **Educate yourself.** Recognize that media are a prominent and important part of the environments in which youth are growing up. As we educate ourselves about the evidence on positive and negative effects of media use, we can learn to provide media guidance to youth, just as we teach adolescents to drive and monitor their driving behavior.

- **Inquire about use.** Professionals should include an assessment of adolescents' media use routinely. In addition to asking about how much time, where, and with whom, ask adolescents what types of media they enjoy, what social media they use, and how they interact with their families around electronic media use.

- **Show interest.** If young people come in listening to music, ask to hear what they are listening to and discuss it with interest and respect. Similarly, you can ask them about their favorite movie, TV show, or video game. If they want to share their social media pages, ask them what they and others are saying/showing, and what those interchanges mean to them. Not only will you be able to assess any areas of concern, but you also will learn a lot about the young person. As today's youth develop independent identities, they move from homogeneous use of the most popular TV, movies, and music to a more personal and individual "media diet" of the music, movies, television, games, and social media that resonate with them.

- **Explore adolescents' concerns.** Ask youth if they have any concerns about their media use. You may be surprised at how many have media-related issues with which they are struggling—from avoiding homework by surfing the Web to concerns about "addiction" to video games to fears about inappropriate messaging or even bullying—and they have no idea to whom they can turn. You can be a caring, knowledgeable, and confidential source of help in the digital realm as you are in other important domains of their lives.

- **Explore parents' concerns.** Because so many parents feel helpless in this area, they may never have expressed their worries or had the opportunity to expand their skill sets in managing their family's media use.

- **Provide realistic solutions.** Be prepared to present evidence-based, balanced, and feasible solutions for media-related concerns or health issues. Do not blame or shame an adolescent, but provide understanding, empathy, and respectful suggestions for how she can take better control of the situation. For example, if poor sleep is a problem because she takes her cell phone to bed, suggest that she give it to a parent for recharging overnight. If obesity appears related to television viewing, suggest not eating while watching television and removing televisions from bedrooms and kitchens.

- **Think about health issues.** Be alert to possible media influences on physical, mental, and social health. Obesity, anxiety, poor school performance, and many other health issues have been associated with the media content youth consume, how much they use, and the ways in which they use media. For example, a young person who plays violent video games may be more apt to throw a punch earlier or not stand up for a victim of bullying because he accepts that the world is violent and only the strong survive. You can address these health risks by discussing your concerns and rectifying misconceptions.

- **Encourage parents to participate.** Adolescents and their parents may need encouragement to continue or start co-viewing television and talking about media use. Watching *Glee,* sports, or music awards and "friending" each other on Facebook can be a great way to build intergenerational connections and discuss potentially negative media content.

- **Teach about consistently observing boundaries.** Professionals may be asked by young people to connect through social networks. You should never "friend" or otherwise connect with teens via social media. This runs the risk of boundary violations, allows youth into the cyber-equivalent of your "personal space," and gives them the impression that they are special. By explaining, for example, *"I am your doctor and care for your health and well-being. Being Facebook friends should include your friends and family, not your doctor, your counselor, or your principal. By keeping these rules, you can be sure to protect your information and others' privacy as well."* You can certainly have a social media presence for your professional practice, through which you can provide information on hours, services, policies, and even health education and other tips. But, be careful not to offer any specific diagnoses or recommendations online for which you may be held liable or discuss specific clients' behaviors in even the most generic ways as these can be Health Insurance Portability and Accountability Act violations. Finally, protect yourself and your time. Social media, even with friends and family, can be a huge time sink and energy drain. To preserve your own health and sanity, you need to protect and keep sacred both your physical and online space.

- **Discuss media multitasking.** The brains of this generation of youth are getting a lot of practice quickly making decisions and absorbing information rapidly. This makes many of them think that they are experts at multitasking. The problem is that our brains haven't evolved as quickly as the technology and their demands. Speed at processing information may be at the expense of accuracy, focused thinking, and reflection, and may have implications for memory and retention. Although they may feel they can handle doing their homework while watching TV, listening to music, texting their friends, and downloading a video, research has consistently proven this theory wrong, even among America's best students. If they wish to excel, they need to focus on their homework, and only their homework.

- **Most importantly, recognize and discuss media as a powerful and almost ever-present health influence in the world of today's adolescents.** Simply by acknowledging, in a nonjudgmental way, that media are part of adolescents' lives, you indicate that balanced, moderate, and focused media use is important to their overall health just as is eating or sleeping right.

•• Group Learning and Discussion ••

What media content plays in our waiting area? Do we model appropriate media use?

How can we incorporate discussions about media in our interactions with adolescents and their families?

Youth tend to hear only about the negative aspects of media use when adults talk to them. How might talking about the positive effects first more strategically position us and parents to address the risks?

What kind of realistic suggestions can we offer parents to participate in and monitor media use? (ANSWERS: Watching media with teens, keeping media out of bedrooms, talking about protecting themselves and others from harassment and exploitation, discussing cyberbullying, addressing the myth of multitasking, teaching time management, modeling and guiding digital citizenship, and reminding them that co-viewing "difficult" content can easily and beneficially substitute for or supplement "The Big Talk" (about sex, drugs, etc).

Continuing Education

If you are applying for continuing education credits, a test is available online. For more details, visit www.aap.org/reachingteens.

■ Suggested Reading

American Academy of Pediatrics Council on Communications and Media. Media violence. *Pediatrics.* 2009;124:1495–1503

American Academy of Pediatrics Council on Communications and Media. Media education. *Pediatrics.* 2010;126:1012–1017

American Academy of Pediatrics Council on Communications and Media. Children, adolescents, substance abuse, and the media. *Pediatrics.* 2010;126:791–799

American Academy of Pediatrics Council on Communications and Media. Children, adolescents, obesity, and the media. *Pediatrics.* 2011;128:201–208

Christakis DA, Zimmerman FJ. Media as a public health issue. *Arch Pediatr Adolesc Med.* 2006;160:445–446

McKetta S, Rich M. The fault, dear viewer, lies not in the screens, but in ourselves: relationships between screen media and childhood overweight/obesity. *Pediatr Clin North Am.* 2011;58(6):1493–1508

Mitchell KJ, Finkelhor D, Jones LM, Wolak J. Prevalence and characteristics of youth sexting: a national study. *Pediatrics.* 2012;129:1–8

Murray JP, Biggins B, Donnerstein E, et al. A plea for concern regarding violent video games. *Mayo Clin Proc.* 2011;86(8):818–820

Rich M, King BE. Center on Media and Child Health: Scientific evolution responding to technological revolution. *J Child Media.* 2008;2(2):183–188

Rich M. Virtual sexuality: the influence of entertainment media on sexual behavior. In: Brown J, ed. *Managing the Media Monster: The Influence of Media (From Television to Text Messages) on Teen Sexual Behavior and Attitudes.* Washington, DC: National Campaign to Prevent Teen Pregnancy; 2008:18–28

Rideout V. *Generation M2: Media in the Lives of 8- to 18-Year-Olds.* Menlo Park, CA: Kaiser Family Foundation; 2010

Strasburger VC; American Academy of Pediatrics Council on Communications and Media. Sexuality, contraception, and the media. *Pediatrics.* 2010;126:576–582

Strasburger VC, ed. Children, adolescents, and the media. *Pediatr Clin North Am.* 2012;59(3, theme issue):533–738

Strasburger VC, Jordan AB, Donnerstein E. Children, adolescents, and the media: health effects. *Pediatr Clin North Am.* 2012;59(3):533–587

Strasburger VC, Wilson BJ, Jordan A. *Children, Adolescents, and the Media.* 2nd ed. Thousand Oaks, CA: Sage; 2009

■ Related Video Content

53.0.1 How Does Media Figure Into the Lives of Kids? Rich.

53.0.2 Media's Effect on Our Youth. Strasburger.

53.1 Replacing the "Big Talk": Media's Potential to Foster Parent-Child Communication. Strasburger.

53.2 Why Vulnerability to the Influence of Media Varies by Developmental Stage. Strasburger.

53.3 Parents' Role in Helping Youth Manage Media. Rich.

53.4 Our Discomfort With Technology Must Not Prevent Us From Discussing Media Use With Our Children. Rich.

18.5 Using Media History as a Way to Connect With and Understand Youth. Rich.

41.2 Media as a Super-peer. Rich.

55.3 Cyberbullying. Rich.

■ Related Web Sites

Center on Media and Child Health (CMCH)

www.cmch.tv

Open access, comprehensive database of scientific research on the effects of media use on the physical, mental, and social health of children and adolescents; *Media Health Matters*, a free online parent newsletter; CMCH Blog and CMCH Twitter feed with regular research updates for clinicians; and a Facebook page for ongoing information and parent discussions regarding media health issues: www.Facebook.com/centeronmediaandchildhealth. (All of these free resources can be linked to your practice Web site via an RSS feed.)

Ask the Mediatrician

www.askthemediatrician.org

Online advice column for parenting in the digital age that can also be linked to your Web site via an RSS feed.

Center for Media Literacy

www.medialit.org

Provides public education to promote and support media literacy education with a focus on developing critical thinking and media production skills.

Common Sense Media

www.commonsensemedia.org

Provides easy-to-use parent reviews of kid-friendliness of movies, TV, and educational apps.

Pew Internet and American Life Project

http://pewinternet.org

A nonpartisan, nonprofit "fact tank" that provides information on the issues, attitudes, and trends shaping America and the world. The project produces reports exploring the impact of the Internet on families, communities, work and home, daily life, education, health care, and civic and political life.

CHAPTER 54

Helping Teens Cope With Divorce

Jo Ann Sonis, LCSW, DCSW

 Related Video Content

54.0 Helping Adolescents and Families Navigate Through Separation and Divorce

■ Why This Matters

Approximately 40% of couples with children divorce. Before the divorce, during the separation and even after divorce, children experience parental conflict. The degree of conflict and how it is managed—rather than parental separation itself—may account for many of the emotional differences between children whose parents have divorced and those whose parents stay together. In fact, high conflict in intact homes has been found to produce effects that are similar to families who divorce.

> **Divorce often disrupts a teen's sense of self-efficacy and security. Professionals can help parents create an environment in which their teen feels safe and in control.**

Following a divorce, children are more likely to live in a household headed by their mother, have less daily contact with their father, and experience a notable detrimental change in their financial situation. With such significant changes in multiple aspects of their lives, it is not surprising that the emotional effects of divorce on teens can take a heavy toll. Interruptions in normal development are reflected in differences in academic learning, social relationships, and separation from their parents. While teens that live in divorcing homes are at emotional risk and some teens may feel devastated by the dissolution of their parents' marriage, others may feel relief to not have to endure daily or ongoing parental conflict.

Professionals can have an important role for teens affected by divorce. We can work with teens to understand and validate their experience and help identify meaningful coping strategies. We can also help parents find ways both to better support teens and to care for themselves.

■ The Teen's Experience

The most important role for the professional is to understand how the teen is experiencing his parent's separation or divorce. Once the professional understands how the teen is feeling and what is most concerning, the clinician can help the teen identify and adopt coping strategies that will allow him to focus on normal developmental tasks. In addition, this knowledge can help us guide parents how to manage the separation in ways that are sensitive to their teen's needs.

It is important to spend some time alone with the teen so you can learn what he is experiencing at home. Remind the teen that this is a confidential conversation unless you are concerned about safety. You might start by asking the following types of questions:

- *Your mother shared with me that she and your father have recently split up and this has been difficult for all of you. How is this affecting you and your relationship with each of your parents?*

This open-ended question can generally assess a teen's comfort in talking about the separation. This may be his first opportunity to put into words how he feels about what is going on at home.

- *Have you ever been in a situation with your parents where one is speaking negatively about the other? Or where another relative was speaking badly about one of your parents? If yes: How did that make you feel?*

This allows a teen to talk about the frustration and helplessness of hearing someone (even, or maybe especially, the other parent) speak negatively about his parent.

- *Do you find yourself feeling that you want to defend either parent to the other? If so, what is that like for you?*

Listen for information about splitting and forming special alliances with one or the other parent. If a teen is feeling pulled into the conflict, you can remind the teen that the conflict is between the 2 adults and not the teen. And you can use this information to guide the parents that they will need to take care to not say things that pull their teen into the adult-only conflict because ultimately it will negatively impact the relationship with both parents.

- *Do you ever worry that they are so angry that someone will get hurt? Have you seen them hurt each other or you or your siblings?*

Several studies have shown that conflict temporarily rises in some families before or at the time of separation. Witnessing domestic violence has detrimental consequences for children and teens. Ensuring that the teen is not at risk for experiencing this level of conflict can be critically important to ensure that the divorce does not lead to additional emotional or physical trauma.

- *Some teens worry about who will take care of them and their brothers and sisters. Others worry whether they will have to move or change schools and whether their family will have enough money. Do you have any of these concerns or any that I haven't mentioned?*

This question normalizes their situation and provides reassurance about common concerns during this time. It is also a way for teens to express questions that they may have but are afraid to ask because they do not want to appear too self-focused at a time of crisis for their parents. Sometimes there are immediate answers and sometimes not; working together the professional, teen, and parents may be able to allay some of the teen's greatest worries.

- *Are you feeling that you have no say in what is happening?*

This addresses the uncertainty and insecurity many teen's face. Divorce often disrupts a teen's sense of self-efficacy and security. Professionals can help parents create an environment in which their teen feels safe and in control as much as possible. This can be achieved by allowing the teen to make age-appropriate decisions, keeping school, sports, and social activities as consistent as possible and working toward solutions such as living within the same school district to minimize disruptions.

- *So how are you coping with all of these changes?*

This opens the door to talking about understandable but unhealthy coping such as avoiding school work to just play electronic games or using drugs or alcohol to zone out. It may also identify teens who try to become perfect "little girls" or "little boys" by withholding their real feelings and suppressing their challenges. This can prevent parents from offering appropriate support or counseling. It is important that children and teens share their feelings in "real time," as they are happening, and try not to spare their parents. Professionals can counsel parents to reassure their teen that they can handle their feelings about the divorce and want to be there to help.

■ Developmental Maturity and Divorce

The impact of divorce is different based on the teen's age and maturity. A young teen will try to make sense of the causes and her own role in the divorce differently than an older teen.

Case 1: Lela is a 13-year-old who was bought in by her mother because she was complaining of intermittent stomach pain. She had stopped playing field hockey and participating in social activities with friends for the past month. After ruling out a major medical reason for the abdominal pain, the pediatrician explored other issues.

> Pediatrician: *"Lela, you told me your stomach pain started about a month ago, was there anything unusual or stressful going on at that time?"*
>
> Lela: *"Well, I guess the only thing different is that my father moved out of our house about 6 weeks ago. I thought that he was coming back since my parents said that their separation was only temporary, but he hasn't come back and we've only seen him once since."*
>
> Pediatrician: *"It must be hard not seeing your dad. Have you asked your mom questions about what is going on with your dad?"*
>
> Lela: *"I told her that I wanted to see him, but she said he needs his space. My parents were fighting a lot before he left because I kept getting in trouble in school and my mom was always yelling at my dad about why he wasn't talking to the teachers, and why she was always the one who had to do everything."*
>
> Pediatrician: *"Do you feel like you had anything to do with their separating?"*
>
> Lela: *"I'm not sure. They were arguing about everything all the time. They really got into it because he forgot to pick me up after a field hockey match and one of my friends had to take me to her house."*
>
> Pediatrician: *"Do you know how that happened?"*
>
> Lela: *"They both blamed each other since they thought the other one was picking me up and I felt like I made things worse. I was really embarrassed in front of all my friends since I was just left there."*
>
> Pediatrician: *"That must have been really hard and embarrassing. It also sounds like you might be worried that somehow you contributed to their breakup."*
>
> Lela: *"Well, I don't know, it just happened after that day at hockey practice."*
>
> Pediatrician: *"I'd like to spend some time talking with your parents about how they can remember to support you as they try to figure out what the next steps for them as a couple are. Is that okay with you? Do you mind if I share with them your worries about causing the separation and how difficult it is for you when they fight?"*
>
> Lela: *"Do you think they'll get mad?"*
>
> Pediatrician: *"No, I think they will feel comforted to get some help for their family during this really difficult time."*

In this discussion, Lela is having difficulty expressing her feelings about her parents' divorce and instead is experiencing the painful loss as somatic pain. By asking the right questions about her experience, the pediatrician can help her express her confusion as more specific feelings such as guilt, sadness, or loss. With this understanding, the pediatrician can meet with the parents and help them to communicate in ways that are more effective with one another and more sensitive to the emotional needs of their daughter. It is important to get permission from the teen about what can be shared with her parents before having this conversation. Possibly due to her developmental age, Lela seems to feel at least partially responsible for her parents' separation. She also expresses embarrassment over being left by her parents at her field hockey game. At this age, teens are highly concerned, even preoccupied, with peer acceptance and feeling self-conscious. An older teen might understand that her parents are "having issues" and not take it personally.

Case 2: An 18-year-old named Doug comes in for a routine physical examination. He discloses that his parents have been divorced for 9 months and that it "has been really hard on him."

> Nurse Practitioner: *"Your parents' divorce has been rough on you; can you tell me more about that?"*
>
> Doug: *"My parents have tried hard to make things as easy as possible for me and my brothers, but I blame my dad for leaving and moving in with some woman who obviously doesn't care about his family. My dad buys us a lot of stuff, but he really doesn't spend much time with us, and, when he does, it's always with his girlfriend. My mom gets upset because she can't buy us things."*
>
> Nurse Practitioner: *"Do you talk with anyone about what is going on?"*
>
> Doug: *"Well, I used to talk with my girlfriend, but we broke up a few months ago."*
>
> Nurse Practitioner: *"I'm sorry to hear that. What happened?"*
>
> Doug: *"She stopped calling me as much as she used to and I thought she was into someone else. She kept saying that she wasn't but I didn't believe her."*
>
> Nurse Practitioner: *"Is it sometimes hard for you to trust people?"*

Doug agrees and goes on to recount anger and disappointment in his father for physically and emotionally abandoning the family. In late adolescence, young people normally begin to recognize parents' flaws, but this may be more pronounced in families of divorce. In addition, the divorce may have made him a bit fearful, anxious, and hypervigilant. Doug wonders if he misread his girlfriend's involvement in cheerleading as a betrayal or abandonment. The nurse practitioner can normalize these feelings and help calm down some of the hypervigilance that some teens feel when they are trying to protect themselves or a parent.

■ Advice to Parents Experiencing Divorce or Separation

- Model appropriate/collaborative behavior to show that parents can work together on behalf of their child(ren) despite their differences with the other parent.
- Friends and peer support systems are extremely important. Put in your greatest effort to not disrupt their lives. For example, if there is weekly scheduled visitation, plan this around after-school or sports activities to ensure they can continue strong peer relationships.

- Attend special events such as graduations, proms, sports competitions, etc.
- Work out a plan for holidays in advance to give time to each parent and his or her respective extended families.
- *Do not* speak negatively about the opposite parent in the presence of the teen.
- If there is joint custody, include both parents in visits with schools and professionals. Consider sending a letter to explain the importance of both parents remaining involved and how communication will be handled between households.
- Avoid trying to be an "ideal parent." Focus instead on spending quality time.
- Divorce can be an opportunity for youth to take advantage of one or the other parent. It is important that parents try to set consistent limits and expectations in both homes.
- When adolescents see their parents under stress, such as when they are going through a divorce, they may withhold their real feelings and suppress their challenges. This can lead to perfectionism and/or prevent parents from offering appropriate guidance and monitoring (see Chapter 48).
- In order to keep communication flowing, it is important that children and teens not feel they need to spare their parents. Parents might consider saying something like, *"Yes, I have been stressed and I notice you're trying to protect me. Sometimes I worry that you're trying so hard to spare me. Please know it is my job to guide you. More than that, one of my greatest pleasures is to parent you—through good and bad times. Please don't take that away by trying to spare me. Let me know what is going on in your life so I can really be your parent."*

■ Conclusion

Divorce is a highly stressful time for many teens, and we can be strong resources and advocates. The developmental age of the teen changes their experience and highlights how different types of feelings may alert us that a family could benefit from counseling to help everyone in the family adjust to the changes. Failing to address these difficulties could lead to ongoing depression, social isolation, educational disruption, difficulty with peer and romantic relationships, and even self-medicating with drugs or alcohol. Professionals who understand the teen experience and work with the family to provide guidance about divorce and address ongoing issues may be able to decrease detrimental outcomes and instead use this challenging period to build resilience and strength.

•• Group Learning and Discussion ••

Break into groups of 3 and work through the following scenarios. First, interview the teen privately and then guide the parent (privately or with the teen depending on your practice style) about how to best help the family navigate through the divorce/separation.

Scenario 1: Brianna is a good student in the 11th grade whose grades have dropped significantly in the last year. In a private interview she shares that her father moved out about 8 months ago, but that the previous year was even worse. Her parents fought nonstop. It seemed that they fought about everything: money, the house being a mess, and mostly about the kids. Brianna really loves her dad and had never known how much her mom didn't. Her mom spends a lot of time crying now. She talks endlessly about how much her husband never really cared about anyone. *"If he cared he wouldn't have walked out."*

Scenario 2: Matt is a 13-year-old who gets straight As and is a star soccer player. He also is the middle school president of "Students for a Better Community." His parents divorced when he was 10. His father needed to take an extra job after his mother moved out of state. He assumed many caretaking roles of his 2 younger siblings. He is charming and answers every question "correctly." As you ask him about his relationship with his father, he says that it is great: *"My father has a lot on his mind. You know being a father and a mother and working all the time too. So, I make sure that all of the other kids fall into line."* When asked about substances he responds, *"Oh no, my father has enough on his mind, I would never cause him any trouble."* When you explore school and friendships, he becomes a bit silent. He averts his gaze as he becomes tearful. It turns out he is bullied in school, and his friends have not been supportive to him because they fear the bully. Instead, they laugh along. When you ask if he has told his father or mother, Matt says, *"Oh no, they have enough to worry about."*

■■■■■■■■ Continuing Education ■■■■■■■■

If you are applying for continuing education credits, a test is available online. For more details, visit www.aap.org/reachingteens.

■ Related Video Content

54.0 Helping Adolescents and Families Navigate Through Separation and Divorce. Sonis.

54.1 Case: A 17-Year-Old Discusses With a Social Worker How Her Parents' Divorce Has Affected Her. Sonis.

54.2 Children of Divorce Can Become Perfectionists to Spare Their Parents. Sonis, Ginsburg.

■ Related Handouts/Supplementary Materials

Don't Spare Me! Help Your Child Understand that You Want to Be There When They Need You, Even if You are Busy or Stressed

Strategies to Protect Your Children and Teens During Your Divorce or Separation

■ Related Resources

American Academy of Pediatrics: Helping Children and Families Deal with Divorce and Separation
http://pediatrics.aappublications.org/content/110/5/1019.full

The Mayo Clinic: Children and Divorce: Helping Kids After a Breakup
www.mayoclinic.com/health/divorce/HO00055

The American Academy of Child and Adolescent Psychiatry: Children and Divorce
www.aacap.org/cs/root/facts_for_families/children_and_divorce

Kids Health: Dealing With Divorce for Teens
http://kidshealth.org/teen/your_mind/families/divorce.html

CHAPTER 55

Bullying

Zachary McClain, MD
Kenneth R. Ginsburg, MD, MS Ed, FAAP, FSAHM

 Related Video Content

55.0 Bullying Must Not Be Viewed as a Routine Part of Growing Up

■ Why This Matters

It has been estimated that bullying affects about 30% of youth either as bullies, as victims, or both. Bullying has the potential to define a youth's childhood and adolescence and, if not addressed, can lead to lifelong struggles with identity and self. Additionally, bullying can be associated with serious consequences, including anxiety, depression, and somatic disorders. In rare cases, bullying has been associated with suicide.

> When the answer to the fundamental question of adolescence, "Who am I?" is "someone others degrade," it can have profound implications on well-being and self-esteem.

As long as one thinks of bullying as an unpleasant, expected rite of childhood, or just "kids being kids," it is difficult to understand why it can be so scarring. To begin to grasp the potential magnitude of the effect of bullying, one has to contextualize it within adolescent development. The fundamental question of adolescence remains "Who am I?" When the answer to that question is "someone others degrade," it can have profound implications on self-esteem and well-being. The other question associated with adolescence is "am I normal?" Adolescence is the time when peers take on great importance partly because peer perceptions largely define what is normal. The implication, therefore, of a peer or peers choosing to define you as so abnormal that you are worthy of bullying can be profound.

Bullying can be addressed successfully. No intervention has been found to eliminate it entirely; however, the types of interventions that work with peers have been shown to be quite successful. These interventions stand in contrast to older style interventions that exclusively targeted the victim or the bully. Professionals have an important role in assessing youth for bullying and then ensuring they get adequate emotional support. They also can join with parents, community programs, and schools to ensure that the interventions being used are consistent with the best evidence, which suggests bullying is most effectively reduced when everyone in the club or school adopts a "no bullying" expectation as standard.

■ Background

Bullying is getting a great deal of attention recently as some extreme (rare) cases have led to serious injury or suicide. Less extreme cases are an all-too-common occurrence and can significantly affect the victim. Numerous studies have shown that bullying is more prevalent among males than females and that it occurs with greater frequency among middle school–aged youth than high school–aged youth,[1] but the focus should turn from pinpointing whom it affects to comprehending that it is a major problem for all US youth. The prevalence of bullying has caused local, state, and federal governments to mandate that school policies address bullying. In 1999, for example, there were no state laws addressing bullying among students, but by 2010 there were 41.[2]

It is essential for the health professional, school counselor, teacher, or youth worker to know that bullying affects well-being in multiple ways. It has been associated with physical injury, physical symptoms (eg, nausea), symptoms of anxiety or depression, difficulty concentrating, poor self-esteem, high rates of school absenteeism, social isolation and loneliness, and poor school performance.[3] Anyone working with adolescents must be vigilant to the subtle signs of bullying in order to break the cycle.

Bullying comes in many forms: physical aggression, verbal abuse, cyberbullying, teasing, name-calling, and rumors. Regardless of its manifestation, bullying is always intended to harm or disturb, occurs repeatedly over time, and involves an imbalance of power.

The National Institute of Child Health and Human Development conducted a national representative survey of almost 16,000 youth in grades 6 through 10 who completed a World Health Organization health behavior survey and found that almost 30% of children reported moderate or frequent involvement in bullying, which provides a national estimate of a staggering 6 million youth involved at that time.[1] The survey also showed that those involved demonstrated poorer psychosocial adjustment than noninvolved youth and that bullying is associated with other problem behaviors such as alcohol use, cigarette smoking, and poorer academic achievement. Additionally, it showed that bullying is associated with poorer relationships with classmates and loneliness. Bullying has paramount effects on an adolescent's feelings of connection with peers and establishment of key social interactions.

There are benefits to a community-wide approach because bullying occurs in areas that are unsupervised by adults. If adults are looking for it and intervening, it is less likely to occur under their watchful eyes. Bullying can occur wherever youth gather, not just at school. When adults are present at "hot spots," it can create a more protected environment.

For the health professional, it is important to know that victims of bullying have significantly more health problems than their bully and non-victimized counterparts. Most notably, victims of bullying have significantly more somatic health symptoms, such as abdominal pain, fatigue, dizziness, and chest pain.[4] One study has shown that victims are more often worried about going to school and more likely to manifest symptoms in order to stay at home during school days. This should not be interpreted as faking, rather as how stress manifests in the body (see Chapter 44). A surprising finding is that victims also have health-related issues not routinely associated with stress, such as ear pain and upper respiratory symptoms.[4] The key message is that health professionals seeing youth for repeated health problems should consider bullying on their differential diagnosis.

■ Bullies, Victims, and Their Audience

The classic portrait of a bully is that of a big tough guy on the playground pushing around a scrawny kid. Truthfully, however, there is no single picture of a bully and a victim. Bullies take many forms. The classic picture involves boys, but we now know that girls, or "mean girls," can bully just as much as boys can. Occasionally, they can be physical bullies, but more often they attack with words and relational aggression, and the nonphysical way they bully can still be damaging to a victim's emotional health. The more complex understanding of the bully's psychology makes it clearer that there cannot be a one-size-fits-all bully-targeted intervention. Regardless, bullies need to be guided to develop strategies that will help them control their misplaced anger, and they need to understand appropriate socialization and expectations of behavior.

Bullies need to be identified, held accountable, and given needed help. It had long been accepted that bullies tend to be unhappy and have a low opinion of themselves. In many cases they may be depressed, angry about their life circumstances, or have suffered traumas of their own. They target other young people to try to make themselves feel better; they thrive by controlling or dominating others. In fact, though, many bullies do not have low self-esteem, and instead have high status and many friends.[5] Some youth hold them in high regard based on their notoriety. Others may admire their toughness and try to emulate them. In fact, some bullies have high self-regard that they use to rationalize their offensive behaviors, believing they have a right to be dominant.

Next, we must consider the victim. Youth vulnerable to bullying can fall into a number of categories, but tend to be seen as "different" by their peers. They are often passive or easily intimidated, but many situational factors, such as being new at a school or shifting alliances, increase one's potential to be targeted. Surviving bullying must not be viewed as a rite of adolescence that builds character. Instead, it increases victims' vulnerability, interferes with their social and emotional development, and can harm school engagement, which is so critical to academic success. Victims may need support to maintain or develop positive self-perceptions and guidance to prevent them from blaming themselves for their experiences.

Victims can be given strategies that will make it less likely they'll be targets. In some cases, avoidance is a good strategy. For example, if a young person knows where a bully lurks, we may advise victims to avoid that area altogether. We can suggest they walk away and ignore the bully, because attention only feeds an aggressor who thrives on eliciting a reaction, but that can be hard advice to follow, especially in a school. In some cases, a few assertive words that demand respect or being left alone can be helpful. It can also be helpful to travel in groups.

Bullying likely would not exist if there were only bullies and victims. Bullies thrive on others seeing what they do, and the audience is integral to the bullying act. The audience comprises a spectrum of spectators. Followers have a positive attitude toward bullying and will play an active role in the act, but are careful to not take the lead. Supporters tend to draw attention to the bullying but don't join in. The disengaged onlookers don't get involved, but watch to see what happens. The true champions of the bullying circle are the defenders who dislike the act and help the victim. In the end, when others stand by and do nothing or somehow get caught up in group dynamics that support the bullying, they implicitly give the go-ahead. Implicit in the motivation for the audience is that adolescents want to feel "normal," and one of the ways they achieve that is by defining someone else as "abnormal." Why challenge a bully if it might draw attention to yourself? Better to stay off the radar screen. The reality, however, is that without bystanders—an audience—bullying will diminish.

Bullying takes many forms as well. Gossip, shifting alliances, and degrading behavior can be common. In middle school culture, alliances quickly rearrange and who's in one day may be out the next. What you wear, how you walk, and who you're seen with in the hallways might all provide ammunition for your "frenemies." If you're at the top of the social order, you might have to do everything you can do to stay there. If you're trying to get to the top, you've got to knock some kids down a few notches to earn your spot. Gossiping and cruel put-downs can serve to make you look better at someone else's expense.

A typical scenario is one where a peer shames another in front a group of kids or betrays a secret that is painfully personal. When carried to an extreme, a peer group might actually shun someone, creating a dynamic that completely isolates the victim, and being ignored or shunned during adolescence can be as damaging to well-being as being actively tormented.

■ Cyberbullying

Cyberbullying is an increasing problem for adolescents.[6] The instant and far-reaching reactions available because of computer and ever-present cell phone access can bring out the worst in peer dynamics. In the past, when a disagreement happened at school, everyone went home and time was able to diffuse much of the tension. Now, texting and social networking keep disagreements alive long after the school day ends, further spreading gossip and fueling the tension exponentially. It feels anonymous and safer because you're not directly confronting the peer. Reputations can be destroyed because messages last forever in the cyberworld. It may be difficult to grasp how being cyberbullied might feel to a teen. After all, at face value they are just words on a computer, and there is no physical injury. In context, however, we must remember that much of a teen's social life exists in cyberspace.

55.3

■ The Olweus Model

There are some promising bullying interventions worthy of attention, many based at least partly on the work of Norwegian researcher Dr Dan Olweus. The Olweus model addresses the behavior of victims and bullies and works to affect the environment in which bullying occurs. It is beyond the scope of this chapter to offer a comprehensive review of bullying intervention programs and strategies, but they all agree that the solution involves more than engaging with the bully and the victim.

In the early 1980s, a group of adolescent boys committed suicide after being bullied by peers. The Norwegian Ministry of Education started a national campaign to counteract bullying, and the Olweus Bullying Prevention Program (OBPP) was born. The primary goals described by the original OBPP were to reduce existing bullying problems at school, prevent the development of new ones, and foster improved peer relations at school.

Central to the Olweus model is that communities and schools create an environment where bullying is not acceptable, and the goals of the OBPP are met through restructuring the school environment. A code of conduct is taught where clearly defined acceptable behavior and core values of empathy and caring are reinforced. Both students and teachers convey the message that there is no tolerance for bullying. An adult presence is felt throughout the hallways, classes, and playgrounds. Students learn that reporting is their ethical responsibility, not an act of cowardice or disloyalty. Everyone in the school setting learns that there is no such thing as an innocent bystander. This is all done while also attending to the emotional needs of both the victim and the bully. Therefore, changes are comprehensive and are made at the individual, classroom, school, and community levels.

The OBPP has been very effective and shown impressive reductions in student self-reports of bully/victim problems.[5,7] The first OBPP implementations took place in the United States in the mid-1990s, and multiple studies have shown its effectiveness in decreasing the prevalence of bullying.[8–10]

■ Practical Points

Just as bullying has many faces, so does the presentation of the youth sitting in front of you. As mentioned previously, bullying can be seen outwardly with evidence of physical injury or physical symptoms, such as nausea, anorexia, abdominal pain, and recurrent symptoms of cough and cold, preventing school attendance. However, bullying can present more subtly. Adolescents can show signs and symptoms of anxiety or depression, difficulty concentrating, poor self-esteem, and poor school performance.

The American Academy of Pediatrics policy statement regarding the role of the pediatrician in youth violence prevention defines bullying for the general pediatrician and highlights it as a growing concern for school-aged children.[11] It also states that it must first be accepted that bullying behaviors are not considered a normative rite of passage and can lead to detrimental consequences. This is the first step for all professionals when confronted with a young person whom you think is affected by bullying—understand that it is not normal.

There have been evidence-based studies that examine annual screening questions for adolescent risk of violence; however, there are not validated screening questions for bullying. A good place to start is with nonjudgmental, open-ended questions like, "How are things going at school?" or "Do you like school?" Follow-up questions may include, "Have you ever been teased at school?" or "Who do you play with at recess?"/"Who do you hang out with at school?" Some professionals may be concerned that they will be "typing" a young person by asking about bullying, implying that they seem like an outsider. In fact, talking routinely about bullying makes it a safe subject to discuss. Do not be afraid to ask, *"Do you feel safe at school/in the neighborhood?"* and to directly ask, *"Have you ever been a victim of bullying in or out of school, or even online?"*

The young person with somatic symptoms can be gently asked whether she has noticed that she is more likely to feel badly when she is stressed. *"Many people, kids and adults, find that stress makes their body feel awful. Everybody's different. Some people get stomachaches, others get really tired, and others get chest pain. It's not faking at all; it is just what our bodies do when we have uncomfortable experiences or emotions. Do you think that your body might be reacting to stress? If yes, what kind of things are stressing you out now?"* (See Chapter 44 for a more detailed assessment strategy.)

In parallel to assessing the young person for behaviors, it is also important to educate parents about the warning signs of bullying, such as if their child is frequently in fights at school, they make frequent trips to the nurse's office, or they flatly don't want to go to school. After assessing the child and educating the family, it is tantamount to refer them to school- or community-based interventions around them, with a focus on interventions in the Olweus model.

•• Group Learning and Discussion ••

If you work within a setting where youth gather, the first question is self-reflection: Do you create an environment where bullying is routinely rejected as part of your culture of safety? (Consider visiting http://www.violencepreventionworks.org/public/index.page.) Do you ensure there are adults present in the "hot spots"?

If you work within a referral or health setting, discuss as a group how bullying might present.

Break into groups of 3, dividing the roles of professional, teen, or parent. You can either work through a bullying case that has presented in your setting or you can use one of the 2 cases below. First, conduct a private interview with the young person and then invite in the parent to partner with you in approaching the bullying environment.

CASE 1

A 15-year-old boy is brought to you by his mother for refusing to go to school in the morning. The mother has received truancy notices because he has missed too many school days. He reports that when he tries to get up and go to school in the morning, his stomach hurts him and he spends at least 1 hour before school in the bathroom. Sometimes he has diarrhea or feels as if he is going to vomit.

In your interview you learn that in school, one of his friends is making comments about him in a teasing manner. His peers support the bullying behavior and often join in on the banter. Although he is feeling targeted and ostracized, he does not want to challenge the group too much for fear of losing friends or their taking sides. In addition, there is another one of his classmates who rides the school bus with him and they get off at the same stop in the afternoon. As he walks home, his classmate follows him closely and makes disparaging comments to him until he reaches his home. The boy is reluctant to inform the administrators at school because he feels this will further make him a target of harassment. He is tearful and appears ashamed as he speaks of these situations. Through tears, he tells you, *"I am different; it's all my fault. They keep calling me a "faggot" and I think they're right."*

(Consider reading Chapter 61 in preparation for this discussion.) Remember that "coming out" is a complex process that occurs over time. Do not feel as if you need to engage the mother on this underlying source of anxiety today. Rather, you should focus on supporting the youth and breaking his sense of isolation first by being universally nonjudgmental and respectful and also by referring him to appropriate support services. One of the best ways of being supportive here is by ensuring close follow-up with you.

CASE 2

A 16-year-old girl, Jen, comes to your office immediately after a fight at school. For 2 months, this girl claims to have been harassed by the individual she fought. Comments were made as she passed her in the hallways that she would simply ignore. The other girl would also post taunting and untrue comments on Facebook and begin rumors about her. At lunch that day, she was approached in the cafeteria by someone in the bully's peer group who told your patient she was fat and ugly; she did not respond. She tried to avoid further conflict by excusing herself and going to the bathroom to decompress. As she was leaving the bathroom, she was encircled by the main bully and a large group of the bully's friends. She dared Jen to hit her, and, after calling her a litany of names, Jen slapped the bully in the face. As a consequence, she will be serving a 4-day out-of-school suspension.

▪▪▪▪▪▪▪ Continuing Education ▪▪▪▪▪▪▪

If you are applying for continuing education credits, a test is available online. For more details, visit www.aap.org/reachingteens.

■ References

1. Nansel TR, Overpeck M, Pilla RS, et al. Bullying behaviors among US youth: prevalence and association with psychosocial adjustment. *JAMA.* 2001;285:2094–2100

2. Olweus D, Limber S. Bullying in school: evaluation and dissemination of the Olweus Bullying Prevention Program. *Am J Orthopsychiatry.* 2010;80(1):124–134

3. Bond L, Carlin JB, Thomas L, Rubin K, Patton G. Does bullying cause emotional problems? A prospective study of young teenagers. *BMJ.* 2001;323(7311):480–484

4. Wolke D, Woods S, Bloomfield L, Karstadt L. Bullying involvement in primary school and common health problems. *Arch Dis Childhood.* 2001;85:197–201

5. Olweus D. Bully/victim problems in school: facts and intervention. *Eur J Psychol Educ.* 1997;12:495–510

6. David-Ferdon C, Hertz MF. Electronic media, violence, and adolescents: an emerging public health problem. *J Adolesc Health.* 2007;41(6 suppl 1):S1–5

7. Olweus D. Bully/victim problems among schoolchildren: basic facts and effects of a school based intervention program. In: Pepler D, Rubin K, eds. *The Developmental and Treatment of Childhood Aggression.* Hillsdale, NJ; Erlbaum:1991:411–448

8. Olweus D, Limber SP. The Olweus Bullying Prevention Program: implementation and evaluation over two decades. In: Jimerson SR, Swearer SM, Espelage DL, eds. *The Handbook of School Bullying: An International Perspective.* New York, NY: Routledge; 2010:377–403

9. Black SA, Jackson E. Using bullying incident density to evaluate the Olweus Bullying Prevention Programme. *School Psychol Int.* 2007;28:623–638

10. Bauer N, Lozano P, Rivara FP. The effectiveness of the Olweus Bullying Prevention Program in public middle schools: A controlled trial. *J Adolesc Health.* 2007;40(3):266–274

11. American Academy of Pediatrics. Role of the pediatrician in youth violence prevention. *Pediatrics.* 2009;124(1):393–402

■ Related Video Content

55.0 Bullying Must Not Be Viewed as a Routine Part of Growing Up. Ginsburg.

55.1 Parents' Unconditional Acceptance Can Help Buffer Young People From Being Bullied. Chaffee.

55.2 Bullying Is Not Acceptable in the Workplace; Neither Is It Acceptable in School. Kinsman.

55.3 Cyberbullying. Rich.

55.4 Am I Normal? A Developmental Perspective on the Roots of Bullying. Sugerman.

55.5 A Culture That Honors Differences Is One That Will Not Allow Bullying. Chaffe.

55.6 How Supporting Your Child's Sense of Self Protects Your Child Now and Throughout Life. Chaffe.

18.15 Case: SSHADESS Screen Reveals Bullying. Lewis.

■ Related Web Sites

The Centers for Disease Control and Prevention (CDC) has injury prevention information and bullying victimizations measures that can be found at www.cdc.gov/violenceprevention/pub/measuring_ bullying.html.

Resources regarding bullying, dating violence, and youth suicide and the home of the Olweus Bullying Prevention Program can be found at www.violencepreventionworks.org/public/index.page.

Youth violence fact sheets and links to the World Health Organization bulletin on bullying can be found at www.who.int/mediacentre/factsheets/fs356/en.

The leading national organization providing crisis intervention and suicide prevention services to lesbian, gay, bisexual, transgender, and questioning youth can be found at www.thetrevorproject.org.

Writer Dan Savage and his partner Terry Miller started the It Gets Better Project to show young LGBT people the levels of happiness, potential, and positivity their lives will reach if they can just get through their teen years. It includes heartfelt, moving video testimonials at www.itgetsbetter.org.

Managed by the United States Department of Health and Human Services, resources on bullying, cyberbullying, risk factors, prevention, and treatment can be found at www.stopbullying.gov.

CHAPTER 56

Unhealthy Relationships

Marina Catallozzi, MD, MSCE
Susan T. Sugerman, MD, MPH, FAAP

 Related Video Content

56.0 Every Teen Deserves to Be ROUTINELY Screened for the Health of His or Her Relationships

■ Why This Matters

Unfortunately, unhealthy relationships and relationship violence are common among adolescents. Relationship violence can be any coercive behavior, including physical, sexual, and mental (or emotional) abuse, perpetrated by someone who is or was involved in an intimate or dating relationship with the victim. The goal of the violence is to establish control over the partner.[1] About 10% of students nationwide report being physically hurt by a boyfriend or girlfriend in the past 12 months.[2] Among adult victims of rape, physical violence, and/or stalking by an intimate partner, 22% of women and 15% of men first experienced some form of partner violence between 11 and 17 years of age.[3] These statistics make it clear that adolescents and the adults in their lives need to understand and talk about adolescent relationship violence (ARV).

> Romantic and sexual connections give adolescents a particularly intense sense of self-worth because they feel wanted, valued, and desirable. Risky relationships can happen to anyone, but particularly to those who want and need external validation.

Adolescents need to have a clear understanding of healthy and unhealthy relationships before they begin to be involved in romantic relationships. They can learn about healthy and unhealthy relationships both by having discussions about these topics with the adults in their lives and by seeing examples of healthy relationships around them.

It is vital that professionals who serve adolescents routinely inquire about the quality of relationships and reinforce with youth how to assess their own relationships. Further, we need to recognize signs of unhealthy relationships and know how to guide youth toward wise decision-making and offer them access to the resources to get help.

■ Background

Some important things to know about ARV include
- Adolescents do not usually identify as victims because the violence is often mutual, even though the power dynamic may not be. This mutual violence can make someone mistakenly feel they are not a victim, or that it is not abuse.
- Adolescent relationship violence is not child abuse because the perpetrator is not a guardian or live-in partner of a guardian, and the parent is not condoning/enabling this violence; in most circumstances, the parent knows nothing about it.

- Past violence can put an adolescent at risk for ARV, including[4,5]
  — Childhood maltreatment or abuse
  — Prior history of sexual abuse
  — Exposure to family violence
  — Exposure to community violence
- Consequences of ARV for adolescents include
  — Mental health issues such as depression, substance use, and suicide
  — Increased sexual risk behavior that can lead to pregnancy and sexually transmitted infections (STIs).

■ Adolescents Are at High Risk for Relationship Violence

Adolescents naturally look to their peers for a sense of value outside of their family. Romantic and sexual connections give adolescents a particularly intense sense of self-worth because they feel wanted, valued, and desirable. In fact, the feelings of an early romantic relationship can bring about temporary changes in the brain similar to the highs seen with drug use. Hormonal changes in a changing body also cause confusion and can contribute to poor decisions driven by new and changing needs. Also, in today's sexualized society, there are not many examples of healthy relationships—just a lot of exposure to sex.

Risky relationships can happen to anyone, but particularly to those who want and need external validation, those who have not been taught to protect themselves in relationships, and those who have been exposed to unhealthy relationships between adults (eg, their parents) or peers. Repeated or prolonged exposure may make it so they won't be able to recognize unacceptable behavior.

No one asks to be abused, and usually unhealthy relationships evolve over time. A strong connection full of flattery and admiration can turn into jealousy and become controlling. The partner who is the victim may still be drawn to the good things that their partner did and may still do in the relationship, so much so that they feel the need to defend the abuser. Thus they isolate themselves from people who can help. It is vital for adolescents to have a strong sense of what is a healthy and what is unhealthy in a relationship as well as continued access to adults who can recognize the signs of abuse and offer to help.

Adolescents Need to Know What *Healthy* Relationships Look Like

People in healthy relationships know who they are and, most important, who they are not. With a sense of their own goals, they are motivated to protect their needs. They are able to find value in and care for their partners and also expect to be treated well. In healthy relationships, people feel better about themselves and more confident about who they were before entering the relationship. *A healthy relationship makes it easier to be more of who you are, not less or different.* Partners in healthy relationships encourage one another to pursue their individual talents and dreams. Adolescents in healthy relationships should find their grades go up, not down. They learn to incorporate their new love interest into their lives, finding ways to balance the desire for personal intimacy with the need to stay connected to the people and activities they care about.

A relationship is only as good as its worst day. It is easy to be happy in a new relationship. How partners get through hard times (both in their relationship and outside of their relationship) is most important. Adolescents have a chance to have a thriving relationship if they can work together to handle problems with mutual compromise and a commitment to problem-solve rather than trying to win every fight.

Here Are Some Characteristics of a *Healthy* Relationship

- Mutual respect
- Trust
- Honesty
- Compromise
- Individuality
- Good communication
- Anger control
- Problem solving
- Fighting fair
- Understanding
- Self-confidence
- Being a good role model **56.1**

Adolescents Need to Know What *Unhealthy* Relationships Look Like

Adolescents who look to others to validate their sense of self are at high risk for getting into relationships with partners who will try to define them by controlling them or even abusing them. Jealousy can be the first sign of an unhealthy relationship. Because jealousy initially makes adolescents feel wanted, some find it "cute" at first. It is a red flag that may be the first sign of a controlling partner.

Some Things That Can Alert an Adolescent or Adult to an Unhealthy Relationship

- Control
- Jealousy
- Dependence
- Dishonesty
- Disrespect
- Hostility
- Intimidation
- Physical violence
- Sexual violence

Adolescents in an *Unhealthy* Relationship May Notice That Their Partner

- Demands to know where they are and who is with them at all times
- Pressures them to do things they don't want to do
- Tells them how to behave, dress, or wear their hair
- Prevents them from doing what they like to do
- Calls them names, insults them, criticizes them
- Makes them feel unworthy or ashamed of themselves
- Blames or punishes them for events out of their control
- Holds them responsible for the abuser's problems
- Threatens to control them by doing something to harm them or their reputation if they don't comply—they may send or post inappropriate photos, spread rumors, etc
- Threatens to hurt them (or even himself/herself) for not doing what they want
- Makes them feel guilty for not setting appropriate limits, like not wanting to have sex
- Controls access to needed support (medical care, access to family, ability to pursue education, etc)
- Uses technology to spy on them or constantly stay in touch

  Adolescents who are in unhealthy relationships need to get help.

■ What Adults (Parents and Providers) Can Do to Support Adolescents

Pointers for Parents

1. **Live by example.** Parents that have a healthy relationship need to let their children see their relationship in action and witness how they handle conflict while still having consideration for each other.

2. **Remember that love is important.** Even though love can mean different things to an adolescent and adult, it is important to remember that romantic attachments can be very intense for adolescents.

3. **Sexuality is a spectrum.** Help adolescents understand that sex can include anything from making eye contact to actual intercourse, and that there are many ways to communicate interest in these activities. Teach adolescents how they can communicate boundaries with their partners.

4. **Waiting is okay.** Being a little bit older and more mature before starting relationships can be protective; don't push adolescents to have boyfriends or girlfriends too soon.

5. **Ask the questions.** Ask the adolescent what he means when he is talking about romantic relationships. This can help you understand how he is approaching a relationship and if it is developmentally appropriate.

6. **...but don't ask too many questions.** If you are too "nosy," adolescents won't share information with you. Make sure to let the adolescent know that you are available to her by providing respectful opportunities for her to share with you. This will encourage her to come to you for advice when she is ready.

7. **It's not about you.** Romantic relationships are a normal way for adolescents to separate from parents, form new attachments, and figure out who they are. If you reject their partner you will alienate the adolescent and they will be less likely to come to you when they are in trouble.

8. **Teach them to demand what they deserve.** Let the adolescent know that healthy relationships involve compromise, but that the most important thing is that a good relationship should make him feel more secure and confident about who he is without changing his identity. Let him know that part of feeling good about who he is involves feeling honored in his relationships, having his own space, and spending time with family and friends.

9. **The older they get, the more they need you.** Instead of leaving the lessons about healthy relationships to the media and popular culture, teach your adolescent about how to have a good relationship by modeling relationship skills. Find local resources if you are not able to do it alone.

10. **Recognize the red flags of unhealthy or violent relationships in your adolescent and get help.**
    — Withdrawal from friends and activities; spending more time alone with their partner
    — Need to obtain permission from the partner to make even simple plans or commitments for fear the partner will be upset
    — Frequent apologies for the other's behaviors
    — Sudden changes in plans for reasons that don't make sense
    — Use of clothing to hide certain body parts (arms, eyes, etc); visible marks or bruises
    — Close friends (or parents) don't like the partner (there's often a good reason)

All of these are signs that the adolescent needs help as soon as possible. Sources of help can include health care providers, counselors, and local resources.

Pointers for Providers

Providers need to know the spectrum of relationship violence. While most of the violence will not be high risk, it is important to intervene before it becomes riskier using the 5 As. The 5 As can be used to figure out how to support adolescents in choosing healthier relationships and how to get out of unhealthy relationships. See Figure 56.1.

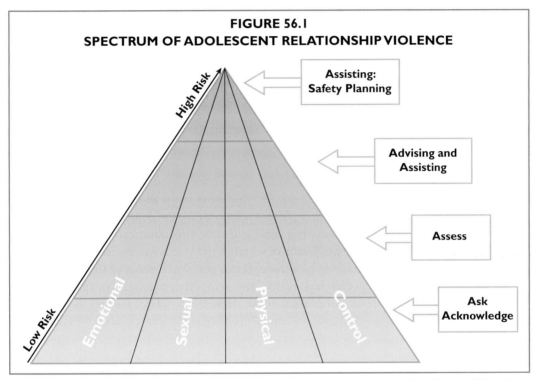

FIGURE 56.1
SPECTRUM OF ADOLESCENT RELATIONSHIP VIOLENCE

Columbia Center for Youth Violence Prevention (CCYVP): Research Program—Understanding Dating Violence (Elizabeth Isakson, Marina Catallozzi, David Bell, Melissa Dupont-Reyes, Leslie L Davidson)

The 5 As of Relationship Violence

- Ask
- Acknowledge
- Assess
- Advise
- Assist

1. **Routinely *ask* about ARV.** It can be hard to make asking about relationships part of your regular history with an adolescent, but it gives you the chance to give anticipatory guidance around healthy relationships and relationship violence. Even if an adolescent is not in a relationship, it is a chance to discuss what he considers a healthy relationship. Some of the things that can make it hard to ask about relationships and violence are the time that it takes, feeling competent in dealing with someone who is in a violent relationship (ie, safety assessment and referral issues), and knowledge of confidentiality and legal issues. Providers can try to create a friendly, supportive, and understanding environment by
   — Universalizing and normalizing the asking: *"I ask everyone this."*
   — Contextualizing the problem and being nonjudgmental: *"Many teens have issues with this."*
   — Remembering that disclosure may not happen the first time you ask.
   — Focusing on behaviors and not the word or concept of "abuse." This avoids value judgment and may elicit more disclosure.

— Avoiding discrimination. This can be a problem for both young men and women and both should be asked.

— Asking *all* adolescents something like

❖ *"Tell me about your relationship...."*

❖ *"Does (he or she) get jealous often?"*

❖ *"Does (he or she) dislike when you spend time with your other friends or family?"*

❖ *"Does your partner check up on you? If yes, how often?"*

❖ *"In your relationship, does your partner threaten or physically hurt you?"*

❖ *"Has anyone forced you to have sexual activities that made you feel uncomfortable?"*

2. *Acknowledge.* When an adolescent discloses information about a violent relationship, remember that violence in adolescent relationships is common but not acceptable. A provider's reaction matters. If there is a specific disclosure, it can be validated with statements like

— "You do not deserve this."

— "You are not alone."

— "It is not your fault."

Simple statements can be a powerful reinforcement for help-seeking behavior.

3. *Assess* **the level of violence to determine what next steps must be taken.** If an adolescent endorses an unhealthy or violent relationship, the degree and frequency of violence must be assessed. If there is a "yes" to a screening question, first assess for fear, as fear can be an important factor in whether the youth will be comfortable taking next steps. The degree of fear (or lack thereof) can give you a sense of the seriousness of the situation from the teen's perspective. Also remember to assess for the risk factors associated with violence for either partner (ie, depression, school failure) as these comorbid conditions are associated with ARV (either leading to violence or as a result of violence).

— If "yes" to physical violence, asses

❖ Duration, frequency, severity

❖ Accessible weapons and/or threats to use weapons

❖ Threats to harm in another way

❖ History of fighting, losing temper quickly

❖ History of hurting animals or other people

❖ If the violence is escalating

— If "yes" to sexual coercion/violence, assess

❖ Duration, frequency, severity

❖ Who decides when and if you will have sex

❖ Are/how are condoms negotiated

❖ Concerns about pregnancy, if the partner wants a pregnancy

❖ Concerns about STIs or history of STIs

— If "yes" to controlling, assess whether the partner ever

❖ Tries to isolate from family and friends

❖ Gets extremely jealous or mean

❖ Forces calls to check in or ask permission

❖ Controls clothing

— Assess what strengths and/or supports the adolescent has

❖ Self-awareness

❖ Self-esteem

❖ Family

❖ School environment

❖ Friends

4. ***Advise*** **the adolescent based on the level of violence and the strengths that are identified and based on where they are on the spectrum of relationship violence.**
   Advise and *assist* differ only in the need for urgency and depend on where the adolescent is in terms of the spectrum of relationship violence and safety. When advising the adolescent, the youth should be given a choice about next steps and resource materials. Phone numbers and Web sites should be shared. It is key to offer close follow-up and to allow the adolescent to come back whenever needed. General safety planning for the future is also critical. Know local laws so that you can call authorities for assistance.

5. ***Assist*** **the adolescent in determining safety risk and accessing help.**
   — An immediate intervention is needed with red flags, such as a threat made by someone with access to firearms, escalating violence, or threats (especially choking, threat of killing/death, suicidality in either partner).
   — Safety planning (determining a safe place with a friend, immediate family, relative, or shelter) is vital. Establish a code word for notification of identified support individuals. A code word is a word that can be subtly but clearly placed into a conversation that conveys the need for assistance or initiates a demand that the youth return home.
   — Where to go for safety immediately in their neighborhood (police precinct, hospital).
   — Program important numbers into their phone, using alias names to avoid raising suspicions.
   — Emergency social service referral.
   — Involving the police.
   — Order of protection.

Taking these steps can make a difference to young people who need to be extricated from a potentially life-threatening situation. However, even just screening for unhealthy relationships and defining healthy ones helps adolescents clarify their own needs and expectations for intimate relationships.

•• Group Learning and Discussion ••

Knowing local resources that can extricate youth from dangerous relationships is a first step toward making your setting a place where adolescents can turn for help. If you are not aware of local services, then familiarize yourself with them prior to this group exercise.

Break into pairs and work through the following scenarios.

Scenario 1: Alex, a 15-year-old patient, is in your office for an annual examination before going away on a bike tour in the summer. Alex has told you that he has had some crushes, but has never dated anyone. His friends are starting to have girlfriends, and his best friend started having sex with his girlfriend. What are some ways that you can discuss healthy relationships with Alex given that he has not yet started dating? What relationships in Alex's life might he look to as an example of a healthy or unhealthy relationship?

Scenario 2: Nicole has returned to your office after starting the birth control pill about 6 weeks prior. When you enter the room there is a male with her who she introduces as her boyfriend. She seems nervous around him and he is reluctant to leave the office. When he does finally leave, she starts responding to his texts. How can you use the 5 As to determine the health of the relationship and determine what kind of help or resources Nicole needs?

▪▪▪▪▪▪▪▪ Continuing Education ▪▪▪▪▪▪▪▪

If you are applying for continuing education credits, a test is available online. For more details, visit www.aap.org/reachingteens.

■ References

1. *Preventing Domestic Violence: Clinical Guidelines on Routine Screening.* San Francisco, CA: Family Violence Prevention Fund; 1999

2. Black MC, Basile KC, Breiding MJ, et al. *The National Intimate Partner and Sexual Violence Survey (NISVS): 2010 Summary Report.* Atlanta, GA: National Center for Injury Prevention and Control, Centers for Disease Control and Prevention; 2011

3. Centers for Disease Control and Prevention. Youth Risk Behavioral Surveillance—United States, 2009. *MMWR.* 2010;59 (No.SS-5)

4. Malik S, Sorenson SB, Aneshensel CS. Community and dating violence among adolescents: perpetration and victimization. *J Adolesc Health.* 1997;21(5):291–302

5. Foshee VA, Benefield TS, Ennett ST, Bauman KE, Suchindran S. Longitudinal predictors of serious physical and sexual dating violence victimization during adolescence. *Prev Med.* 2004;39:1007–1016

■ Related Video Content

56.0 Every Teen Deserves to Be ROUTINELY Screened for the Health of His or Her Relationships. Catallozzi, Bell.

56.1 A Concrete Flow Sheet That Explains Healthy Versus Unhealthy Relationships to Teens. Sugerman.

56.2 Case Example: Helping a Teen Navigate an Unhealthy Relationship. Sugerman.

56.3 Discussion on Healthy and Unhealthy Relationships. Campbell, Ginsburg.

56.4 Case Example: Be Vigilant for Signs of Control. Catallozzi.

56.5 Healthy Relationships Include Communication About Your Sexual Needs. Clark.

56.6 Assessing the Health of Sexual Relationships. Chaffee.

56.7 Case Example: Talking About Relationships as Part of a Sexual Health Visit. Sugerman.

56.8 Young Men Also Need Positive Messages About Relationships. Bell.

36.5 Case Example: Supporting Balanced Parenting: Guiding a Teen to Navigate Through an Unhealthy Relationship. Sugerman.

■ Related Handouts/Supplementary Materials

Relationship Requirements (from the heart and the head)

Pointers for Parents: Fostering Healthy Relationships

■ Related Web Sites

Centers for Disease Control and Prevention. Teen Dating Violence

www.cdc.gov/ViolencePrevention/intimatepartnerviolence/teen_dating_violence.html

Columbia Center for Youth Violence Prevention (CCYVP)

https://sites.google.com/site/ccyvp11

LoveIsRespect.org

www.loveisrespect.org

National Dating Abuse Helpline

800/331-9474 (or text "loveis" to 77054)

CHAPTER 57

Emotional, Physical, and Sexual Abuse

Angela Diaz, MD, MPH

 Related Video Content

57.0 Emotional, Physical, and Sexual Abuse

■ Why This Matters

Childhood emotional, physical, and sexual abuse are widespread phenomena that often have devastating lifelong effects.

Childhood abuse is predominantly a prepubertal phenomenon,[1] but its effects usually start expressing themselves in adolescence and persist into adulthood.[2] Common consequences include disability, suffering, and limitations in the quality of life, which can be serious and severe.[3,4] Physical and sexual abuse has been associated with[2,3]

- Poor self-esteem
- Alcohol and drug abuse
- Eating disorders and obesity
- Risky sexual behaviors and teen pregnancy
- Depression, anxiety, suicidality, and a myriad of other sequellae

Adolescents deserve to be safe. People who have been traumatized can heal. We need to ask the questions to protect those who are not safe, and to facilitate healing in those who have been hurt.

> **Do not ask about abuse as part of the sexual history; ask about it in the context of relationships, safety, and environmental risks. You do not want to send the message, even by inference, that sexual abuse is part of the teen's sexuality.**

■ Background

My own research and many other studies show that teens with a history of abuse are more likely than their peers with no history of abuse to be depressed and suicidal, to run away from home, to smoke cigarettes, to use alcohol and drugs, and to engage in other high-risk behaviors, including using alcohol and drugs to make sex easier.[5]

Abuse is seen in all cultural and racial groups and in all socioeconomic groups.[6] However, children with disabilities are at increased risk, especially those with mental or emotional disability, blindness or deafness, and other disabilities that might be viewed as impairing the child's credibility as an accuser. The younger the victim or the more cognitively or emotionally impaired they are, the less able they may be to identify and describe their experiences.[7]

Although the full prevalence of childhood physical and sexual abuse is unknown, lifetime prevalence of abuse reported from nonclinical population-based studies has ranged between 20% and 54% for women and between 5% and 19% for men.[1, 8-14] Estimates vary widely because disclosure is sensitive to the way in which questions are framed and to study methodologies.[12,13] Childhood sexual abuse is not a diagnosis or a disorder. Rather, it is a range of complex and widely varied experiences. Activities covered by the term "child sexual abuse" include sexual intercourse or attempted intercourse, oral-genital contact, fondling of genitals or other parts of the body directly or through clothing, exhibitionism, exposing children to adult sexual activity or pornography, as well as the use of the child for commercial sexual exploitation such as trafficking or pornography. Thus victims' experiences will be widely varied in extent, intensity, frequency of episodes, duration of abuse over time, number of perpetrators, the relationship of any perpetrator to the victim, the response of a non-abusing parent and other significant family members to the disclosure, and the impact.[12,14]

Identification of abuse can contribute to prevention, lessen disability, and improve future functioning and success in life.[4,15] Reporting can be protective as it mobilizes child protection services and can facilitate entry to helpful interventions.[16] Reporting also lets children know that their abuse is considered wrong and will not be tolerated by caring adults. Physicians and other child care professionals are mandated by law to report childhood abuse whenever they suspect its presence in children and adolescents younger than 18 years.[17-19]

■ The Importance of Asking About Abuse

A visit to a health care provider or other professional presents a natural opportunity for identifying abuse, because we are accustomed to asking personal questions in the context of the visit and youth expect this and are usually prepared to answer.[20-22] The physical environment of the practice setting can help make it easier for teens to talk about sensitive, highly personal issues such as abuse. Having posters, pamphlets, and other materials that address sensitive issues signals the teen that the professional is willing to talk about any experience or question no matter how difficult.

Asking about abuse should be part of the general history taking; therefore, the provider will need to become comfortable asking highly sensitive questions rather than relying on physical signs, symptoms, and information volunteered during the general medical history. Physical signs of abuse will be rare when the abuse occurred earlier in life. Even if the abuse is ongoing, it is uncommon for there to be physical evidence, especially in adolescents. Providers may also be prompted to ask about abuse when caring for young people who present with a sexually transmitted infection or pregnancy at a very young age, unexplained emotional changes, or deterioration in social or school functioning. Adolescents may volunteer a history of abuse during a visit without being asked, but this is relatively uncommon. Because abuse is such a common phenomenon with lifelong negative sequelae, and the physical examination and medical history will identify very few victims, providers should routinely ask every adolescent directly about abuse.

A pediatrician once asked me, *"Why should I ask about abuse and trauma at each visit."* I replied, *"How often do you check the ears during a routine exam of an adolescent? In routine care without ear complaints, you identify ear infections at a rate of one in a gazillion, yet we see abuse in as many as one in every 4 adolescents."* ▶ 18.9

■ Approach to Asking About Abuse

My approach to screening is based on my experience in working with many hundreds of adolescents who have a history of childhood emotional, physical, and sexual abuse and other sexual trauma, as well as on my research with teens with a history of abuse and the abuse literature.

How Should You Ask About Childhood Emotional, Physical, and Sexual Abuse?

When an adolescent comes for her visit with a parent, I first talk about confidentiality with both the teen and her parent. I point out that if there is abuse (or risk of harm to self or others), I cannot keep confidentiality because I am a mandated reporter. With the parent in the room, I will take a general history and avoid questions related to sensitive issues (see Chapter 14). When the parent has left the room and I am alone with the teen, I preface my history taking by saying, *"I am going to be asking you some questions—they are questions I ask every teen."*

Do not ask about abuse as part of the sexual history. Ask about abuse in the context of relationships, safety, and environmental risks. You do not want to send the message, even by inference, that sexual abuse is part of the teen's sexuality. Although abuse can impact a teen's feelings about sexuality, abuse is an act of coercion not a chosen behavior. Later, during the sexual history, clarify and educate about the clear distinctions between voluntary sexual behavior and coercive, nonvoluntary sexual activity. Helping teens distinguish between sexual feelings and choices and any sexual abuse experiences they have endured is the first step in helping them address the harm they have suffered while allowing them to develop a healthy sense of identity and sexuality.

Ask in a nonjudgmental way. Be conscious of your body language to avoid the implication of shame or stigma or inadvertently communicating that you'd prefer the answer to be "no" (see Chapter 15). Use language that is developmentally and culturally appropriate and that the teen understands. Avoid clinical language. Be sensitive to the differences between the early, mid-, and late adolescent and adjust your language accordingly. It is not enough to ask, *"Have you ever been sexually or physically abused?"* Many teens will not understand this term and many abuse victims may have been coerced in such a way that they don't yet define their experience as abuse. Always ask in an open-ended and nonjudgmental way, even when you may have strong feelings about how terrible the teen's experience may have been. To further reduce stigma, communicate that you are not asking about abuse because of something unique you are picking up from this particular adolescent. The abuse victim will already have cognitive distortions, and many may feel that they are abnormal compared to other teens.

Ask about abuse in the context of how a teen relates to his family. *"Who do you live with?"* *"Do you get along well with your parents?"* and *"Do you communicate with them?"*

You may hear responses that vary from, *"I don't communicate with them at all,"* *"I communicate well but not about personal things,"* or *"I communicate with them freely."* It is common for teens in general to communicate well with one parent and not the other.

Ask about abuse in a direct and specific manner. I start by asking about emotional abuse.
- *"Has a parent or other adult said things to you that make you feel hurt?"*
- If so, *"Who?"* and *"What did they say?"*

It is not unusual to hear a response of, *"I was told I will never amount to anything,"* or *"I was told I am a prostitute,"* or *"I was told I am fat,"* and so on. After asking about the facts, I will ask about the impact that the emotional abuse has had on the teen. I will ask, *"How did it make you feel?"* and then explore sequelae, such as low self-esteem, anger, isolation, anxiety, depression, self-harm, drinking, or substance abuse. This is true also when I ask about physical and sexual abuse.

Ask about physical abuse using straightforward, simple, and descriptive language that every teen will understand. I do not ask, *"Have you been physically abused?"* A teen is likely to simply say, *"No."* He or she may think or say, *"I was hit because I did something wrong."* After all, that's how the abuser usually justifies his or her actions—as something the teen deserves. Teens often respond best to specific questions.

- *"How are you punished?"*
- "Has anyone ever punished you by hitting you with a belt, slapping you, punching you, pulling your hair?"
- "Do you ever get hit with an object like a stick?"
- "Did you ever have to go without eating as a punishment?"
- "Did you ever get put in a closet or left in the dark?"

It is helpful to develop knowledge of the patient's culture; in some cultures physical punishment is accepted as a form of discipline. However, all culture groups view child sexual abuse as abhorrent.

When learning more about a teen's physical abuse, I also explore

- "Who did it?"
- "When was the last time?"
- "How often does this happen?"

Ask about sexual abuse in a specific and clear way.

- "Has anyone ever touched your body in a way that made you feel uncomfortable or when you did not want them to?"
- "Has anyone ever touched your breasts when you did not want them to? Your vagina? Your penis? Buttocks? Anus? Or any other part of your body?"
- "Has anyone ever asked you to touch them in a sexual way or do something you did not want to do?"
- "Has anyone ever forced you to perform any sexual act on your body or on theirs when you did not want to?"

I ask the question in a somewhat redundant way: *"Has anyone ever forced you…"* and then I add, *"When you did not want to?"* This gives a chance for a teen whose perceptions are confused or conflicted to identify her or his conflicting feelings. This is essential as coercion can be very subtle. A teen will sometimes say, *"I wasn't forced…but I did not want to."* With any positive answer, I will pursue the issue in more depth, exploring the specifics. *"Who did it?" "When was the last time?" "How often does this happen?" "Was it your father? Mother? Brother? Sister? Uncle? Aunt? Grandparent? Neighbor? Teacher? A stranger?"*

With an open-ended style, I ask the adolescent to describe what happened, staying with the facts and her or his interpretation. I ask the teen to describe what occurred and if the abuse progressed over time. I remain attentive to both the teen's and my own reactions. While it is important to be empathetic, you should not respond with alarm or a statement like, *"Oh, my God!"* That will tell the teen victim that you are not prepared to hear what she or he needs to tell you.

■ Cognitive Distortions Are Common in Abuse Victims

Often a teen will say, *"It was my fault."* I respond by saying, *"It is the responsibility of the adult to not cross those boundaries, regardless of what you as a child said or did, even if you ran around naked."* I may add, *"Children may take off their clothes and run around naked; it's normal and natural. Children also sit on adults' laps. It doesn't mean they are asking to be touched inappropriately."* It is not uncommon to hear an adolescent say, *"I feel terrible, my friends haven't had this happen, it only happened to me. I'm damaged. I'm bad."* You can say, *"In reality, abuse happens to many, many people."*

■ A Victim May Have Very Dissonant Experiences— Love and Hate, as Well as Guilt and Anger

The sexual abuser may have said, *"You like it,"* or *"This feels good, no?"* or *"You want this."* The abused adolescent's inner reality was that he or she did not want it or like it and it did not feel right, but their feelings are never validated leading to dissonant and conflicting feelings. Friends, unaware of the abuse, may have said, *"What a wonderful family you have."* This may lead the adolescent to feel that something must be wrong with his own perceptions of his family. To further complicate the abused adolescent's feelings, sexual abuse victims may experience arousal during abuse, which can lead to feelings of guilt and confusion. If this is disclosed, I say, *"People are born with their body's ability to react— this doesn't mean you wanted your body to react,"* or *"The human body reacts automatically to being touched, you cannot control whether you react or not react. It just happens."*

■ It Is Important to Have Resources Available to Counsel Patients and Address Their Concerns

You should be knowledgeable about the reporting mandates in your state, as you are a mandated reporter of neglect and abuse. At the very least, if the abuse is recent or ongoing, you are mandated to make a report to child protective services. If the abuse has stopped and the perpetrator was never reported, is still a risk to the patient, or is a risk to other children, the abuse needs to be reported to child protective services. If one child is being abused in a household, other children are at risk. You also must assess what the teen needs physically and emotionally to heal.

In situations where we must make a report, we will try to mobilize whatever resources are available to us. If you work with a social worker or other staff who assist with patient care, this is the time to involve them.

In my setting, we are careful to explain the process and why we must report, and to prepare the adolescent for the potential reactions of family members. Typically, we inform the adolescent that a report must be made to keep the adolescent and other children safe and because health care providers are mandated reporters. We are careful to explain that the report is not being made because of anything the adolescent has done. Very clearly we state that he or she is not being reported—it is not something that the teen did wrong.

The most difficult situation is reporting abuse by a family member. First, we assess what supports the adolescent has and will try to invite a supportive person to come in. This might be a parent or caregiver, an older sibling or other relative, or a close friend. We are careful to then assess whether calling in the report will put the adolescent at increased risk. We always work out a safety plan with the adolescent, and we will work to engage a supportive parent or caregiver. Once we have worked out a safety plan, we will often call a parent who is not involved in the abuse to say that we are reporting. Before we call, we make sure the teen is saying this parent is not abusing them and that, based on our assessment, we believe this parent is not *directly* complicit. We explain the child protective service investigation process, which may vary from state to state. It is important that you familiarize yourself with the process in your locality. Most importantly, we will take the time needed to help restore a sense of safety and balance to the adolescent.

In my practice, we always make a plan for the adolescent to return for follow-up, even though the child protective service is responsible for the investigation. This should be something you consider in terms of how your practice operates and what resources you have available, whether on-site or through networks and collaborations. In my experience, even when an adolescent expresses feeling betrayed when told I must make a report, the adolescent will return to the practice for care. This is why it is helpful, when available to you, to widen your circle of helpers and create allies and collaborators who can provide a team-based approach.

The next step is to assess what the teen may need by way of support and counseling. Not all victims of abuse want to be referred to counseling, and just referring them is unlikely to be successful unless they are extremely motivated and ready. Be aware that you don't have to do everything in one interview. You can let the adolescent know that disclosing was one step and that she can keep the conversation open with you. If the teen is not ready for a referral and is not in an acute crisis after disclosing, you can schedule another visit for a routine follow-up just to check in and see how she is doing.

Talking to a safe parent or any safe and trusted adult in the teen's life can be helpful, but it is essential that you first assess her or his relationship to the teen and to the abuser. Many non-abusing parents whose children disclose abuse find it hard to believe that their spouse or other trusted adult is an abuser. They may blame the teen or suggest that the teen is lying. This will only reinforce the teen's shame and sense that he does not deserve to be listened to or protected. This may increase the likelihood that the teen will not seek counseling services. You can assure a non-offending parent/caring adult that teens who disclose abuse should be believed. By believing a victim, a parent/caring adult can help in the first steps to healing. When a parent does not believe the victim, the victim's emotional responses to the abuse are always more complex and potentially more damaging than when the parent shows understanding. I want to stress that if a teen says they have been abused, a parent should believe them (see Chapter 37). ▶ 18.7, 57.1

Parents of Children Who Have Been Sexually Abused Should Be Strongly Encouraged to Get Help for Themselves

This can be done through a support group or psychotherapy. Some parents and children will benefit from family therapy. It is important to remember that parents may themselves have been victims of sexual abuse, and it is not uncommon for child abuse to co-occur along with domestic partner abuse. Counseling can address the pervasive sense of guilt that some parents may feel for not recognizing the abuse earlier.

■ Closing the Interview

Any teen who discloses abuse to you has made herself vulnerable. It is essential you acknowledge the important step the patient has taken.

Before the teen leaves the office, it is important to help make the young person whole enough to walk out and go on. Let the teen know she is not to blame and that whatever feelings may emerge, they are valid. Tell the teen that she may have an emotional response sometime later that day or in the future, and that, if this happens, not to panic. Predicting a possible response lessens its negative impact if it should occur.

Let the teen know she can call you to talk or for a referral "to someone who can help," being sensitive that this not be seen as a "hand-off" (see Chapter 33). Make sure that the young person understands there are resources that will help and knows how to reach you. Disclosure may result in the teen feeling a strong bond with you, and she may well need help transitioning to another service, such as a social worker or other therapist. Again, explain that you are not a therapist, but remain open and engaged so that the teen does not experience feelings of being passed off to someone else after opening up to you. It is important to facilitate a bond to the person who will help the teen take the next steps. Let the teen know, if it is possible, that this therapist is someone you trust and someone who is very competent and helpful.

This is just the beginning—we can connect the young person to services or continue to monitor those who are not ready for that step. Many teens will say, *"I'm fine."* I respond, *"You may say you are fine now, but, unless you deal with this, it may come up when least expected. Unless you process this, you will always have the potential to react. It is important that you work through this in order for you to heal."*

I always remind the young person, *"You can always come back to continue this conversation,"* and I thank the young person for his or her courage and openness.

Commercial Sexual Exploitation of Children (CSEC)

Commercial sexual exploitation of children (CSEC) is a preferred term to describe "child prostitution." Commercial sexual exploitation of children encompasses anyone younger than 18 years engaged in systems of prostitution and sexual exploitation and represents a form of sexual abuse, child sexual exploitation, or statutory rape. There is a movement away from the term "prostitution" as it implies the child is responsible for being sexually exploited and children cannot consent to their own abuse.

▶ 57.2

Exploited children and youth are hidden among us. They attend our schools and community programs, and come to our health care settings, often for emergency services or for treatment of illnesses or sexually transmitted infections and pregnancy. We must use these contact points as an opportunity to extricate youth from these abusive situations.

CSEC includes:
Commercial
- Street prostitution
- Pornography
- Stripping
- Erotic/nude massage
- Escort Services
- Phone-sex lines
- Private parties
- Gang-based prostitution
- Interfamilial pimping
- Forms of Internet-based exploitation

Survival Sex

Red Flags/Risk Factors
- Truancy—young person stops going to school
- Sudden changes in appearance (nails, hair, clothing)
- Has access to cash (taking friends shopping, out to eat)
- History of arrest for drug possession or sale, theft, possession of weapons, or prostitution
- Older boyfriend/partner
- Several mental health symptoms
- Severe post-traumatic stress disorder, anxiety, other traumatic symptoms (eg, disassociation)
- History of sexual abuse and/or exposure to domestic violence
- Early sexual initiation and/or knowing a great deal about sex
- Acting more mature than age
- Non-English speaking, with "boyfriend/guardian" answering all questions
- Any situations in which teen is not allowed privacy with a professional or to speak for herself
- AWOL from foster care home (repeatedly)
- Multiple and concurrent sexually transmitted infections and/or pregnancies,
- Sexualized behavior (ie, knows more about reproductive health than would expect for age)

Steps for making CSEC a priority in your setting
- Ask in-person and on intake forms, "Have you ever exchanged sex for money, housing, or drugs?"
- Collaborate with other agencies who work with at-risk or identified CSEC victims (human service agencies, schools, juvenile justice, police, local district attorney's, sexual assault response team/sexual assault centers/child advocacy centers).

Commercial Sexual Exploitation of Children (CSEC), continued

Resources

- Safe Horizon Anti-Trafficking Program and Hotline http://www.safehorizon.org/index/what-we-do-2/antitrafficking-program-13.html
- 1-800-621-HOPE (4673)
- National Center for Missing and Exploited Children http://www.missingkids.com
- Polaris Project with NATIONAL HOTLINE 1-888-373-7888
- http://www.polarisproject.org/

Contributed by Tonya A. Chaffee, MD, MPH, FAAP

●● Group Learning and Discussion ●●

A major barrier to professionals asking about abuse is their discomfort with the reporting rules and regulations, as well as with making appropriate referrals for healing. Given the prevalence of abuse in every sociodemographic group, it is our responsibility to routinely assess youth for abuse history. Therefore, a group assignment to lower barriers might include

1. Reflecting on whether unconscious biases might make us more or less likely to routinely screen for abuse in different populations.
2. Agreeing to routinely set the stage for trustworthy communication in the beginning of every relationship so parents and teens understand privacy rights and limitations of confidentiality. This will eliminate the potential for a teen experiencing betrayal after you report.
3. Clarifying state reporting laws.
4. Posting the phone numbers for reporting.
5. Practicing filling out reporting forms.
6. Assembling a list of local healing professionals with expertise in counseling abuse victims.

▪▪▪▪▪▪▪▪ Continuing Education ▪▪▪▪▪▪▪▪▪

If you are applying for continuing education credits, a test is available online. For more details, visit www.aap.org/reachingteens.

■ References

1. Finkelhor D, Ormrod RK, Turner HA. The developmental epidemiology of childhood victimization. *J Interpers Violence.* 2009;24(5):711–731
2. Trickett P, Putnam F, Noll J. Child Abuse Team/Mayerson Center: Longitudinal Study on Childhood Sexual Abuse Summary. http://ohiocando4kids.org/Sexual_Abuse_Longitudinal_Study Accessed June 26, 2013
3. Sickel AE, Noll JG, Moore PJ, Putnam FW, Trickett PK. The long-term physical health and healthcare utilization of women who were sexually abused as children. *J Health Psychol.* 2002;7:583–597
4. Berkowitz CD. The long-term medical consequences of sexual abuse. In: Reece RM, ed. *Treatment of Child Abuse: Common Ground for Mental Health, Medical, and Legal Practitioners.* Baltimore, MD: Johns Hopkins University Press; 2000:54–64

5. Labor N, Medeiros D, Carlson E, et al. Adolescents' need to talk about sex and sexuality in an urban mental health setting. *Soc Work Ment Health Vol.* 2005;3:135–153

6. Finkelhor D. Epidemiological factors in the clinical identification of child sexual abuse. *Child Abuse Negl.* 1993:17:67–70

7. Westcott H, Jones D. Annotation: the abuse of disabled children. *J Child Psychol Psychiatry.* 1999;40:497–506

8. Finkelhor D. Current information on the scope and nature of child sexual abuse. *Future Child.* 1994:4(2):31–53

9. Finkelhor D, Hotaling GT. Sexual abuse in the National Incidence Study of Child Abuse and Neglect: an appraisal. *Child Abuse Negl.* 1984;8(1):23–32

10. Schoen C, Davis K, Collins KS, Greenberg L, DesRoches C, Abrams M. *The Commonwealth Fund Survey of the Health of Adolescent Girls.* New York, NY: The Commonwealth Fund; 1997

11. Schoen C, Davis K, DesRoches C, Shekhdar A. *The Health of Adolescent Boys: Commonwealth Fund Survey Findings.* New York, NY: The Commonwealth Fund; 1998

12. Hulme PA. Retrospective measurement of childhood sexual abuse: a review of instruments. *Child Maltreat.* 2004;9(2):201–217

13. Hulme PA. Psychometric evaluation and comparison of three retrospective, multi-item measures of childhood sexual abuse. *Child Abuse Negl.* 2007;31(8):853–869

14. Putnam F. Ten-year research update review: child sexual abuse. *J Am Acad Child Adolesc Psychiatry.* 2003;42(3):269–278

15. Battaglia TA, Finley E, Liebschutz JM. Survivors of intimate partner violence speak out: trust in the patient-provider relationship. *J Gen Intern Med.* 2003;18(8):617–623

16. Sgroi S. *Handbook of Clinical Intervention in Child Sexual Abuse.* New York, NY: The Free Press; 1982

17. Johnson CF. Child maltreatment 2002: recognition, reporting and risk. *Pediatr Int.* 2002;44(5):554–560

18. United States Department of Health and Human Services, Administration for Children and Families, Administration on Children, Youth and Families, Children's Bureau. Mandatory Reporters of Child Abuse and Neglect: Summary of State Laws. https://www.childwelfare.gov/systemwide/laws_policies/statutes/manda.pdf. Accessed June 26, 2013

19. United States Department of Health and Human Services, Administration for Children and Families, Administrations on Children, Youth and Families, Children's Bureau. What Is Child Abuse and Neglect? Child Information Gateway; 2008 http://www.childwelfare.gov/pubs/factsheets/whatiscan.pdf. Accessed June 26, 2013

20. Diaz A, Manigat N. The health care provider's role in the disclosure of sexual abuse: the medical interview as the gateway to disclosure. *Child Health Care.* 1999;28(2):141–149

21. Ong LM, de Haes JC, Hoos AM, Lammes FB. Doctor-patient communication: a review of the literature. *Soc Sci Med.* 1995;40(7):903–918

22. Simeonsson RJ. Family expectations, encounters and needs. In: Bambring M, Raub H, Beelman A, eds. *Early Childhood Intervention: Theory, Evaluation, and Practice.* Berlin, Germany: De Gryuter; 1996:196–207

■ Related Video Content

57.0 Emotional, Physical, and Sexual Abuse. Diaz.

57.1 A Homeless Teen Shares a Tragic History of Abuse. Youth.

57.2 The Making of a Girl. The GEMS Project.

18.7 The Goal Is Not to Get the Most Detailed History, It Is to Get the Most Therapeutic History for the Youth at That Time: A Case of Abuse That Revealed Itself Over Time. Ginsburg.

18.9 Incorporating a Screen for Abuse Into the SSHADESS Screen. Diaz.

■ Related Handout/Supplementary Material

Hidden Among Us: Sexually Exploited and Trafficked Youth

■ Related Web Sites

Break the Cycle: Empowering Youth to End Domestic Violence

www.breakthecycle.org

Commercial Sexual Exploitation and Domestic Trafficking

GEMS (Girls Educational & Mentoring Services)

www.gems-girls.org

National Sexual Violence Resource Center

www.nsvrc.org

New York City Alliance Against Sexual Assault

Hotlines

www.svfreenyc.org/survivors_hotline.html#3

Get Help

www.svfreenyc.org/survivors.html

Rape, Abuse, and Incest National Network

www.rainn.org

CHAPTER 58

Youth Violence

Kenneth R. Ginsburg, MD, MS Ed, FAAP, FSAHM

 Related Video Content

58.0 Youth Violence

■ Why This Matters?

Violence is the third leading killer of youth aged 14 to 21, though for marginalized and underresourced communities the toll is disproportionately higher.[1,2] Mortality represents only the tip of the iceberg, with more than 150 injuries for every death.[1,2] Violence is produced through the complex interaction of multiple factors, including family breakdown, economic disparities, and the ever-present supply of weapons, and teens have to navigate a culture that sometimes glorifies and normalizes violence. Although we may not be able to address these larger issues, we must not allow the fear of futility to prevent us from doing our part.

> **Injured youth may be ashamed for a variety of reasons, ranging from their antisocial behavior to their frustration over not winning the fight. At the least, they may fear for their safety. While this vulnerability may make them receptive to guidance, it may also make them particularly sensitive to a perceived slight.**

We can position ourselves to make a difference by optimizing those precious few moments in our offices where we can assess youth for risk and point them toward healthier futures. If we become familiar with community resources available to adolescents in crisis, then our role as assessors can be lifesaving.[3]

The research base does not exist to describe precisely which office-based strategies prevent future injury. This chapter hopes to increase your comfort level with assessing youth at risk for violence and in offering brief behavioral change strategies. Ultimately, our youth deserve the rigorous outcome studies that will point us toward those interventions likely to produce the best outcomes.

■ Approaching Youth Violence in Our Offices

This chapter is divided into 3 interrelated sections. The first section offers an overview on approaching violence from a strength-based perspective. The second discusses strategies for assessing youth for current and future risk for violent injury. The third section offers brief behavioral interventions.

Addressing Risk While Building on Strength and Avoiding Shame

The traditional approach to "at-risk" youth is to assess their risk and then educate them on consequences. This approach may work for some highly motivated youth prepared to change. However, it may frustrate others because it leaves them without the tools to navigate their world or resources to change their environment. Still others may feel offended, judged, and ultimately alienated.

Youth injured as a result of violence may be ashamed for a variety of reasons, ranging from their antisocial behavior to their frustration over not winning the fight. At the least, they may fear for their safety. While this vulnerability may make them receptive to guidance, it may also make them particularly sensitive to a perceived slight. If a young person experiences shame during an interaction, an opportunity for change may be missed and the increased tension may make the youth more reactive. Reactivity may increase the likelihood she will continue the cycle of violence and retaliation.

When we focus our clinical energies only on addressing worrisome behaviors, we run the danger of only conceptualizing youths' lives in terms of risk. While well-intentioned, this strategy can reinforce shame. Instead, we must recognize the context of their lives and listen attentively for what they are doing right. A person affiliated with gangs seeks protection and understands loyalty, a drug-affected youth may be masking a deep sensitivity, and any teen who has shared negative behaviors has the capacity and desire to engage helpful people. When we recognize these points of competency, we position youth to build new capabilities. A ripple effect may follow that will counteract some of the forces that drive the young person to engage in risk behaviors (see Chapter 25).

Next, when we work with youth, we must move beyond telling them what behaviors to avoid and reinforce for them what to do. Stress is the driving force toward many unhealthy behaviors. Although these behaviors lessen uncomfortable feelings, they can be destructive in the short (eg, violence) or long term (eg, drugs). We must guide youth to develop positive coping strategies that can both reduce stress and keep them safe. Many strategies described in Chapter 31 on coping may be helpful here, but, in the case of violence, prevention also consider alternative strategies to cope with a violent world. For example, gangs may confer safety in a very real sense, but so might participation in a program that keeps youth away from gang territories or conflicts.

Assessment

We can assess youth for developing problems before crises strike. However, adolescents will not—and perhaps should not—disclose personal information without first knowing you are trustworthy. See Chapter 14 for a full discussion on setting the stage for a trustworthy relationship.

A comprehensive psychosocial assessment includes several opportunities to ascertain violence risk (see Chapter 18). Many teens have a challenging relationship with their parents, but it is important to determine when the relationship is reaching crisis proportions. It is always important to ask, *"Is your home a safe place for you?"* Substances are important to explore because drug use and dealing contribute sharply to violent injuries.[4] Violently injured youth are also at greater risk for the development of mental health problems such as depression and post-traumatic stress disorder, and poor mental health has been associated with an increase in violent behavior.[5] Also explore whether the young person has been bullied because that may increase his chances of being either a victim or perpetrator of violence. When exploring sexuality, always assess for the health of relationships. Ask, *"Does he treat you well?"* followed by, *"Does he get jealous?"* (See Chapter 56.)

The Violence Screen

While there are validated screens to assess violence-related attitudes and behaviors[6] and there has been some research into which questions may predict violent activity,[7,8] we still have much to learn about which questions are most effective in a clinical setting. Here is an overview of topics you can tailor to meet the needs of your youth.

The Injury Setting

It is critical to know whether an injured teen is in the midst of a cycle of retaliation. *"What's going to happen now, is this over?"* or *"Are you going to get even?"* or *"Are people still after you?"* When asking these questions, avoid use of the words "fear," "afraid," or "worried" as they might force a false bravado. In an emergency department setting, the intent to retaliate was measured by asking, *"Not all fights are over after someone gets hurt. Do you think you will hurt someone because of this fight?"* The response identified youth at risk to carry a weapon, assault someone, and be assaulted within the next 8 weeks.[8] Remember that if a life is threatened, you are required to report the threat to appropriate authorities.

A Routine Setting

Violence Exposure

Teens can be exposed in the home, school, or on the streets. The youth inured to violence, or who sees it as the appropriate way to handle stress or conflict, is at risk. A teen disciplined violently may know no other way to raise her own children and will not be prepared to handle disagreement. (Use every available opportunity to reinforce with parents that "discipline" means "to teach," it does not mean "to punish," and absolutely does not mean "to hurt.") Finally, ask *"Do you ever get in fights?"* and *"Have you ever been injured in a fight?"*

Perception of Safety

Learning whether the teen feels safe can reveal a great deal about his risk and what steps may be taken to lower that risk. *"Do you feel safe at school?"* *"Are there a lot of fights at your school?"* *"Do people bring weapons to school?"* Most importantly, learn what he does to make himself feel safer. Start with an open-ended question such as, *"What do you do to keep yourself safe?"* Adolescents may respond in one of 2 manners. The first reassures you they are safe because they describe the safety of their neighborhood or the steps they take to stay out of trouble. Other youth lead with, *"Don't worry about me."* These youth are not prepared to divulge their behavior. I tend to respond with, *"Is someone watching your back, or do you carry something for protection?"* Some youth respond, *"No, I can fight for myself, people have learned not to mess with me."* Others divulge gang affiliation or weapon carrying. When youth remain silent, consider asking, *"Do you think a knife or gun would make you safer…do you carry one?"* Many youth believe a weapon will protect them and do not even consider that it increases their risk. Their goal of self-protection should be acknowledged before being guided to consider that weapon carrying may make them more likely to be killed. (See Promoting Positive Behaviors.)

Threshold for Fighting

You can learn about a teen's volatility by exploring what it takes to get her to fight. *"What do you usually do when you are really mad or frustrated?"* *"Do you get in fights?"* *"Are you able to walk away from fights…how do you do that?"* Next ask, *"What makes you mad enough to fight?"* Because youth reach their threshold for fighting at different points, someone who wishes to escalate a conflict may push until he forces a response. First, a person may call another a name or insult, or disrespect that person. Then the person moves on to insult a mother, family member, or gang member. If the person is still resistant to fighting, the instigator may invade the person's body space; teens call this "getting in my face," or "if he steps up to me." Finally, if the "victim" has not successfully de-escalated the situation, the instigator touches, pushes, or "puts his hands on me." Adolescents may not feel able to walk away once touched. If they do, they may be seen as unable to stand up for themselves, leading to victimization. An advantage of programs instituting zero tolerance is that potential victims can say "you're not even worth it," let off steam verbally, and then walk away with their pride intact by shifting blame to the program.

Promoting Positive Behaviors

Discussions have to consider both cognitive development and state of crisis. In both, the case of a young adolescent or one in crisis, it is best to keep the flow of conversation concrete. The key to helping concrete thinkers grasp consequences of behaviors is to break down abstract concepts into multiple concrete steps. Instead of delivering messages in one bolus—lecture style—process one idea at a time. Probing questions followed by appropriate silence allows teenagers to be guided to their own realization of consequences. The teen is guided through each step until she arrives at the desired abstract realization; she will "own" the solution. (See Chapter 28.)

Taking Social Context Into Account When Devising a Safety Plan

Adults often suggest teenagers should change their behavior to reach success or safety. Even when the teenager is in full agreement that the proposed change is beneficial, he still has to worry about how that change will be received by peers. Therefore, suggestions should be accompanied by a plan to "save face," or maintain pride. As examples, leaving town will be interpreted as cowardice, and improving school behavior may be seen as selling out. Ask, *"How do you think this will play with your friends, will they back you?"* Then, each proposed change should be matched with a face-saving strategy, including shifting the blame to parents or disciplinarians: *"My mother said if I get suspended one more time I will...."* or *"Principal Smith says if I cut class again he'll expel me; that would kill my mother, she has high blood pressure."* In the case of a teen who needs to leave town quickly for safety, make sure she has a place to go and a good excuse for travel other than fleeing violence (eg, *"I have to go down to take care of my grandmother; she's real sick."*).

Prior to any intervention, consider who he most wants to please (eg, grandmother), or for whom he serves as a role model (eg, 7-year-old brother). You will be better prepared to bring out the best in an adolescent when he realizes his better behavior matters to someone.

Examples of Brief Interventions

Following are examples of how you might proceed based on the psychosocial screen. Always combine guidance with appropriate referrals and parental involvement.

If the teen is in the middle of a cycle of retaliation

1. If your community has street-savvy violence reduction specialists, try to engage them to break the cycle of violence.
2. Consider suggesting the teen leave town until tensions subside. Expect resistance as the teen worries about his social context and refuses to "punk out." If his life is in danger, work to "create" a viable out-of-town crisis that emergently needs attention (eg, a sick relative). Don't tell anyone but his parents that it is fabricated, this can be dangerous if not handled carefully.
3. An adolescent about to engage in retribution may be unaware of the peril because of her inability to grasp future consequences while in crisis. The decision tree is one style of producing an abstract realization of future consequences. Discuss her plans while sketching out each resulting step. Ask open-ended question such as, *"Well, what would happen if the knife were taken from your hand, and instead you were stabbed in the back?"* (See Chapter 28, page 227, for an example of a lifesaving decision tree.)

▶ 28.2

If the youth seems vulnerable to violence escalation

You have asked what makes the teen mad enough to fight. Below are suggestions of responses for each violence threshold.

1. If she responded she fights "if someone calls me a name," recognize this teen is at highest risk, may have an impulse disorder, or may be reactive due to a history of toxic stress.
   — Try to get her to realize that the person is calling her names not because she believes it, but because she is trying to get her angry.
   — Ask, *"Who wins if she is trying to get you to fight and you do fight? Not who beats who, but who really wins?"*
   — Talk about the strength of walking away.
   — Teach how deep, slow breathing is calming. Teach how it allows people to think things through wisely instead of jumping into situations (see Chapter 31).

2. If she responded, *"If someone calls my mother a name."*
   — Does the person know your mother?
   — Could you use a sense of humor to help out in this situation?
   — Suppose you defend your mom's honor but get hurt, have you helped her? How will she feel if you get killed just because someone called her a name?

3. If she answered, *"If someone gets in my face or steps up to me* [invades body space]."
   — Don't let yourself be cornered. Keep a leg in front of you and stand at an angle to help protect your space.
   — Ask whether giving street respect—"my fault" or "my bad, excuse me"—might de-escalate the situation.
   — Turn or sit down to avoid the chest-to-chest posture that escalates tension.

4. If she stated, *"Only if someone hits me,"* recognize this teen has a high threshold. *"Great, I am so glad you try to avoid fights. But, I want you to understand a few things to make sure you can stay safe."*
   — Fighting clean (using fists only) means the fight will probably stay that way. Pulling out a weapon may begin the cycle of retaliation.
   — Try not to be around when fights happen—that gets you into the cycle of escalation and retaliation just for being a bystander.
   — If you are in a fight, try to break even. If you win big, they may keep coming after you. If you can break even, the anger may be used up.

If the teen is considering obtaining a weapon for safety

Tell him how pleased you are that he values his life, but tell him you worry that if he carries a gun, he may be in greater danger. Ask for permission to think this through with him. Acknowledge you do not live in his world, and it is up to him to decide if what you say makes sense. The following role-play should be done calmly and in slow motion so the teen can remain thoughtful, rather than reacting viscerally or feeing threatened.

1. Have the teen take the role of a person with a gun.
2. You take the role of the teen you are with, who may or may not carry a gun.
3. Discuss how the best option is to keep walking or avoid the conflict entirely.
4. Assume that the cycle of escalation has reached the point where a physical conflict is going to occur.
5. While standing close (don't actually invade his space), state
   — *"Suppose a fight is about to happen. You're a guy with a gun and I'm pretending I'm you. You don't know whether I have a gun or not. What would happen if I took a swing at you like this?"* (Take a slow-motion swing toward the patient, without actually coming into contact with him.)

6. The teen will respond in 1 of 2 ways

    a. *"I'll swing back at you."*

    If he says this, say, *"Exactly! I'm going to get hurt, but I'm going to live."*

    b. *"I'm going to shoot you."*

    Respond, *"Will you really shoot me if we've stayed clean* (meaning no weapons) *up to now?"*

    Most youth will say, *"No—I'd probably still fight clean."*

    Some youth will say, *"You don't know what you're talking about. Where I come from, if you swing at someone, you're dead."*

    If he makes the latter statement, you must trust him because he is the expert on navigating his life. Respond by saying, *"You know your neighborhood better that I do. We need to keep thinking about how to keep you alive."*

7. Assuming he said the fight would stay clean, state

    — *"What if we're in each other's face and a conflict is about to happen, and I do this."* (Reach for something at your right hip. The youth will know that means you are reaching for a gun.)

    In virtually all cases, he will say, *"I would shoot you first."*

    Respond, *"Exactly. Do you see carrying a weapon made me much more likely to be killed? Even if I had a reputation for packing a weapon, do you see that you might have killed me because you wouldn't even have taken the chance that I would fire first?"*

This new abstract understanding may be so inconsistent with the way he has been thinking that he may need to repeat the scenario to think through his other fears, such as being mugged or being the victim of a drive-by shooting. In the case of a mugging, you can clearly demonstrate that a criminal needs to kill the victim who has a weapon, but not the unarmed victim. In the case of a drive-by shooting, the presence of a weapon is not protective.

If they know what the right behaviors are but feel they will not be able to escape danger if their friends are involved

Teenagers often have the desire to avoid risk behaviors but simply cannot escape their social context.

1. It is an important learned skill to replace risky activities and behaviors with safer ones. Learn what the teen does with his friends—both the positive and the negative. For example, if he either plays basketball or smokes marijuana when there is nothing else to do, talk about always carrying a ball. This allows him to maintain friendships while avoiding negative behaviors. As obvious as this skill seems, it may be new to younger teenagers.

2. However, if it comes down to a major conflict with friends, often the teenager cannot avoid the situation. It is developmentally difficult for a youth to say to his friends, *"I disagree with your behavior."* However, it is normal to say, *"My mother's a b----."* For this reason, teenagers should be prepared to shift the blame to their parents. The adolescent should create a code word with his parents (see Chapter 41, page 335). If the parent receives a call in which the teen uses the code, it signals the parent to demand the teen returns home immediately. *"What do you mean you're calling now, you were supposed to be home hours ago!"* If the teen is not able to extricate himself, he escalates, *"You're lucky I even called. I'll be home when I feel like it!"* In response, parents then demand to know exactly where he is and arrange for him to be picked up *immediately.*

If you are at a loss or the teenager states, "How can you know what it's like for me?"

Frequently teenagers reject our guidance or we are at a loss to suggest strategies for survival in an adolescent world so different than the one we grew up in. Youth are often not subtle when we don't understand their lives, and they will tell us, *"You just don't get it."* This signals that it is best to just listen. Active listening helps people develop their own solutions. In these cases, I state, *"I know you're in trouble, but I don't know the right thing to say. It is up to you to figure out how to stay alive. I do know that there are 2 possible roads you're headed down: one is to make and follow your dreams and the other might be serious trouble."* At this point, the ladder diagram is a technique that can break an overwhelming situation into smaller steps, allowing consideration of how each choice can lead toward alternative futures (see Chapter 29). **29.0**

If it is clear that the teenager's behavior is a reaction to stress, or he is so stressed he can't think clearly and may react rashly

When a teen is filled with rage, catecholamines are surging through his body. He is in fight or flight mode and is unlikely to come up with rational protective decisions. A first step is to use up acute stress hormones to allow oneself to maintain an ability to think clearly through crises. Try to determine if his primary feeling is "fear" or "rage." If he can acknowledge fear, guide him to run it out (or play it out through sports). Even consider having the teen run in place before trying to counsel him. **31.3.1** If he acknowledges rage, then suggest he mimics fighting or overcoming a challenge by shadow punching, using a punching bag, hitting pillows, or lifting weights. A routine exercise regimen is central to stress-reduction plans to help adolescents deal with long-term ongoing stressors (see Chapter 31).

●● Group Learning and Discussion ●●

The key to violence interventions is to stay uniformly even-tempered to give the teen the opportunity to become calm himself so he can think through the situation. Your body language and words should both convey safety to prevent the teen from becoming reactive (see Chapter 15). This stands in sharp contrast to the "straight talk/tough love" approach that can backfire by making the youth more reactive.

Prior to meeting, assign a group member to explore whether there is a local program that provides street-level interventions to quell the cycle of violence by working directly with youth to interrupt plans for retaliation.

Break into pairs and work through the following scenarios:

Scenario 1: Dom is brought into your office. He is sweating, he has large pupils, and he won't sit down to talk to you. He will only say, *"I can't stay here, I have to take care of business."* (Hint: He can't listen until he works through his stress hormones.) After he becomes calm, you learn that someone in his neighborhood attacked his cousin, and that his cousin is hospitalized. Dom is a good student and wants to be a firefighter like his dad. He doesn't have a weapon, but says that it won't be hard to get one.

(Consider decision trees, ladder diagrams and, above all, listening.)

Scenario 2: Molly is a 14-year-old girl who has a black eye and scratches over her face. You ask what happened, and she says that she got into a fight with some "B." When you asked her what made her mad enough to fight, she says that this girl insulted her family and then *"got all up in my face."* Molly tells you that she doesn't have time to talk right now, she has to go home. Molly has a "crew" of other girls in the neighborhood. You suspect that Molly is going to get even. You ask her. She says, *"I'm no punk, she's*

•• Group Learning and Discussion, continued ••

going to have to learn a lesson." Molly is caught up in the drama and perils of the neighborhood but has good values and dreams of being a nurse. She is a good older sister. Because her mother works 3 jobs, she largely raises her younger siblings. You know the other girl. She is known to carry weapons outside of school.

▪▪▪▪▪▪▪ Continuing Education ▪▪▪▪▪▪▪

If you are applying for continuing education credits, a test is available online. For more details, visit www.aap.org/reachingteens.

▪ References

1. Centers for Disease Control and Prevention. *Web-based Injury Statistics Query and Reporting System (WISQARS)* [online]. http://www.cdc.gov/injury/wisqars/index.html. Accessed July 22, 2013

2. Centers for Disease Control and Prevention. National Center for Injury Prevention and Control Youth Violence: Facts at a Glance. http://www.cdc.gov/violenceprevention/pub/YV_datasheet.html. Accessed July 22, 2013

3. Cunningham R, Knox L, Fein J, et al. Before and after the trauma bay: the prevention of violent injury among youth. *Ann Emerg Med.* 2009;53:490–500

4. Ellickson P, Saner H, McGuigan KA. Profiles of violent youth: substance use and other concurrent problems. *Am J Public Health.* 1997;87(6):985–991

5. Boney-McCoy S, Finkelhor D. Is youth victimization related to trauma symptoms and depression after controlling for prior symptoms and family relationships? A longitudinal, prospective study. *J Consult Clinical Psych.* 1996;64:1406–1416

6. Dahlberg LL, Toal SB, Swahn M, Behrens CB. *Measuring Violence-Related Attitudes, Behaviors, and Influences Among Youths: A Compendium of Assessment Tools.* 2nd ed. Atlanta, GA: Centers for Disease Control and Prevention, National Center for Injury Prevention and Control; 2005

7. Sege R, Stringham P, Short S, Griffith J. Ten years after: examination of adolescent screening questions that predict future violence-related injury. *J Adolesc Health.* 1999;24:395–402

8. Wiebe DJ, Blackstone MM, Molen CJ, Culyba AJ, Fein JA. Self-reported violence-related outcomes for adolescents within eight weeks of emergency department treatment for assault injury. *J Adolesc Health.* 2001;49:440–442

▪ Related Video Content

58.0 Youth Violence. Ginsburg.

22.0 Trauma-Informed Practice: Working With Youth Who Have Suffered Adverse Experiences. El Centro staff, Covenant House staff.

23.0 De-escalation and Crisis Management: Wisdom and Strategies From Professionals Who Serve Youth Who Often Act Out Their Frustrations. Youth-serving agencies.

23.1 De-escalation if Someone Wants to Leave to "Get Even." Covenant House.

23.2 Why Youth Act Out...and What They Really Need. YouthBuild youth.

28.2 Helping a Young Person Own Her Solution: A Case of Using a Decision Tree to Prevent Violent Retaliation. Ginsburg.

29.0 Gaining a Sense of Control: One Step at a Time. Ginsburg.

31.3.1 Stress Management and Coping/Section 2/Taking Care of My Body/Point 4: The Power of Exercise. Ginsburg

31.3.2 Stress Management and Coping/Section 2/Taking Care of My Body/Point 5: Active Relaxation. Ginsburg.

37.0 Delivering Upsetting News to Parents: Recognizing Their Strengths First. Ginsburg.

45.1 Dealing With Grief by Living Life More Purposefully. Ginsburg.

55.0 Bullying Must Not Be Viewed as a Routine Part of Growing Up. Ginsburg.

56.0 Every Teen Deserves to Be ROUTINELY Screened for the Health of His or Her Relationships. Catallozzi, Bell.

SECTION 8

Serving Special Populations

The strength-based strategies offered throughout this work have been written in general terms that will apply to most youth. This section addresses unique populations so that you can better meet their specific challenges and concerns.

There are many youth subpopulations deserving of focused attention; however, we have limited discussion to the following:

- Youth with chronic disease and disabilities (see Chapter 59)
- Youth in transition from pediatric to adult care (see Chapter 60)
- Sexual and gender minority youth (see Chapter 61)
- Immigrant youth (see Chapter 62)
- Military-affiliated youth (see Chapter 63)
- Foster youth (see Chapter 64)
- Youth infected with HIV (see Chapter 65)
- Street and homeless youth (see Chapter 66)

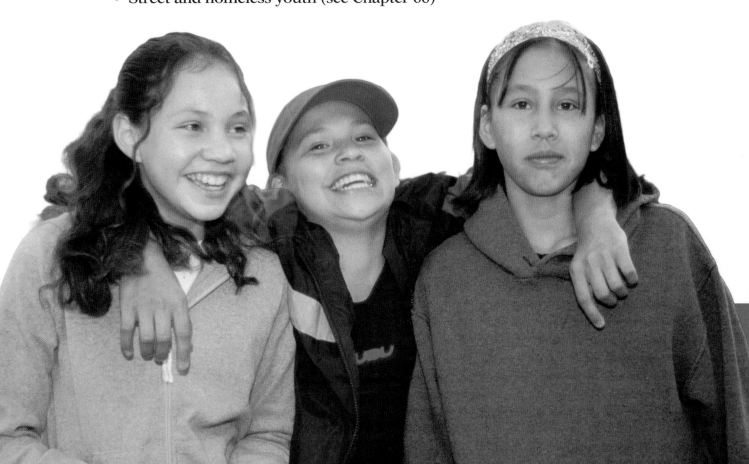

These chapters will likely leave out a subpopulation of particular interest to your practice setting. If this is the case, we suggest that as a group learning and discussion exercise your colleagues discuss how the core principles covered throughout this work could best be applied to meet that group's needs and expectations.

CHAPTER 59

Teens With Chronic Illness and Special Health Care Needs: A Person-Centered Approach to Communication

Jonathan R. Pletcher, MD, FAAP
Karyn E. Feit, LCSW
Lisa K. Tuchman, MD, MPH
Nadja G. Peter, MD

 Related Video Content

59.0 An Overview of Working With Teens With Chronic Disease and Special Health Care Needs

■ Why This Matters

It has been well documented over the past 20 years that not only do 30% to 35% of all youth experience adolescent development with special health care needs, but that this proportion will only increase. Nearly half of teens with special health care needs can be said to have moderate to severe chronic illness or physical and/or emotional disability. This means that more than 1 in 10 youth will face the challenges of adolescence while experiencing intermittent hospitalization, and visits with multiple medical and therapeutic specialists. Additionally, their underlying health condition may affect their mobility and, therefore, their ability to access community and neighborhood resources. Depending on the condition, chronic illness may alter pubertal growth and development, which in turn impacts socialization with both adults and peers. Teens living with chronic conditions also may have to endure the daily discomfort and potential side effects of their ongoing medical treatment plan. In spite of these challenges many, if not most, of these teens are high functioning and productive members of their families and communities.

> **While the existence of a chronic illness can affect all aspects of personal identity, it does not need to be the defining characteristic of how others view the teen, or the teenager's self-perception.**

▶ 59.1

Like many aspects of adolescent health and development, healthy relationships with adults and social groups are instrumental to their success.

Although this population represents a minority of all teens, they account for most primary care office visits and inpatient stays. Parents and teens often rely on providers to offer guidance and support as they negotiate the journey from dependence to independence for the teen. While the existence of a chronic illness can affect all aspects of personal identity, it does not need to be the defining characteristic of how others view the teen, or the teenager's self-perception.

A diagnosis-centered or deficit-oriented approach to thinking and communication places emphasis on the teen as fragile, and minimizes the importance of essential adolescent experiences such as risk-taking and exploration. If the provider focuses solely on medical issues, it minimizes the teen's capacity to discuss issues related to normal maturation, such as sexuality, substance use, emotional distress, or safety concerns. While the role of the clinician includes fostering adherence to medication and self-care routines, it is advisable to integrate these messages into a person-centered approach that respects the needs and strengths of individuals across domains.

■ What This Means in Practice

Language Matters

It is vitally important to treat and respect teens who endure a disability or who have a chronic illness in the same way one does all teens. This means thinking and speaking in person-first language. "Labeling" an individual by their diagnosis leads to stigmatization and is dehumanizing. For example, consider the following statements:

- Joseph is autistic and he is retarded.
- Felicia is a "sickler" who always needs pain meds.
- Joyce is a wheelchair-bound paraplegic.

These commonly used descriptors may inadvertently paint a stereotypic picture where Joseph can easily be assumed to be dependent on others, and he likely will not develop the capacity to have a career let alone achieve higher education. Felicia may be thought to be addicted to narcotics, which must impact her ability to enjoy healthy relationships. And poor Joyce is probably stuck in her house all day with little community engagement. Now consider the following:

- Joseph is a high school senior. With some school and family support for mild intellectual disability and autism diagnosed when he was a child, he has learned to adapt and advocate for accommodations that will serve him well when he starts college next year. He hopes to have a career as a data manager.
- Felicia is an incredibly resilient 19-year-old young lady with sickle cell disease. She is actively engaged with developing alternative pain management strategies since she has decided that she does not want to depend on pain medication. She is, in part, motivated by her plans to get married next year and possibly become a parent.
- Joyce is an active 15-year-old who was born with spina bifida. She uses a wheelchair so well that she started a basketball team for young women who use wheelchairs. She is frequently featured in the newspaper for speaking at local community events where she advocates for opportunities for teen athletes with physical disabilities.

It is very easy to use the brief former descriptions, particularly in busy clinical settings. However, by taking a few extra seconds to offer a person-first description of each individual's special needs, much time and effort is saved in the long run. While a clinician might not greet a patient as a "sickler," thinking and using similar language in the workplace is evident to teens. These messages often get unintentionally transmitted and can cause irreparable damage to a relationship. It is important to remember that disability, chronic illness, and even special needs are cultural and societal concepts. Many conditions that were once considered significant disabilities are no longer considered that due to advances in technology (eg, eyeglasses, hearing aids, adaptive learning devices), as well as advances in public policy (eg, Americans with Disabilities Act and Individuals with Disabilities Education Act).

Certain words should be explicitly discouraged. Specifically, "retarded," "MR," and "mental retardation" should be replaced with intellectual or cognitive disability. Not only is the older terminology diagnostically inaccurate, these words are commonly used pejoratives in our culture. These terms simply have no place when we are trying to form a connection with youth.

Equity Matters

Several reports from young adults affected by chronic illness and physical disability reveal that health professionals are not as likely to ask about their mood, sexual behavior, or substance use. The focus of visits tends to be on perceived acute medical needs associated with their diagnosis. This finding may contribute to the significant health disparities that exist for young adults with special needs, including increased risk of depression. Further, individuals with physical and cognitive disability are at increased risk of being victims of bullying or of physical or sexual abuse. Additionally, teens with a chronic condition must cope with additional anxiety over the loss of their physical integrity and possibly their lives. They often become more aware of their bodies and have been shown to possess a more negative body image compared to their healthy peers. Thus clinicians should be prepared to screen and respond to concerns of depression, anxiety, suicidal thoughts, abuse, eating disorders, sexual activity, and substance use.

Confidentiality 14.4

To ensure all aspects of health and well-being are addressed, it is just as important to discuss confidentiality and its limits with teens with special health care needs as it is with any teen. Reviewing the value of a confidential private discussion with parents may be met with more resistance than is typical. Many parents respond to an empathy statement followed by pertinent information:

> *"I understand that you have had to be there with your daughter through hospital-izations and very scary times. That can make it more difficult to leave her alone with a health care provider.* Pause and wait for acknowledgment. *Based on my experience, teenagers who have medical concerns can really benefit from the same discussions regarding mood and safety as all teens."*

If possible, this discussion and process should be in place during early adolescence. It should be a routine part of every office visit, as there is often a lengthy agenda to cover. Many clinicians use written or computer-assisted questionnaires to ask sensitive questions. If this occurs, special care must be taken that it is completed confidentially by the teen (and not the parent). These questionnaires should also be reviewed at the beginning of the confidential portion of the visit. A real and everyday pitfall is discovering that a teen is suicidal or sexually active just as she is leaving the office.

Genuineness is a key concept for clinicians. This means being who you appear to be and not pretending to be able to do something you cannot. Asking open-ended questions can serve to elicit the teen's agenda(s). A question that is open but not too ambiguous signals that they have the floor to state why they are seeking care at this time. You might ask,
- *"How can I help you today?"*
- *"Tell me what you have come to see me about."*

- *"What would you like to discuss today?"*
- *"What can I do for you?"*

Supporting Parents 36.4, 59.4

For teens with a chronic illness, increased reliance on parents can happen just at a time when unaffected peers are developing increasing independence. Parents might assume ownership over their adolescent's medical care, even though that can facilitate static dependence. Providers can help teens, parents, and caretakers to decide when a teen can begin developing the skills to more actively care for herself or himself, including increasing participation and autonomy in health care decision-making. Understandably, some parents may be anxious and more protective as their teens struggle through trial and error to develop self-care skills. Coaching parents and caretakers about how and when to begin transitioning control of medication management and decision-making for their teen can be an effective way of supporting the adolescent's emerging autonomy. The type and level of support provided to parents can be based on whether or not the mutually identified self-care goals are being met by the teen. Just as in working with all teens, it is advisable to ask for permission in offering advice or a recommendation that the parent may not expect. When appropriate, it is also important to inform and listen to the teenager about how you are supporting his parents. This is particularly relevant in maintaining the centrality of the patient-provider relationship.

Peer Support 59.5

Many studies have been published that explore whether support group interventions can improve the psychological well-being of chronically ill youth. Support groups in general have been shown to reduce isolation, foster a sense of identity, bridge gaps in traditional services, nurture empowerment, and facilitate the giving and receiving of support. The social integration into a peer group that occurs naturally during adolescence is potentially thwarted by chronic illness. Data exist that chronically ill teens not only have fewer friends in their social networks but also less intimate relationships and tend to be more socially marginalized than their healthy peers. Learning how other teens adapt and cope with the challenges of their chronic illness can help teens feel connected with peers, develop tried and true peer strategies for managing illness, and lessen the stress from being different than adolescent peers who are not coping with an additional challenge. The REACH OUT curriculum is one peer group intervention that allows youth to learn healthy coping strategies and practice these strategies with group support.

Promoting Adherence 59.2

In a culture that is accustomed to immediate gratification, the inability for youth to see immediate health improvements can be an additional stressor. The least effective ways to help teens with medication adherence is to wag our fingers and hope that they blindly take our word for what is best. What often works better is identifying the reason for resistance in an open and honest manner. Fostering an open and nonpunitive relationship can help teens feel comfortable discussing their reasons for non-adherence. By asking appropriate follow-up questions in a supportive manner, we can encourage them to become accountable for their decisions and help them to find ways to communicate about how we can be helpful. If we ask patients about ways we can make them feel more comfortable talking about difficult subjects, they usually answer, *"Don't judge me. Don't tell me what to do. Don't change the subject about what things were like for you. And don't share my personal business with anyone unless I tell you it is okay."*

While the provider's goal is usually to promote adherence, the teen's goals may differ. However, common ground can usually be found by facilitating a discussion on the patient's longer-term goals. This can lead to a discussion regarding how keeping up with self-care and medication routines can increase the likelihood that they will be ready to take advantage of future opportunities. If the teen is particularly resistant to adhering to standard medical regimens, we should attempt to understand their reasons. These may include personal beliefs regarding illness, vulnerability, or safety and efficacy of a given regimen. In fact, I once heard the statement, *"To tell you the truth, I come to doctors for a diagnosis, and then I go to my herbalist for treatment."* This disclosure went a long way to building trust and mutual understanding. Some questions that might be helpful to elicit health beliefs include

- *"What do you think might be happening to you?"*
- *"Do you have any ideas or theories about these health problems yourself?"*
- *"What do you think might happen if you did not get medical treatment?"*
- *"What kinds of medical treatments have you tried?"*
- *"Could you describe for me what works best for you?"*

Another approach is to attempt to identify barriers to trust and communication. It is not uncommon for teens with special needs to have been traumatized in medical settings. They may have had negative past experiences with medications or treatments. Alternatively, adhering to medical recommendations may not be possible given the realities of an individual's daily life or available resources. Many may be living in poverty or other extreme conditions.

With the mutual goal of improving or maintaining health, the patient and provider can negotiate the health care plan. It is often helpful for the provider to ask for patients' advice. This places the teens at the center, recognizing they are the experts of their own lives and how their health problem affects them. Sample questions include

- *"What do you think might be the best plan of action?"*
- *"What were you hoping might be able to be done for this?"*
- *"What do you think is a reasonable goal for our next visit?"*

Answers to these questions can be used to build a common agenda and ensure that there are clear goals with mutual buy-in.

■ Case Example

The following excerpt from a patient visit with a social worker demonstrates one way to help teens identify resistance and move toward making positive health decisions.

> Social Worker: *"Hi Suzanne, my name is Jessica and I have been asked by Dr Joseph to speak with you today about your managing the challenges of living with lupus. I have heard from some of my other patients that missing school and having to remember to take medicines are some of their biggest challenges. What would you say are the 2 most difficult things for you about having lupus?"*

Try to get to the root of the resistance by normalizing the problems faced by other youth who are in similar situations.

> Suzanne: *"Well, for one thing, no one really knows what it is like to feel pain all the time or not be able to go out with friends because I am having a flare."*

> Social Worker: *"When you try and explain things to your friends, what do you say?"*

Here the social worker is gauging Suzanne's cognitive and developmental skills while trying to further understand her recognition of the barriers to her medical treatment.

Suzanne: *"I don't really know. I just tell them I don't feel good, but then I end up getting angry and frustrated and things just get worse and worse until I just feel like giving up. Sometimes I just stop taking my medication altogether because I don't even think it helps, even though my rheumatologist tells me it does. I don't think that people can understand unless they are going through it themselves."*

Here, Suzanne gives the social worker a lot of information. She identifies some of her usual coping and feelings of helplessness about her situation. She additionally identifies several specific indicators about the reasons she sometimes chooses not to take her medications.

Social Worker: *"You may be right, it is really hard to understand how someone else is feeling if you haven't walked in their shoes. When you feel like giving up and you don't take your medications for an extended period, let's say a month, what happens?"*

Social worker is validating her feelings of helplessness and trying to help Suzanne see the consequences of failing to take her medications without lecturing her.

Suzanne: *"I usually have a flare and I end up in the hospital. I fall behind in school and have already had to repeat the ninth grade."*

Social Worker: *"So, even though you don't see immediate results from taking your medications, you seem to be able to describe what has happened when you stopped taking your medications."*

Reflecting back what Suzanne described while emphasizing her ability to describe the consequences of her actions.

Suzanne: *"Yeah, it makes sense, but sometimes it is hard to remember what it was like being in the hospital when I am home with my friends."*

Social Worker: *"I think I understand what you are saying. When you are feeling okay for a while, you forget what it was like to be getting treatment in the hospital and missing out on some fun things at home and school. When you start feeling like that, it's like you feel as though you don't really need to take your medications. Can you think of some way that would help you to remember that you don't want to return to the hospital?"*

Checking for clarification and reaching for realistic ways Suzanne can take her medication when she doesn't feel bad by remembering what it was like when she does.

Suzanne: *"I guess if I kept the cards from the hospital up around my room it might remind me what can happen if I stop taking my medications. That's something I could try."*

■ Promoting Normal Development: Reproductive Health in Teens With Chronic Conditions

Reproductive health is an integral component of physical, social, and emotional well-being. Most adolescents with chronic conditions can be expected to experience similar normative stages of physical and emotional development, including puberty, desire for romantic relationships, and envisioning future parenthood. There may be specific risks of hormonal contraception, sexually transmitted infections, and pregnancy depending on disease processes or therapeutic regimens. A significant subset of youth with intellectual disability or developmental delay will experience the same physical maturation as their age-matched peers with a mismatch in expected emotional and cognitive development. Youth with severe neurodevelopmental disability often have difficulty during puberty with unpredictable mood swings and emotional outbursts, severe pain with menstruation, challenges with hygiene, and regulating normal sexual urges in socially acceptable ways. Finally, awareness of the prevalence of sexual abuse against women with developmental disabilities will often prompt discussions regarding screening and contraception.

Because reproductive health questions can be sensitive, it is important to realize most youth and parents will not initiate these discussions, despite having concerns. Another barrier to communication is that medical regimens and needs may "outrank" reproductive health during brief medical visits in the minds of parents and providers. Therefore, it becomes important to initiate reproductive health discussions, providing an opportunity for parents and teens to ask questions and providing a safe venue for ongoing discussion as the youth matures and issues arise. Practical ways to address reproductive health issues include the following:

- Discussions about reproductive health should take place at least every yearly physical examination. Do not forget to ask about pubertal development, menses, and how they are affecting the youth.

- For some teens with chronic illness, menstrual challenges, such as difficulty wearing a sanitary napkin and knowing when to change it, are common issues. Resources can be provided, such as picture boards and incorporating self-care goals into an individualized educational plan (or IEP).

- Discuss boundaries in relationships. Crushes or sexual feelings for another person are normal and happen to everyone. Sometimes they can be mutual, but sometimes they are one-sided, which can be confusing. While difficult, most teens during adolescence experience unreciprocated feelings. It provides an opportunity to discuss respect for the feelings of others and that crushes are personal. Remind youth that, in time, they will likely be attracted to someone who has similar feelings for them.

- Do not assume a youth is not involved in romantic relationships because they have a chronic condition. Offer the same opportunity for a confidential discussion as is offered to all youth. Ask about relationships and whether they have become intimate with a partner. Ask if there are questions about birth control, condoms, or future parenthood. Not only will you identify essential health information and opportunities to prevent significant problems, but you will gain important insights and reinforce trust with your patient.

- Disclosure in relationships is an important issue if a chronic illness is transmissible (eg, HIV or hepatitis) or requires daily ongoing care (eg, cystic fibrosis or diabetes). As adolescence progresses to young adulthood, how the chronic illness affects fertility or how it could be passed on to offspring might also affect disclosure. A key factor affecting one's ability to disclose disease status is acceptance of one's own medical condition.

- Acceptance is necessary to adapt to an illness while tolerating the unpredictability of the disease while staying engaged in a meaningful life. The need for psychosocial support for youth with chronic conditions as they negotiate acceptance might only come to light during discussions regarding complex relationship dynamics.

■ Setting the Stage for Transition

As we consider transition to adult care, we must also include attention to increased independence in the educational, vocational, emotional, and social domains. Teens with special needs are often excluded from social and work-related opportunities. Therefore, every provider should be accustomed to discussing the teen's roles and responsibilities at school, at home, and in the community. Therefore, starting in late childhood or early adolescence, every visit should include a discussion regarding school participation. This includes asking about educational and prevocational plans and progress. Enjoyable activities and hobbies should be encouraged, particularly if they are compatible with group or community settings. Asking about friends and adult supports, and encouraging these connections, also can serve several functions. Youth living with chronic illness should be offered the opportunity to engage with others who may share many of their fears and concerns. Support groups may be offered in schools, hospitals, or outpatient facilities. It may be helpful to find more general support groups when a youth is first diagnosed with a disease because there is often a process of adjustment when it is difficult to acknowledge the reality of living life with an illness that may not ever go away. For instance, it may be hard for a teen recently diagnosed with cancer to attend a cancer support group. It may be easier for him to attend a general group for teens with chronic illness. Transition is discussed in much more detail in Chapter 60.

■ Conclusion

A person-centered approach to thinking about and communication with youth who have special health care needs is an invaluable method of promoting youth development in spite of significant challenges. This allows providers to assist in healthy identity formation that is not based on medical diagnosis or disability. Rather, we can play an integral role in promoting healthy and sustainable relationships, community engagement, and achievement through education. Ultimately this approach leads to shared agendas and outcomes with adolescents through optimized self-care, self-advocacy, and adherence to medical treatment. These processes set in motion during adolescence can have a lasting and positive impact toward improved health throughout life.

●● Group Learning and Discussion ●●

The key point in this chapter is that while some youth have special needs related to a health condition, they remain adolescents first and deserve the same comprehensive care as all teens. This can be challenging for 2 reasons. First, time may be at a premium because their visits likely need to cover issues specifically related to their condition. Second, their parents may assume tighter control over the visits, either because of (perhaps justified) higher levels of worry or because of negative past experiences.

Break into groups of 3, dividing roles between clinician, parent, and teen. Practice discussions that explain why the teen needs a private relationship that covers all of the routine and expected topics of adolescent development. Then, after the "parent" has left the room, practice a discussion that considers the condition in the much broader context of development. Consider asking the young person how she might be wiser or stronger precisely because of her condition. When the parent returns, ask how they think their child has grown or benefited from the challenges of navigating her condition.

■■■■■■■■ Continuing Education ■■■■■■■■■

If you are applying for continuing education credits, a test is available online. For more details, visit www.aap.org/reachingteens.

■ Suggested Reading

Abraham A, Silber TJ, Lyon M. Psychosocial aspects of chronic illness in adolescence. *Indian J Pediatr.* 1999;66:447–453

Blum RW. Sexual health contraceptive needs of adolescents with chronic conditions. *Arch Pediatr Adolesc Med.* 1997;151:290–296

Buhlmann U, Fitzpatrick SB. Caring for an adolescent with chronic illness. *Prim Care.* 1987;14:57–68

Cromer B, Enrile B, McCoy K, Gerhardstein M, Fitzpatrick M, Judis J. Knowledge, attitudes and beliefs related to sexuality in adolescents with chronic disability. *Dev Med Child Neurol.* 1990;32:602–610

DiNapoli PP, Murphy D. The marginalization of chronically ill adolescents. *Nurs Clin North Am.* 2002;37(3):565–572

Druss B, Pincus H. Suicidal ideation and suicide attempts in general medical illness. *Arch Intern Med.* 2000;160:1522–1526

Greydanus DE, Rimsza ME, Newhouse PA. Adolescent sexuality and disability. *Adolesc Med.* 2002; 13:223–248

Hallum A. Disability and the transition to adulthood: issues for the disabled child, the family, and the pediatrician. *Curr Probl Pediatr.* 1995;25:12–50

Lotstein DS, Inkelas M, Hays RD, Halfon N, Brook R. Access to care for youth with special health care needs in the transition to adulthood. *J Adolesc Health.* 2007;43:23–29

Louis-Jacques J, Samples C. Caring for teens with chronic illness: risky business? *Curr Opin Pediatr.* 2011;23:367–372

Maslow GR, Haydon AA, Ford CA, Halpern CT. Young adult outcomes of children growing up with chronic illness: an analysis of the National Longitudinal Study of Adolescent Health. *Arch Pediatr Adolesc Med.* 2011;165(3):256–261

Newacheck PA, Taylor WR. Childhood chronic illness: prevalence, severity, and impact. *Am J Pub Health.* 1992;82:364–371

Pacaud D, Crawford S, Stephure DK, et al. Effect of type 1 diabetes on psychosocial maturation in young adults. *J Adolesc Health.* 2007;40(1):29–35

Patterson J, Blum RW. Risk and resilience among children and youth with disabilities. *Arch Pediatr Adolesc Med.* 1996;150:692–698

Pless IB, Power C, Peckham CS. Long-term psychosocial sequelae of chronic physical disorders of childhood. *Pediatrics.* 1993;91(6):1131–1136

Schopler JH, Galinsky MJ. Support groups as open systems: a model for practice and research. *Health Soc Work.* 1993;18(3):195–207

Stevens SE, Steele CA, Jutai JW, Kalnins IV, Bortolussi JA, Biggar WD. Adolescents with physical disabilities: some psychosocial aspects of health. *J Adolesc Health.* 1996;19(2):157–164

Suris JC, Parera N, Puig C. Chronic illness and emotional distress in adolescence. *J Adolesc Health.* 1996; 19:153–156

Suris JC, Resnick MD, Cassuto N, Blum RW. Sexual behavior of adolescents with chronic disease and disability. *J Adolesc Health.* 1996;19:124–131

Zindani GN, Streetman DD, Streetman DS, Nasr SZ. Adherence to treatment in children and adolescent patients with cystic fibrosis. *J Adolesc Health.* 2006;38:13–17

■ Related Handout/Supplementary Material

REACH-OUT: A Support Group for Teens Living with Chronic Illness

■ Related Video Content

59.0 An Overview of Working With Teens With Chronic Disease and Special Health Care Needs. Pletcher.

59.1 Helping Youth and Parents Understand That Alongside the Challenges of Having a Chronic Disease Often Comes Long-standing Strengths. Pletcher, Peter.

59.2 Youth With Chronic Disease and Adherence to Medications and Treatment Plans. Peter.

59.3 Adolescents With Chronic Disease May Suffer From PTSD. Tomescu.

59.4 Guidance for Parents: It Is Your Role to Be Protective, But Seeing Your Child With Chronic Disease as "Fragile" Can Unconsciously Undermine Your Child's Progress. Pletcher.

59.5 Helping Youth With Chronic Illness Navigate Peer Relationships. Pletcher.

59.6 Youths' Ability to Care for Themselves and to Trust You Is Impacted by Experiences of Bias and Discrimination. Pletcher.

59.7 Caring for Youth With Chronic Illness: The Importance of Understanding How They Use Traditional Healing and Complementary Medicine. Pletcher.

59.8 Caring for Youth With Chronic Illness: Helping Youth Better Describe the Timing and Quality of Their Symptoms. Pletcher.

59.9 Caring for Youth With Chronic Illness: Overcoming Challenges to Optimal Communication With Teens and Families. Pletcher.

59.10 Caring for Youth With Chronic Illness: Hygiene and Wellness. Pletcher.

59.11 Working With Youth With High-Functioning Autism. Zucker.

59.12 Teen Testimony: A Story of Strength and Resilience in the Face of Managing Cystic Fibrosis. Youth.

4.3 Older Children and Adolescents Are Capable of Participating in Health Decisions. Peter.

14.4 Setting the Stage for a Long-term Partnership: Focus on Youth With Chronic Disease. Pletcher.

18.3 A Strategy for Incorporating a Comprehensive Psychosocial Screen Into the Office Visit. Pletcher.

18.18 Case: 11-Year-Old Girl With Chronic Disease and Depression. Peter.

24.0 Among the Hardest Things We Do—Delivering Bad News. Ginsburg, Reirden, Arrington-Sanders, Garofalo, Hawkins, Pletcher.

25.6 Helping Youth With Chronic Disease Own How Adversity Has Built Their Resilience. Pletcher.

36.4 A Focus on Parenting Teens With Chronic Diseases: Balancing Protection With the Need for Youth to Make and Recover From Mistakes. Pletcher.

39.3 Adolescents With Chronic Disease Need Parents Who Care for Themselves. Pletcher.

42.2 Teen Testimonial: Survival, Resilience, and Overcoming Depression. Youth, Ginsburg.

60.4 Preparation for Transition Begins Early: A Visit With an 11-Year-Old. Peter.

60.5 Discussing Transition With a Mid-adolescent With Chronic Disease. Peter.

■ Related Web Sites

Kidshealth.org, Nemours

http://kidshealth.org/teen/your_mind/problems/deal_chronic_illness.html#

The Center for Children With Special Needs, Seattle Children's Hospital

http://cshcn.org/teens

Starlight Children's Foundation

www.starlight.org

CHAPTER 60

Transitioning From Pediatric to Adult Care

Nadja G. Peter, MD

Karyn E. Feit, LCSW

Jo Ann Sonis, LCSW, DCSW

Oana Tomescu, MD, PhD

Jonathan R. Pletcher, MD, FAAP

 Related Video Content

60.0.1 Transition Is a Process, Not a Transfer
60.0.2 Helping Families Create a Framework for Transition—Fostering Growing Independence in Health Care (and Life)

■ Why This Matters

An estimated 30% of adolescents have one or more chronic medical conditions that will continue to require care in adulthood. Most young people with chronic illness will transfer care from pediatric to adult health care providers. The aim of a successful transition is for the young person to feel ready and comfortable, and to be able to develop a meaningful and sustained relationship with his or her new adult provider. Though transitioning medical care is important, young people with chronic illness are simultaneously managing many transitions (eg, starting college or work, leaving foster care, moving to independent housing, transitioning off of an insurance plan, developing relationships). For young people, health care is only one of many priorities. Understanding the broad social, economic, and emotional challenges that affect a young person's transition to adult care can better ensure success. Providers can work together with youth to help them fit health care into their changing, busy lives and orchestrate a transition that can lead to **60.1** a sustained partnership with an adult care provider to ensure continued excellent care.

> **Transition is a process, not an event. The actual transfer of care is the culmination of many years of preparation.**

■ Transition Is a Process ▶ 60.0.1

Transition is a process, not an event. The actual transfer of care is the culmination of many years of preparation. This process ideally starts during childhood. Transition occurs through a gradual transfer of decision-making authority, responsibility for daily care, arranging appointments, and management of insurance issues from the parent/caregiver, to joint responsibility that allows for increasing involvement of the young person and, ultimately, if able, full responsibility of all aspects of his or her health by the young adult with his or her adult provider. Ideally, the process of transition should align with other areas of the young person's development. For example, a 10-year-old who can responsibly do her own homework and make her own snack can likely also remember to take her daily medication with some supervision. The most important first step toward transition is engaging children and teens in feeling that their health is important and that they are capable of caring for themselves.

■ Policies and Guidelines

The shared management model developed at the University of Washington (see Related Web Sites) outlines 4 stages of role shifts for the child, parent, and health care provider. Initially, the child is the "receiver" of health care and gradually becomes the "doer," then the "manager," and ultimately the "CEO" of their own health care team. The timing of these role transitions depends on the developmental stage of the child and his physical and cognitive abilities. Almost all patients, even those with developmental delays, can progress through some of these stages. Health care providers can model these role transitions during the medical visits. For example, instead of directing all questions to the parents or caretaker, providers can ask a 10-year-old to explain what he understands of his medical history, what medications he should be taking, and if he is actually remembering to take his medications. This helps parents to know that they too can ask their child to step up and start being responsible for some of his own medical care. Another important step to ensure a successful transition is for the provider to meet alone—by at least 12 years of age—with their patients. This allows for a brief check-in on confidential issues that may impact care and also allows patients time to ask questions that they might be afraid or embarrassed to ask in front of their parents. For example, *"I heard that most people with spinal muscular atrophy die before 20, is that going to happen to me?"* or *"I went to a movie with my friends and I started coughing up all this mucus. I read on the CF Web site that I can take 2 Benadryl with a Red Bull to temporarily stop the secretions so I don't gross out my friends. Is that okay?"* The time spent privately with young people may address some of their most salient questions.

The provider may also want to check in with their patient's parents/caretakers to see if they have any concerns. In privacy, a parent may ask, *"I know you want me to give him more responsibility, and I'm letting him do his own sugars and corrections. He's doing a pretty good job—well, except for last Saturday night when he took extra insulin so he could sleep late. But, on the whole, I'm really proud of him, but is it okay if I still check his glucose at night to be sure he doesn't go too low?"* Moments like this allow parents to get guidance from providers without embarrassing (or "outing") their teen or taking away from their teen's emerging confidence. ▶ **36.4**

Providers can also help parents who, out of fear of losing their child, have difficulty thinking about their child's future, are not sure how to raise a teen with special health needs, or are simply too busy with their child's day-to-day health needs to think about the future. Providers can help these parents take a moment to plan ahead and ensure that the parents boost all of their social supports by providing education for grandparents, babysitters, siblings, teachers, and coaches. Also, being sure parents know about links to parent groups, advocacy organizations, and peer groups can be very helpful. Help parents remember that their child will benefit tremendously by having supportive relationships outside their family with peers and supportive adults. By supporting peer connections, parents can positively impact all aspects of their child's emotional development and overall well-being (see Chapter 8). ▶ **60.0.2, 60.2**

■ Practical Issues That Affect Transition to Adult Care   ▶ 60.3

Insurance plans and benefit packages often change after age 18 years, and again after age 21 years. With recently passed legislation, there is more flexibility, sometimes up to age 26 years, but not in all cases. In addition, even if patients have insurance, their benefits packages are often different. It may be extremely helpful for the parent and young person to meet with a social worker or case manager familiar with insurance issues before the young person turns 18 to discuss insurance options and apply for any relevant programs that require registration prior to his or her 18th birthday.

Understanding the Adult Health Care System

As a young person enters the adult health care system, it can be important to discuss the differences in how the practices approach patient care. It is important to emphasize that these are simply differences. They are neither good nor bad. Pediatric practices may be more nurturing and the adult practices may be more focused on patient autonomy. There are advantages and disadvantages to both systems. For some patients, a brief pre-appointment visit to the new office will greatly increase comfort. Young people who are learning to make their own appointments will need support to learn how to manage a phone menu, get referrals, and order prescription refills. Youth who have been lifelong patients in a pediatric practice may have learned shortcuts and ways to self-advocate (such as knowing the "back line"). Though this will not be possible at first in their new practice, as they become established as a patient, they will become more comfortable and get to know different ways to communicate effectively.

Importance of the Summary Letter

There are several ways to arrange the actual transfer of care. If at all possible, it is ideal to have a young person schedule a visit with her new provider prior to the official transition of care. If there is no transition program available, this can sometimes be done as a consult to the adult provider. It can be helpful for the pediatric provider or team to help a young person make the call for that first appointment so any problems can be immediately addressed. If young people or their parents/caregivers will make the appointment themselves, it is important to provide them with names and numbers of potential new providers. Patients are more likely to go to a new provider that is specifically recommended by their old provider. A simple, *"'He's a great doctor. I've sent several other young people to see him and they have been very happy,"* can be a huge encouragement during a challenging transition.

To ensure continuity of care, one of the most important things a pediatric provider can do is to provide a clinical summary and letter of introduction to the adult provider. Having the young patient sign a release of protected health information to the adult provider will allow the pediatric provider to send a letter to the adult provider in advance of the first visit. Adult providers prefer a 1- to 2-page summary highlighting the patient's health history, including a problem list, medical history, surgical history, other procedures, medication list, allergies, ancillary services, and contact information. The most important piece of information to ensure continuity of care is the current plan of care. It is also helpful to include any information that you have found helpful in communicating with your patient, such as the role of family members, cultural considerations, and the use of any adaptive equipment. Finally, alerting the new provider to other barriers that impact care can diminish glitches that may arise early in care. Some families have trouble with transition because of costs related to transportation or co-pays. Difficulty getting time off of work can lead to missed or cancelled appointments.

Transitioning care can be time-consuming. To make the process easier and go more smoothly, electronic medical records can be used to create a template for a transition summary. In addition, many states have downloadable transition planning guides and checklists through the Title V programs of their departments of health. Several programs have templates or information available online to help with this process (see Related Web Sites). One program even has online videos that teach young people how to refill prescriptions or make their own appointments.

■ Special Challenges

Certain patient populations may have more significant problems transitioning. Some of these are youth with very rare conditions, youth with multisystem illnesses or multiple chronic illnesses, youth with severe developmental disabilities, youth in the foster care system or who lack social support systems, youth or families with severe or undertreated mental health problems, and families who are questioning their child's self-care skills. It is important to identify these issues early, as additional planning may be necessary. For example, for a youth with a rare condition, an adult provider may need to be educated on the condition prior to transfer. For youth with multiple conditions, and multiple health care providers, the order of transitioning may need to be decided. For youth with developmental disabilities it will be important to assess their social support system beforehand, make sure they are optimally involved in available community systems, and also address issues of guardianship or power of attorney prior to transition. If a major mental health problem is identified at the time of planned transition, it might be better to postpone transition until treatment is begun and a plan for future treatment is in effect. While some young people are ready to assume more of their own care, their parents may feel worried. Reassure these parents that their teens may still be learning how to take care of themselves, but that continued support can further improve their self-care skills. While most young adults want to find the adult provider that is the "expert" regarding their health concerns, many have found that it is more important to find the adult provider who wants and has the capacity to learn about their unique diagnoses and complexities even though they may not be an expert at the outset.

■ Concluding Thoughts

In summary, the actual transfer of care from the pediatric to the adult health care system should be the culmination of a long transition process. The transition process should begin many years before the actual anticipated transfer year and consist of the gradual transition of health-related tasks, decision-making, and communication/advocacy from the parent/caregiver to the patient. Incorporating simple transition-related guidance into each visit will prepare children, adolescents, and their parents/caretakers for the later successful and positive transition to adult care.

•• Group Learning and Discussion ••

- Discuss as a group what policies and procedures you have in place to aid the transition process.
- When do you start discussing transition? Do you tend to wait until it is imminent, or do you treat it as a developmental process?
- Reflect on whether you tend to be only problem-focused with teens with special medical concerns. If so, what might your practice consider to make it feasible to give these youth the same comprehensive care other youth receive?
- If you currently use a transition checklist, is it used uniformly? If not, assign a group member to explore the suggested resources and download checklists and tools that match your practice.
- Do you have adult practices to which you routinely transition your patients? What do you do to make these transitions go more smoothly for the teen, family, and adult provider?
- Then discuss cases of transition that have been particularly challenging in your practice. Consider cases where the parents' hypervigilance and worry (likely well-earned) have made it difficult for them to give their adolescent increasing autonomy in preparation for transition and increased self-care. Strategize ways that you could help the parent feel more secure allowing these necessary steps toward both transition and independence. If time allows, break into groups of 3 (clinician, teen, and parent) and role-play the strategies you have discussed.

■■■■■■■■ Continuing Education ■■■■■■■■

If you are applying for continuing education credits, a test is available online. For more details, visit www.aap.org/reachingteens.

■ Suggested Reading

American Academy of Pediatrics Committee on Bioethics. Informed consent, parental permission, and assent in pediatric practice. *Pediatrics.* 1995;95:314–317

Callahan TS, Winitzer RF, Keenan P. Transition from pediatric to adult-oriented health care: a challenge for patients with chronic disease. *Curr Opin Pediatr.* 2001;13:310–316

Cappelli M, MAcDonald NE, McGrath P. Assessment of readiness to transfer to adult care for adolescents with cystic fibrosis. *Child Health Care.* 1989;18:218–224

Crosnier H, Tubiana-Rufi N. Transition from pediatric to adult care for diabetic adolescents in the Paris-Ile-de-France area. *Arch Pediatr.* 1998;5:1327–1333

Dickey SB, Deatrick J. Autonomy and decision making for health promotion in adolescence. *Pediatr Nurs.* 2000;26:461–467

Kieckhefer G, Trahms CM. Chronic illness in children: supporting the development of children as they move from compliance toward shared management. *Pediatr Nurs.* 2000;26(4):354–363

Kieckhefer G. Keeping the AFOs on: a developmental approach to engaging children and families in shared management, a presentation on March 26 at the 2010 Duncan seminar by Gail M Kieckhefer, PhD, PNP, ARNP, Family and Child Nursing and MCHB Pediatric Pulmonary Center, University of Washington. http://www.seattlechildrens.org/pdf/GK-handouts.pdf. Accessed June 26, 2013

Lotstein DS, Inkelas M, Hays RD, Halfon N, Brook R. Access to care for youth with special health care needs in the transition to adulthood. *J Adolesc Health.* 2007;43:23–29

Reiss J, Gibson R. Health care transition: destination unknown. *Pediatrics.* 2002;110:1307–1314

White PH. Access to health care: health insurance considerations for young adults with special health care needs/disabilities. *Pediatrics.* 2004;110:1328–1335

■ Related Video Content

60.0.1 Transition Is a Process, Not a Transfer. Peter.

60.0.2 Helping Families Create a Framework for Transition—Fostering Growing Independence in Health Care (and Life). Pletcher.

60.1 Health Care Transition Is Only One of Many Transitions in Late Adolescence. Peter.

60.2 Preparing Our Children to Become Their Own Health Care Decision-Makers. Peter.

60.3 Addressing Barriers to a Smooth Transition Process. Peter.

60.4 Preparation for Transition Begins Early: A Visit With an 11-Year-Old. Peter.

60.5 Discussing Transition With a Mid-adolescent With Chronic Disease. Peter.

60.6 Case: Preparing a Late Adolescent With Chronic Disease for the Insurance Issues Associated With Health Care Transition. Feit.

36.4 A Focus on Parenting Teens With Chronic Diseases: Balancing Protection With the Need for Youth to Make and Recover From Mistakes. Pletcher.

■ Related Web Sites

The following Web sites offer information for teens, parents, and clinicians about transition of care. Some sites also include transition checklists that will help teens and parents keep track of their progress, highlighting areas that need focused attention.

The Children's Hospital of Philadelphia
The Children's Hospital of Philadelphia offers the handouts listed below on its site: www.chop.edu/service/transition-to-adulthood/resources-for-patients-and-families.html

Care Binders
A care binder is an organizing tool for families who have children with special health care needs. Care binders help you keep track of important information about your own or your child's health and care. To create your own care binder, choose one of the following:
- Care Binder for parents
- Care Binder for young adults

Tips for Parents and Caregivers
First Steps to Teach Children About Their Health Ages 4-6

Next Steps to Help Children Understand Their Health Ages 7-10

Preparing Children to Take Charge of Their Health Ages 11-13

Guiding Youth to Take Charge of Their Health Ages 14-17

Transitioning Young Adults from Pediatric to Adult Healthcare Ages 18-21

Tips for Patients to Take Charge of Their Health
It's Your Health: What You Need to Know Ages 11-13

It's Your Health: What You Need to Know Ages 14-17

It's Time: Are You Ready to Transition to Adult Healthcare? Ages 18-21

Taking Charge of Your Health – A Guide for Teens and Young Adults Brochure

Taking Charge of Your Health – A Guide for Teens and Young Adults

Emergency Information Wallet Card

Tips for Young Adults With Intellectual Challenges

From Pediatric to Adult Medical Care

Beyond High School Graduation

Planning for Education and Training After High School

Get Ready. Get Set. Let's Go To Work!

Moving into a Home of Your Own

Got Transition?

www.gottransition.org

Healthy Transitions

http://healthytransitionsny.org

Seattle Children's

http://teenology101.seattlechildrens.org/adolescent-transition

Adolescent Health Transition Project

http://depts.washington.edu/healthtr/resources/tools/checklists.html

Health Care Transition

http://hctransitions.ichp.ufl.edu

Florida HATS

www.floridahats.org/?page_id=608

CHAPTER 61

Sexual and Gender Minority Youth

Nadia L. Dowshen, MD, FAAP, AAHIVS

Linda A. Hawkins, PhD, LPC

Renata Arrington-Sanders, MD, MPH, ScM, FAAP

Daniel H. Reirden, MD, FAAP, AAHIVMS

Robert Garofalo, MD, MPH

 Related Video Content

61.0 Working With LGBT Youth Has a High Yield Because We Can Help Them Overcome Stigma, Shame, and Isolation…and Show Them That It Can Get Better

■ Why This Matters

Approximately 10% of individuals identify as lesbian, gay, bisexual, transgender, or questioning/queer (LGBTQ) and, therefore, all youth professionals will likely care for sexual and/or gender minority youth regardless of where they practice. Unfortunately, many LGBTQ youth are at higher risk for poor health outcomes, including contemplating and attempting suicide, drug abuse, and sexually transmitted infections (STIs), including HIV. It is important to distinguish that these health risks are not due to an individual's sexual orientation or gender identity, but rather result from the stress and isolation they face because of their identity. You have the power to make a difference by overcoming that isolation and being at least one person in their life who supports them no matter who they are. For this reason, you may find supporting LGBTQ youth to be one of the most satisfying aspects of your practice with teens, and will likely find it among your highest yields in impacting on the life trajectories of adolescents.

> Showing youth that you are supportive of all gender and sexual identities by creating a safe, inclusive space can make a huge impact on making all youth comfortable with trusting you with any concern or difference.

▶ 61.1

■ Background

In order to understand sexual and gender identity development, one needs to distinguish between the following constructs: sexual orientation, sexual behavior, and gender or gender identity.

Sexual orientation refers to one's pattern of physical and emotional attractions to others. While, traditionally, one's sexual orientation has been described as homosexual or heterosexual, adolescents may be more comfortable with newer terminology like questioning, queer, or bisexual. These terms may also help to address the current thinking that, for some individuals, sexual identity may not be best captured by the traditional homosexual-heterosexual dichotomy, but rather lie somewhere in between these 2 categories. It is important to note that the term *queer*, while considered by many to be derogatory, has been reclaimed by many youth to describe sexual orientation or gender identity that does not conform to societal norms.

Sexual behavior refers to the way one chooses to express sexual feelings. Sexual behavior often does not correlate with sexual orientation, especially among adolescents. In other words, heterosexually identified youth may have same-gender sexual experiences and homosexually identified youth may have opposite-gender sexual experiences.

Gender identity is a personal and culturally defined construct based on one's perception of being male or female. Much like sexual orientation, gender identity can occur across a wide continuum, and its complexity is not necessarily well captured as a binary structure. Transgender youth, for example, are individuals whose gender identity is discordant to some extent with their biologically or anatomically defined sex assigned at birth. Although a person may be born anatomically female, they may have a male gender identity (ie, female-to-male transgender individual or transgender man).

■ Creating a Safe Space From the Front Door 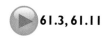 61.3, 61.11

Providing a safe and open environment starts well before a youth enters your office.

- Create a space respectful to all youth regardless of sexual orientation and/or gender identity.
- Consider displaying gay-positive/-friendly messages in windows and on posters in the waiting area and in examination rooms/offices. Forms and patient education materials that include options or messages that are open to different sexual and gender identities may go a long way to making youth feel comfortable.
- Registration/front desk staff should be trained and comfortable providing nonjudgmental, respectful service regardless of gender, sexual, or cultural identity and physical appearance. For example, transgender youth may often go by a name that is different from their legal birth name. If physical appearance differs from what is considered gender typical or changes over time, staff should not stare or ask unnecessary question. We all know not to do this for other physical differences, but sometimes we need a reminder to maintain the same neutral stance with these youth (see Chapter 12).

Setting the Stage 61.2

Ultimately, LGBTQ teens want the same things as other youth when it comes to interactions with professionals. Professionals can make sexual and gender minority youth comfortable by setting the stage appropriately for nonjudgment, respect, and honesty (see Chapter 14). Be explicit about the fact that you take care of and support all youth with different dreams, challenges, and identities.

- Remind youth that honesty in communication in both directions between youth and provider can lead to the strongest partnership to promote health and well-being.
- Ask what teens want to be called (initially and when parents are out of the room).
- Explain that you will use professional language, but that youth can always speak however they are most comfortable talking about anything.

Discussing Sexual Health and Sexuality 61.5

- When taking a sexual history, be specific and expansive. Explain any terms you use and ask for detail if there is something a youth says that you do not understand. Consider using the ABO (attraction, behavior, orientation) framework to ensure completeness. See Box 61.1 for examples of specific questions to ask.
- Use language that is inclusive rather than exclusive and ask questions that are open-ended and nonjudgmental.
- Consider asking about whether youth have questions about any sexual behaviors or activities whether they have experienced them or not.

Box 61.1. Questions to Consider When Taking a Developmentally Tailored Sexual History: Using the Attraction/Behavior/Orientation (ABO) Framework

Attraction

All young people develop sexual feelings and have to make decisions about sexual behaviors as they grow up. Have you ever had a crush on or a romantic relationship with a boy or girl? Are you romantically or sexually attracted to men (boys), women (girls), or both?

Are you having sexual feelings? Attractions? Are you comfortable with those attractions? What do I mean by attractions? I mean you look at someone and you get turned on, or they take your breath away.

Are you dating someone? Tell me about who you are dating and what your relationship is like.

Behavior

What about your friends? Have any of your friends started to have sex? What do you think about that? Can you explain how you will make decisions about when to have sex?

Have you ever had any physical contact, like kissing or touching in private areas, with a boy or a girl? If touching, above or below the waist? Clothes on or off? Has any of this ever happened, even against your will?

Do you or have you ever had vaginal sex? Oral sex? Anal sex?

Do you have sex with men (boys), women (girls), or both?

How do you protect yourself against sexually transmitted infections (STIs) and pregnancy?

Do you use condoms for anal or vaginal sex? How many times out of 10 do you use them?

Do you have sex with anyone other than your boyfriend or girlfriend? In those situations, how often are you using condoms?

Has anyone ever pressured you or forced you into doing something sexually that you didn't want to do?

Have you ever needed to trade sex for money, drugs, or a place to stay?

Orientation

How would you describe your sexual orientation? Many young people aren't sure or prefer not to use a label and that's okay too. For example, do you consider yourself heterosexual (straight), gay, lesbian, or bisexual?

How to Get Help

If you have questions about sex or sexual orientation, what adult in your life can you talk to? It's important for you to know that doctors and nurses have a responsibility to help young people stay healthy, which means avoiding unwanted pregnancy and STIs. Not having sex is the only 100% safe way to do this. If you ever do decide to have sex, explain to me how you could get to a doctor or nurse to discuss preventing pregnancy and STIs.

- Recognize the distinction between behavior/attraction/orientation and avoid assumptions.
  — Address family planning issues for lesbian women. Many young women who have female partners may have had or will have male partners. Also, many lesbian women will consider pregnancy and parenting, and professionals should be prepared to discuss options.
  — Don't jump immediately from a male patient identifying as gay to HIV testing. Many young gay men may not be at high risk for HIV infection and, therefore, HIV testing should be approached the same way as for other youth as part of routine screening.
- When asking youth about sexual orientation, you may want to remind them that adolescence is a time where people are often exploring their attractions, and that some people may have a label for their identity like gay, bi, or straight, and others may not yet or never want to have a label and that's okay too.

In a Medical Setting: Physical Examination and Touch 61.13

- Assess for abuse/forced sex prior to examination.
- Always explain why and how you are going to examine sensitive areas.
- Physical examination of private areas can be particularly traumatic for youth who do not identify with their anatomy (eg, examining the penis and testicles of a transgender young person who was assigned male sex at birth but identifies as female).
- Consider whether you need to do sensitive parts of the examination the first time you meet a patient. Often, it is not necessary that day to do a full physical examination. By offering the option to defer sensitive parts of the examination, the provider may build trust in the therapeutic relationship.
- Suggest strategies to make youth most comfortable with invasive or sensitive physical examination. For example, a youth may want to listen to music or hold someone's hand during a pelvic examination.
- Screening should be done based on anatomy and behavior, not sexual orientation or gender identity.
  — Routine testicular examinations should be done for transgender women and cervical cytology, when indicated, should be done for transgender men.
  — Consider performing ano-rectal STI screening for all individuals who have receptive anal sex regardless of gender/sexual orientation, if you can access a certified laboratory.
- Consider offering self-examination or specimen collection when possible if it makes youth more comfortable (ie, self-collected anal or vaginal swabs for gonorrhea/chlamydia testing).

■ Mental Health

Remember that mental health issues among sexual and gender minority youth often present as a result of the trauma, isolation, and stigma that they experience as a result of not receiving universal acceptance.

- Address depression and suicidality for all youth when they present with physical symptoms.
- Assess for bullying for all youth. LGBTQ youth are more likely to be the victims of verbal and physical harassment.
- It is helpful to connect youth with adult LGBTQ mentors and peer support. These can be powerful tools to break isolation.

■ The Coming Out Process 61.7–61.10; 61.21

"Coming out" or disclosing one's sexual orientation or gender identity to family, friends, and communities is a consistent challenge for LGBTQ youth. You can support youth through their coming out process by helping them consider the following:

- When deciding who to tell, first think about who in your life you can trust with this information and who will provide the support you need.
- Remember to think about safety and consider whether now is the right time to tell if it may lead to physical violence or losing housing or financial support.
- It is particularly important for adolescents to understand that peoples' feelings will change over time, and that a bad initial reaction doesn't mean that person will remain unsupportive.
- Consider helping youth to plan for the process by using techniques like role-playing.
- Formulate a backup plan if reactions are different from expected.

Addressing Parents' Concerns 61.14

When parents learn that their child may be lesbian, gay, bisexual, or transgender, even those that want to be supportive will often have concerns. Worries may include thoughts or questions like, *"Did I do something to cause this?" "What about having children?" "It's going to be hard for him/her."* When addressing these concerns, it can be helpful to focus on the positive and provide resources for support. Remind parents that they are the most important people in their child's life, and that the love and caring they have already shown are powerful things (see Chapter 37).

Studies have shown that when parents support their LGBTQ children, the youth have better physical and mental health outcomes. Ultimately, you can reassure parents that, while sexual and gender minority youth will face challenges because of their identities, those challenges can build their resilience. Above all, reinforce that, with love and support, they will be able to fulfill their hopes and dreams.

■ The Bottom Line and Knowing Yourself as a Provider 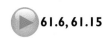 61.6, 61.15

Remember that it is not your job to uncover youths' identities, but rather to be open and supportive so that when they are ready to seek help they know that they can trust you. It doesn't mean that you have failed in any way if a youth never comes out to you. In fact, showing youth that you are supportive of all gender and sexual identities by creating a safe, inclusive space can make a huge impact on making all youth comfortable with trusting you with any concern or difference whether related to being LGBTQ or not.

As professionals we all have strengths and weaknesses and aspects of care that test our limitations or our comfort level. If you don't feel that you can provide comprehensive, nonjudgmental care for LGBTQ youth, work to find other resources in your community. Then use your trusting relationship to guide the youth toward those resources. In some communities, those resources are lacking, making it even more important that you can connect the young person to national or regional organizations and to trustworthy online resources.

•• Group Learning and Discussion ••

Prior to meeting, please have a member of your group assemble a list of local support services for sexual and gender minority youth. If none exist, assemble a list of national hotlines.

Break into groups of 3 and work through your choices from among the following scenarios.

1. Melody is a 17-year-old girl coming for routine care. Take a standard sexual history using the ABO framework.

2. Zach is a 16-year-old young man. He became sexually active about a year ago and has had both male and female partners. He is not sure that he wants to label himself, but would like to discuss his feelings with peers. There is no one at his school that he can imagine helping him think this through.

3. Haley is a 15-year-old young woman who has known from an early age that she was attracted to girls. She is in love with 17-year-old Shakira, and they seem to have a healthy relationship. She wants to tell her parents, but has no idea how they would react. The subject of same-sex attraction has never come up explicitly at home except when her 14-year-old twin brothers call female athletes "Lesbos" and, when they fight, they call each other equally offensive homophobic terms. Her mother is in the waiting area. She would appreciate your guidance and facilitation in speaking to her mother.

4. Diamond is a 17-year-old whose gender identity is not clear to you. Have a conversation to learn how best to address and interact with this adolescent. **61.20**

5. A couple you have known since their son was a toddler comes in today for a private conversation. They are nearly certain their son is gay. Their friends also suspect this and have advised them to have him see a psychiatrist or priest to see if he can be "fixed" before this goes too far. They come for your advice.

▪▪▪▪▪▪▪▪ Continuing Education ▪▪▪▪▪▪▪▪

If you are applying for continuing education credits, a test is available online. For more details, visit www.aap.org/reachingteens.

■ Related Video Content

61.0 Working With LGBT Youth Has a High Yield Because We Can Help Them Overcome Stigma, Shame, and Isolation…and Show Them That It Can Get Better. Youth, Dowshen, Reirden, Hawkins, Garofalo.

61.1 LGBTQ Youth Are Not "At Risk"! They Have Been Isolated and Marginalized; They Can Thrive When We Break Their Isolation. Garofalo, Reirden.

61.2 Setting the Stage for ALL Youth: Honesty, Non-judgment, and Respect. Dowshen.

61.3 Using Inclusive Language With All Youth to Create a Safe Space for LGBT Youth. Reirden.

61.4 Avoiding Labels—Talking About Sex in a Developmentally Appropriate Manner. Arrington-Sanders.

61.5 Taking a Sexual History Without Making Assumptions. Dowshen, Arrington-Sanders, Reirden.

61.6 Your Respect and Presence Are More Important to Your Ability to Provide Care to LGBT Youth Than Your Sexual or Gender Identity. Arrington-Sanders, Garofalo.

61.7 Creating a Safe Space for Coming Out. Hawkins.

61.8 "Coming Out" Is a Lifelong Process: How to Support LGBT Youth When They Come Out to You. Hawkins.

61.9 "Coming Out": Disclosure Is on the Youth's (Not the Professional's) Time Line. Garofalo, Reirden.

61.10 The Ideal Coming Out Experience. Youth.

61.11 Be Prepared to Provide Care to a Population That May Be Invisible to You. Be Open. LGBT Youth Will Let You Know When They Are Ready to Talk About Sexual Orientation or Gender Identity. Garofalo, Reirden.

61.12 Providing Appropriate Screening and Prevention Messages for Sexual Minority Youth: Make Decisions Based on Behavior, NOT Identity. Garofalo, Reirden

61.13 How to Make Sexual and Gender Minority Youth More Comfortable With the Physical Examination. Arrington-Sanders.

61.14 The Role of Parents of LGBT Youth: Encouragement, Love, and Support. Youth, Arrington-Sanders, Garofalo.

61.15 The Importance of Role Models for LGBT Youth. Garofalo.

61.16 Being LGBT Is Just One Part of a Young Person's Identity. Garofalo.

61.17 Being Humble: It's OK to Make Mistakes, But Ask in a Respectful Way When Unsure About What Language to Use to Make LGBT Youth Comfortable. Youth, Hawkins.

61.18 LGBT Youth Guidance: It's OK if You Don't Feel Comfortable or Have All the Answers, But Know Your Resources to Get Us the Help We Need. Youth.

61.19 It Can Get Better for LGBT Youth: The Keys to Resilience. Youth.

61.20 Youth Testimony: "This Is How to Address Me" (and Much More): Guidance From a Young Transgender Person. Youth.

61.21 Advice for Coming Out to Peers and Community. Hawkins.

11.7 Who Should Get Tested for HIV and Other STIs? Reirden, Garofalo.

11.12 Avoiding Labels: Exploring Attractions, Behaviors, and Orientation. Hawkins, Arrington-Sanders.

12.1 Creating an LGBTQ-Friendly Space. Dowshen, Arrington-Sanders, Hawkins.

34.3 Preparing Youth to Disclose Difficult Personal Information to Parents. Reirden, Hawkins

■ Related Web Sites

LGBT YOUTH

GLBT National Health Center Youth Talkline
www.glnh.org/talkline

OutProud, the National Coalition for Gay, Lesbian, Bisexual & Transgender Youth
www.outproud.org

The Trevor Project: Suicide Prevention Helpline for Gay and Questioning Youth
www.thetrevorproject.org

YouthResource: A Web Site by and for GLBTQ Youth
www.youthresource.com

It Gets Better Project
www.itgetsbetter.org

Advocates for Youth
www.advocatesforyouth.org

PROFESSIONALS, PARENTS, AND FRIENDS

Gay and Lesbian Medical Association (GLMA): Directory of LGBTQ Friendly Health Care Professionals
www.glma.org

Gay, Lesbian and Straight Education Network (GLSEN)
www.glsen.org

National Gay and Lesbian Task Force: Youth Issues
www.thetaskforce.org/issues/youth

National Youth Advisory Council (NYAC)
www.nyacyouth.org/index.php

Parents, Families and Friends of Lesbians and Gays (PFLAG)
http://community.pflag.org

Safe Schools Coalition
www.safeschoolscoalition.org/safe.html

Family Acceptance Project
http://familyproject.sfsu.edu

Gender Spectrum
http://genderspectrum.org

CHAPTER 62

Reaching Immigrant Youth

Dzung X. Vo, MD, FAAP

 Related Video Content

62.0 Serving Immigrant Youth

■ Why This Matters

Immigrant youth experience many health disparities related to social determinants of health, including minority ethnicity or race, non-majority cultural background, linguistic barriers, and larger societal biases.[1,2] In addition, immigrant youth juggle unique developmental challenges, including developing a racial/ethnic identity and a strategy for managing acculturation. Both of these tasks have profound effects on adolescent behaviors and health.[2,3] By adapting and acculturating to a new culture and society, immigrant youth and families demonstrate tremendous strengths. Professionals working with immigrant youth and families should become familiar with the process of racial/ethnic identity development and acculturation, which, in turn, can help them develop a nuanced understanding of the stressors immigrant youth and families face.

> Recognize and build on strengths that may help immigrant youth adapt successfully, such as courage and persistence, multilingualism and cultural flexibility, and family or community connectedness.

■ Case

Jen is a 13-year-old Chinese American female admitted for malnutrition, low heart rate, and low temperature secondary to anorexia nervosa. She had been having increasing conflicts with her parents over the past year. She began restricting her diet over the past 3 months, down to about 400 kilocalories/day, and lost weight from 110% to 75% of suggested body weight. She endorsed body image dissatisfaction and desire to lose weight. She was described by her parents as increasingly withdrawn, oppositional, and irritable.

Jen's parents emigrated from China (they are first-generation immigrants), and Jen was born and grew up in the United States (second-generation immigrant). Although Jen lived with her parents, she felt emotionally distant from them. *"They don't understand me; they just want me to be the good little Chinese girl."* She told her admitting physician, *"I don't feel Chinese. I hate Chinese food and I barely even speak Chinese. I just want to be like everyone else."*

For their part, Jen's parents felt confused by their daughter's mood and behavior, stating, *"I don't understand why she's acting that way."* and *"Why would she be stressed? She doesn't have anything to be stressed about."* Jen's parents' first language is Cantonese, and they spoke limited English. They felt she was being "disobedient" as a result of "bad influences." They were reluctant to see a mental health counselor, feeling *"counseling is for crazy families"* and *"they wouldn't understand our culture anyway."*

■ Issues With Immigrant Youth

The case illustrates many of the important themes in reaching immigrant youth, including identity development, acculturation, and acculturative stress. Providers should communicate with immigrant youth in a way that explores possible areas of stress related to cultural issues, while also remembering that individual adolescents within immigrant groups are heterogeneous and have unique developmental trajectories. All youth, including immigrant youth, want to be seen and understood as individuals, not just as members of a particular racial/ethnic or cultural group.[1] Two important models of identity development—(1) racial/ethnic identity (REI) development and (2) acculturation theory—can help providers understand possible areas of stress or strength for immigrant youth.

One of the key developmental tasks of adolescence is identity development, exploring the questions, *"Who am I?"* and *"Where do I fit into the world?"* The REI development models describe the process of developing one's sense of belonging to one's group, and asks, *"How do I identify with and relate to my group?"* Phinney's[4] REI model proposes a 3-stage progression.

1. **Unexamined.** In this stage, adolescents have been exposed to ethnic identity issues but have given minimal consideration to their own ethnic identity.
2. **Identity search (exploration).** This stage is sometimes triggered by an event such as an experience of overt discrimination or racism, which forces the adolescent to consider issues of ethnicity, identity, privilege, and racism. Identity search is an intense process of immersion in one's own culture and may involve rejection of the dominant culture.
3. **Achieved identity.** Youth may eventually come to a deeper understanding and appreciation for their ethnic identity and how they fit in with their ethnic group. Achieving this understanding requires coming to terms with cultural differences between their ethnic group and the dominant society, and the lower or disparaged status of their group in the society. The meaning of an achieved identity can vary by individual. For some youth, achieved identity can involve a higher degree of involvement with one's own ethnic group and traditions, while other youth may feel confident in their own ethnic identity without necessarily maintaining ethnic involvement, language, or customs.

For many adolescents, REI development is not linear and unidirectional. Rather it is a dynamic process that can continue in cycles, involving ongoing life experiences and further rethinking of the role and meaning of one's ethnic identity.

Acculturation is a related but distinct concept to REI development. Acculturation is "the dual process of cultural and psychological change that takes place as a result of contact between 2 or more cultural groups and their individual members."[5] Traditional models of acculturation are unidimensional, progressing from "less acculturated" to "more acculturated," with the end result of acculturation being complete assimilation into the dominant society and culture.

More recent literature on acculturation proposes a more complex, multidimensional process. Berry[5] proposes 4 acculturation strategies that derive from 2 basic issues facing immigrants. The issues involve the distinction between (1) a relative preference for maintaining one's heritage culture and identity (which is similar to REI theory) and (2) a relative preference for participating in the larger society. Generally positive or negative orientations to these 2 issues lead to 4 possible acculturation strategies.

1. **Integration.** Youth maintain their own heritage, culture, and identity and also seek involvement in the larger society and culture.
2. **Assimilation.** Youth prefer involvement in the larger society, turn their back on involvement with their heritage culture, and become absorbed into the dominant society.
3. **Separation.** Youth value holding on to their original culture and generally avoid interaction with others outside of their culture.
4. **Marginalization.** Youth have little possibility or interest in maintaining their heritage culture (often for historical reasons of enforced cultural loss) and little interest or possibility in involvement with the larger society (often for reasons of racism or discrimination.) An example of this would be Southeast Asian American immigrant youth who feel marginalized from their families because of acculturative dissonance between the youth and their families (ie, the youth may not be fluent in their language of origin or be familiar with traditional cultural practices). These youth may also be marginalized from the mainstream American community because of their appearance or other cultural factors, and this dual marginalization may place them at higher risk for health risk behaviors.

Racial/ethnic identity and acculturation have important implications for adolescent health and behavior.[2-5] Higher levels of ethnic identity have been associated with improved markers of mental health. Less acculturated youth may be at higher risk for social isolation and mental health problems. On the other hand, more acculturation among youth has been linked to higher likelihood of health risk behaviors, including substance use, sexual behaviors, and obesity-related behaviors—a pattern referred to as the "healthy immigrant effect."[6] Acculturative stress associated with cultural conflict can be a major stressor for immigrant youth. For example, acculturative dissonance (acculturation gaps or discrepancies between parents' and children's acculturation) may disrupt family relationships and increase risk for significant family conflicts[2,7] Emerging research suggests that bicultural self-efficacy, meaning the ability of an individual to function effectively in multiple cultural contexts, and an integrated acculturation strategy may be protective for optimal psychological and sociocultural adaptation and functioning.[2,3]

■ Working With Immigrant Youth 12.2

Professionals working with immigrant youth and families should consider adopting the following strategies in history-taking and counseling:

- **Strength-based counseling.** Recognize and build on strengths that may help immigrant youth adapt successfully, such as courage and persistence, multilingualism and cultural flexibility, and family or community connectedness.
- **Cultural humility.** Providers should refrain from making assumptions and judgments about immigrant youth and should also be aware of and manage their own (perhaps unconscious) biases (see Chapter 19).
- **Screen all adolescents equally** for health risk and protective factors. Some providers may not feel it necessary to screen certain immigrant groups for health risk behaviors. In a study on Chinese and Vietnamese immigrant youth, the immigrant youth felt providers assumed they did not engage in certain health behaviors such as sex and substance use, and the youth wanted their providers to ask them about these health behaviors.[1] (See Chapter 18.)
- **Immigration history.** Providers should ask about the youth and family's immigration history, with particular attention to generational status of parents and youth, and possible histories of trauma and marginalization associated with migration. Immigrant and refugee families may have fled conflict and war in their countries of origin. In addition, immigrant and refugee youth and families may face barriers to education, employment,

and health care related to their immigration documentation status. This severe stress and trauma may have profound effects on the families and youth, as well as on the providers listening to traumatic stories (see Chapter 67).

- **Assess REI development and acculturation.** Asking about markers of identity and acculturation can help providers understand immigrant youth better. Useful questions include, *"Where were you born?" "Where were your parents born?" "What does being* (insert ethnic group) *mean to you?" "What language do you speak at home?" "What language do you prefer to speak?"* and *"What ethnic group(s) do you prefer to hang out with?"*

- **Assess and address acculturative stress.** Ask about potential threats to identity development and acculturation, including real and perceived discrimination and racism. Screen for symptoms of mood and mental health complications, keeping in mind that mental health symptoms may present differently in different cultural contexts (eg, with physical vs psychological symptoms). Provide validation and anticipatory guidance about acculturative stress, discrimination, and racism. Provide treatment or referrals for stress management and mental health treatment if indicated. Potential questions to ask and messages to provide include

  — *"Some young people who are also* (insert ethnic group) *have told me that they have been bullied, harassed, called names, or treated unfairly just because they are* (insert ethnic group). *Has this ever happened to you?"* Then listen deeply, without judgment, and allow the youth to tell his story.

  — If the youth describes experiences of discrimination: *"I am sorry to hear that you have had to experience that kind of treatment. What you experienced is a kind of racism or discrimination. It is not your fault, and no one should ever have to experience that. It must be really stressful. How are you coping with it?"*

  — If the youth does not describe experiences of discrimination: *"I am glad to hear that you haven't experienced that kind of treatment. I wish I could tell you that you never will experience racism and discrimination in this country. Unfortunately, I know from my own experience and the youth I work with that there is real racism and discrimination in this country. I also know that experiences with racism and discrimination can be very upsetting. Please know that if you ever have these experiences in the future, this is a safe space to talk about it and get support. Is there anyone else in your life who you would feel safe talking to about these issues if they ever come up for you in the future?"*

- **Acculturation gaps.** Try to get a sense of not only the youth's acculturation, but also the acculturation of his parents/caregivers, and possible acculturation gaps. Ask about potential linguistic and cultural barriers within the family. Ask about family conflicts, and explore whether or not they have a cultural component. Provide guidance around acculturation gaps and parenting for both parent(s) and youth, using culturally specific messages or materials if appropriate (eg, see Lee[8]). Develop and maintain referral resources for culturally competent family therapy in your community, and refer if necessary for significant family conflicts that affect functioning and mental health.

- **Confidentiality and language interpretation.** Confidentiality and the limits of confidentiality are cornerstones of adolescent psychosocial interviewing (see Chapter 14). Professional language interpretation is considered the best practice for reducing linguistic barriers for immigrants. However, acculturation may affect adolescents' views on confidentiality and interpretation. In our study on Asian American youth in Philadelphia, we found less-acculturated youth were more likely to want to translate for their families, less likely to want their health information to be kept confidential, and more likely to intentionally mistranslate in order to protect their families from potentially upsetting information.[1] Nonetheless, providers should discuss and maintain appropriate confidentiality with all youth, and treat all youth equally.

- **Promote positive REI development, bicultural self-efficacy, and integrated acculturation.** This can be done by acknowledging and reinforcing markers of bicultural self-efficacy and integration, such as multilingualism, and involvement in multicultural activities and social networks. Providers may also encourage participation in community youth development programs that promote connectedness and positive racial/ethnic identity development.

Improving the Health of Immigrant Youth

Youth providers, in their roles as advocates, educators, and researchers, can make a difference for the health of immigrant youth in many ways beyond individual clinical care.

- **Systems advocacy.** Advocate for and use quality professional language interpretation services, culturally competent services, and elimination of disparities and barriers that affect immigrant youth.
- **Make health care settings immigrant friendly.** This can include visual markers, such as multilingual signs, and images and representations of diverse youth and families in posters and other materials.
- **Training.** Teach health care trainees about disparities, cultural humility and cultural competence, identity development, and acculturation.
- **Research.** Move beyond assumptions of homogeneous ethnic groups, and document disparities among ethnic subgroups. Contribute to research that documents disparities and promotes health equity. In framing and reporting research, be mindful not to perpetuate harmful stereotypes that can increase stigma among marginalized communities, and highlight the role of social determinants of health in racial/ethnic disparities. Contribute to the growing research on racial/ethnic identity and acculturation, especially as it pertains to adolescent health and behaviors.

•• Group Learning and Discussion ••

In order to create a practice more receptive and helpful for immigrant youth, consider discussing the following issues:

1. What ethnic minorities and/or immigrant youth walk through our doors?
2. As each of them looks at our posters and public health materials, will they see people who look like them?
3. Do we have access to a language line or translator so their parents can be fully and respectfully included?
4. Do we use youth as translators for their parents? If so, what are the implications for privacy? What are the implications for trusting the accuracy of the translation?
5. Do we hold a cognitive bias that immigrants tend to be "good" kids or, conversely, "troublemakers?" How might this affect our interactions with these youth?
6. How can we discuss and support positive REI development and acculturation in our youth?

■■■■■■■■ Continuing Education ■■■■■■■■

If you are applying for continuing education credits, a test is available online. For more details, visit www.aap.org/reachingteens.

■ References

1. Vo DX, Pate OL, Zhao H, Siu P, Ginsburg KR. Voices of Asian American youth: important characteristics of clinicians and clinical sites. *Pediatrics.* 2007;120(6):e1481–e1493

2. Vo DX, Park MJ. Racial/ethnic disparities and culturally competent health care among youth and young men. *Am J Mens Health.* 2008;2(2):192–205

3. Berry JW, Phinney JS, Sam DL, Vedder P. Immigrant youth: acculturation, identity, and adaptation. *Appl Psychol.* 2006;55(3):303–332

4. Phinney JS. Ethnic identity in adolescents and adults: review of research. *Psychol Bull.* 1990;108(3):499–514

5. Berry JW. Acculturation: living successfully in two cultures. *Int J Intercult Relat.* 2005;29(6):697–712

6. Flores G, Brotanek J. The healthy immigrant effect: a greater understanding might help us improve the health of all children. *Arch Pediatr Adolesc Med.* 2005;159(3):295–297

7. Le TN, Stockdale G. Acculturative dissonance, ethnic identity, and youth violence. *Cultur Divers Ethnic Minor Psychol.* 2008;14(1):1–9

8. Lee E. *Ten Principles on Raising Chinese American Teens.* San Francisco, CA: Community Youth Center; 1988. http://www.evelynlee-mentalhealth.org/ten_principles.asp. Accessed June 26, 2013

■ Related Video Content

62.0 Serving Immigrant Youth. Vo.

62.1 Serving Across Cultures. Trent.

12.2 Creating an Immigrant Youth-Friendly Space. Vo.

CHAPTER 63

America's Children: The Unique Needs and Culture of Military Youth

LTC Keith M. Lemmon, MD, FAAP

 Related Video Content

63.0 Supporting Military-Affiliated Youth

■ Why This Matters

Military children and adolescents occupy a special place in the heart of the nation. This unique population of American youth represents the legacy of the nation's warriors who have given so much to the country over the last decade in the wars in Iraq and Afghanistan. Military children and teens serve and sacrifice on behalf of the nation as much as their parents do. They just do it in a different way.

> **Military children and teens serve and sacrifice on behalf of the nation as much as their parents do. They just do it in a different way.**

Soldiers, sailors, airmen, and marines risk their lives routinely to protect the interests of the United States. They spend long tours away from their homes and their loved ones. They are exposed to dangerous and potentially life-threatening circumstances on a routine basis. Their children often grow up without their physical presence and influence. For military members, serving is voluntary. For children and adolescents, on the other hand, their entrance into the odyssey of military life and the service and sacrifice required of them is involuntary. This special population has a unique culture and is exposed to specific types of adversity.

Military children and adolescents come from a diverse cross-section of the American population. Many live on military installations across the United States and around the world. Military children, especially those from the reserve component, are also found in the school rooms, playgrounds, and our offices everywhere.

Military-dependent children face a host of unique stresses. During peace time, military children move frequently, are commonly stationed away from extended family support, and have parents who have highly demanding jobs often requiring regular travel for training or missions. During wartime, military children face the prospect of multiple deployments of their father or mother into a hostile combat zone; deal with a physical absence during a deployment and a possible emotional absence in the lead up to and recovery from a deployment; and continually deal with the specter of a combat injury, death, or even suicide as a potential outcome of a parent's military service. They also must deal with frequently altered family roles and increased stress in the nonmilitary family member who remains at home.

■ Military Child and Adolescent Culture

Many military children may be bearing complex psychosocial burdens that are not readily visible to the culturally naive observer.[1] Providing care for children in military families requires "appropriate knowledge, understanding and appreciation of cultural distinctions" as outlined in the 1999 American Academy of Pediatrics policy statement on culturally competent care.[2] In order to deliver effective care to military youth, a more in-depth understanding of what it means to be the child of a military service member is imperative. Unfortunately, there have been no sociological studies systematically outlining the specific cultural components of military children. As in other cultures, there are wide variations of individual members, but a general understanding of the norm is a helpful place to begin. Having served in the military since 1989; raising my own children on military bases and communities across the country; and dealing daily with the physical, emotional, and behavioral health needs of the children and adolescents of other military service members, I have gathered some observational insight into the basic components of military youth culture.

There are both positive and negative aspects to military youth culture. Many military children get to live in and integrate into diverse geographical areas of the world that other US children will never get to see. This may help them be more open-minded and tolerant of other cultures, races, classes, and religions. Military children, especially those who live on a military installation, express an enhanced sense of physical security while, at the same time, feeling uneasy about being surrounded by instruments of war. Being a military family member provides a significant advantage to getting children's basic needs met, especially during a time of financial insecurity affecting the rest of the country. Military children's parents receive regular, predictable income for their service, along with the benefits of free and readily accessible health care and prescriptions, discounted and tax-free food and commodities at post exchanges and commissaries, as well as free on-post housing or tax-free housing allowances. Community services on military installations are usually comprehensive with excellent child care, after-school programs, recreational facilities, and programs for military children and their families. This often helps children experience an enhanced sense of community that can mitigate the challenging aspects of military culture.

Military children realize early that the needs of the military service often come before their own needs. It is not that military parents want this, but it is a mandate and a principle of what it means to serve in the military. Mission first is a founding tenet of military service. Most military parents do an excellent job of tempering this requirement with providing for the physical and emotional needs of their children, but there are times when it is out of their control. Most military kids move frequently during the course of their parent's military career and state that these frequent moves help them develop the ability to make friends easily. This may not be true for children who are introverted or have a social or developmental challenge. After experiencing a few moves and the negative emotions that accompany leaving comfortable friends and environments behind, some children adapt by turning inward and avoiding the social risks necessary to make new friends. Older military children and adolescents are often perplexed when faced with the question of where are they from. They're not sure whether to answer with where they were born, where their extended family has its roots, or where they spent the most time during a particular assignment. Some military children look at this as a positive aspect of their life experience, while others have trouble integrating this into their sense of identity and belonging.

Military children receive frequent reinforcement that the work that their parent does is meaningful; this often flavors how children of service members consider options for what to do with their lives. Since military service is not particularly lucrative, military kids generally see their parents' work as a means to serve in devotion to something greater than oneself rather than working to acquire wealth. This can result in internal conflict, guilt, or shame, as the military child navigates the normal egocentric stages of childhood when it is normal to be focused on themselves rather than on self-sacrifice.

Military children receive their parents' benefits until they are 21 years old unless they are enrolled as full-time students, in which case they receive them until 23 years of age. At that time, after a lifetime of relying on the comprehensive benefits of their military parents, they must transition to the civilian world. Many military children choose to join the military themselves, which can sometimes be a less challenging transition than entering the civilian world.

The military still has a predominantly authoritarian leadership style as its default, especially among the enlisted and noncommissioned officer ranks. This leadership style is adaptive for much of the difficult work service members must perform, but can have a negative effect when carried over into parenting. This is not to say that all, or even most, military children are raised with an authoritarian style. In fact, some military parents might compensate for the stresses of a military lifestyle by erring toward more permissive parenting. Military children, like most children, will likely benefit from an authoritative (or balanced) parenting approach (see Chapter 36).

It is increasingly clear that there are some significant and lasting effects of having a family member engaged in prolonged and recurrent military deployments. Research demonstrated that parental distress in the at-home caregiver and the active duty member, as well as cumulative length of parental combat-related deployments, independently predicted increased child depression and externalizing symptoms among 6- to 12-year-old military-dependent children. Although behavioral adjustment and depression levels were comparable to community norms, anxiety was significantly elevated in children of both currently deployed and recently returned service members. These findings seem to indicate that parental combat deployment has a cumulative effect on children that remains even after the deployed parent returns home, and that is predicted by psychological distress of both the active duty and at-home caregiver.[3] Among 101 Army families, 32% of children of deployed soldiers scored at "high risk" for psychosocial problems on the Pediatric Symptom Checklist (2.5 times higher than the national norm).[4] In a large retrospective cohort study, it was found that mental and behavioral health visits increased by 11% in military children when a parent deployed, behavioral disorders increased 19%, and stress disorders increased 18%.[5]

■ Maintaining Family Connections Through Deployment 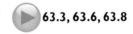 63.3, 63.6, 63.8

Multiple deployments have caused a generation of military children to be physically separated from at least one of their parents for significant portions of their growing years. It is important that parents know that although they cannot change the basic reality of this aspect of military life, they *can* take steps to decrease the impact on their children. Military resources such as family readiness and support groups offer important ongoing support. Your role may be to offer brief suggestions and then confirm families are connected to existing supportive resources[6] (see Related Web Sites for some suggestions) and behavioral health specialists when appropriate.

This section will offer some suggestions on how to maintain connections during deployment. They derive from military families who have offered their insight, wisdom, and experience through informal interviews and group discussions. Their ideas may serve as talking points between you and families. The suggestions here are not meant to substitute for those from military professionals.

The goal for families has to be to maintain a continual connection and meaningful communication despite very real external challenges. It's naïve to believe deployment will have no impact at all. The goal is to minimize that impact.

■ Reducing the Stress and Maximizing the Benefits Associated With Communication

Technology allows communication at levels that would have been previously unimaginable. Separated parents can often be involved in making family decisions and in keeping up, to some degree, with family events. However, precisely because these communications are so highly anticipated and sometimes their timing is unpredictable, they can also be stressful.

The home-based parent should take care not to make the communications something children would rather avoid. While it's important to have the deployed parent involved in family functioning, it's important these touch points not be used only as opportunities to discuss the tough issues. They should be moments to impart guidance, not punishment. Parents should encourage children to focus mostly on the things in their lives that make them proud and to also get advice about any concerns occupying their minds.

Parents report that deployed parents sometimes have difficulty finding the right words or setting the right tone in conversations because switching mentalities from being a soldier in a war zone to being a parent is sometimes quite difficult. Even though they want desperately to be "present," they may have trouble getting the conversation started. Sometimes their frustration may become masked as inattention or even anger. The weight of parental guilt they feel in their inability to have a "normal" conversation with their family may damage their self-image as an effective parent or attentive spouse and, therefore, have later implications for reintegration into the family. Families suggest there are steps they can take to make it easier for the distant parent to comfortably engage with his or her children.

- The home-based parent can "drop seeds" to the deployed parent regarding what to talk about. An advanced e-mail can prep the deployed parent on topics of interest, major milestones, struggles, or accomplishments. This may help the deployed spouse avoid the discomfort and shame associated with an inability to connect with his or her children.

Spouses have also shared that they struggle knowing how much to share long distance. They want to include their husbands or wives but don't want to upset them. In fact, they may be guided not to upset their spouses with information that may distract them from the mission, especially if there is no action they can take. Home-based spouses know that, if they concern their spouses but leave them unable to fix the problem, they may be rendered frustrated and powerless. This recurring dilemma places pressure on the home spouse and leaves the distant spouse worrying if something important is being withheld.

- Families may consider agreeing prior to departure what the deployed parent needs to know. That way, each individual can specify the level of detail important to him or her. This takes some of the weight off the caregiver at home who is concerned about worrying the deployed parent. Even if this understanding is made prior to deployment, situations can change on a daily basis, and the home parent should remain open to the cues that a given conversation needs to remain lighter. Parents might first create an advance "code word" that suggests that a check-in is desired, but it's not a good time for a deep conversation. If the code word is activated, the conversation can remain light and reassuring, while avoiding straying into harder topics the deployed parent is not in the frame of mind to address.

The pressure of making the most of the few minutes may sometimes be too much for children and teens who may feel shy or awkward trying to summarize their week or express their emotions on the spot. They propose creating a communications center to alleviate this problem.

- The communications center consists of a bulletin board and a supply of pens, markers, post-it notes, and a calendar. The caregiver encourages children to make notes on the communications center so they can share them during the call to the deployed parent. The notes can be about sports, grades, or just important stories or feelings. When the parent calls, the children collect their notes and are reminded of what they wanted to talk about. This may be particularly useful when communications are sporadic or unpredictable. In those cases, the excitement can leave the family not knowing where to start, and then feeling frustrated at the end of the contact.

Another barrier to effective communication during deployment may be a parent's inability to use words to express affection. Many caring and responsive parents express their love through their presence or physical interactions. Consider the father who can be a jungle gym for his young children, a point guard on the basketball court, fully present at school meetings and dance recitals, but who is never quite capable of finding the words to express his emotions. During deployment, distance prevents presence and it may be that only words are useful. Therefore, it may be helpful to hold conversations prior to deployment about the importance of learning to use language to express love and offer reinforcement. A person raised without these words may find this suggestion a serious challenge. Nevertheless, it may be helpful to think about developing this skill set.

■ Building Memories

- Perhaps before deployment, the service member can record DVDs or write letters to be brought out during special events like graduations, birthdays, and sporting events, and even the daily routines like bedtime. Simple "I love you" recordings, messages, and notes can be left unrelated to any event as reminders to children of the unconditional and ever-present parental love. It may also reassure them that the parent is gone because he or she is serving the nation, not because he or she wants to be away.
- Equally as important is for the "home team" to prepare memories to share with the returning parent. Watching videos of a winning goal will never match being there, but it does allow families to relive moments together. Even recording favorite television shows or major professional games can allow the family to experience those missed opportunities together. Finally, annotated photo albums can serve as tools for telling richer stories later.

These memory tools will be invaluable for returning parents because they will reinforce how closely parents were held even while they were away. They also may be helpful for the "home team" to have a project to focus on together. Important conversations can be held about the deployed parent while working on the projects. Opportunities for listening and talking may abound while working on the projects, allowing the caregiver insights into how the children are coping with the separation.

■ Parental Roles in Discipline During Deployment

One of the impacts that deployment has on family life is that the distant parent cannot participate in day-to-day discipline. Discipline is such a central part of parenting that this produces frustration in both spouses. The challenge is to find an appropriate and productive role in discipline for the deployed spouse.

Why Is It Hard for Deployed Parents to Be Involved in Discipline?

Most discipline is not about major infractions, it is about the daily guidance parents use to mold their children. Discipline happens every time a parent notices and reinforces the positive and directs away from negative behavior. Discipline loses its effectiveness if the young person cannot clearly associate the consequence she receives with the action she took. For this reason, the most obvious reason that the deployed parent cannot be optimally involved is that he simply is not present.

The deployed parent's ability to be involved in discipline is limited by more than geographical distance. Many deployed parents are under extreme stress and exposed to trauma that they cannot share, making it difficult to find the right words or set the right tone in conversations. Deployed parents are also likely immersed in a hierarchical communication style. This communication style may be counter to what is beneficial and effective in family relationships: listening empathetically, conveying mutual respect, considering other's feelings or stresses, compromise, negotiation, expressing vulnerabilities and fears, and providing comfort and emotional support.

Next, it may be asking too much of the home-based spouse to include the deployed spouse, especially for issues that may require more heavy-handed discipline. First, the home-bound spouse may be conflicted about upsetting the deployed spouse. Although the deployed spouse should likely be informed about major infractions that concern safety, if she becomes knowledgeable but left unable to fix the problem, she may become frustrated in her powerlessness. The answer to this dilemma is not easily found and likely needs to be decided on a case-by-case basis.

One final difficulty that involvement with discipline poses for the deployed spouse is that it can position him or her as "the heavy," potentially interfering with maintaining the best family connections possible during separation. The interaction time is so limited that it is important that it is optimized. Children should not dread the contact. As tempting as it may be to say, *"Wait until we Skype with your father on Wednesday night!!"* parents should be guided against using the contact as a threat. Again, there are case-by-case exceptions where both parents' involvement is appropriate.

What Can Be the Role of Deployed Parents While They Are Away?

Despite the concerns listed above, it remains important that deployed parents *do* remain involved in discipline. The answer may be found in the meaning of the word "discipline"— to teach. The deployed parent can remain involved in teaching and guiding—the most important aspects of discipline.

They can focus their energy on the positive parenting that ultimately promotes desired behaviors and reduces the need for that part of discipline requiring consequences or punishments. During calls, texts, and Skyping the deployed parent can remember to mention how important his child/adolescent is to him; stay focused and interested in what the youth wants to talk about; stay abreast of their activities, games, and major school events; and provide positive reinforcement. For example, a deployed father might say, *"Mom mentioned how helpful you've been cutting the grass. She says it looks even better than when I do it! Thanks bud, I really appreciate it."*

Preparing for Deployment

A key to discipline is that adolescents learn that they earn freedom and privileges through demonstrated responsibility and actions. This means that discipline can be discussed in advance of any problem; in fact, the best discipline can prevent problems. When parents lay out clear expectations that are associated with privileges, youth learn what it takes to earn privileges and what it takes to be able to keep them. Consequences can be immediate because when a young person shirks responsibilities or breaks the prearranged rules, he loses the associated privileges. The lessons are efficient because consequences are always tied directly to behaviors; they are "fair" because they are understood in advance.

The military family that makes the effort to schedule a meeting and create a written contract with their older child or adolescent about privileges and expectations will have the benefit of both parents exerting joint discipline even through deployment. The written contract records understandings and all parties signal agreement with their signatures. The teen understands that *"In order to get XXX, my parents need to me to do YYY"* or, conversely, they understand that both parents have stated, *"In order for us to feel comfortable with XXX, we need to know that you will do YYY."* If these kind of agreements are made as a family in advance of deployments, and perhaps revisited every 3 months while deployed or at least during mid-deployment leave, the separated parent will be "present" with every major disciplinary opportunity.

When an adolescent is pushing for relaxed privileges, the non-deployed parent can refer to the written agreement, remind their adolescent that all 3 of them (both parents and adolescent) agreed to these conditions, and remind the adolescent that they all agreed to reassess significant changes during mid-deployment leave. In the case of negative behavior, rather than needing to summon the authority of the distant parent with potentially alienating statements like, *"You're lucky your mother isn't here,"* or *"Wait until your father gets on the phone,"* the home parent will be able to say, *"Both us agreed that we expect you to XXX, and that the consequence would be YYY if you were not able to show responsibility."* This will never replace the actual presence of a parent, but it can produce a tangible reminder of the distant parent's concern and desire to be involved.

■ Discussing "Parentified" Adolescents During Deployment

Military families have to acclimate to frequent and sometimes prolonged separations in which at least one parent is absent from the role as caregiver. In response, older children and adolescents may take on additional roles within the home, including child care activities. In some cases, they may even care for the emotional needs of the remaining parent who is enduring additional stressors. This may have both positive and negative implications for healthy development. It may also affect the reintegration experience for the returning parent.

The phenomenon of children taking over parental or adult roles is called "parentification." There is scant literature on the subject specific to the military child and less specific to the military parent returning to a household in which a teen has been parentified. It is not likely that your interaction can prevent an adolescent from taking on adult roles in the setting of a household with a functionally single parent caring for multiple children. There is simply a need for older children to offer their assistance. Rather, this brief discussion will offer some points you may want to raise to increase the likelihood of a positive outcome.

Adolescents who take on household tasks to aid in its function are likely to reap some important benefits. First, they can earn a genuine sense of contribution as well as pride in their displayed competencies. Second, there may be benefits to their character development, as they understand the importance of being a role model to their younger siblings. These young people also may display maturity beyond their years. Above all, they can learn how family members care for each other and how families function best when responsibility is shared. Current literature discusses the potential benefits for the parentified child. A promising finding is that parentified children may develop increased posttraumatic growth and resiliency, although more research is needed to confirm results.[7] Additionally, for those adolescents with major stressors in their lives, such as having an ill parent or family instability, parentification has been shown to be predictive of better coping skills and less substance use.[8]

On the other hand, literature on parentification also reveals concerns about negative outcomes such as increased substance use,[9] risk for mental illness,[10] poor relationship functioning,[11,12] and youth internalizing and externalizing behaviors.[11] In the parentified child, there are concerns that there may be a disruption to the normal developmental process of individuation (understanding oneself as an individual independent and apart from one's family). Of particular concern are those children who have had to care for the emotional needs of their parents.[11,13]

The literature on the military connected child reveals that adolescents generally have a more difficult time with reintegration than do younger children.[14,15] This is likely multifactorial and tied at least somewhat to the normal developmental struggle for independence all adolescents must pass through. It may be particularly challenging to have gained more independence during a parent's absence only to lose some of it on his or her return. The loss of that independence may come from returning parents treating the adolescent in a pattern similar to the way the adolescent was treated a year ago (a long time developmentally in the life of adolescents).

Adolescents indicate that the difficulty of reintegration stems from the returning parent's lack of appreciation for the teen's maturation and lack of recognition of newly established family routines and responsibilities.[12] It is worth considering that a child who was functioning as an adult in the household will be particularly resistant to being disciplined or monitored by a parent who has been absent for a prolonged period. The parentified adolescent may experience the reintegration of the deployed parent as an unwelcomed step backward on his road to independence.

Talking Points to Consider

Below are examples of ways to breach the topic of parentification.

- *"It's going to be tough managing a household with your (husband/wife) gone for a year. Tell me about your plans for managing this period. I know your oldest child is X years old, do you think she will be helpful?"*
- *"This will give her a wonderful opportunity to contribute to your family, and she should feel great about this. Teens love opportunities to demonstrate their maturity and take a lot of pride in their adult skills."*
- *"I want to see her get all of the benefits from helping out and not any of the potential problems. Sometimes kids who take on extra household roles may experience some problems. Would you like to discuss this for a minute or 2 so you can think this through a bit to make sure you can get all the help you need while decreasing the chances that there will be any problems?"*

If permission to engage is granted, consider any of the points below if they are relevant to the family.

- *"It is still important for teens to have some time with their friends. He may be so eager to please you or to prove to himself that he is an adult that he may sacrifice some of those good and important times with friends. I don't want him to resent that later. It is good for him to learn to put family first, just make sure that he still allows himself to have some kid time too."*

- *"This is a time where some downtime is essential to adolescents because it can be the time where they figure out who they want to become. So make sure he has some of that quiet time to just figure things out."*

- *"Sometimes I worry that kids who feel they have to be 'strong' to help out might also feel that it is babyish to go their parents for help. In their effort to please their parents, they might forget about themselves and fail to turn to their parents for the support they still need. So make sure he is clear how much you appreciate his help, but also that he understands that he remains your child and that you will always be there for him too."*

- *"Sometimes kids who take on extra roles in the house go out of their way to also protect you. It seems you are really close and he's wise enough to know how many extra stresses you are under. It is important for him to know that he is already helping you by taking on so many extra responsibilities at home. He shouldn't feel as though it's his job also to take care of you. Let him know that you have friends too, and let him see you taking care of yourself. Yes, taking care of yourself really is the best thing you can do to take care of your kids."*

- *"Sometimes teens have the toughest time when their parent returns from deployment. It's tough for them to suddenly have an extra parent giving them rules, monitoring their behavior, and disciplining them when necessary. At the same time, it is important they receive all of this support. It may be that some kids who have taken on extra roles in the household will be particularly resentful of being told what to do. That's why it's so important that, as helpful as your son is while your spouse is away, he still knows you are in charge. Never stop monitoring him or having him check in with you. At the same time let him know that, as long as he keeps demonstrating responsible behavior, he will continue earning your trust. That will make it easier on your spouse when he/she returns."*

■ Avoiding Perfectionism   63.1

The military insists on very high standards because there is literally no room for error. Consequently, parents may hold their own children to exceedingly high goals and expectations. Between this and military youths' strong desire to not create additional stress on their parents, they may be at increased risk for perfectionism (see Chapter 48).

■ Conclusion

The circumstances created by wars have traditionally brought about significant advances in medical knowledge. It is likely that one of the more important health advances to come from the current war will be a more sophisticated understanding of psychological trauma and its aftermath. Much work is being done to better understand combat stress, post-traumatic stress disorder, and traumatic brain injury in service members and veterans. It is imperative that military youth advocates ensure that the related effects experienced by children and adolescents are characterized as well. Understanding how combat-related psychological stress in military members is experienced by youth living in military families is a critical concept yet to be fully understood. Military-affiliated children of future conflicts deserve to benefit from the lessons learned from these years.

Understanding military youth culture and the contexts these adolescents navigate is the first step to effectively serving these youth. Then we can contribute to their healthy development by helping their families navigate deployment while maintaining family connection, using effective discipline strategies, and avoiding parentification.

●● Group Learning and Discussion ●●

1. Discuss whether you are aware of military-affiliated youth in your practice setting. (Please consider that National Guard and Reserve youth likely are seen in your center and have special needs.)

2. Discuss what screening questions you should consider asking to check in to be sure military youth are managing the additional stressors of military-affiliated life. (It is important to ask these questions without assuming these youth are not coping well. In fact, despite their added stressors, most military youth are quite resilient.)

3. Break into pairs and practice the following conversations you might have with military parents:
    a. Taking care of themselves as a first step of being able to care for their children and teens
    b. Maintaining connection during deployment
    c. Handling discipline during deployment
    d. Avoiding parentification

Continuing Education

If you are applying for continuing education credits, a test is available online. For more details, visit www.aap.org/reachingteens.

References

1. Lemmon K, Chartrand M. Caring for America's children: military youth in time of war. *Pediatr Rev.* 2009;30(6):e42–e48

2. American Academy of Pediatrics Committee on Pediatric Workforce. Culturally effective pediatric care: education and training issues. *Pediatrics.* 1999;103:167–170

3. Lester P, Peterson K, Reeves J, et al. The long war and parental combat deployment: effects on military children and at-home spouses. *J Am Acad Child Adolesc Psychiatry.* 2010;49(4):310–320

4. Flake E, Davis B, Johnson P, Middleton L. The psychosocial effect of deployment on children. *J Dev Behav Pediatr.* 2009;30:271–278

5. Gorman G, Matilda E, Hisle-Gorman E. Wartime military deployment and increased pediatric mental health and behavioral health complaints. *Pediatrics.* 2010;126(6):1058–1066

6. Esposito-Smythers C, Wolff J, Lemmon KM, Bodzy M, Swenson RR, Spirito A. Military youth and the deployment cycle: emotional health consequences and recommendations for intervention. *J Fam Psychol.* 2011;25(4):497–507

7. Hooper LM, Marotta SA, Lanthier RP. Predictors of growth and distress following childhood parentification: a retrospective exploratory study. *J Child Fam Stud.* 2008;17(5):693–705

8. Stein JA, Rotheram-Borus MJ, Lester P. Impact of parentification on long-term outcomes among children of parents with HIV/AIDS. *Fam Process.* 2007;46(3):317–333

9. Chase ND, Demming MP, Wells MC. Parentification, parental alcoholism, and academic status among young adults. *Am J Fam Ther.* 1998;26(2):105–114

10. Jones R, Wells M. An empirical study of parentification and personality. *Am J Fam Ther.* 1996; 24:145–152

11. Peris TS, Goeke-Morey MC, Cummings EM, Emery RE. Marital conflict and support seeking by parents in adolescence: empirical support for the parentification construct. *J Fam Psychol.* 2008;22(4):633–642

12. Valleau P M, Bergner RM, Horton CB. Parentification and caretaker syndrome: an empirical investigation. *Fam Ther.* 1995;22(3):157–164

13. McMahon TJ, Luthar SS. Defining characteristics and potential consequences of caretaking burden among children living in urban poverty. *Am J Orthopsychiatry.* 2007;77(2):267–281

14. Chandra A, Lara-Cinisomo S, Jaycox LH, et al. Children on the homefront: the experience of children from military families. *Pediatrics*. 2010;125(1);16–25

15. Huebner AJ, Mancini JA. *Adjustments among Adolescents in Military Families When a Parent is Deployed*. West Lafayette, IN: Military Family Research Institute at Purdue University; 2005

■ Related Video Content

63.0 Supporting Military-Affiliated Youth. Lemmon.

63.1 Addressing Perfectionism in Military Youth. Youth, Lemmon, Ginsburg.

63.2 Military Youth: Service, Resilience, and Leadership. Lemmon.

63.3 Military Families: The Importance of Staying Connected. Lemmon.

63.4 A Plea to Military Parents: Caring for Yourself Is the Best Way to Help Your Children Thrive. Lemmon.

63.5 Seeking Help Can Be an Act of Strength. Lemmon.

63.6 Maintaining Family Connections During Deployment. Ginsburg.

63.7 What Can I Do to Help Military Youth Navigate Through Adolescence? Lemmon.

63.8 Military Youth Coping With Separation: When Family Members Deploy. Youth.

■ Related Handouts/Supplementary Materials

Maintaining Connection...during Deployment with Your Teenager

Staying Connected...to your School-Aged Child

■ Related Web Sites

American Academy of Pediatrics Deployment Support Web Site
www2.aap.org/sections/uniformedservices/deployment/index.html

MilitaryKidsConnect.com
https://www.militarykidsconnect.org

Military One Source
www.militaryonesource.mil

Military Child Initiative
www.jhsph.edu/mci

Military Child Education Coalition
www.militarychild.org

National Military Family Association (NMFA)—Operation Purple Camps
www.militaryfamily.org/our-programs/operation-purple

CHAPTER 64

Foster Care Youth: Engaging Foster Care Youth Into Care

Tonya A. Chaffee, MD, MPH, FAAP

 Related Video Content

64.0 Meeting the Unique Needs of Foster Care Youth

■ Why This Matters

Approximately 50% of the estimated 408,000 children and youth in foster care are adolescents. Adolescents are more likely to have been in foster care for longer periods, lived in multiple placements, and resided in institutional or group settings. Each year approximately 28,000 teens "age out" of foster care. Of these young people, 25% suffer from post-traumatic stress disorder and approximately 50% are living with a chronic medical condition.

> **We need to be able to provide a compassionate, caring, informed environment to allow teens to talk about their experiences, get help from us when needed, and develop insight into the hidden strengths that can emerge from this type of adversity.**

Care providers, including physicians and social service workers, are sometimes the most constant adult influences in a foster teen's life. As we provide care for these youth, we must bear in mind the multiple disruptions and traumas and the subsequent health and emotional challenges that these youth face. We need to be able to listen with compassion and empathy and provide a safe environment allowing these vulnerable teens to talk about their experiences, get help when needed, and gain insight into the hidden strengths that can emerge from their adversity.

■ Establishing Trust and Respect

Foster care youth are among the most vulnerable adolescent populations. By the nature of being placed in foster care, these youth have some history of neglect, abuse, or a family crisis that lead them to be placed in the foster care system. These past traumatic experiences can often manifest as behavioral and emotional challenges. Further, the traumas may have created mistrust and fear toward adults, flavoring their interactions with the many adults involved in their lives (including social workers, therapists, attorneys, and health care clinicians). How we communicate with foster care youth will often play a key role in how youth perceive social services and the health care world now and in the future.

Given the preexisting traumatic circumstances and chaos of their past, it is essential to first establish a trustworthy and respectful relationship. To have the greatest ongoing impact, this needs to be our main agenda of the visit, above any other plans or tasks of the visit (eg, immunizations, medication refills, or addressing behavior problems). A critical first step toward building a strong professional-teen relationship is respecting how a youth presents himself at the visit, including recognizing that current or past undesirable behaviors may represent attempts at self-protection.

■ Confidentiality

Foster care youth have many adults directly or indirectly involved in their lives, including but not limited to foster care parents, social workers, counselors, probation officers, attorneys, court-appointed child advocates, as well as others who often know a great deal about their lives. This can make confidentiality and consent issues very challenging and contribute even more to the challenges of establishing trust. Therefore, confidentiality must be discussed, clearly defined, and fully honored by all team members (see Chapter 14).

■ Establishing a Medical Home

Foster care youth often have transient and changing living situations either due to their foster care living situation (eg, lack of permanent housing and/or group home) or because their own behaviors have led to changes in their living situation. This can make establishing a medical home even more difficult. As with all adolescents, the concept of a medical home needs to be addressed to ensure consistent care. However, in this case, extra flexibility is warranted because of the challenges of their changing living situations.

A critical step of building a medical home is to have foster youth stay connected to your practice. This requires being easily available, even during their numerous changing life events. This will likely involve your practice needing to display more than routine flexibility and enhanced strategies for follow-up. For example, youth may miss appointments because of meetings with their case workers or because their foster parents were not able to leave work to bring them to the office. Recognizing that these youth cannot control these circumstances, they need to be rescheduled as soon as possible. A personal contact stating that their absence was noticed might reinforce the importance you hold to your connection.

■ Health Decision-making

Foster care youth often lack parents or a consistent permanent supportive adult to help them in their daily lives. Because of this, many have already learned to make complex health decisions independently (eg, reproductive health issues). In addition, many youth often know their health histories better than many non–foster care youth. It is helpful to learn how much youth understand about their own health and how they have made health decisions in the past, and to recognize and reinforce the good health decisions they have already made.

■ Case

Tom is a 15-year-old who has been placed into his fourth foster care placement in the past year. He has been in foster care for 3 years, when his mother was incarcerated for drugs. His father died when he was 1 year old, and Tom doesn't know anything about him. He was initially placed with a relative but removed due to behavior problems. He was then placed in several different group homes in different counties. He was recently arrested for shoplifting and was in juvenile hall for 3 months. He was placed into this current group home after release from juvenile hall. He comes for his scheduled appointment with you for a physical examination to gain placement into this group home.

You enter the room and he is sitting with a group home counselor who gives you forms to fill out, but you notice there are no health records. The counselor says Tom needs a refill on his asthma medications and needs a referral for an eye examination.

Tom is sitting in the chair listening to music on an MP3 player with ear pieces on and not looking at you. You begin the visit by reaching your hand out to shake his and asking him what he is listening too. He mentions the band name. You ask him who his favorite bands are, and he shares this with you. You then ask him if he knows why he is at the clinic today and what he would like to talk about. He states he doesn't know and doesn't really care. You respond that you understand and still want to give him excellent care. Then you ask the counselor to honor your patient's privacy and wait in the waiting room so you can speak directly with Tom.

You recognize that he doesn't want to be at the visit, so rather than address the forms or other medical issues first, and in order to connect with him, you allow him to set the agenda for the visit. In doing so, you first acknowledge that it's okay to not want to engage with you (because he doesn't know or trust you yet), but you also let him know you are interested in getting to know him and respect his feelings about the purpose of the visit. You also let him know that he has your complete attention, and that he deserves to get the best care possible and you are there to ensure that he does. You also emphasize that even though there are forms to fill out, and many people know about his past personal life, you will keep any information discussed during the visit and future visits confidential (including information on the forms) unless his safety is a concern. He can decide what others need to know or not know.

Tom then tells you that he had an emergency department visit for his asthma 1 week ago because he ran out of meds and wasn't given anything when he was released from juvenile hall. Given that he has opened up and starting talking about this health issue, you acknowledge it must be hard to manage his asthma alone, particularly around refilling his medications and the recent change in his living situation. You explain that you want to work with him to help him avoid future emergency department visits for his asthma and commend him on how much he already knows about his asthma. You set up a plan for future refills so that he can get the medication he needs by himself. He agrees to follow up in a couple of weeks to see how his asthma is doing. You explain that you will be the person to coordinate his care around his asthma and any other health problems he may be concerned about. You give him your contact information so he can communicate with you without having to make an appointment. That way he can call if he prefers to check in by phone if any other circumstances come up and he wants to talk.

With this first visit, Tom has learned that you respect what he wants to talk about and what he doesn't want to talk about. You also showed him that you are impressed by his decisions around his asthma care. You also open the door to future discussions, by phone or in person, that can address whatever agenda he brings to you. Building trust with a stepwise approach allows a young person to "test you" and see if you are actually deserving of their trust. Given the series of disappointments with adults throughout his life, it makes sense that Tom's trust of you should build incrementally.

■ Aging Out

Yearly, more than 20,000 foster care youth will "age out" of foster care. Outcomes for youth who have "aged out" of care are poor. Between 25% and 45% had not completed high school, 20% to 50% are unemployed, and approximately 25% had experienced homelessness after leaving foster care. Professionals who work with foster care youth can support "preparation for adulthood." By gaining their trust, we can help youth to stay engaged in school; gain marketable work skills; plan for safe, stable, and affordable housing; teach basic life skills, such as completing a job application; encourage keeping positive connections to supportive peers and adults; plan for adequate access to health care; and learn how to access essential legal documents pertaining to their personal, family, medical, and educational histories. Youth with supportive coaching and strong connections can forge successful transitions out of foster care with our continued support.

■ Conclusions

Supporting youth who are living in foster care can be one of the most meaningful and influential roles a professional can have in an adolescent's life. The main focus of care should be on gaining trust and living up to the trust given to you. Creating consistent relationships, including a medical home, can provide stability and the forum to slowly address the complex set of skill sets a young person needs to achieve before "aging out" of foster care. Finally, by communicating deep respect for these resilient youth, we can help them become aware of and embrace their own strengths.

●● Group Learning and Discussion ●●

The overriding message in this chapter is that trustworthy relationships matter, especially to foster youth. Further, it underscores that forming a consistent relationship holds the potential of significantly impacting on their health and well-being precisely because stability is often lacking in the lives of foster care youth.

Your ability to impact on the health and well-being of foster care youth may be enhanced if you have a clearer idea of what navigating the foster care system in your area is like. Your practice group should consider inviting a representative of the foster care system, a youth advocate, and/or foster care youth to a session to inform your practice about the system that serves local youth.

Finally, discuss what extra procedures could be put into place within your practice group that could lower access barriers for foster youth and increase the likelihood that you would be able to maintain connections with them, despite the frequent change in circumstances they might endure.

■■■■■■■ Continuing Education ■■■■■■■■

If you are applying for continuing education credits, a test is available online. For more details, visit www.aap.org/reachingteens.

■ Related Video Content

64.0 Meeting the Unique Needs of Foster Care Youth. Chaffee.

64.1 Interview With a 21-Year-Old Foster Care "Graduate" Who Is Now a Foster Care Advocate. Auerswald, Youth.

64.2 Foster Care: A Missed Opportunity to Build Self-sufficiency? Hill.

64.3 Being Attentive to the Proper (and Improper) Use of Psychotropic Medicine in Foster Care Youth. Chaffee.

64.4 Helping Foster Care Youth Overcome Labels. Chaffee.

64.5 Helping Foster Care Teens Pursue Their Dreams to Serve and Improve the Lives of Children and Youth. Chaffee.

57.2 The Making of a Girl. The GEMS Project.

■ Related Handout/Supplementary Material

Hidden Among Us: Sexually Exploited and Trafficked Youth

■ Related Web Sites

American Academy of Pediatrics
Information on foster care children and adolescents
www2.aap.org/fostercare/FosteringHealth.html

Information on effects of child abuse
http://aappolicy.aappublications.org/cgi/content/full/pediatrics;122/3/667

Specific information on consent and confidentiality issues with foster care children and adolescents
www2.aap.org/fostercare/PDFs/FosteringHealth/Ch6_Medical_%20Consents.pdf

Child Welfare Information Gateway: Protecting Children and Strengthening Families
Foster Care Advocacy and Education
www.childwelfare.gov

The **Annie E. Casey Foundation,** as part of its Welfare Strategy Group, explores best practices and policies to support young people in foster care. Downloadable reports can be accessed at www.aecf.org/KnowledgeCenter/ChildWelfarePermanence/FosterCare.aspx.

CHAPTER 65

Youth Infected With HIV

Nadia L. Dowshen, MD, FAAP, AAHIVS

Linda A. Hawkins, PhD, LPC

Renata Arrington-Sanders, MD, MPH, ScM, FAAP

Daniel H. Reirden, MD, FAAP, AAHIVMS

Robert Garofalo, MD, MPH

 Related Video Content

65.0 Our Critical Role in Helping Youth Navigate Living With HIV

■ Why This Matters

There are more than 1 million people living in the United States with HIV/AIDS. While the number of new infections has stabilized in general, adolescents and young adults make up more than one-third of new cases, and rates of new infections are rising in this age group. Additionally, the increasing numbers of youth infected with HIV perinatally who are surviving to adolescence and adulthood have unique health care and psychosocial needs. Professionals who work with adolescents need to be ready to address HIV prevention, screening, and diagnosis. We know that early diagnosis and linkage to appropriate care can improve health outcomes for these youth.

> **HIV is one of very few chronic diseases left in the world where automatic support after diagnosis, from one's friends, family, and community, is not guaranteed. When people feel isolated and stigmatized, they often cannot begin to engage in behavior change or take action to improve their health. The more we can do to remove shame and blame, the easier it will be for youth living with HIV to begin healing.**

■ Prevention and Screening 65.1

The first step in providing excellent HIV/AIDS prevention and screening for adolescents is setting the stage for a confidential space to address sexual health in an open and nonjudgmental way (see Chapter 14). Having conversations about sex and sexuality with adolescents is not easy, and it takes practice. When taking a sexual history, consider using the attraction, behavior, orientation (ABO) approach in order to be complete. See page 533 in Chapter 61 for examples of questions to ask.

HIV testing should be approached as a routine screening practice as recommended by the Centers for Disease Control and Prevention and the American Academy of Pediatrics. Routine, rather than risk-based, screening is now recommended because studies have shown that individuals often do not report their risk factors to health care professionals (ie, unprotected sex or sharing needles for intravenous drug use). While HIV disproportionately affects youth of color and young men who have sex with men, an individual's risk behavior may have no relationship to sexual, gender, or cultural identity. Approaching HIV screening by informing patients that this testing is recommended routinely as a normal part of adolescent health care will show youth that you are not making judgments about their risk and may decrease barriers to testing and treatment. Whenever a young person agrees to HIV testing, it is always important to communicate a plan for how you will follow up on results.

■ Delivering HIV Test Results 24.0, 65.3

Delivering HIV test results in a way that is sensitive and educational takes practice. Whether the result is positive or negative, it is helpful to assess the patient's expectation of the result. When delivering a negative result, professionals should take this opportunity to provide education. Ask youth what they feel they have done well to keep themselves healthy sexually and what they think they could do better. If they reveal risky behaviors, professionals may want to use a harm reduction approach by helping them identify ways they can reduce risk, even if they are not ready to change or stop the behavior entirely.

Hopefully, we will never or rarely have to deliver positive HIV test results. However, we all need to be prepared (see Chapter 24).

- When preparing to give a positive result, it is important to be in touch with and keep your own emotions in check before meeting with the patient. Remember that while this is difficult news, this is often not the hardest thing going on in the young person's life and you don't want to make it more of a catastrophe than the adolescent would otherwise perceive or be prepared to address.
- Make sure that you sit on the same level as the youth and that you are physically not blocking an exit from the room.
- Be calm but matter of fact when you speak, and pause to allow the youth to react.
- Without diminishing the pain and sadness that may go along with this diagnosis, it is important to convey a message of hope. We know that if HIV-positive individuals get appropriate medical care, like with other chronic diseases such as diabetes, they can lead long, productive, healthy lives.
- It may be particularly helpful in this situation to provide support in the form of appropriate touch. For example, putting your hand on the adolescent's shoulder can be comforting and reminds the youth that they are worthy of love and respect. This is particularly important because the youth is living with a disease still associated with shame and stigma and are often made to feel untouchable.
- Allow time for the patient to react and ask any questions. Explain to the youth that she may initially want to disclose her diagnosis to 1 to 2 people who she knows will be supportive and trust to keep the information private.
- Remember that listening may be more important than talking. The patient will guide you about her needs.
- Finally, assess for safety and establish a plan for close follow-up and to connect the patient to an appropriate HIV care provider in her community as soon as possible.

■ Shame and Stigma Associated With HIV 65.8

HIV is one of very few chronic diseases left in the world where automatic support after diagnosis, from one's friends, family, and community, is not guaranteed. Unfortunately, shame and stigma are still a major part of this disease. When people feel stressed and isolated as a result of stigma, they often cannot begin to engage in behavior change or take action to improve their health. The more we can do as professionals to remove shame and blame, the easier it will be for youth living with HIV to begin healing.

■ Confidentiality and Disclosure of HIV Diagnosis 34.3, 65.7

Confidentiality and disclosure issues are particularly important for youth living with HIV/AIDS because of stigma still associated with the disease.

- The consequences of disclosure can be devastating, so remember to review who is and is not aware of the diagnosis (ie, partners, parents, friends, other professionals, and staff).
- When discussing disclosure, help the youth to consider potential benefits (ie, emotional support, help with medication, lifting and sharing burden) and risks (ie, safety, housing, losing relationships).
- Disclosure to sexual and romantic partners can be particularly complicated. It is best to disclose when possible, but safer sex to protect the youth and partner(s) may be the goal in situations where the risk to one's safety of disclosing may be too high.
- Consider strategies like role-playing to provide support around when and how to tell.

■ Tips for General Care for Youth Living With HIV/AIDS 65.5

- As a non-HIV care provider, it is appropriate to check in about relationships and disclosure. For example, *"How is HIV fitting into your life right now?"*
- Talk about safer sex practices, and remember that the goal is for youth to have healthy sexual lives where they are protecting themselves and their partners.
- Check in about HIV specialty care and whether there are any problems or issues with provider communication.
- Ask what you need to ask, but not more. Remember that HIV is a chronic disease, not an identity. When a youth living with HIV visits a medical provider, they want relevant health issues related to their HIV status to be addressed. However, they also want to be treated just like any other teen and to be asked about other aspects of their life and health.
- Assess all medical complaints calmly and without alarm as you would with any patients. Provide reassurance if the complaint is not related to HIV. If you don't know or you are concerned clinically about whether the complaint is related to HIV, ask the specialist.

■ Medication Adherence/Readiness 65.9

While adhering to medication during adolescence is a common challenge for youth living with many different chronic diseases, youth living with HIV/AIDs face particular barriers related to the disease and treatment. Most individuals will need to start antiretroviral therapy (ART) within a few years of their HIV diagnosis and will need to stay on these medications for the rest of their lives. People living with HIV/AIDS need to take their medication every day at the same time in order to maintain viral suppression. Even just a few missed doses can lead to the development of resistance. Most of the time, youth will need to start or continue taking medication when they feel healthy; this can be a difficult concept for adolescents to understand, depending on their stage of cognitive development. Additionally, youth often do not want to take medication because it is a reminder of their disease, and the shame and stigma that goes along with it. Further, they worry it could potentially result in unintended disclosure of their diagnosis to others if their medications are found. These issues need to be addressed before starting medications. Other strategies that may help prepare youth for starting medication or improving adherence include practicing what it will be like to take medicine every day at the same time by taking a daily multivitamin, having a support system, taking the patient's daily routine into account when choosing specific medications, and reminders (ie, alarms, text messages, pill boxes). It is key to check in about adherence regularly without judgment or expectation.

■ Role of Spirituality/Religion

Spirituality and religion often play key roles in the lives of youth and may be particularly important in helping young people and their support networks cope with living with a chronic disease. Professionals can support young people living with HIV/AIDS by acknowledging that spirituality and religion can be powerful tools as part of the healing process. Unfortunately, some communities of faith may not be prepared to provide the kind of guidance and support that young people need, especially when dealing with a disease that is still associated with stigma and shame. Helping young people to find supportive faith communities or individual spiritual leaders or practices can be important in helping HIV-positive youth live happy and healthy lives.

●● Group Learning and Discussion ●●

(Consider reviewing chapters 14 and 24 prior to this group learning experience.)

Break into pairs and work through the following scenarios. Assume that you have "set the stage" for a trustworthy relationship prior to this discussion. You may choose to offer a brief "booster" on privacy rights before the discussions.

1. Offer HIV prevention education to a 16-year-old girl with a lifetime history of 7 sexual partners and infrequent condom use. She receives regular medroxyprogesterone injections to prevent pregnancy.

2. Deliver a positive HIV test result to an 18-year-old man who reports having sex with both males and females and having primarily same-sex attractions. He has not disclosed these attractions or experiences to anyone. His father is in the waiting area, and he does not know how his father would react to any of this news.

3. Discuss medication adherence with a 17-year-old young man who has been on ART for 8 months. Remember to ask about his adherence in an open-ended way, and then proceed with discussion after he shares that he "usually" remembers to take his medication.

■■■■■■■ Continuing Education ■■■■■■■■

If you are applying for continuing education credits, a test is available online. For more details, visit www.aap.org/reachingteens.

■ Suggested Reading

American Academy of Pediatrics Committee on Pediatric AIDS. Adolescents and HIV infection: the pediatrician's role in promoting routine testing. *Pediatrics*. 2011;128(5):1023–1029

Branson BM, Handsfield HH, Lampe MA, et al. Revised recommendations for HIV testing of adults, adolescents, and pregnant women in health-care settings. *MMWR Recomm Rep*. 2006;55(RR-14):1–17; quiz CE11-14

Centers for Disease Control and Prevention Division of HIV/AIDS Prevention. *HIV Among Youth*. Atlanta, GA: National Center for HIV/AIDS, Viral Hepatitis, STD, and TB Prevention; December 2011:2 http://www.cdc.gov/hiv/youth/pdf/youth.pdf. Accessed June 26, 2013

■ Related Video Content

65.0 Our Critical Role in Helping Youth Navigate Living With HIV. Garofalo, Dowshen, Hawkins.

65.1 Who Should Be Tested for HIV? Garofalo, Dowshen, Arrington-Sanders.

65.2 Testimony and Wisdom From a Young Man Living With HIV. Youth.

65.3 Giving a Young Person a Positive HIV Test Result. Garofalo, Dowshen, Hawkins, Reirden.

65.4 Working With Youth Living With HIV: Identifying Personal Strengths and Social Supports. Dowshen, Hawkins.

65.5 HIV in the Context of Real Life: From Harm Reduction to Romantic Relationships. Garofalo, Dowshen, Arrington-Sanders.

65.6 Helping Youth Living With HIV Manage Disclosure and Safer Sex With Sexual Partners. Reirden, Arrington-Sanders, Dowshen, Hawkins, Garofalo.

65.7 Helping Youth Living With HIV Navigate Disclosure of Their Diagnosis. Reirden, Hawkins.

65.8 Shame and Stigma as a Toxic and Persistent Force in Serving HIV-Positive Youth. Reirden, Hawkins, Dowshen, Arrington-Sanders.

65.9 Helping Youth Living With HIV Manage Their Medications. Reirden, Dowshen, Arrington-Sanders, Garofalo.

11.7 Who Should Get Tested for HIV and Other STIs? Reirden, Garofalo.

24.0 Among the Hardest Things We Do—Delivering Bad News. Ginsburg, Reirden, Arrington-Sanders, Garofalo, Hawkins, Pletcher.

34.3 Preparing Youth to Disclose Difficult Personal Information to Parents. Reirden, Hawkins.

CHAPTER 66

Serving Homeless and Unstably Housed Youth

Colette (Coco) Auerswald, MD, MS, FSAHM

 Related Video Content

66.0 The Life Cycle Model of Youth Homelessness

■ Why This Matters

Homeless and unstably housed youth are a largely invisible, diverse, stigmatized, and high-risk population. Though the population is widely held to be sizable, current estimates of the size of the population are poor.

■ Family Background and Development

Though homeless youth are diverse, they often share the experience of significant family dysfunction in their childhood homes, including physical, sexual, and emotional abuse; neglect and abandonment; and/or parental drug abuse. Homeless adolescents, like other youth, are faced with the challenges of accomplishing the developmental tasks of adolescence, including adjusting to changing body, developing a sense of self-identity, negotiating adult relationships with former caretakers/parents, developing economic independence (education/work), and forming mutually supportive friendships and intimacy. However, youth must accomplish these tasks hampered by the dysfunctional environments in which they were often raised, without the support and resources of adult caretakers and without a stable roof over their heads. Youth often have a poor educational history with a history of school failure or expulsion being common. Furthermore, they may not have successfully completed the essential developmental tasks of childhood, including the ability to develop appropriate attachments and trusting relationships. Though facing many challenges, investigators have also emphasized the resilience and resourcefulness of homeless and unstably housed youth.[1]

Foster youth and youth with a history of involvement in the juvenile justice system are disproportionately represented among homeless youth. Furthermore, sexual minority youth, including lesbian, gay, bisexual, queer, transgender, questioning, and intersex youth, are overrepresented on the street, often because of marginalization by their home community and/or family rejection. However, many unstably housed and homeless youth

> **Just as youth are mentored into street life, extrication from the streets may require mentoring. In order for youth to become "mainstream smart," they need to be exposed to the skills required to thrive in the mainstream.**

fall outside of these categories. In some large metropolitan areas, many homeless youth have travelled far before finding themselves homeless. However, in most cities and in rural areas, unstably housed and homeless youth are generally from the local community.

■ Risky Behaviors and Morbidity and Mortality of Homeless Youth

Homeless youth are more likely than non-homeless youth to be exposed to violence and be involved in behaviors that put them at risk, including survival sex (exchanging sex for drugs, money, shelter, or protection) and substance abuse. These behaviors are, in turn, reflected in a high prevalence of psychological disorders (eg, depression, anxiety, and post-traumatic stress disorder), HIV, chlamydia, gonorrhea, hepatitis B and C, and a high mortality rate.

■ The Life Cycle of Youth Homelessness 66.0

Although most studies have lumped homeless youth together in one category, other studies suggest that youth's risks, service utilization, and outcomes differ greatly, varying by geographic area, demographic characteristics, and homelessness history. In fact, homelessness may present quite differently in different cities or among different subgroups of youth. Some cities serve as destinations for homeless, runaway, and marginalized youth. These locations are more likely to have a distinct street culture. In other cities, youth homelessness may present primarily as youth "couch surfing" between acquaintances' houses or "squatting" in abandoned buildings. Within each city, there are likely to be distinct subcultures of unstably housed youth. What all homeless and unstably housed youth have in common, unless they are safely sheltered, is the necessity to meet basic survival needs. Youth often need to choose among a host of illegal and dangerous means to survive, including panhandling, stealing from stores or people, dealing drugs, and survival sex.

An understanding of the life cycle of youth homelessness can help inform the clinical and service approach to youth (Figure 66.1). This model was developed from ethnographic research and has been tested epidemiologically in larger samples of youth.[2–7] The model is based on ethnographic work conducted in San Francisco and thus likely most closely applies to locations where a street culture exists. However, the key points that pertain to potential points of intervention are worthy of consideration in every location.

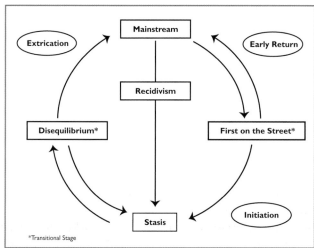

FIGURE 66.1
THE LIFE CYCLE OF YOUTH HOMELESSNESS

From Auerswald CL, Eyre SL. Youth homelessness in San Francisco: a life cycle approach. *Soc Sci Med.* 2002;54(10):1497–1512. With permission from Elsevier.

Research regarding homeless and housed adults and adolescents has demonstrated that to understand individuals' decisions regarding behaviors, we must understand that the social context of people's lives shapes norms, expectations, and opportunities to engage in or avoid risk. Engaging in risky behaviors may represent effective short-term coping behaviors to a youth's environment. The model of the life cycle of youth homelessness may assist professionals in better understanding the sociocultural context of the decisions of homeless youth, including decisions regarding risky behaviors.

The Mainstream Stage: Pre-Street Life

Youth on the street who describe their life prior to living on the street almost uniformly recount catastrophic family dynamics. Street youth describe themselves as not having a choice. Given their predicament at home, street life can be a reasonable option.

First-on-the-Street Stage

Youth who are first-on-the-street are immigrants to the street culture and environment. They are acutely preoccupied with how to meet their basic needs in their new surroundings. One consequence is that experienced street residents, other street youth, or homeless adults easily identify newcomers by their demeanor and their naïveté. Some may reach out to help, while others prey on those new on the street. The social ties of first-on-the-street youth, though they may be dysfunctional, may be the only remaining ties to the mainstream world. Further, they may be seen as essential to survival.

The first-on-the-street stage is an example of a transitional state, a temporary state of transition from one status to another within society. The first-on-the-street youth will be driven out of this transitional state by the need to meet his basic needs and by the need for connection with others on the street.

Initiation Stage

Initiation to street life is a process of acculturation to street life—its resources and economy, language, and drugs it is often facilitated by street mentors. During the initiation to the street stage, mentors introduce youth to the street culture and economy and teach them "street smarts," the skills required to protect themselves and their possessions. Motivated by the need to survive, the process of becoming part of the street economy is rapid.

Stasis Stage

During the stasis stage, youth are integrated into street culture and the street economy. This stage is defined by the seeming contradiction between the youth's belief that street youth form a community and the descriptions of the harsh and conflictual reality of the life of the homeless. Stasis is further characterized by distrust for people and institutions in the mainstream, or non-homeless, world. This distrust is often well-founded in past negative experiences of abuse or lack of follow-through by prior providers. Similarly, youth in stasis are often very wary of and avoid shelters because of the stigma associated with shelter use, the rules imposed on shelter clients, and the lack of safety perceived by youth in those shelters shared with older adults. Youth in stasis generally have social ties primarily to other homeless youth or adults.

Disequilibrium Stage

The chaos in which youth live frequently precipitates episodes of disequilibrium, minor or major disasters that threaten a youth's ability to continue to survive on the street. Examples of disequilibrium episodes include being robbed, arrested, or assaulted; becoming ill; or exposure to particularly harsh weather. Our research has suggested that youth in disequilibrium may be at increased risk for initiating very high-risk behaviors.[7]

Disequilibrium is another example of a transitional state. Youth in disequilibrium will most often return to the street; however, the crisis may motivate them or give them the opportunity to attempt to leave the street.

Extrication Stage

Youth in the extrication stage are attempting to leave street life. Obstacles are many. Youth in extrication appear to be more likely to seek medical services, perhaps as a first step to leaving the street.[4] Our research suggests that many street-based youth are actively engaged in trying to leave street life. Research in Los Angeles suggests that most youth return home within the first 18 months.[8]

Recidivism Stage: The Return to Street Life

Attempts at extrication may fail because youth did not have the appearance, hygiene, credentials, social connections, skills, or address to reenter mainstream life. Ongoing substance abuse may also pose a significant obstacle to leaving street life. Lacking other options, some youth may return to the street. Youth homelessness is often intermittent, with youth cycling in and out of homelessness.

■ Youth Presenting to Care 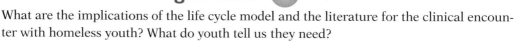 12.9, 66.5

What are the implications of the life cycle model and the literature for the clinical encounter with homeless youth? What do youth tell us they need?

> *"If a homeless youth shows up in clinic, it's a big deal. Providers should pay attention and listen."* (Homeless youth focus group participant)

Overall Points

- Many, if not most, youth can and will leave the street, particularly if they access services. The earlier youth leave the street, the more likely they will successfully and permanently exit homelessness.
- Youth on the street are diverse and may differ based on their life cycle stage. Therefore, a stage-based, customized approach to interventions with street youth may be most effective at reducing their risk. The approach to reducing the risk of a runaway who has been on the street for a couple of weeks is necessarily different from the approach to a youth who is integrated into street culture.
- The life cycle model focuses on removal from the street as the primary intervention to decrease rates of risky behaviors that increase youth's risk of contracting HIV or suffering other negative outcomes. Obtaining housing first is an appropriate goal for youth at all stages, regardless of risk behaviors.
- Unstably housed and homeless youth who may be most open to intervention and outreach are those in transitional stages (eg, first-on-the-street and disequilibrium) and extrication, stages that offer a window of opportunity for removal from street life.
- The life cycle model suggests the steps required for extrication. To leave the street, a youth must reverse the process of initiation by finding a niche in the mainstream economy, achieving a mainstream identity, forming ties with healthy peers, and leading a less substance-dependent existence. Just as youth are mentored into street life, extrication may also require mentoring in order for youth to become "mainstream smart" by being exposed to the skills required to thrive in the mainstream.
- For youth at all stages, helping youth create and/or maintain social network contacts in the mainstream can protect youth from high-risk behaviors and its consequences.

Youth Presenting in a Service Agency or Clinic

- A youth presenting to care for an immediate need, even an illness, represents a **window of opportunity** to reconnect to services and maybe, ultimately, to family or housed contacts.
- **It may be difficult to identify a youth as homeless.** Being homeless is a stigmatized identity. Youth, especially youth of color, may not identify as "homeless," but may be more likely to identify as "unstably housed." Youth who do not identify as homeless may be less likely to access services intended for homeless youth, such as drop-in centers or clinics for the homeless, and may be less likely to comfortably connect with outreach workers. **66.2**
- The appendix[3,4,7] at the end of this chapter is a proposed **screening tool** for identifying homeless youth that can be used in a written form or that can guide clinical screening by a provider.
- Given their needs to prioritize survival needs, youth may need to access services on a **drop-in basis.** Youth need to be praised for reaching out for care and not punished for missing appointments.
- Providers should **attend to a youth's immediate and basic needs first.** The therapeutic alliance a provider can develop by honoring these immediate needs will give him or her the credibility to address long-term goals over time.
- Though a **nonjudgmental stance** is important with all youth, it is particularly important with homeless youth, who have been labeled with a stigmatized social status (being homeless) and may be engaged in stigmatized activities in order to meet their needs (panhandling, survival sex, selling drugs, sleeping in public places). Particular attention should be paid to body language, since youth on the streets often absorb scorn and judgment through others' body language (see Chapter 15). For this reason, youth are very sensitive to verbal or nonverbal cues of stigmatization given by the reception or front office staff when being welcomed to a facility.
- The provider must be familiar with **local and state consent and confidentiality laws for the care of adolescents.** Though most states require parental permission for most medical services and procedures, youth in many states may be able to consent to sensitive health services. These might include reproductive health care (eg, sexually transmitted infection [STI] treatment, contraception, abortion), mental health care, and substance abuse treatment. Mature minor statutes in some states may also allow youth to consent for care.
- The provider should be familiar with their **local youth-friendly referral sources for care,** including mental health services, emergency housing, STI/HIV care, respite care for families, and foster care services.
- Youth in stasis may not be interested in services to leave the street. A **harm reduction** approach to these youth to minimize the impact of their life circumstances on their behavioral and physical health is appropriate.[9] A harm reduction approach does not require a youth to abandon his main coping strategy until a new coping mechanism is in place. The priority in a harm reduction approach is to decrease the negative consequences of a behavior. For example, a harm reduction approach to injection drug use may offer active users a needle exchange program.
- **Access to care for youth younger than 18 years.** Youth may refuse care if it is offered on the condition that parents are contacted.
- **Access to care for youth 18 years of age and older** may be complicated by lack of health insurance and the financial repercussions of being billed for services.
- **Youth may lack the skills or modeling for obtaining primary health care.** A youth's reserved or hostile attitude may be a response to prior negative interactions or abuse at the hands of responsible adults. A positive interaction and flexible environment may

allow youth to establish continuity of care with a provider, which is highly valued by youth who likely have few stable supportive relationships in their lives.

- Youth may be willing to access **emergency housing or shelter services** in order to recover from an acute illness.
- Supporting youth to exit the street requires a multidisciplinary team to address the youth's multiple needs.[10]
- Box 66.1 offers some advice from youth to clinicians providing care to homeless and unstably housed youth.

Box 66.1. Advice From Youth for Providers Caring for Homeless and Unstably Housed Teens

- Listen.
- Be sensitive.
- Don't assume.
- Be supportive.
- Be respectful.
- Expect the unexpected.
- Understand that people may come with an attitude. Be flexible.
- Walk with truth and love.
- Enjoy yourself!
- Communicate.

■ Approaching Homeless Youth

- Homeless youth often have a strong history of abuse and exploitation and may lack experience with caring adults who have only their best interests in mind. Therefore, it is critical to connect with these youth in a way that demonstrates your trustworthiness (see chapters 14 and 15).
- When working with these young people, it is particularly important to consider boundaries. First, many of these youth have a history of exploitation and other inappropriate interactions with adults. Second, precisely because your caring might be a relatively rare experience, the teen may become reliant on you. Many of these youth have had far too much experience with abandonment or adults letting them down, so they must be clear about what you can and cannot offer. When we offer them the support that empowers them to take independent action, our interactions remain therapeutic (see Chapter 20). **▶ 66.12, 66.13**
- Many of these adolescents experience a high level of demoralization that stifles their ability to even consider change. A strength-based interview approach that allows you to elicit the teen's strengths and then authentically reflect those strengths back to the youth may be a first step toward the adolescent gaining the confidence to consider positive behavioral change (see Chapter 25).

- Homeless youth may have the highest levels of sensitivity to social injustices and a genuine commitment to improving others' lives. Further, they may be models of resilience, regarding life's stressors as their most consistent teachers. Eliciting these points can be a starting point of strength-based communication.

  To view testimony from homeless youth that demonstrates wisdom, strength, and a commitment to repairing the world, see videos 66.7, 66.16, and 66.17.
  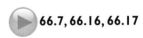 **66.7, 66.16, 66.17**

- Don't assume that the youth are runaways. Understand that the streets may be perceived as the best or safest option. Homeless youth often have had a history of sexual exploitation or abuse and physical trauma in their homes. Escaping to the streets often feels like the best option.

■ Appendix. Unstable Housing Status Screening Tool

In the last 6 months, have you stayed one or more nights in any of these places because you could not stay in your home or you did not have a home?

- A shelter _____
- Outdoors _____
- A squat _____
- With a stranger or someone you did not know well _____
- A car _____
- On public transportation _____
- A single-room occupancy (SRO)/hotel _____
- Jail _____
- One or more of these places, but I don't want to say which _____

Scoring: If participant indicates only one of these choices, ask if this was for one night or more (eg, "You said you stayed outdoors in the past 6 months. Was this for one night, or more than that?").

*If participant stayed **0 or one night total** in any place or combination of places, participant is not to be considered unstably housed.*

*If participant stayed **more than one night** in any place or combination of places, participant is to be considered unstably housed.*

•• Group Learning and Discussion ••

Prior to the group session, explore what homelessness looks like in your location. Assign one person to check in with a local homeless serving agency and ask whether there is a street culture, or whether homeless youth in your area are more likely to be unstably housed through "couch surfing" or squatting. Find out whether there are youth-specific shelters or whether adolescents are incorporated into the adult system. Assign another person to compile a list of local services to complement the national hotlines and resources listed here.

Then break into pairs to work through the following scenarios:

- A 17-year-old young man, Ezekiel, comes to your setting. He is addicted to heroin and tells you that he is in a hurry and only has half an hour before he needs to be on the other side of town. (You suspect he needs to get his next injection, as he seems a bit sweaty.) He is coming to you for a (sore throat: medical scenario) (forms to apply for disability: nonmedical scenario). He does not want to answer any questions about how he is surviving and states, *"I'm doing what I have to do....that's all."* He cleans his "works" (needles and syringes) with bleach occasionally. He has no desire to stop heroin or get off the streets now. (The number for the needle exchange facility is 555-1111; the number for a family planning and sexual health center is 555-2222. Your goal is to be welcoming while avoiding judgment, and to engage in harm reduction.)

- Kim is a 19-year-old woman who has been on the streets for almost 3 years. She came from an abusive environment where she feared for her life. She has been engaged in survival sex, but now has lived with the same guy for 6 months. She earns her rent by "entertaining" his friends. She has a black eye and a large bandage on her forehead and cigarette burns on her forearm. She tells you she fell down the steps and doesn't respond to questions about the burns. You believe she is in disequilibrium. She has a 4-year-old daughter who she adores but who is in foster care. As you talk to her, you learn about the 16-year-old who she befriended last week. The girl was frightened and new to the streets. She walked the girl to the bus stop and used nearly all of her money to buy a ticket to a town across the state where the girl's aunt was ready to receive her. The experience reminded her of how badly she wants to get a GED and be a counselor who can help kids "straighten out their lives…. *"You know, show kids that someone cares."* The number to the youth shelter or women's shelter is 555-3333. (If you live in a town without a youth shelter, you give her The Covenant House Nine Line, 800/999-9999, which will connect her with emergency and shelter services.)

■■■■■■■ Continuing Education ■■■■■■■

If you are applying for continuing education credits, a test is available online. For more details, visit www.aap.org/reachingteens.

■ References

1. Rew L. A theory of taking care of oneself grounded in experiences of homeless youth. *Nurs Res*. 2003;52(4):234–241

2. Auerswald CL, Eyre SL. Youth homelessness in San Francisco: a life cycle approach. *Soc Sci Med*. 2002;54(10):1497–1512

3. Hickler B, Auerswald CL. The worlds of homeless white and African American youth in San Francisco, California: a cultural epidemiological comparison. *Soc Sci Med*. 2009;68(5):824–831

4. Carlson J, Sugano E, Millstein SG, Auerswald C. Service utilization and the life cycle of youth homelessness. *J Adolesc Health*. 2006;38:624–627

5. Auerswald C, Sugano E, Cruz E, Ellen J. Very high risk behaviors and the life cycle of youth homelessness: are youth in crisis at highest risk [abstract]? *Pediatric Academic Society Annual Meeting*. Washington, DC; 2005

6. Valente A, Auerswald C. Social network effects on sexually risky and exploitative behaviors in street youth in San Francisco differ by gender. Sunbelt XXXI Conference of the International Network for Social Network Analysis (INSNA). St Pete Beach, FL; 2011

7. Parriott AM, Auerswald CL. Incidence and predictors of onset of injection drug use in a San Francisco cohort of homeless youth. *Subst Use Misuse*. 2009;44(13):1958–1970

8. Milburn NG, Rosenthal D, Rotheram-Borus MJ, et al. Newly homeless youth typically return home. *J Adolesc Health*. 2007;40(6):574–576

9. Harm Reduction Coalition. http://harmreduction.org. Accessed June 26, 2013

10. Slesnick N. *Our Runaway and Homeless Youth: A Guide to Understanding*. Westport, CT: Praeger Publishers; 2004

■ Related Video Content

66.0 The Life Cycle Model of Youth Homelessness. Auerswald.

66.1 Tips for Serving Unstably Housed Youth. Auerswald.

66.2 Not All Unstably Housed Youth Would Describe Themselves as Homeless. Auerswald.

66.3 Testimony From Youth With a History of Unstable Housing: How We Deserve to Be Treated. Youth.

66.4 Testimony From the Executive Director of Covenant House PA. Hill.

66.5 Testimony From Youth With a History of Unstable Housing: What Makes a Difference in Whether We Will Make It. Youth.

66.6 Passing the Test: Earning the Trust of Homeless and Marginalized Youth. Bailer, Covenant House PA staff.

66.7 Homeless and Marginalized Youth: Young People Who Have Been Tested by Life Bring so Much to the World. Covenant House PA staff.

66.8 Staff Diversity: Creating a Safe Environment Where ALL Youth Feel Safe. Covenant House PA staff.

66.9 What Does Success Look Like When We Work With Homeless and Marginalized Youth? Auerswald, Covenant House PA staff.

66.10 Facilitating Homeless and Marginalized Youth to Believe in Their Potential to Achieve Success. Covenant House PA staff.

66.11 Never Make Promises to Homeless and Marginalized Youth That You Cannot Keep. Hill.

66.12 Homeless Teens: Boundaries, Rules, and High Expectations Can Be Welcomed by Underparented Youth. Hill, Covenant House PA staff.

66.13 The Importance of Understanding Boundaries (and Your Own Buttons) When Working With Marginalized Youth. Hill.

66.14 The Truth May Unfold Slowly for Youth With a History of Adults Failing Them. Hill.

66.15 Testimony From a Young Woman With a History of Unstable Housing: My Path Toward Becoming a Youth Advocate. Youth.

66.16 Testimony From a Young Man With a History of Unstable Housing: "Pain Is Like a Teacher"—Recovery and Resilience. Youth.

66.17 Testimony From a Young Man With a History of Unstable Housing: "We Need Both Truth and Love." Youth.

66.18 Testimony From Youth With a History of Unstable Housing: Don't Assume We Are Drug Addicted...But Do Understand Why We Might Use Drugs. Youth.

12.9 Youth With a History of Homelessness or Unstable Housing Share What They Need From Youth-Serving Agencies. Youth.

23.0 De-escalation and Crisis Management: Wisdom and Strategies From Professionals Who Serve Youth Who Often Act Out Their Frustrations. Youth-serving agencies.

57.2 The Making of a Girl. The GEMS Project.

61.20 Youth Testimony: "This Is How to Address Me" (and Much More): Guidance From a Young Transgender Person. Youth.

■ Related Handout/Supplementary Material

Hidden Among Us: Sexually Exploited and Trafficked Youth

Self-care for Providers

Throughout this text, we challenge the false assumption that teens are beyond reach and hope to have enhanced your skill set at being able to engage deeply and effectively with youth. However, engagement involves an investment of energy, and you will become depleted unless you invest in yourself to restore that energy. Engagement also opens you to a deeper degree of vulnerability as you bear witness to pain, trauma, and inexplicable disparities; this exposure makes you susceptible to burnout. A key to burnout prevention is to process your emotions in a way that allows you to both express your thoughts and feelings and maintain balance. The bottom line is that you need to actively invest in your own care with the same level of commitment you give to the youth you serve.

Our goal is to enhance your ability to reach youth so that you can serve with a great deal of satisfaction over a lifetime.

"Healer, Heal Thyself: Self-care for the Caregiver" (Chapter 67), builds the case for the importance of caring for yourself and offers concrete strategies to do so.

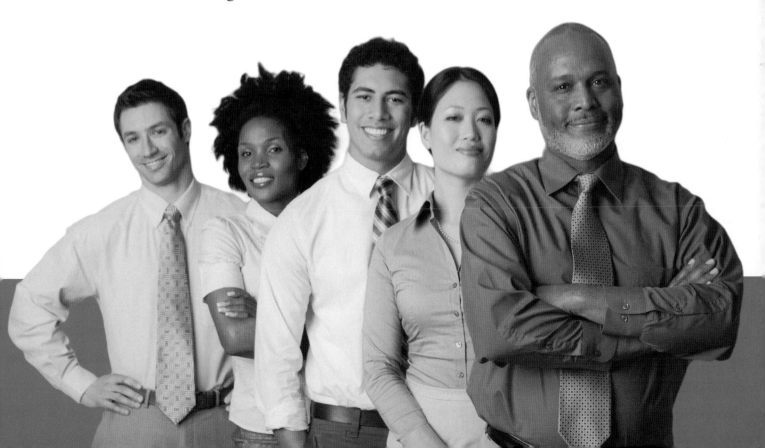

In "Getting Out of the 'Fast Lane'— More 'Miles to the Gallon'?" (Chapter 68) Dr Jenkins, one of the most respected and beloved leaders in pediatrics and adolescent health and medicine, discusses how to remain satisfied and continue to contribute late into your career and even after formal retirement.

"Have I Really Made a Difference? Trusting That Our Presence Matters" (Chapter 69) reminds us that although we sometimes wonder if we have made a difference, we need to trust that our guidance can have a lasting effect—even after our visits are a distant memory.

CHAPTER 67

Healer, Heal Thyself: Self-care for the Caregiver

Oana Tomescu, MD, PhD

 Related Video Content

67.0 Healer, Heal Thyself: Self-care for the Caregiver

■ Why This Matters

Throughout this text, we have suggested that you foster the kind of connection with teens that positions you as a positive force in their lives. We have encouraged you to look beyond the presenting concerns and uncover the deeper psychosocial factors that affect their well-being. In making this suggestion, we are essentially asking you to expose yourself to pain. Reaching out to youth on this deeper level will expose you to the hardships they encounter as they navigate their lives. Although the strength-based model will help you witness compassion and resilience amidst the suffering, your deeper engagement will leave you vulnerable to the uncertainties of the human condition. This vulnerability, if not properly managed, can lead to maladaptive coping strategies that distance you from your emotions and from those very people you are trying to help. This detachment, a state called "burnout," will limit your effectiveness and, more importantly, decrease your job satisfaction and affect your own happiness.

> **If you see self-care as selfish or seeking help yourself as a waste of time, then feel free to reframe it as a selfless act—"I care for myself, so I can be stronger for others. I invest in my wellness, so I can serve for a lifetime."**

This chapter is about managing the distress experienced when caring for others. I explore the concept of the *wounded healer*[1] and highlight several wellness strategies that I hope will augment your self-care toolkit. The only way you will be able to have the emotional reserve to care for others over a lifetime is if you are as compassionate with yourself as you are with others, and as committed to your own wellness as you are to the well-being of the teens and families you serve.

■ Wounded Healers

The Emotional Cost of Being a Caregiver

The terms "compassion fatigue" and "secondary trauma" describe a psychological state that is considered a natural consequence of helping distressed people.[2] Bearing witness to another person's suffering takes an emotional toll on caregivers, and this is true whether caregivers are family members, lay people, or professionals. Family caregivers experience similar rates of depression and anxiety as those in their care.[3–5] Psychological distress is also common among professional caregivers: whether the population studied is occupational health advisors, human resources advisors, therapists and family liaison officers,[6] mental health nurses,[7] or physicians during different levels of training and in various specialties.[8]

Like any physical wound that can fester if untreated, it is hypothesized that prolonged states of unrelieved distress can lead to a deeper state of dysfunction called burnout.[9,10] Burnout is composed of 3 psychological domains: depersonalization (feeling disconnected from others), emotional exhaustion (no longer being able to care or feel), and having a low sense of personal accomplishment (negative self-worth).[11] Burnout has been shown to negatively impact caregiver empathy, provider-patient communication, medical errors, and general quality of care.[12–17] Burnout has also been associated with a higher prevalence of mood disorders, suicidal ideation, substance abuse, and work disability.[18–21] Burnout essentially represents a disconnected state: When we are burned out, we lose the ability to connect with others (depersonalization and emotional exhaustion) and with ourselves (negative self-worth). We feel numb and depleted and can come to believe that we have lost the gift we were given as healers.

Every caregiver knows these results viscerally. We care for others during times of suffering due to physical and/or emotional illness, and guide them as they navigate a traumatic and sometimes abusive world. It is difficult and, at times, even emotionally scarring to see another person in physical or psychological pain. It is natural to share that person's suffering and to experience it to some degree ourselves. We also experience many other intense emotions when we care for others: anger at the condition, frustration at not being able to do more, and fear about the ultimate outcome. In different circumstances, we may also experience intense positive emotions, like happiness, joy, and a sense of relief. We often feel responsible for those in our care: when treatment plans don't work or cause harm, when it is clear the illness is "winning," or when their environmental stressors seem insurmountable. The intensity and consistency with which we experience these natural emotions is what leads to distress, burnout, and dysfunction. Experiencing these emotions without self-awareness can harm us. When this happens, even if subtle, we become less effective healers. Our challenge as caregivers is to learn how to stay connected with the people in our care without letting these emotions destroy us.

We must begin to recognize that all of these emotions stem from our capacity to love. Even the negative emotions like anger, frustration, and fear originate from a deep-seated love we have for the person in our care. Avoiding these natural emotions only serves to suppress their origin (love), which over time can become numbing. We must also stop being afraid of the word "love." It is our capacity to love that enables us to be genuinely empathetic and fully present with others. The word "love" in English sometimes implies enmeshment or even sexual attraction, whereas in so many other cultures and languages, it refers to the feeling we have for another human being—the appreciation for and connection with their very humanity. We must love with appropriate boundaries, with the understanding that our presence facilitates, but does not guarantee, healing: Those in our care must do the heavy lifting. While we might have different levels of comfort with the word "love," if it could be understood in a way that made it feel universally safe, we would embrace it (see Chapter 20).

■ Other Stresses of Professional Caregivers

The work culture of professional caregivers can be unduly taxing. Many of us work in environments that normalize, and indeed reward, overextending oneself beyond one's physical and/or emotional capacity. There is often a mismatch between conflicting demands and allotted time, resources are often insufficient, and the threat of malpractice is prevalent.[22] Organizational factors that result in decreased work satisfaction and high stress include work-life interference, productivity-based compensation, perceived time pressures, and lack of control over administrative issues.[22–25]

Aside from these external stressors, there are also internal qualities among professional caregivers that can predispose to a heightened perception of stress. Caregiver personality and temperament play a large part. The obsessive personality trait is common among physicians.[22,26] In balanced amounts, this trait can have positive effects on commitment and conscientiousness. However, excessive amounts of obsession, a form of perfectionism, can result in an unrealistic need to control the environment and in overcommitment at work. Perfectionists can become overly reliant on external feedback for affirmation and may also suffer from an "imposter" syndrome, waiting to be discovered as less capable than their peers. The mismatch between the nature of the caregiver's job and the caregiver's personality has been hypothesized to augment stress and burnout.[22]

Why we chose a career that requires bearing witness to another's suffering in an environment fraught with external pressures is a significant question we must each answer at some point in our lives. We each have our own reasons, conscious and quite likely subconscious as well. Many of us have entered our respective fields with at least *some* knowledge of the stressful nature of the work environment and the personal challenges we will have to address during our career. We each bring our unique personalities and past experiences with us on this path, and these often subconscious issues can affect how we interact with those in our care. Despite our differences, however, if we were all to meet together and share what brought us to this healing path, I deeply believe we would all reflect on our journey and say that we are here to care for others, to help people in need, to serve humanity, to heal, and to love.

■ Caregiver Physical and Emotional Health

According to many published studies, caregivers do not make adequate time for their own care. Among a sample of lay caregivers, 83% had engaged in age-appropriate preventative health practices, but only 63% continued to adhere to these guidelines during the follow-up term of the study.[27] More burdened family caregivers seem to neglect self-care and have increased rates of depression and health problems when compared to their less burdened counterparts.[28,29] Studies involving physicians reveal very limited medical and emotional self-care. Only a minority of doctors studied engaged in preventive services.[30] One in 4 doctors surveyed reported seeking medical advice when symptoms arose,[31] and only 1 in 3 had identified their own primary care physician, preferring instead to ask colleagues for medical advice or to self-manage their illnesses.[32] Furthermore, suicide is disproportionately high among physicians, especially among female doctors, yet, as a group, doctors are even less likely to tend to their emotional health.[33] Reasons for this poor self-care have been explored.[34] Some physicians reported feeling pressure to portray an unrealistically healthy image, while others stated that they did not want to be a burden to colleagues by taking time off to seek medical attention. Physicians also stated that once symptoms arose, they experienced alternating states of panic (due to knowledge of the worst-case scenario) and denial (that illness cannot happen to them), and that this oscillation delayed them from coming to medical attention.

These studies tell us that we can become lost in the care of others. Caregiving can become so all-encompassing that we forget to think about our own health. Additionally, medical knowledge can be paralyzing to some caregivers when symptoms of illness emerge. These trends apply to both our physical and emotional health. We do not regularly have our own health care team to turn to for help, we postpone being evaluated in a timely manner when physical and emotional symptoms arise, and we forgo preventive health services in both of these domains. We need our physical health to be able to engage in the rigorous demands of our work, but we also need our emotional health to be able to heal others. Our challenge is to tend to our own health with as much nurturing energy as we pour into the care of others.

■ Wellness Strategies

Much has been published about caregiver wellness strategies. Spending time with family and friends, religious or spiritual activity, self-care, setting limits around work, and adopting a healthy philosophical outlook are all common wellness strategies cited in various studies.[35–37] We all know how beneficial habits like regular physical exercise, healthful eating, and adequate sleep are to our general health. We try to spend as much time as possible with friends and family and to engage in our hobbies for their positive effects on our state of being. The rest of this chapter explores other wellness strategies to add to your self-care toolbox.

Cultivate Awareness/Mindfulness

We often multitask our way through our days. We plan our day while driving, check e-mail during meetings, and have several applications open at the same time on our computers. When our minds become accustomed to doing several things at once, we lose the ability to experience one thing at a time, to be fully grounded in any given moment or, in other words, to be *aware.* Have you ever gotten home and sat down to dinner only to realize you cannot actually sit still? Have you tried to watch TV to "get your mind off your day" and discovered that you must, *at the same time*, also read the newspaper or play solitaire or search the Web aimlessly in order to keep your mind occupied *enough*? You now need several applications open and running to feel "comfortable." It is as if your engine is stuck in fifth gear and you cannot slow down. Like a car, you need to be able to transition into slower speeds in order not to crash. We must acknowledge that the pace to which we have become accustomed is dangerous. Running all day at full speed makes us efficient, but at what cost? We often lose awareness of the world around us. Our minds are either looking ahead making plans or trying to process past events. We are not grounded in the present moment, noticing the people in front of us, or the cues they are sending. We are, in essence, disconnected.

Dr James Gordon[38] writes that "awareness allows us to see where we are; to stand for a moment outside ourselves; to appreciate in a powerful, personal way how the world around us affects us; to observe the thoughts, feelings and sensations that arise in us." Work in neurobiology has shown that self-awareness improves our connection to others. Being aware of our own emotional and physical states activates the insula and anterior circulate cortex, which are the parts of our brains that function in reading other people.[39] Mindfulness, which can be defined as the nonjudgmental awareness of the present moment, has its roots in Buddhist traditions, and with the work of Dr Jon Kabat-Zinn[40–42] and many others, mindfulness is becoming part of mainstream healing.[43] Mindfulness has been explored as the core of relationship-centered care, and this connection between personal awareness and effective patient care has been likened to what is called the "art of healing."[44–50]

How do we cultivate awareness of the present moment? How do we retrain our minds to be able to focus on only one thing at a time? Not just the task that lies in front of us to complete, but precisely the more subtle nuances of our emotional and physical states. The first step is coming to awareness that you are multitasking. Identify it when it occurs. Name it: "I am multitasking right now." Don't try to change it; just notice your patterns. As you become aware of these fast-paced times, begin asking yourself when during your day is it most important for you to be mindful and fully aware. Begin to choose the moments in your day when you will not multitask. For instance, being fully present with the people you encounter may be most important to you. On a different day, being present with yourself during a self-care activity could be your focus. Come up with strategies to slow yourself down before these critical moments. Inhale fully for at least 5 seconds; pause and then allow yourself to exhale for another 5 seconds *before* starting your next task. In this brief interlude, picture your mind, which may be still focused on your last activity or has already run ahead to other matters, reconnecting with your body. Consciously noticing a physical detail in your current environment, such as the wood grain of the next patient's door or the color of the floor tile on which you are standing, can also help ground you in the present moment. Prepare yourself to focus on just this next activity and then begin. Do this before entering your own front door in order to be fully present with your loved ones. Do this multiple times during the day to slow yourself down. Being present and aware takes practice, so consider exploring different ways to cultivate mindfulness: yoga, meditation, deep-breathing techniques, personal narrative writing, religious and spiritual practice, and personal psychotherapy can all help you become more aware (see Chapter 32, page 255). **32.5, 67.6**

Become Aware of Your Energy Balance

As we acknowledge the draining nature of our work, we also need to realize that much of the work of caring for others is incredibly fulfilling and, in fact, sustaining. A key self-care strategy is assessing our energy balance on a day-to-day basis. Conceptualize yourself as a *vessel of energy*, a beautiful dynamic entity through which energy flows in and out, depending on your moment-to-moment experiences. At any given moment, your energy gauge reads like a gas tank: full, half full, almost empty. Learn to assess this energy gauge daily and, more importantly, learn to identify which experiences sustain your energy and which drain it. Once you have identified the sustaining experiences, learn to maximize the energy exchange in these experiences: Like a thirsty sponge, open your pores and soak it all in. For instance, when a teen or family gives you positive feedback, how often do you allow yourself to slow down and be fully present and receptive? Learning to be fully present in these moments increases the energy exchange.

Draining experiences, once identified, need not be shunned. In fact, many things that drain us are unavoidable: forms, insurance company claims, and all the nitty-gritty of our work. Other encounters, perhaps with an angry or demanding youth or parent, while draining, can be informative and are often necessary to understand the type of care the teen needs. We cannot avoid these experiences, but rather by being aware that they are draining and *why* they drain us, we can learn to minimize their effect on us. Learning to identify what drains and restores you is a key to finding this balance every day. Therefore, assess your energy gauge frequently. Make time every day for what sustains you, both at work and also in your life outside of work.

Find Meaning in What You Do

When caregivers can make sense of their caring role, they are better able to sustain their connection with others without becoming distressed or burned out.[51,52] Finding meaning in traumatic experiences has been studied as a coping strategy in the management of stress,[53–55] is associated with increased personal growth,[56,57] and has been linked to well-being.[58] Interestingly, whether caregiver exposure to traumatic events results in negative consequences or beneficial personal growth seems to be modulated by regular personal reflection and a healthy lifestyle.[6]

Ask yourself again why you chose this caring path. Take the time to explore how helping others makes you feel. Contemplate what you have learned and how you have grown on your journey. Become proactive in your personal reflection through techniques such as narrative writing, meditation, psychotherapy, Balint groups, art, or music. No matter what methods resonate best with you, the key is to make sure you prioritize time for this type of reflection. The more aware you are of your personal philosophy of caring for others, the more you will notice moments throughout your day that reinforce your mission. These moments are the ones that will provide you with the most sustaining energy possible; you just need to learn to identify them and then take them in, like a deep breath of fresh air.

Seek Balance in Your Identity

The concept of work-life balance is well known to us all. Making time for our families and friends and our "outside work" interests and hobbies sustains us and fills our energy tanks. It allows us to step away from the suffering we witness and reconnect to the rest of the world. Making time for our "outside" interests is an adaptive strategy that enables us to stay balanced and to remember that we are also human ourselves. When we forget, or choose to ignore, this basic tenet, barriers emerge that lessen our capacity to connect with others and, thus, lessen our ability to heal them. Seeing those in our care as "other" is a maladaptive coping strategy that results from repeatedly witnessing illness and suffering. It protects us from the very cold realization that life is ephemeral and unpredictable and that we, or our loved ones, can be stricken at any moment. We thus create the "other" phenomenon: These bad things cannot happen to me; they only happen to others. In this way, we distance ourselves subconsciously. Soon, we can no longer connect and, at its most dangerous, we begin to blame others for the problems and illnesses that afflict them. By keeping our identities balanced, we can fight this potentially damaging socialization process. We are not only caregivers, but also husbands, wives, parents, friends, artists, writers, animal lovers, foodies, and movie buffs. We are not separate from the others in our care.

▶ 20.2

Seek balance in your identity and seek a healthy work-life balance as well. It is important to separate home from work so that you have a protective boundary to allow you to recharge and appreciate those with whom you share your life. Otherwise, you may make the relationship-damaging mistake of thinking that the needs of your family and friends are somehow shallow or unimportant compared to the tragedies you deal with at work. Although you need a healthy separation, make sure your identity is fully integrated. Ask yourself: Are you as compassionate at home as you are at work, and vice versa? Are you as calm at work as you are at home? Are there different personas you use to get through your day? Work toward becoming more integrated, balanced, and whole.

Process Your Emotions

Many emotions arise as we care for others. In the moment when we are present with those in our care, it is innately human to experience the same emotions they are feeling. In fact, in order to create the "safe place" in which youth can unload, we must be empathetic and present with the emotions they experience. However, because we are there to help, we cannot lose ourselves in their emotions; we must remain balanced and objective. Therefore, in the moment, in order to maintain healthy boundaries and a therapeutic relationship, we have to subjugate our own emotional reactions. To be clear, we should be warm, empathetic, and authentically caring, while not allowing ourselves to become so emotional we lose our ability to make professional judgments or position the teens or family members to feel they need to take care of us (see Chapter 20).

While we cannot—and should not—fully experience our emotions in the moment with the adolescent, we must make time to do this at some other point. What happens when we let these traumatic emotions build up inside? Emotions begin leaking out in odd and inappropriate circumstances: breaking a glass leads to uncontrollable crying or getting cut off by another driver results in spewing of uncharacteristic anger and hate. Essentially, we lose control over our emotions. When this happens, a natural tendency is to begin to avoid all emotions, to try to hold them in because it becomes too painful to have them emerge. We try to lock them away inside of a figurative box, building what is the equivalent of a repository of emotions. Indiscriminate in what it holds, this box becomes the storage compartment for all our emotions: "positive" ones like joy and love, as well as the "negative" ones like anger, fear, and hate. Soon this box becomes too scary to open and we lose the ability to feel any emotion at all. We feel "numb" or "dead inside." We lose the ability to connect with others and, in effect, become disconnected from our natural selves.

Dr Ken Ginsburg teaches about this, and he calls this container the "leaden box." Lead is heavy and shielding. Lead is also impermeable. We have all built such a box at one time or another. Processing emotions that are locked in a leaden box is very difficult. It is truly scary to think of opening the lid for fear of the chaos that can emerge: years of traumatic experiences lie in wait, eager to explode. However, Dr Ginsburg teaches that instead of a lead box full of chaotic emotions, we can choose instead to visualize a Tupperware container: one large Tupperware container full of smaller ones that each store the emotional content of one encounter. We have the choice to open just one small container at a time and to deal with just that single moment. What was the emotion we felt? Why was this so painful for us? How has it affected us since the experience? What were we meant to learn?

Dr Ginsburg suggests that we "burp" our Tupperware regularly, that we deal with these emotions closer and closer to when we experience them. Allowing yourself to process these subjugated emotions will help you understand the youth and families you serve better and will make it easier to connect with them at the next encounter. Over time, you will become less afraid of emotions because they are not as painful and chaotic to experience. Over time, you will begin to feel that you have more space available to be present with all of the people you serve. This is the Tupperware model of emotion processing. However you choose to visualize these subjugated experiences, make a commitment to your emotional health. Realize that you need to experience the emotions you generate during your daily interactions. The labels "positive" and "negative" are just your perception: Every emotion is necessary to your learning. Store the emotion away in the moment to maintain some objectivity, but come back to it as soon as you can and let yourself experience it fully. Learn from it, and then let it go.

Processing your emotions may not be as simple as visualizing them in smaller, more organized, brightly colored boxes. You still need tools and strategies to handle each emotion safely and with confidence that you will not be overwhelmed. Explore different ways of experiencing the content of each small container. You may try writing about the encounter or talking to someone you trust. At times, expressing your emotions through music, poetry, or art may give you the outlet you need. Exercise, especially intense cardiovascular exercise like running or dancing, can be incredibly conducive to experiencing intense emotions like anger. Letting yourself laugh or cry is another way to "burp" your Tupperware. These same methods that help you experience emotions can also be used to practice mindfulness, gain awareness of your energy balance, and explore your personal philosophy. Experiment with different techniques and find ones that resonate most with you.

67.2

Cultivate Compassion Toward Yourself

For many of us, being kind and compassionate toward ourselves is much more difficult than cultivating compassion for others. However, when we become closed to our own suffering, it is infinitely harder to remain open to the suffering of others. Cultivating self-compassion, therefore, is the key to becoming more compassionate toward those in our care. Ask yourself: Are you as patient with yourself when you make a mistake as you would be with another person? What is the tone of your *inner voice* during your mental exchanges? Do you say things like, *"I am such an idiot for taking this route; what is wrong with me today?"* There are times when our inner voice can become negative and, in fact, quite destructive. It happens differently for each of us, but it is likely we have all experienced this. Our inner voice, though, does not have to be critical or disapproving. In fact, our inner voice can, and should, be an incredible source of strength and guidance for us. The first step to harnessing this guidance is gaining awareness of how your inner voice speaks to you. Begin listening to it. Is it always disparaging? What does it usually say to you, and when do you hear it most frequently? If you have an inner voice that is unsympathetic, make an active decision to be more compassionate to yourself. Talk back to it using a gentle and loving tone, and ask it to be kinder. Your conscious awareness and natural kindness can recondition your inner voice to speak to you with love. Every time it speaks harshly, gently remind it to be kinder. Over time, your inner voice can change its tone, and this internal support system will begin to guide you in ways that are loving and compassionate.

If your inner voice seems unyielding to your effort to calm it, then you may consider professional guidance. Yes, you deserve support just as much as the youth and families you serve. Just as you guide youth to accept help without shame or stigma, free yourself from the shackles that tell you that as a caregiver you should be able to find the answers yourself. If you see self-care as selfish or seeking help yourself as a waste of time, then feel free to reframe it as a selfless act—*"I care for myself, so I can be stronger for others. I invest in my wellness, so I can serve for a lifetime."* Remember most of all that every healing effort starts with the health of the caregiver. ▶ **67.4**

■ Parting Thoughts

It is a gift to be able to care for another human being, even a calling or a personal path. We have all accepted this gift and know that caring for another can be both incredibly gratifying and overwhelming. Our innate ability to care, to connect, and to love is what puts us at risk; this double-edged sword can leave us wounded, unless we are active in our own healing process. Make a commitment to your own self-care. Develop daily strategies that allow you to be more mindful, that sustain your energy balance, and that help you find meaning in your work. Remember that you are not superhuman: Keep your identity integrated and whole, process your emotions regularly in ways that feel safe and supported and, most of all, cultivate loving-kindness and compassion toward yourself.

•• Group Learning and Discussion ••

This chapter hopes to initiate reflection and then personal action. That reflection holds the potential to catalyze the hard work of self-care we all need to do as individuals. However, our work environments can support or undermine our ability to adequately process our emotions and experiences, and ultimately to care for ourselves. Use this chapter as a launching pad to discuss how your practice setting could be healthier for the caregivers. Also process why attention to preventing burnout will, in fact, increase the quality of service you can all offer.

▪▪▪▪▪▪▪▪ Continuing Education ▪▪▪▪▪▪▪▪

If you are applying for continuing education credits, a test is available online. For more details, visit www.aap.org/reachingteens.

▪ References

1. Fox RC. The human condition of health professionals. Distinguished lecture series: University of New Hampshire; November 19, 1979; Durham, New Hampshire

2. Figley CR. Compassion fatigue: towards a new understanding of the cost of caring. In: Hudnall Stamm B, ed. *Secondary Traumatic Stress: Self-care Issues for Clinicians, Researchers and Educators.* 2nd ed. Baltimore, MD: Sidran Press; 1999:3–28

3. Golant M, Haskins NV. Other cancer survivors: the impact on family and caregivers. *Cancer J.* 2008;14(6):420–424

4. Pitceathly C, Maguire P. The psychological impact of cancer on patient's partners and other key relatives: a review. *Eur J Cancer.* 2003;39:1517–1524

5. Hodges LJ, Humphris GM, Macfarlane G. meta-analytic investigation of the relationship between psychological distress of cancer patients and their carers. *Soc Sci Med.* 2005;60:1–12

6. Tehrani N. Compassion fatigue: experiences in occupational health, human resources, counseling and police. *Occup Med.* 2010;60:133–138

7. Edwards D, Burnard P, Coyle D, et al. Stressors, moderators and stress outcomes: findings from the All-Wales Community Mental Health Study. *J Psych Ment Health Nurs.* 2000;7:529–537

8. Ramirez A, Addington-Hall J, Richards M. ABC of palliative care: the carers. *Br Med J.* 1998;316:208–211

9. McManus IC, Winder BC, Gordon D. The causal links between stress and burnout in a longitudinal study of UK doctors. *Lancet.* 2002;359:2089–2090

10. Association of Professors of Medicine. Predicting and preventing physician burnout: results from the US and the Netherlands. *Am J Med.* 2001;111:170–175

11. Maslach, C. Burned out. *Hum Behav.* 1976;5:16–22

12. Travado L, Grassi L, Gil F, et al. Physician-patient communication among southern European cancer physicians: the influence of psychosocial orientation and burnout. *Psychooncology.* 2005;14(8):661–670

13. Williams ES, Manwell LB, Konrad TR, et al. The relationship of organizational culture, stress, satisfaction and burnout with physician-reported error and suboptimal patient care: results from the MEMO study. *Health Serv Manag Res.* 2007;32(3):203–212

14. Shanafelt TD, Bradley KA, Wipf JE, et al. Burnout and self-reported patient care in an internal medicine residency program. *Ann Intern Med.* 2002;136(5):358–367

15. Thomas MR, Dyrbye LN, Huntington JL, et al. How do distress and well-being relate to medical student empathy? multicenter study. *J Gen Intern Med.* 2007;22(2):177–183

16. Ratanawongsa N, Roter D, Beach MC, et al. Physician burnout and patient-physician communication during primary care encounters. *JGIM.* 2008;23(10):1581–1588

17. West CP, Huschka MM, Novotny PJ, et al. Association of perceived medical errors with resident distress and empathy. *JAMA.* 2006;296:1071–1078

18. Brown SD, Goske MJ, Johnson CM. Beyond substance abuse: stress, burnout, and depression as causes of physician impairment and disruptive behavior. *J Am Coll Radiol.* 2009;6:479–485

19. Willcock SM, Daly MG, Tennant CC, et al. Burnout and psychiatric morbidity in new medical graduates. *Med J Aust.* 2004;181:357–360

20. Dyrbye LN, Thomas MR, Massie FS, et al. Burnout and suicidal ideation among US medical students. *Ann Intern Med.* 2008;149:334–341

21. Wilter JH. Stress, burnout and physician productivity. MGMJ. 1998;May/June:32–37

22. Riley GJ. Understanding the stresses and strains of being a doctor. *Med J Aust.* 2004; 181(7):350–353

23. Linzer M, Visser MRM, Oort FJ, et al. Predicting and preventing physician burnout: results from the US and the Netherlands. *Am J Med.* 2001;111:170–175

24. Williams ES, Konrad TR, Linzer M, et al. Physician, practice, and patient characteristics related to primary care physician physical and mental health: results from the physician worklife study. *Health Serv Res.* 2002;37(1):121–141

25. Keeton K, Fenner DE, Johnson TR, et al. Predictors of physician career satisfaction, work-life balance, and burnout. *Obstet Gynecol.* 2007;109(4):949–955

26. Lawrence J. Stress and the doctor's health. *Aust Fam Physician.* 1996;25:1249–1256

27. Matthews JT, Dunbar-Jacob J, Sereika S, et al. Preventative health practices: comparison of family caregivers 50 and older. *J Geron Nurs.* 2004;30(2):46–54

28. Perlick DA, Rosenheck RA, Miklowitz DJ, et al. Prevalence and correlates of burden among caregivers of patients with bipolar disorder enrolled in the Systematic Treatment Enhancement Program for Bipolar Disorder. *Bipolar Disord.* 2007;9:262–273

29. Perlick DA, Rosenheck RA, Miklowitz DJ, et al. Caregiver burden and health in bipolar disorder: a cluster analytic approach. *J Nerv Ment Dis.* 2008;196:484–491

30. Kay M, Mitchell G, Del Mar C. Doctors do not adequately look after their own physical health. *Med J Aust.* 2004;181(7):368–370

31. Pullen D, Lonie CE, Lyle DM, et al. Medical care of doctors. *Med J Aust.* 1995;162:481–484

32. Gross C, Mead L, Ford D, et al. Physician, heal thyself? Regular source of care and use of preventative health services among physicians. *Arch Intern Med.* 2000; 160, 3209–3214

33. Center C, Davis M, Detre T, et al. Confronting depression and suicide in physicians: a consensus statement. *JAMA.* 2003;289(23):3161–3166

34. Thompson W, Cupples M, Sibbett C, et al. Challenge of culture, conscience and contract to general practioners' care of their own health: qualitative study. *BMJ.* 2001;323:728–731

35. Shanafelt TD, Novotny P, Johnson ME, et al. The well-being and personal wellness promotion strategies of medical oncologist in North Central Cancer Treatment Group. *Oncology.* 2005;68:23–32

36. Weiner E, Swain G, Wolf B, et al. qualitative study of physicians' own wellness-promotion practices. West J Med. 2001;174:19–23

37. Quill TE, Williamson PR. Healthy approaches to physician stress. *Arch Intern Med.* 1990;150:1857–1861

38. Gordon JS. *Manifesto For a New Medicine.* Reading, MA: Perseus Books; 1996:107

39. Hanson R, Mendius R. *Buddha's Brain: The Practical Neuroscience of Happiness, Love and Wisdom.* Oakland, CA: New Harbinger Publications, Inc.; 2009:126, 177–190

40. Kabat-Zinn J. *Full Catastrophe Living: Using the Wisdom of Your Body and Mind to Face Stress, Pain and Illness.* New York, NY: Delta Trade Paperbacks; 1990

41. Kabat-Zinn J. *Wherever You Go There You Are: Mindfulness Meditation in Everyday Life.* New York, NY: Hyperion; 1994

42. Kabat-Zinn J. *Coming to Our Senses: Healing Ourselves and the World Through Mindfulness.* New York, NY: Hyperion; 2005

43. Gazella KA. Bringing mindfulness to medicine: an interview with Jon Kabat-Zinn. *Altern Ther.* 2005;11(3):57–64

44. Novack DH, Epstein RM, Paulsen Randall H. Toward creating physician-healers: fostering medical students' self-awareness, personal growth, and well-being. *Acad Med.* 1999;74(5):516–520

45. Novack DH, Suchman AL, Clark W, et al. Calibrating the physician: personal awareness and effective patient care. *JAMA.* 1997:278(6):502–509

46. Connelly J. Being in the present moment: developing the capacity for mindfulness in medicine. *Acad Med.* 1999;74(4):420–424

47. Connelly JE. Using mindfulness in clinical medicine. *Perspect Biol Med.* 2005;48(1):84–94

48. Schmidt S. Mindfulness and healing intention: concepts, practice and research evaluation. *J Altern Compliment Med.* 2004;10(S1):S7–S14

49. Epstein R. Mindful practice in action (I): technical competence, evidenced-based medicine and relationship-centered care. *Fam Syst Health.* 2003;21(1):1–9

50. Epstein R. Mindful practice in action (II): cultivating habits of mind. *Fam Syst Health.* 2003;21(1):11–17

51. Quinn C, Clare L, Woods RT. The impact of motivations and meanings on the wellbeing of caregivers of people with dementia: a systematic review. *Int Psychogeriatr.* 2010;22(1):43–55

52. Sorrells-Jones J. Caring for the caregivers: a wellness and renewal project. *Nurs Admin Q.* 1993;17(2):61–67

53. Pearlin LI, Mullan JT, Semple SJ, et al. Caregiving and the stress process: an overview of concepts and their measures. *Gerontologist.* 1990;30:583–594

54. Baumeister RF, Vohs KD. The pursuit of meaningfulness in life. In: Snyder CR, Lopez SJ, eds. *Handbook of Positive Psychology.* New York, NY: Oxford University Press; 608–618

55. Folkman S, Moskowitz JT. Positive affect and the other side if coping. *Am Psychol.* 2000;55:647–654

56. Shakespear-Finch J, Gow K, Smith S. Personality, coping and posttraumatic growth in emergency ambulance personnel. *Traumatol Online J.* 2005;11:325–334

57. Paton D. Posttraumatic growth in protective services professionals: individual, cognitive and organizational influences. *Traumatol Online J.* 2005;11;335–346

58. Zika S, Chamberlain K. On the relation between meaning in life and psychological wellbeing. *Br J Psychol.* 1992;83:133–145

■ Related Video Content

67.0 Healer, Heal Thyself: Self-care for the Caregiver. Tomescu.

67.1 How "Choreographed Conversations" Can Prevent Burnout While We Still Give Youth What They Need. Ginsburg.

67.2 The Tupperware Box: A Model for Releasing Trapped Emotions. Ginsburg.

67.3 Burnout Prevention Tips From Professionals Who Serve Marginalized and Traumatized Youth. YouthBuild Philadelphia.

67.4 We Do Not Serve Others Well When We Are Not Centered. Singh.

67.5 Deep Boundaried Connections Restore Our Own Energy. Singh.

67.6 Mindfulness Allows Us to Remain Fully Present Even Amidst Our Exposure to Suffering. Vo.

20.2 Toxic Boundaries: How Seeing People as "Other" Disrupts Our Connections and Diminishes Us. Ginsburg.

32.4 Getting Practical: Bringing Mindfulness Into Your Life. Vo.

32.5 Mindfulness as a Tool to Increase Your Clinical Effectiveness. Vo.

32.7 Mindfulness as a Means to Increase Self-acceptance, Diminish Shame, and Defeat Self-hatred. Vo.

34.4 Professional and Parent: Insight From Having 2 Roles With Teens. Ford.

68.1 Dr Jenkins on Self-care, Boundaries, and Burnout Prevention. Jenkins.

CHAPTER 68

Getting Out of the "Fast Lane"—More "Miles to the Gallon"?

Renée R. Jenkins, MD, FAAP

 Related Video Content

68.0 An Interview With Dr Renée Jenkins on "Dialing Down"…But Still Doing Things That Matter

■ Why This Matters

Our self-image is often closely aligned with our professional responsibilities. For those of us who serve others, our work often defines us. In addition, our passion for the impact on others' lives invigorates and sustains us. Practically speaking this means that the prospects of slowing down, and ultimately retiring, can be greeted with apprehension, ambivalence, and even avoidance. We should anticipate these understandable feelings and plan for this stage of life with the same level of care and thoughtfulness we paid to earlier phases of our careers.

In fact, one's potential impact may be at its very greatest late in one's career after being well seasoned through experience. However, a passive approach in a changing landscape may leave your "productivity" measured by outdated standards. Active planning may allow us to slow down while still making the most substantial contributions of one's career.

Just as self-care and introspection were critical to preventing burnout, they are also essential to our maximizing our impact long after leaving the "fast lane." As you thoughtfully prepare for the later years of your career, you should also be planning for a satisfying and fulfilling retirement. We may not go to the same "jobs" after retirement, but our service to others can continue throughout our life span.

> If I have learned nothing else over this long career, 2 points resonate. First, one can barely even imagine how our students and mentees will impact the world. Second, even youth who don't always seem to be listening hold tightly onto the positive energy we share. They don't need us telling them what to do; they need us to believe in their potential.

■ Preparation

Life course transitions can be divided into first through fourth ages, very much like the 3 stages of adolescence. Childhood and young adulthood comprise the first 2 ages, and the third age is 55 to 79 years, which commonly encompasses plans for, and ultimately, retirement, before the fourth age of dependency and decline. Given the current life expectancy of a retiree of an average 65 years of age, both men and women can look forward to about 16 and 18 more years, respectively. In more recent times, this population is seen as healthy, active, mellowed, and wiser by life's experiences and has time to take a more long-term and considered view of life.

As a professional, there is also a developmental process to consider, especially if one is in an academic environment. There is a progression from early career (ie, junior faculty status in academics), to mid-career, to late career, then retirement. In a practice or agency setting, the pathway has been described as an early skill-building stage, a mid-career stage, a mature professional stage, and a late career stage. The sense of dynamism and growth are the pivotal characteristics of the process, but the support in coping successfully with each stage varies according to the stage and the environment in which this growth takes place. Many more opportunities are available during the early phases of one's career as formal skills and assimilating to the career culture are commonly agreed-on goals. But the goals are less clear than previously and diverge into more possibilities as the age cohort moves forward.

Preparation for the later career stages has focused for the most part on financial planning, with not as much preparation given to psychological and emotional changes related to successfully shifting and/or disengaging from the more intense lifestyle of the mid-career professional. More sources are becoming available to help people anticipate and plan for these changes, with a focus on a more creative and productive set of roles.

Nancy Schlossberg's[1] book, *Revitalizing Retirement: Reshaping Your Identity, Relationships, and Purpose,* emphasizes the need for individuals to assess their changing role so they can continue to feel that they matter. Mattering implies the need to feel noticed, appreciated, and depended on. The institution has to see the value of senior faculty/staff in the roles they play in mentoring and preserving institutional culture and reputation.

There are organizations and medical schools that recognize the importance of drawing from the wisdom of well-seasoned professionals as we build a new generation of compassionate caregivers; there are others who might be paying too little attention to preserving the culture of the organization and more to "efficiency."

There is a growing demographic of aging professionals and faculty, and we must recognize that they could use more explicit planning as they transition to the "third age." This planning must address more than financial well-being; it must address the psychological, physical, and emotional issues inherent in maturing. This period must be seen as an opportunity for renewal and redirection, rather than stagnation and decline.

■ A Personal Journey

I turned 65 this year and have a Medicare card, and it doesn't feel like I thought it would. I have a lot of energy, of course not as much as I had 10 years ago, but I'm clinically active, recently started a new administrative role, and am becoming the local "go-to" person on mentoring faculty. As a member of the "baby boomers" coalescing to form the "grey tsunami," I now realize, as well as from getting pressured by my family, that slowing down and spending more time with them should be moved up in priority for someone my age. So now I'm thinking about it, and I probably should have been doing so about 5 years ago.

So how do I move on and take the next step? Again, Schlossberg's[1] book helps by describing alternative retirement paths:

Continuers—These folks essentially dial time down doing the same type of work, but with less time commitment. They may even volunteer, for example, working one clinic a week per month. It's safe doing what you know (and love!) and choosing not to try new things.

Easy gliders—This group takes each day as it comes. They might have invested very little planning but prioritize recreation and a lot of unscheduled time. The problem is that it can eventually lead to boredom.

Adventurers—These people move in new directions, retiring from one career and going to another (eg, painting, writing). They settle in and commit to new interests.

Searchers—This is the group of people who try a lot of different things, never really landing for very long on anything.

Retreaters—These people vegetate. Some get lucky, but most hope something will come to them; they're not searching.

I'd love to be an adventurer, but I feel mostly like a continuer, at least for now. But I'm giving myself a couple years to figure it out. I plan to return to Schlossberg's[1] book, perhaps taking a deeper dive next time, allowing myself time and space (and a little guidance) to figure this out. I may consider a few sessions with a career coach, and I will definitely review reputable Internet resources like the University of Hawaii site on preretirement (www.hawaii.edu/retirees) and connect with universities and nongovernmental organizations with "third age" and senior faculty programs.

In the meantime, I will revel in the advancement and successes of those that I have mentored and supported. I cannot imagine ever choosing not to continue mentoring others, because I know that any impact I might have had as an individual is magnified multifold by the contributions made by others I have had even a small role in nurturing. I will continue to celebrate the spark in the medical students embracing pediatrics and adolescent medicine as career choices, because I *know* they are headed for a gratifying career. Above all, I will continue to admire and advocate for the young people, my adolescent patients, who rise above all the barriers set in their way and arrive in young adulthood thriving. They are models of resilience, and it has been a privilege to be in their lives.

I can take a step back and choose to travel in a different lane. It may not be as "fast," but I know it will be productive. I will continue to plant seeds, because if I have learned nothing else over this long career, 2 points resonate. First, one can barely even imagine how our students and mentees will impact the world. Second, even youth who don't always seem to be listening hold tightly onto the positive energy we share. They don't need us telling them what to do; they need us to believe in their potential.

Perhaps I am looking most forward to the extra time I will have to thoroughly enjoy my family.

And oh yes…I hope to learn that it is not selfish to take good care of myself as well.

•• Group Learning and Discussion ••

Consider taking an opportunity to reflect within your practice group whether you are taking full advantage of the expertise and wisdom of *all* members of the group. People have different gifts to offer at varied stages of their career. Have recent changes in your practice or business model narrowed how you define a contribution to your practice?

Continuing Education

If you are applying for continuing education credits, a test is available online. For more details, visit www.aap.org/reachingteens.

■ Reference

1. Schlossberg NK. *Revitalizing Retirement: Reshaping Your Identity, Relationships, and Purpose.* Washington, DC: American Psychological Association; 2009

■ Related Video Content

68.0 An Interview With Dr Renée Jenkins on "Dialing Down"…But Still Doing Things That Matter. Jenkins.

68.1 Dr Jenkins on Self-care, Boundaries, and Burnout Prevention. Jenkins.

■ Related Web Site

University of Hawaii at Mānoa
http://manoa.hawaii.edu/retirees

CHAPTER 69

Have I Really Made a Difference? Trusting That Our Presence Matters

Kenneth R. Ginsburg, MD, MS Ed, FAAP, FSAHM

 Related Video Content

69.0 Have I Really Made a Difference? Trusting That Our Presence Matters

■ Why This Matters

Caring makes us vulnerable to pain. If we expose ourselves to others' suffering while feeling a sense of futility, in time it simply won't feel worth it. Eventually we may shut ourselves off from compassion, thereby minimizing our potential to facilitate healing.

Believing that what we do matters is a core element of burnout prevention. Three key strategies are needed to help prevent burnout. First, we need appropriate boundaries that allow us to feel intensely, but to do so in a way that is both safe for us and therapeutic for the teens we serve. Next, we need to commit to self-care, including having strategies to manage the emotions that arise in the process of caring for others. Perhaps most importantly, we have to trust that caring is worth it.

> **Bask in the knowledge that the seeds you plant sometimes take root. You'll only rarely see the flower that blooms, but it blooms nonetheless.**

■ Trusting We Make a Difference

We do this because we are committed to the health and well-being of youth and believe passionately that building strong youth secures our future. We put in long hours, often give more than expected, and sometimes absorb pain to our own detriment, because we believe it will matter. If only we could be sure that our investment of time, energy, and passion would pay off.

We all sometimes end our days and wonder if we made a difference. Did I listen well enough to hear what she was trying to say? Was she listening? Did she understand why I was worried? Is he ready to follow through? Does her feeling safe and secure in my office really matter when she returns home to a life of chaos? Does him deciding to make the most of his life while in my presence matter, when he has to do what it takes to survive the deadly streets?

Rest assured that we all wonder whether or not our caring made a difference. Even the adolescent medicine specialists who have contributed to this work certainly sometimes question whether our efforts matter. We have shared with you our best techniques and some of our most moving experiences. Perhaps you have heard these anecdotes and too humbly wondered if you could match their effectiveness. Remember, we had the luxury of choosing them as our anecdotes! They have become our standard stories precisely because they offered us the rare opportunity to witness success right in front of our eyes. Please know that on most days, just like you, we go home and silently wonder whether what we did mattered.

Fortunately, we witness enough "aha moments" and see enough kids moving forward that we persevere. Those of us in practice long enough have had the privilege of seeing the impact of our involvement years later. Perhaps the most gratifying moments—or those that at least serve as the greatest reinforcement—come when we later encounter youth that earlier we didn't even know were listening. They tell us of a seed we planted. They tell us that we were the ones who helped them understand that they were acceptable just as they were. Or, they tell us that they stopped doing drugs, not really because we informed them of their dangers (they had heard all of that before), but because we allowed them to voice that they were using drugs to numb their intense pain. More importantly, we made them feel good about having feelings and competent in finding ways to express rather than hide their emotions. They bring us their own children to show us that they want to create a better life for their offspring than they were given. Then they cry as they say that just as we believed in them, they will believe in their children.

There is no technique that will always be effective, and most don't produce immediate results. But, it is worth knowing that a respectful stance rooted in eliciting, reflecting, and building on the existing strengths of youth will at least do no harm. The risk-based approach that focuses on failures or potential dangers can engender shame. Shame reinforces existing negative self-perceptions that can increase stress and lead to a cycle of dangerous choices. A strength-based compassionate approach may not produce immediate change, but it may light a spark. Genuinely trusting that the teen is the expert in her own life may empower her to craft solutions. At the least, it may make her more receptive to the next caring professional who will be there to serve when she is ready to move forward.

Take a breath.

Remind yourself that one of the greatest gifts you can give yourself is to restore your spirit with the knowledge that you do matter. The greatest gift you can give the youth you care for is to commit to serving them for a lifetime—to do what it takes proactively to stem your own burnout. A first step is to let go of the need to find immediate daily gratification in this job and instead to celebrate the integrity of your work, trust the value of your mission, and bask in the knowledge that the seeds you plant sometimes take root.

You'll only rarely see the flower that blooms, but it blooms nonetheless.

▦▦▦▦▦▦▦ Continuing Education ▦▦▦▦▦▦▦

If you are applying for continuing education credits, a test is available online. For more details, visit www.aap.org/reachingteens.

■ Related Video Content

69.0 Have I Really Made a Difference? Trusting That Our Presence Matters. YouthBuild Covenant House Youth, Ginsburg, Diaz, with other faculty.

18.7 The Goal Is Not to Get the Most Detailed History, It Is to Get the Most Therapeutic History for the Youth at That Time: A Case of Abuse That Revealed Itself Over Time. Ginsburg.

Index

A

ABO framework. *See* Attraction/behavior/orientation (ABO) framework
Absolute respect and unconditional love, 154–155
Abstract thinking, 56, 225
Abuse. *See* Violence
Acculturation, 540
    gaps, 542
    strategies, 540–541
    theory, 540–541
Acculturative dissonance, 541
Acculturative stress, 541
ACE study. *See* Adverse Childhood Experiences (ACE) study
Acquired immunodeficiency syndrome (AIDS). *See* Human immunodeficiency virus (HIV)
Action stage of behavioral change, 20, 21, 210
Active listening, 505
Active relaxation, 247
Acupuncture, 370
Acute dissociation, 44
Acute stress disorder, 44, 354
ADD-H: Comprehensive Teacher Rating Scale (ACTeRS), 390
Addictions treatment, 247
Addressing Mental Health Concerns in Primary Care: A Clinician's Toolkit, 347, 359, 385, 398
ADHD. *See* Attention-deficit/hyperactivity disorder (ADHD)
ADHD: What Every Parent Needs to Know, 398
Adolescence, 363, 376. *See also* Adolescents
    activities, interests, and identity formation, 63–64
    cognitive development, 56–58
    experimentation, 94
    fundamental questions, 13
    identity development, 58–59
    identity formation, 540
    independence, 3, 288–289
    modularity theory, 56–58
    moral development, 59
    multicultural and global perspectives, 59–60
    physical development, 55–56
    psychosocial development, 112
    "storm and stress," 25, 56, 283
    stress, 255
    teen brain, 57
    theory-theory, 58
Adolescent-friendly environment, 92, 99–102
Adolescent independence, 288–289
Adolescent pregnancy. *See* Teen pregnancy and parenting

Adolescent relationship violence (ARV), 479–487
    characteristics of healthy relationships, 481
    5 As of relationship violence, 483–485
    goal of violence, 479
    handouts/supplementary materials, 486
    parents, 482
    red flags, 482
    signs/symptoms of unhealthy relationships, 481
    spectrum of relationship violence, 483
    statistics, 479
    Web sites, 487
Adolescent SBIRT algorithm, 431
Adolescent-specific bias, 168
Adolescent world, 53, 63–67
Adolescents. *See also* Adolescence
    AMA classification, 91
    assumptions about health care providers, 113
    expert as to their own well-being, as, 25–30
    exposure to violence, 41
    independence, 288–289
    key characteristics, 94
    making their own decisions, 225–229
    owning their solutions, 225–229
    powerlessness, 112
    risk factors, 94
    signs, need to be referred, 222
    toxic images, 13, 14
    trauma, and, 429
    unmet needs, 91
Adrenaline, 42
Adult professionals. *See* Youth-serving professionals
Advance information, 134
Adventurer, 595
Adverse Childhood Experiences (ACE) study, 40–41
Adversity, 40
Affirmations, 427
Agent of change, 21
"Aha moments," 598
AIDS. *See* Human immunodeficiency virus (HIV)
Alcohol and drug use. *See* Substance use and abuse
Allostatic load, 39
Amygdala, 57
Anchoring bias, 167
Anorexia nervosa, 413. *See also* Eating disorders
Anosognosia, 417
Antidrug public service announcement (PSA), 456
Anxiety, 349–360
    acute stress disorder, 354
    CBT, 357
    defined, 349
    destigmatizing, 349–350
    DSM-5 diagnostic criteria, 350
    GAD, 350–351

Anxiety, *continued*
    medical evaluation, 356
    OCD, 353
    panic disorder, 353
    psychosocial screening/structured screening, 355
    PTSD, 354–355
    related resources, 358–360
    separation anxiety disorder, 351
    social anxiety disorder, 352
    specific phobias, 354
    SSHADESS Screen, 355
    supportive treatment, 357
    tips/guidelines, 356
Apology, 128–129, 191–192
Appeasement, 45
Art of healing, 584
ARV. *See* Adolescent relationship violence (ARV)
Ask-Tell-Ask, 428
Assumptions, 128
Attachment needs, 42
Attention-deficit/hyperactivity disorder (ADHD), 387–398
    brain, 390
    deer hunter/lookout metaphor, 391, 392
    deficit of attention, 391
    differential diagnosis, 393
    DSM-5 diagnostic criteria, 388–389
    exercise, 395
    heredity, 392
    highlighting positives, 392–393
    hyperactivity and impulsivity, 389
    inattention, 388
    key features, 393
    management strategies, 394–395
    medication, 394
    nutrition, 395
    organizational strategies, 394
    related resources, 398
    screening tools, 390
    sleep, 395
    Web sites, 398
    wellness strategies, 395
Attentive listening, 115. *See also* Listening
Attitude of curiosity, 256
Attraction/behavior/orientation (ABO) framework, 533
Atwood, Margaret, 63
AUDIT, 426
Authoritarian parents, 294
Authoritative parents, 294
"Autopilot" mode, 254
Availability bias, 167
Avoidance, 245, 247
Awareness, 256, 584

B
Bad news, delivering to adolescents, 195–199
    contributing to world, 198–199
    debrief, 198
    follow-up plan, 198
    parental involvement, 198
    tips/guidelines, 195–198
Bad news, delivering to parents, 303–307
Balanced parents, 294
Barriers to forging therapeutic connections, 156
Basic principles of resilience theory, 49–50
Beginner's mind, 256
Behavior change, 126
Behavioral change, 19–23
Bells of mindfulness, 256
Belonging, 238, 239, 240–241
Bias, 165–171
    adolescent-specific, 168
    body language, 146
    cultural diversity, and, 145–147
    microaggression, 147
    personal reflection, and, 169
    questions to ask yourself, 263
    stop, ask, and reconsider, 169
    types, 167–168
Black hole of trauma, 44
Blamelessness, 221
Blowing bubbles, 245
BMI. *See* Body mass index (BMI)
Body aches and pains. *See* Somatic symptoms
Body language, 113–116
    bad news, delivering, 196
    bias, 146
    body space, 115
    de-escalation, 189–190
    fear, 114–115
    gaze, 115
    judgment, 115
    openness/desire to serve, 115–116
    power, 114
    tone of communication, 122
Body mass index (BMI), 417
Body memories, 44
Body-mind connection, 265, 367–368
Body movement therapies, 220, 322
Body scan, 256
Body space, 115
Body stance, 114
Boundaries, 125, 153–163
    absolute respect and unconditional love, 154–155
    crises, 192
    ethical standards (professional associations), 162–163
    gifts (tokens of appreciation), 157–158
    homeless youth, 574
    immediacy, 158
    importance of, to teens, 295
    personal limits, 159–160
    rescue fantasy, 156

self-reflection, 156
sharing you own experiences, 155
24/7 availability, 158
Brain
    ADHD, 390
    awareness, 584
    extreme stress, 43
    fight–flight–freeze response, 42
    hand model, 255
    integration of multiple complex functions, 43
    key points, 57
    mindfulness, 254
    passive entertainment, 324
    somatic symptoms, 370
    stress response, 219, 220
    toxic stress, 38
Break problem down to manageable pieces,
        231–235
Breakfast, 323
Breaking bad news, 195–199, 303–307
Breaking up a fight, 189
Brief experience with success, 231
Brief psychosocial screen, 141
*Bright Futures: Guidelines for Health Supervision of
        Infants, Children, and Adolescents*, 12
Bronfenbrenner, Uri, 59, 60
Building competence, 226
*Building Resilience in Children and Teens: Giving
        Kids Roots and Wings*, 246, 297
Bulimia nervosa, 413. *See also* Eating disorders
Bullying, 471–478
    audience, 473
    cyberbullying, 474
    forms, 472
    Olweus model, 474
    opening questions, 475
    overview, 471–472
    somatic health symptoms, 472, 475
    victim, 473
    Web sites, 478
Burnout, 581, 582
Burnout prevention, 159, 160, 579

C

Calcium, 323
"Care versus cure" rehabilitative approach, 369
Caregiver wellness strategies
    assess your energy balance, 585
    cultivate awareness/mindfulness, 584
    cultivate compassion toward yourself, 588
    find meaning in what you do, 585
    process your emotions, 586–587
    seek balance in your identity, 586
    work-life balance, 586
*Caring for Children With ADHD: A Resource Toolkit
        for Clinicians*, 398

Case studies
    break problem into manageable pieces, 233–234
    chronic illness/special health care needs, 515–516
    Circle of Courage, 239–240
    demoralized youth, 205–206
    divorce, 465–466
    foster care youth, 558–559
    helping adolescents own their solutions, 227–228
    immigrant youth, 539–540
    mindfulness, 28, 253–254
    nurturant-authoritative approach, 28
    self-determination theory and autonomy
        support, 26–28
    substance abuse, 431–435
    trauma-informed practice, 181–183
Catastrophic thinking, 243
Cause-and-effect lectures, 225
CBT. *See* Cognitive behavior therapy (CBT)
Chaperones, 101
Character, 32–33, 135
Check-in rule, 335
Childhood abuse, 489–498
    asking questions, 490, 491–492
    child sexual abuse, defined, 490
    children with disabilities, 489
    closing interview, 494–495
    cognitive distortions, 492
    common consequences of abuse, 489
    confidentiality, 491
    dissonant and conflicting feelings, 493
    follow-up visit, 493–494
    prevalence of abuse, 489
    reporting abuse, 493
    sexual exploitation, 495–496
    support and counseling, 494
    Web sites, 498
*Childhood Depression: What Parents Can Do To
        Help*, 347
Choreographed conversation, 226, 305
Chronic hyperarousal, 42
Chronic illness/special health care needs, 511–521
    case example, 515–516
    confidentiality, 513
    health care plan, 515
    language, 512–513
    medication adherence, 514–515
    negative body image, 513
    opening questions, 513
    parents, 514
    REACH OUT curriculum, 514, 519
    reproductive health, 516–517
    setting stage for transition, 517–518
    support groups, 514, 518
    Web sites, 521
Circle of Courage, 237–242
    belonging, 238, 239, 240–241
    case study, 239–240
    generosity, 238, 239, 241
    independence, 238, 239, 241
    mastery, 238, 239, 240
    parents, 240

Clinical mindfulness-based interventions, 253
Cliques, 328–330
Closed body language, 115
Code words, 335
Codes of ethics (professional organizations), 162–163
Cognitive behavior therapy (CBT)
    anxiety, 357, 360
    depression, 344
    negative thoughts, 322
    stress, 220, 244
Cognitive development, 56–58
Cognitive disability. *See* Chronic illness/special
        health care needs
Cognitive errors, 166, 169
Columbia Center for Youth Violence Prevention
        (CCYVP), 483, 487
Coming out process, 535
Commercial sexual exploitation of children
        (CSEC), 495–496
Commission bias, 167
Communicating with adolescent, 119–199
    bias. *See* Bias
    boundaries. *See* Boundaries
    breaking bad news, 195–199
    brief psychosocial screen, 141
    core principles, 121–131
    crisis management, 187–194
    cultural humility, 145–151
    initial interview, 134–135
    overview, 119–120
    paperwork/advance information, 134
    psychosocial interview, 141–142
    resilience framework/principles, 133–138
    SSHADESS Screen, 140–141
    trauma-informed practice, 173–186
Communities That Care model, 10
Community-based youth development strategies,
        14–15
Community-level professional-parent partnership,
        279
Compassion fatigue, 581
Competence, 32, 33, 135
Complex post-traumatic stress disorder (PTSD), 44
Concrete mindfulness practices, 256
Concrete operational thinking, 56
Concretely, thinking, 225
"Conditioned mode," 221
Condoms, 86–87
Confidence, 32, 33, 135, 203
Confidentiality, 93, 106
Confirmation bias, 167
Connected Kids, 337
Connection, 32, 34, 135
Conners Parent and Teacher Rating Scales, 390
Contemplation stage of behavioral change, 20, 210
Continuer, 595
Continuing education credits, 6
Continuum of readiness for change, 428
Contract for Life, 335
Contribution, 33, 34, 136
Control, 32, 33, 34, 136

Conversion disorder, 362, 373
Coping, 32–34, 33, 136, 244–245. *See also* Stress
        management and coping
Coping style, 245
Core principles of positive youth development,
        15–16
Counseling, 269
Counseling, standards of practice, 162
Counselors, 269
Covenant House Pennsylvania, 50
CRAFFT, 430, 431
Creativity/creative activities, 180, 248, 324
Crisis management, 129–130, 187–194
    absolute respect, 189, 192
    apology, 191–192
    assess ongoing risk, 193
    avoid defensiveness, 192
    body language, 189–190
    boundaries, 192
    breaking up a fight, 189
    debrief, 193
    expectations, 306
    get rid of audience, 188
    giving something, 192
    goals, 187
    listening, 190
    precrisis planning, 189
    psychosis/drug use, 188
    referral, 193
    safety, 188
    tone of voice, 191
    what to say/don't say, 191
Cross-cultural perspectives of adolescence, 59
Crowds, 328
CSEC. *See* Commercial sexual exploitation of
        children (CSEC)
Cultural anthropologists, 59
Cultural competence, 145, 148
Cultural humility, 128, 145–151. *See also* Immigrant
        youth
Cyberbullying, 474

D

DARN-C, 428
Dash, Leon, 439
Dated "dating" language, 73
Dating abuse. *See* Adolescent relationship violence
        (ARV)
Daydreaming, 44
De-escalation, 189–190. *See also* Crisis management
Death. *See* Grieving youth
Debrief
    bad news, 198
    crisis management, 193
Decision tree, 227
Decisional balance, 20, 244
Deep breathing, 220, 247, 322
Deer hunter/lookout metaphor, 391, 392
Defensive position, 114
Delayed gratification, 158

Delivering information, concrete step-by-step technique, 226, 228
Demoralization, combating, 203–208
Demoralized youth, 127
Depression, 339–348
    counseling therapies, 344
    healing strategies, 343
    medical evaluation, 342
    psychopharmacological interventions, 344, 371
    related resources, 347–348
    SSHADESS Screen, 340–342
    stigma and shame, 343
    suicide, 344–345, 348
    supportive treatment, 343–344
    vegetative symptoms, 339
Developmental trauma disorder, 44
Dialectical behavioral therapy, 322
Diary, 369
Direct professional-parent partnership, 278
Directive counseling style, 210
Disabled youth. *See* Chronic illness/special health care needs
Discipline, 288, 297
Disengaged parents, 294
Disengagement strategies, 245
Dissociated behavioral sequences, 44
Dissociated emotions, 44
Dissociated knowledge, 44
Dissociation, 43–44, 46
Divorce, 463–469
    advice to parents, 466–467
    case studies, 465–466
    handouts/supplementary materials, 468
    questions to ask teen, 464
    related resources, 469
Dopamine, 57
Draining experiences, 585
Drawing, 384
Driven to Distraction: Recognizing and Coping with Attention Deficit Disorder (Hallowell et al), 390
Driving. *See* Teen driving
Drop, distract, dismiss, and ignore, 222
Drug use/abuse. *See* Substance use and abuse
DSM-5
    ADHD, 388
    anxiety, 350
    eating disorders, 413
    trauma, 44
Dweck, Carol, 406
Dyscalculia, 401
Dysgraphia, 400, 402
Dyslexia, 400
Dyspraxia, 401

E

Easy glider, 595
Eating disorders, 413–423
    anosognosia, 417
    atypical presentation, 414
    DSM-5 diagnostic criteria, 413
    family-based treatment, 418–419
    goal weight, 417
    handouts/supplementary materials, 422
    healthy weight, healthy state, 417–418
    interview, 416
    males, 415
    medical assessment, 416–417
    nutritional needs, 418
    obesity, 415
    overview, 413–414
    professionals, 420
    related resources, 423
    SCOFF questionnaire, 414
    screening, 414–415
    Web sites, 422
Eating meditation, 256
Ecological systems theory, 59, 60
Effects of adversity, 37–47. *See also* Trauma and toxic stress
El Centro de Estudiantes, 50, 179
Elaborating, 213
Electronic media use, 455–461
    antidrug PSA, 456
    benefits of media use, 456–457
    hints/tips, 457–459
    media multitasking, 459
    parents, 457
    super-peer theory, 455
    Web sites, 461
Elicit-provide-elicit, 215
Emotion-focused coping strategies, 245
Emotion-focused engagement coping, 245
Emotional, physical, and sexual abuse. *See* Childhood abuse
Emotional tension, 248–249
Empathy, 269, 371
Engagement, 579
Epinephrine, 42
Erectile dysfunction, 85
Erikson, Erik, 58
Ethical standards (professional organizations), 162–163
Evidence-based mindfulness-based interventions, 254
Exercise (physical activity), 247, 323–324
Expectations, 50, 284, 306, 311
"Exploratory mode," 221
Exploring goals and values, 214
Express empathy, 213
External locus of control, 202
Eye contact, 115

F

"Faking it," 368
Family tension, 310
Fear, body language, 114–115
Fear-conditioned, 43
Female stress responses, 45
Fight–flight–freeze response, 42
Fighting, 189. *See also* Youth violence
First impressions, 134
5 As of relationship violence, 483–485
Fixed mindset, 406
Flashbacks, 44
Focused thinking, 202
Folate, 323
Following, guiding, gently directing, 211
Food advertisements, 456
Formal cognitive operations, 56
Forum for Youth Investment, 31
Foster care youth, 557–561
    aging out, 559–560
    case study, 558–559
    confidentiality, 558
    establishing trust and respect, 557–558
    handouts/supplementary materials, 561
    health decision-making, 558
    medical home, 558
    Web sites, 561
4-H philosophy, 12, 31, 50
4 to 8 breathing, 247
FRAMES
    advice, 215
    empathy, 216
    feedback, 215
    menu, 216
    responsibility, 215
    self-efficacy, 216
Framing effect, 168
Friends Are Important: Tips for Parents, 337
Friendships and peers, 327–337
    adolescent years, 332
    check-in rule, 335
    cliques, 328–330
    code words, 335
    crowds, 328
    early years, 331
    handouts/supplementary materials, 337
    manipulation, 334
    maturity, 330
    peer navigation skills, 333–335
    saying "no," 334
    school-aged years, 331–332
    shifting blame to save face, 335
    Web sites, 337
Fundamental questions of adolescence, 13

G

GAD. *See* Generalized anxiety disorder (GAD)
Gaining a sense of control (one step at a time),
    231–235
Gangs. *See* Youth violence
Gay and lesbian youth. *See* Sexual and gender
    minority youth
Gaze, 115
GDL laws. *See* Graduated driver licensing (GDL)
    laws
Gender identity, 532
Gender-neutral language, 73
Generalized anxiety disorder (GAD), 350–351
Generation gap, 25
Generosity, 238, 239, 241
Genital arousal, 101
Genuineness, 513
Gifts (tokens of appreciation), 157–158
Ginsburg, Ken, 587
GLAD-PC. *See* Guidelines for Adolescent
    Depression in Primary Care (GLAD-PC)
Good news/bad news approach, 304–305
Gordon, James, 584
Graduated driver licensing (GDL) laws, 450
Grey matter, 57
Grieving youth, 375–386
    common grief manifestations, 381
    early adolescence, 377
    family functioning, 376
    guide youth toward help, 380
    guilt, 378
    length of grieving period, 378–379
    life skills, 379
    making sense of a loss, 376
    older adolescents, 377
    parental involvement, 381–382
    related resources, 385–386
    sleep disruption, 378
    stages of grief (adult model), 376
    steering teens toward positive strategies,
        383–384
    tips/hints, 379–381
    unpredictability, 378
    withdrawal from activities, 378
Group learning and discussion, 6
Group rules and norms, 297
Growth mindset, 406
Guidelines for Adolescent Depression in Primary
    Care (GLAD-PC), 345

H

Hall, G. Stanley, 25, 56
Hallowell, Edward (Ned), 390
Hand model of brain, 255
Hand motions, 114
Handling others' pain, 160

Handouts/supplementary materials
    childhood abuse, 498
    chronic illness/special health care needs, 519
    divorce, 468
    eating disorders, 422
    foster care youth, 561
    friendships and peers, 337
    helping adolescents own their solutions, 229
    homeless youth, 578
    military youth, 555
    mindfulness, 259
    monitoring, 301
    perfectionism, 412
    professional-parent relationship, 291, 301, 318
    relationship violence, 486
    resilience theory, 138
    7 Cs of resilience, 36
    sexuality, 79
    stress management, 252
    trauma-informed practice, 186
Headache, 361, 367
Healing environment, 49
Health care professionals. *See* Youth-serving
    professionals
Health realization, 220–221
Healthy coping strategies, 317
Healthy disengagement strategies, 245
Healthy environment, 12
Healthy high achievers, 405
Healthy lifestyle, 220, 221. *See also* Lifestyle choices
Healthy relationships, 481
Healthy Teen Network, 441
Healthy thinking patterns, 244
Healthy weight, healthy state, 417–418
HealthyChildren.org, 385
Help-seeking, 267
Helping adolescents own their solutions, 225–229
Heroes, 406, 408
Heuristics, 166
Hidden Among Us: Sexually Exploited and
    Trafficked Youth, 496
HIV-infected youth. *See* Human immunodeficiency
    virus (HIV)
Hobbies, 324
Homeless and unstably housed youth, 569–578
    advice for providers, 574
    boundaries, 574
    couch surfing/squatting, 570
    disequilibrium stage, 571–572
    extrication stage, 572
    family background and development, 569–570
    first-on-the-street stage, 571
    handouts/supplementary materials, 578
    initiation stage, 571
    life cycle of homelessness, 570–572
    mainstream stage (pre-street life), 571
    recidivism stage (return to street life), 572
    risky behaviors and morbidity, 570
    stasis stage, 571
    strength-based interview approach, 574
    trustworthiness, 574
    unstable housing status screening tool, 575
    youth presenting in a service agency, 573–574
Honesty, 105
Human immunodeficiency virus (HIV), 563–567
    ABO approach, 533, 563
    confidentiality and disclosure issues, 565
    delivering HIV test results, 564
    medication adherence/readiness, 565–566
    prevention and screening, 563
    shame and stigma, 564
    spirituality and religion, 566
    tips for general care, 565
Hyperactivity and impulsivity, 389
Hypervigilance, 45
Hypochondriasis, 362

I

"I understand," never say, 123
Identity
    achievement, 58
    development, 58–59
    diffusion, 58
    foreclosure, 58
    moratorium, 58
    statuses, 58
IEP. *See* Individualized education plan (IEP)
Immediacy, 158
Immigrant youth, 539–544
    acculturation gaps, 542
    acculturation strategies, 540–541
    acculturative stress/acculturative dissonance, 541
    assess REI development and acculturation, 542
    case study, 539–540
    confidentiality, 542
    cultural humility, 541
    immigration history, 541–542
    linguistic barriers, 542
    office space, 543
    promote bicultural self-efficacy/integrated
        acculturation, 543
    REI development, 540
    research, 543
    strength-based counseling, 541
    systems advocacy, 543
Importance ruler, 213, 214
Impostor syndrome, 583
Inattention, 388
Independence, 3, 238, 239, 241, 288–289
Indirect professional-parent partnership, 278–279
Individualized education plan (IEP), 400
Individuals with Disabilities Education Act, 400
Information exchange, goal of, 225
Initial interview, 134–135
Instant vacations, 248
Intake forms, 134
Integration, 26
Intensive group support strategies, 265–266
Internal locus of control, 232
Internalization, 26

Interviewing technique (Circle of Courage), 237–242
Intimacy, 82
Iodine, 323
Iron, 323
It Gets Better Project, 478, 538
"It Gets Better" Web video, 65

J

Journaling, 248, 384. *See also* Diary

K

Keep teens talking (keys to disclosure), 297
Kelty Mental Health Resource Centre, 256, 259

L

Labels, 264–265
Ladder technique, 232, 505
Large problem/small pieces, 231–235
Leaden box, 587
Learning disabilities/differences, 393, 399–404
    ADHD, and, 393, 401
    comprehensive assessment and evaluation, 402
    IEPs, 400
    "lazy," "stupid," 402
    neuropsychological or psychoeducational
        testing, 402
    parents, 402–403
    professionals, 403
    red flags, 401
    related resources, 404
    specific disabilities, 400–401
Lecturing, 202, 225, 226, 286
Left-brain thinking, 221
Legitimate authority, 296
Lerner, Richard, 10, 31, 50
Level of engagement. *See* Boundaries
LGBTQ youth. *See* Sexual and gender minority
        youth
Life course transitions, 593–594
Lifestyle choices
    nutrition, 323
    physical activity, 323–324
    recreational activities, 324
    sleep, 322–323
Limb pain, 361
Listening
    bad news message, 197
    body language, 115
    crisis management, 190
    parent, 286
    respectful, 122
    youth violence, 505
Little, Rick, 10, 31, 264
Locus of control
    external, 202
    internal, 232

Loss of loved one. *See* Grieving youth
Love, 154, 582. *See also* Unconditional love
Loving-kindness, 154, 256
Loving-kindness meditation, 256
Low mood, 221, 222
"Lying," 46

M

Maintenance stage of behavioral change, 20, 21,
        210
Male adolescent-friendly space, 99–102
Male genital examination, 100–101
Male sexuality, 81–88. *See also* Sexuality education
    condoms, 86–87
    erectile dysfunction, 85
    intimacy, 82
    LGBT youth, 83–84, 87
    lubrication, 87
    orgasm, 85
    parental role, 82
    penis size, 84
    premature ejaculation, 85
    sexual arousal, 85
    understanding female sexuality, 83
    understanding mechanics, 82
Manageable steps, 231–235
Marcia, James, 58, 59
Marginalized adolescents, 111–113
Marijuana, 425
Marriage and family therapy, code of ethics, 162
Massage, 370
Mastery, 238, 239, 240
MBSR. *See* Mindfulness-based stress reduction
        (MBSR)
Media. *See* Electronic media use
Media multitasking, 459
Medical errors, 166
Medical ethics, 162
Meditation, 249. *See also* Mindfulness
Mental health
    ADHD, 387–398
    anxiety, 349–360
    depression, 339–348
    eating disorders, 413–423
    ethical code, 162
    LGBTQ youth, 534
Mental imagery, 220, 322
MI. *See* Motivational interviewing (MI)
Microaggression, 147
Micronutrients, 323
Military children and adolescents, 545–555
    communication with deployed parent, 548–549
    discipline, 550–551
    handouts/supplementary materials, 555
    maintaining family connections through deploy-
        ment, 547–548
    memory tools, 549
    military youth culture, 546–547
    parentification, 551–553
    perfectionism, 553

reintegration, 552
Web sites, 555
Mind-body connection, 265, 367–368
Mindful qualities, 256
Mindfulness, 26, 253–259
    awareness, kindness, curiosity, 256
    beginner's mind, 256
    brain, 254
    case study, 28, 253–254
    formal mindfulness practice, 256
    handouts/supplementary materials, 259
    informal mindfulness practices, 256
    most important aspect, 257
    providers, 257, 584–585
    psychoeducation on brain, body, and stress, 255
    referral, 257
    relaxation, and, 247
    setting stage, 255–256
    strength-based approach, 256
    Web sites, 259
    what is it, 253
Mindfulness-based stress reduction (MBSR), 254
Mindfulness of breathing, 256
Mindless state, 254
Minerals, 323
Modularity theory, 56–58
Monitoring strategies, 295–297, 301
Mood, 221–222
Mood stabilizers, 371
Moral development, 59
MOST of Us, 14, 17
Motivational interviewing (MI), 74, 209–218
    adult professional as facilitator, 209
    assumptions, 209
    behavior change, 126
    DARN-C, 428
    elaborating, 213
    elicit-provide-elicit, 215
    exploring goals and values, 214
    express empathy, 213
    following, guiding, gently directing, 211
    FRAMES, 215–216
    guiding principles, 212
    importance ruler, 213, 214
    interviewing tools, 212–215
    OARES/OARS, 216, 427
    philosophical approach, 211
    querying extremes, 214
    recognizes that change is driven by teen, 210,
        264
    stages of change, 210
    substance abuse, 427–428
    support self-efficacy, 210
    teen pregnancy, 443
    Web site, 218
    weighing pros and cons, 244
    youth, ambivalence to change, 211
Motor vehicle accidents. See Teen driving
Multicultural and global perspectives. See Cultural
        humility; Immigrant youth
Multitasking, 585

Munchausen syndrome/Munchausen syndrome by
        proxy, 362–363
Music therapy, code of ethics, 162

N

Nag-free zone, 289
National Campaign to Prevent Teen and Unplanned
        Pregnancy, 79, 441
National Center for Missing and Exploited
        Children, 496
Negative coping strategies, 243
Negative thinking/thoughts, 220
Neurotransmitters, 368
NICHQ Vanderbilt Assessment Scale and Follow
        Up, 390
Non-steroidal anti-inflammatory medications, 370
Non-stigmatizing environment, 93
Nonjudgmental body language techniques, 115
Nonverbal learning disorder, 401
Norepinephrine, 42
Normal dissociation, 44
Nurturant-authoritative approach, 26, 28
Nutrition, 323

O

OARS
    affirmations, 427
    open-ended questions, 427
    reflective statements, 427, 428
    summary statements, 427
OBPP. See Olweus Bullying Prevention Program
        (OBPP)
Obsessive compulsive disorder (OCD), 353
Obsessive personality trait, 583
OCD. See Obsessive compulsive disorder (OCD)
Office-based mindfulness training, 255–257
Office space, 92, 100, 262, 532, 543
Office staff, 262
Old thoughts, 221
Olweus Bullying Prevention Program (OBPP), 474
Omega-3 fatty acids, 323
Omission bias, 167
Open body language, 115
Openness/desire to serve, body language, 115–116
Optimal functioning, 221
Order effect, 167–168
Orgasm, 85
Other specified feeding and eating disorders
        (OSFED), 413, 414
Outercourse, 74
Overcoming shame and stigma, 261–272
    address risk while recognizing strength, 264
    bias, 263
    body-mind connection, 265
    depression, 343
    HIV, 564
    labels, 264–265
    office space, 262

Overcoming shame and stigma, *continued*
    office staff, 262
    overview, 268
    parents, 266–267
    persuade teen to seek help, 267–269
    recognize teen as expert, 264
    somatic symptoms, 368
    trustworthiness, 263

P

Pain management, 370
Panic attack, 353
Paperwork, 134
Parent
    adolescent health, 277
    adolescent independence, 288–289
    adolescent relationship violence, 482
    adolescent substance abuse, 435, 438
    adolescent trauma and toxic stress, 45
    Circle of Courage, 240–241
    disabled youth, 514
    disciplinarian, as, 288, 297
    electronic media use, 457
    grieving adolescents, 381–382
    guide and monitor, as, 287
    health care professionals, and. *See* Professional-
        parent relationship
    importance, 285
    keep teens talking, 297
    learning disabilities, 402–403
    LGBTQ youth, 535
    listening, 286
    nag-free zone, 289
    professionalization of parenting, 316
    reached limit of patience, 309–313
    rejection by teen, 285–286, 309, 311
    repair relationship with child, 312
    role model of appropriate coping strategies, as,
        317
    role model of balance and well-being, as, 316
    rules, 298
    self-care, 315–318
    selfless parenting, 315–316
    sex education, 74–77, 82
    shame and stigma, 266–267
    stay engaged through troubled times, 311
    style of parenting, 294
    teen driving, 450–451, 452–453
    teen parenting, 441
    upsetting news, receipt of, 303–307
    values education, 286–287
Parent-child driving contract, 451–452
Parent-completed Child Behavior Checklist, 390
Parent-teen tension, 310
Parental self-care, 315–318
"Parentification," 551–553
Parenting style, 294
Pastoral counselors, code of ethics, 162
Pathological dissociation, 44

Peer navigation skills, 333–335
Peers, 3, 42, 298. *See also* Friendships and peers
Perfectionism, 317, 405–412
    academic pressures, 406
    adaptive/maladaptive, 405
    definition of success, 409
    fear of disappointment, 407
    growth mindset/fixed mindset, 406
    handouts/supplementary materials, 412
    healthy high achievers, contrasted, 405
    heroes, 406, 408
    model self-acceptance, 408
    opportunities for self-discovery, 409
    permissive style of parenting, 407
    praise, 406, 408
    seeking professional help, 410
    sensationalism of success and failure, 406
    unconditional acceptance, 409
Permissive parents, 294, 297, 407
Personal questions, 105
Phenomenological variant of ecological systems
        theory, 60
Philosophical framework, 3–4
Phobia, 354
Physical activity, 247, 323–324
Physical development, 55–56
Physical disability. *See* Chronic illness/special
        health care needs
Physical environment (office space), 92, 100, 262,
        532, 543
Physical function and pain. *See* Somatic symptoms
Physical reconditioning, 370
Physical stresses, 221
Phytonutrients, 323
Pierce, Chester M., 147
Pilates, 370
Pittman, Karen, 10, 25, 31
Poetry writing, 384
POSIT, 426
Positive stress, 38
Positive youth development (PYD)
    constructs, 50
    programs, 10, 12, 14–16, 31
Post-traumatic stress disorder (PTSD), 41, 44,
        354–355
Poverty, 440
Power, body language, 114
Powerlessness, 112, 231
Praise, 406, 408
Prayer, 249
Precontemplation stage of behavioral change, 20,
        210
Prefrontal cortex, 219, 254
Pregnancy. *See* Teen pregnancy and parenting
Prejudice, 146
Premature closure, 167
Premature ejaculation, 85
Preparation stage of behavioral change, 20, 210
Present moment, nonjudgmental awareness, 255,
        256

Privacy, 106, 269. *See also* Confidentiality
Problem-focused coping strategies, 245
Problem-focused engagement coping, 245
Procedural checklists, 166
Professional organizations (codes of ethics),
    162–163
Professional-parent relationship, 107, 273–318
    community-level professional-parent partner-
        ship, 279
    delivering upsetting news to parents, 303–307
    direct professional-parent partnership, 278
    general framework, 276
    handouts/supplementary materials, 291, 301,
        318
    indirect professional-parent partnership,
        278–279
    overview, 273–274
    parents' resilience reaches its limits, 309–313
    preparing parents, 283–291
    promoting balanced parenting, 293–301
    rules and boundaries, 298
    self-care for parents, 315–318
Professionalization of parenting, 316
Progressive muscle relaxation, 220, 322
Prolonged dependency and attachment needs, 42
Protective factors, 9, 10
Providers. *See* Youth-serving professionals
Pseudoseizure, 362
Psychoanalysts, standards of ethics, 163
Psychoeducation, 180, 255
Psychological distress, 321. *See also* Anxiety;
    Depression
Psychologists, code of conduct, 163
Psychosocial and behavioral problems, 9
Psychosocial interview, 141–142
PTSD. *See* Post-traumatic stress disorder (PTSD)
Pubertal maturation, 55
Punching bag, 505
PYD constructs. *See* Positive youth development
    (PYD)
PYD programs. *See* Positive youth development
    (PYD)
Pyridoxine, 323

Q

Qigong, 322
Querying extremes, 214

R

Race and ethnicity. *See* Immigrant youth
Racial/ethnic identity (REI) model, 540
RAP. *See* Recurrent abdominal pain (RAP)
REACH OUT curriculum, 514, 519
Read-back protocols, 166
Readiness, importance and confidence rulers, 214
Reality, 222
"Receiver mode," 221
Recreational activities, 324

Recurrent abdominal pain (RAP), 369
Reducing shame and stigma. *See* Overcoming
    shame and stigma
Referral
    crisis management, 193
    mindfulness, 257
    substance abuse, 429
    when needed, 222
Reflective statements, 427, 428
REI model. *See* Racial/ethnic identity (REI) model
Relapse, 210
Relationship literacy, 73
Relationship violence. *See* Adolescent relationship
    violence (ARV)
Relaxation techniques
    active relaxation, 247
    mindfulness. *See* Mindfulness
    progressive muscle relaxation, 220
Repetitive thoughts, 221
Rescue fantasy, 156
Resilience research, 10
Resilience theory, 137
    basic principles, 49–50
    7 Cs model, 31–36, 135–136
    expectations, 14, 306
    face time, 134–135
    parents, and, 284
Respectful listening, 122
Respecting youth, 154
Responsiveness, 293, 297
Retirement paths, 595
Retreater, 595
Revisualize a problem into manageable steps,
    231–235
*Revitalizing Retirement: Reshaping Your Identity,
    Relationships, and Purpose* (Schlossberg),
    594
Right-brain thinking, 221
Risk factors, 9, 94
Role-playing, 226
Root cause analyses, 166
Rules and boundaries, 297, 298
Ruminative (mindless) state, 254

S

Safe Horizon Anti-Trafficking Program and
    Hotline, 496
SAMHSA. *See* Substance Abuse and Mental Health
    Services Administration (SAMHSA)
Sanctuary model, 176
Savage, Dan, 65, 478
Saying "no," 334
SBIRT, 430, 431
Schemas, 146
Schlossberg, Nancy, 594
School counselors, ethical standards, 163
SCOFF questionnaire, 414
SDT. *See* Self-determination theory (SDT)
Searcher, 595
Secondary trauma, 581

Self-awareness, 146, 584, 585
Self-care
    parents, 315–318
    professional caregivers, 581–591
Self-determination theory (SDT), 26
Self-efficacy, 32, 33
Self-hypnosis, 220
Self-identified crowd affiliation, 328
Self-regulatory techniques, 220, 322
Self-validation, 72
Selfless parenting, 315–316
Sense of reality, 222
Separate realities, 222
Separation and divorce. See Divorce
Separation anxiety disorder, 351
Serenity prayer, 247
Serotonin reuptake inhibitors, 371
Service with respect and without judgment,
        105–106
7 Cs model of resilience, 31–36
    character, 32–33
    competence, 32
    confidence, 32
    connection, 32
    contribution, 33
    control, 33
    coping, 33
    handouts/supplementary materials, 36
    historical overview, 31–32
    integrating, into your practice, 135–136
Sex education. See Sexuality education
Sexual abuse, 490. See also Childhood abuse
Sexual and gender minority youth, 531–538
    ABO framework, 533
    coming out process, 535
    discussing sexual health and sexuality, 83–84,
        87, 533–534
    health risks, 531
    "It Gets Better" Web video, 65
    mental health, 534
    office space/staff, 532
    parents, 535
    physical examination, 534
    providing support, 535
    setting stage, 532
    terminology/definitions, 531–532
    Web sites, 538
Sexual arousal, 85, 101
Sexual awakening, 82
Sexual behavior, 532
Sexual exploitation, 495–496
Sexual orientation, 531–532
Sexuality education, 69–88
    adult professional, role of, 70–74, 81–87
    code of ethics, 162
    females, 69–80
    handouts/supplementary materials, 79
    males, 81–88. See also Male sexuality
    parental involvement, 74–77, 82
    suggested reading, 80, 88
    Web sites, 79

Shadow punching, 505
Shame, 261. See also Overcoming shame and
        stigma
Shared decision-making, 125
Shifting blame to save face, 335
Shutting off stress response, 220
Signs of youth in need of help, 222
Skipping meals, 323
Sleep hygiene, 248, 322–323
Social anxiety disorder, 352
Somatic symptoms, 361–373
    care versus cure approach, 369
    conversion disorder, 362
    diary, 369
    differential diagnosis and evaluation, 366–367
    empathy, 371
    hypochondriasis, 362
    individual and family therapy, 370
    inform teen what to tell others, 369
    medications, 370–371
    mind-body connection, 367–368
    Munchausen syndrome, 362–363
    ongoing treatment plan, 371
    pain management, 370
    physical reconditioning, 370
    related resources, 373
    returning to school, 370
    routines, 369
    shame and stigma, 368
    SSHADESS Screen, 363–366
    treatment team, 369
    understanding teen's symptoms, 365–366
Spatial violations, 115
Special populations
    chronic illness and disabilities, 511–521
    foster care youth, 557–561
    HIV-infected youth, 563–567
    homeless youth, 569–578
    immigrant youth, 539–544
    military-affiliated youth, 545–555
    sexual and gender minority youth, 531–538
    transition to adult care, 523–529
Speechless terror, 44
SSHADESS Screen
    activities, 140
    anxiety, 355
    communicating with adolescent, 140–141
    depression, 340–342
    drugs/substance abuse, 140
    emotions/eating/depression, 140
    home, 140
    safety, 140–141
    school, 140
    sexuality, 140
    somatic symptoms, 363–366
    strengths, 140
Staged conversations, 74
Stages of change model, 19–20, 210
Standards of practice (professional organizations),
        162–163
Steepled hands clasped together, 115

Stereotypes, 146
Stigma, 261. *See also* Overcoming shame and
    stigma
Stomachache, 361, 369
"Storm and stress," 25, 56, 283
Street youth. *See* Homeless and unstably housed
    youth
Strength-based approach, 1–52
    basic principles of resilience theory, 49–50
    behavioral change, and, 19–23
    community-based strategies, 14–15
    core principles of positive youth development,
        15–16
    effects of adversity, 37–47. *See also* Trauma and
        toxic stress
    goals, 13
    interviewing (Circle of Courage), 237–242
    overview (content), 1–2
    psychosocial assessment, 139–143
    PYD programs, 10, 12, 14–16, 31
    7 Cs model of resilience, 31–36
    strategies (agent of change), 21
    strategies (strength-building skills), 21–22
    youth violence, 499–500
Strength-based communication strategies, 13
Strength-based interviewing (Circle of Courage),
    237–242
Strength-based psychosocial assessment, 139–143
Strength-building skills, 21–22
Stress, 243. *See also* Trauma and toxic stress
Stress continuum, 38–39
Stress management and coping, 243–252
    assessing stressor, 243–244
    coping, 244–245
    handout/supplementary material, 252
    primary prevention, 250
    secondary prevention, 250
    stress reduction plan, 246–249
Stress-management techniques, 321–322
Stress reduction plan, 246–249
    active relaxation, 247
    avoid stress when possible, 247
    categories, 246
    contribute, 250
    dealing with emotions, 248
    emotional tension, 248–249
    exercise, 247
    identify and address problem, 246
    instant vacations, 248
    let some things go, 247
    proper nutrition, 248
    sleep hygiene, 248
    tackling problem, 246–247
    taking care of my body, 247–248
Stress response, 219–220
Stretching exercises, 370
Stroking chin (or other part of face), 115
Students Against Destructive Decisions Contract
    for Life, 335, 452, 454
Substance Abuse and Mental Health Services
    Administration (SAMHSA), 386, 429, 430

Substance use and abuse, 425–438
    Ask-Tell-Ask, 428
    basic principles, 426
    case study, 431–435
    community resources, 429–430
    CRAFFT, 430, 431
    DARN-C, 428
    motivational interviewing, 427–428
    OARS, 427
    parental involvement, 435, 438
    recovery, 430
    referrals, 429
    related resources, 438
    risk factor, 427
    SBIRT, 430, 431
    trauma-informed approach, 429
    warning signs, 427
    Web sites, 426, 438
Suicide, 344–345, 348
Summary statements, 427
Super-peer theory, 455
Supplementary materials. *See* Handouts/supple-
    mentary materials
Survival sex, 495, 570

T

Tai chi, 322, 370
Teacher Report Form (TRF) of the Child Behavior
    Checklist, 390
Teaching problem-solving, 226
Teen brain, 57
Teen dating violence. *See* Adolescent relationship
    violence (ARV)
Teen driving, 449–454
    common driving errors, 449
    fatal crashes, 449
    frame situation to be about safety, 296
    graduated driver licensing (GDL) laws, 450
    monitoring technologies, 452
    on-the-road experience, 452
    parent-child driving contract, 451–452
    parents, 450–451, 452–453
    talking points, 451
    3 seconds to avoid crash, 451
    Web sites, 454
Teen fathers, 443
Teen pregnancy and parenting, 439–447
    addressing misconceptions, 443
    having young people own their solutions, 443
    motivational interviewing, 443
    overview, 439–440
    parental involvement, 441
    poverty, 440
    pregnancy prevention programs, 441
    reinforcing positive, 442–443
    starting conversation, 441–442
    teen fathers, 443
    teens who are already parenting, 444
    Web sites, 447

Teens. *See* Adolescents
Television viewing. *See* Electronic media use
Tend and befriend, 45
Tender-point release, 370
Tension headache, 367
Theory-theory, 58
Tolerable stress, 38
Toxic messages, 13, 14
Toxic stress, 38–39
Transition to adult care, 523–529
 continuity of care, 525
 handouts/supplementary materials, 528–529
 meeting alone with teen, 524
 parents, 524
 policies and guidelines, 524
 role transitions, 524
 special challenges, 526
 summary letter/clinical summary, 525–526
 understanding adult health care system, 525
 Web sites, 529
 years of preparation/culmination of a process, 523–524, 526
Transtheoretical model of behavioral change (TTM), 19–20, 126, 244
Trauma and toxic stress, 37–47
 ACE study, 40–41
 behavioral and emotional manifestations of trauma, 175–177
 brain development, 39
 DSM-5 diagnostic criteria, 44
 exposure to violence, 41
 failure of integration, 43–44
 parental/adult protective measures, 45
 psychophysiological pathways to problems, 41–43
 sentinel article, 37
 signs/symptoms, 45–46, 174–177
 stress continuum, 38–39
 tend and befriend, 45
 vocabulary, 38–39
Trauma-informed practice, 173–186
 case studies, 181–183
 connection with caring adult, 175
 effects of toxic stress and trauma, 174–177
 handouts/supplementary materials, 186
 interpersonal interactions, 180
 interview and assessment, 178–180
 preventing re-traumatization, 181
 sanctuary model, 176
 signs/symptoms, 174, 177–178
 substance abuse, 429
 support and treatment, 180–181
 trauma-informed strategies, 184
 unconditional love, 179
Trauma-informed strategies, 184
Traumatic reenactments, 44
Traumatic stress, 39
Tricyclic antidepressants, 371
Trustworthy relationship, 103–109
TTM. *See* Transtheoretical model of behavioral change (TTM)

"Tupperware box," 160
Tupperware model of emotion processing, 587
Turbo brain, 390
24/7 availability, 158

U

UFED. *See* Unspecified feeding and eating disorders (UFED)
Unconditional love, 154, 179, 284, 311
Unconscious bias. *See* Bias
Undermining messages, 14
Unhealthy disengagement strategies, 245
Unhealthy relationships. *See* Adolescent relationship violence (ARV)
Uninvolved parents, 294
University of Hawaii at Manoa, 596
Unmet needs, 91
Unspecified feeding and eating disorders (UFED), 413, 414
Unstably housed youth. *See* Homeless and unstably housed youth
Upsetting news/bad news, 303–307

V

Values education, 286–287
Verbal wrestling, 297
Vignettes. *See* Case studies
Violence. *See also* Youth violence
 bullying, 471–478
 childhood abuse, 489–498
 dating abuse, 479–487
Violence exposure, 41
Violence screen, 500–502
Visceral bias, 168
Visual and auditory processing disorders, 401
Vitamins, 323

W

Walking meditation, 256
War. *See* Military children and adolescents
Wellness strategies, 246. *See also* Caregiver wellness strategies
When Children Want Children (Dash), 439
White matter, 57
Work-life balance, 586
Wounded healers, 581–584

Y

Yoga, 220, 322, 370
Youth for leadership, 50
Youth in need of help, signs, 222
Youth-serving professionals, 275, 579–598
 adolescent-friendly environment, 92, 99–102
 assumptions, 128
 bias. *See* Bias
 body language, 111–117

boundaries. *See* Boundaries
burnout prevention, 159, 160, 579
chaperones, 101
confidentiality, 93, 106
eating disorders, 420
facilitator, as, 156
genuineness, 513
handling others' pain, 160
honesty, 105
late career stages/retirement, 593–596
learning disabilities, 403
male adolescent-friendly space, 99–102
mindfulness, 257
non-stigmatizing environment, 93
parents, and. *See* Professional-parent
    relationship
personal questions, 105
physical environment (office space), 92, 100
private conversation with each teen, 93
recruitment, 100
retirement years, 593–596
self-care, 581–591
self-reflection, 156
service with respect and without judgment,
    105–106
sexuality education, 70–74, 81–87
trusting that our presence matters, 597–598
trustworthy relationship, 103–109
wellness strategies. *See* Caregiver wellness
    strategies
wounded healers, 581–584

Youth violence, 499–507. *See also* Violence
    assessment, 500–502
    cycle of retaliation, 501, 502
    rage, 505
    shift blame to parents, 504
    social context, 502, 504
    strength-based perspective, 499–500
    stress, 505
    teen's perception of safety, 501
    teen's threshold for fighting, 501–502
    vulnerability to violence escalation, 503
    weapons, 503–504
    when teen says "you just don't get it," 505
    where teen wants to do right thing, 504
Youthbuild Philadelphia, 50

Z

Zinc, 323
"Zoning out," 46